Lippincott Certification Review

Family Nurse Practitioner & Adult-Gerontology Nurse Practitioner

AL RUNDIO, PHD, DNP, RN, APRN, ACNP-BC, ANP-BC, CARN-AP, NEA-BC, FNAP, FIAAN, FAAN
Associate Dean for Nursing & CNE
Clinical Professor of Nursing
Drexel University
Philadelphia, Pennsylvania

WILLIAM J. LORMAN, JD, PHD, RN, MSN, APRN, PMHNP-BC, CARN-AP, FIAAN
Vice President, Chief Clinical Officer
Livengrin Foundation, Inc.
Assistant Clinical Professor
College of Nursing and Health Professions
Drexel University
Philadelphia, Pennsylvania

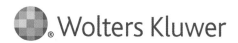 . Wolters Kluwer

Philadelphia • Baltimore • New York • London
Buenos Aires • Hong Kong • Sydney • Tokyo

Acquisitions Editor: Nicole Dernoski
Product Development Editor: Maria M. McAvey
Developmental Editor: Julie Vitale
Production Project Manager: Kim Cox
Design Coordinator: Holly Reid McLaughlin
Manufacturing Coordinator: Kathleen Brown
Marketing Manager: Linda Wetmore
Prepress Vendor: S4Carlisle Publishing Services

9 8 7 6 5 4 3 2 1
Printed in China

Library of Congress Cataloging-in-Publication Data
Names: Rundio, Al, editor. | Lorman, William J., editor.
Title: Lippincott certification review: family nurse practitioner &
    adult-gerontology nurse practitioner/[edited by] Al Rundio, William J.
    Lorman.
Description: Philadelphia: Wolters Kluwer Health, [2017] | Includes
    bibliographical references and index.
Identifiers: LCCN 2016023600 | ISBN 9781496306586
Subjects: | MESH: Family Nurse Practitioners–standards | Geriatric
    Nursing—methods | Nursing Care—methods | Aged | Licensure,
    Nursing—standards | Examination Questions
Classification: LCC RC954 | NLM WY 18.2 | DDC 618.97/0231076—dc23 LC record available at
https://lccn.loc.gov/2016023600

Dedication

Al Rundio

I dedicate this book to my family.

To my wife, Sadie, and my children, Jamie and Heather, and my grandson, Gunnar.

Their love and support for all that I do has been unwavering. They are a constant presence in my life.

I also dedicate this book to my two very *best* friends, Logan and Luke.

Logan and Luke are our two papillons. A dog's love is unconditional. If human beings possessed what dogs innately do, the world would be a much better place.

William J. Lorman

I dedicate this book to my mother, who has taught me to appreciate life and who, in her twilight years, has stressed the importance of quality of life. Because of her, I strive to give every patient I treat the best possible care so they can continue to live a fulfilling life even in the presence of restrictive physical and mental conditions.

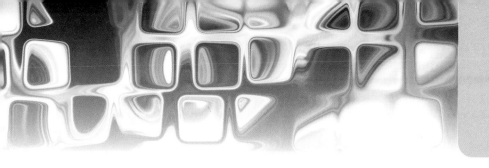

Contributors

Kristen A. Altdoerffer, DNP, CRNP, RN
Assistant Clinical Professor
College of Health and Human Professions
Drexel University
Philadelphia, Pennsylvania

Patrick C. Auth, PhD, PA-C
Program Director
Physician Assistant Department
College of Nursing and Health Professions
Drexel University
Philadelphia, Pennsylvania

Kathleen Bradbury-Golas, DNP, RN, FNP-C, ACNS-BC
Assistant Professor, Graduate Nursing
Felician College
Lodi, New Jersey
Family Nurse Practitioner
Virtua Atlantic Shore Family Practice
Northfield, New Jersey

Ryan J. Clancy, MSHS, MA, PA-C
Clinical Instructor
Physician Assistant Department
Drexel University
Philadelphia, Pennsylvania

Brenda L. Douglass, DNP, APRN, FNP-C, CDE, CTTS
Assistant Clinical Professor
College of Nursing and Health Professions
Drexel University
Philadelphia, Pennsylvania

Ellen D. Feld, MD, FACP
Medical Director, Associate Clinical Professor
Physician Assistant Department
College of Nursing and Health Professions
Drexel University
Philadelphia, Pennsylvania

Julie Kinzel, MEd, PA-C
Assistant Clinical Professor
Physician Assistant Department
College of Nursing and Health Professions
Drexel University
Philadelphia, Pennsylvania

William J. Lorman, JD, PhD, RN, MSN, APRN, PMHNP-BC, CARN-AP, FIAAN
Vice President, Chief Clinical Officer
Livengrin Foundation, Inc.
Bensalem, Pennsylvania
Assistant Clinical Professor
College of Nursing and Health Professions
Drexel University
Philadelphia, Pennsylvania

AtNena Luster-Tucker, DNP, MBA, FNP-C
Assistant Clinical Professor
College of Nursing and Health Professions
Drexel University
Philadelphia, Pennsylvania

Ann McDonough Madden, MHS, PA-C
Clinical Instructor, Physician Assistant
Physician Assistant Department
Drexel University
Philadelphia, Pennsylvania

MaryKay Maley, DNP, APN, FNP-BC, RN-BC
Assistant Clinical Professor
Nursing Department
College of Nursing and Health Professions
Drexel University
Philadelphia, Pennsylvania

Ann S. McQueen, MSN, CRNP, FNP-BC, GNP-BC, RNC
Assistant Clinical Professor, MSN Program
Family Nurse Practitioner Track
College of Nursing and Health Professions
Drexel University
Philadelphia, Pennsylvania

Jennifer L. Mondillo, MBA, MSN, CRNP, PhD (candidate)
Co-Track Director, Family Nurse Practitioner Track
College of Nursing and Health Professions
Drexel University
Philadelphia, Pennsylvania

Kymberlee Montgomery, DrNP, CRNP-BC, CNE, FAANP
Chair, Nurse Practitioner Department
College of Nursing and Health Professions
Drexel University
Philadelphia, Pennsylvania

Owen C. Montgomery, MD
Associate Professor and Chairman
Department of Obstetrics and Gynecology
College of Medicine
Drexel University
Philadelphia, Pennsylvania

Catherine J. Morse, PhD, CRNP-BC, CCRN
Associate Chair of Nurse Practitioner Programs
Associate Clinical Professor
College of Nursing and Health Professions
Drexel University
Philadelphia, Pennsylvania

Catherine Nowak, MS, RN, PA-C
Assistant Clinical Professor
Director of Clinical Rotation
Physician Assistant Department
Drexel University
Philadelphia, Pennsylvania

Claire E. Pisoni, MPAS, PA-C
Clinical Instructor
College of Nursing and Health Professions
Drexel University
Philadelphia, Pennsylvania

Al Rundio, PhD, DNP, RN, APRN, ACNP-BC, ANP-BC, CARN-AP, NEA-BC, FNAP, FIAAN, FAAN
Associate Dean for Nursing & CNE
Clinical Professor of Nursing
College of Nursing and Health Professions
Drexel University
Philadelphia, Pennsylvania

Megan E. Schneider, MMS, MSPH, PA-C
Clinical Instructor
Physician Assistant Department
College of Nursing and Health Professions
Drexel University
Philadelphia, Pennsylvania

Joanne Schwartz, PhD, CRNP, CNE
Assistant Professor
College of Nursing and Health Professions
Drexel University
Philadelphia, Pennsylvania

Diana D. Smith, MHS, PA-C
Director of Didactic Curriculum
Physician Assistant Department
Drexel University
Philadelphia, Pennsylvania

Mary L. Wilby, PhD, CRNP, ANP-BC
Assistant Professor
Adult-Gerontology NP Track Coordinator
School of Nursing and Health Sciences
La Salle University
Philadelphia, Pennsylvania

Reviewers

Kathleen Maguire, BSN/BS, JD, RN
Director of Certification
Managing Editor, Journal of Forensic Nursing
Elkridge, Maryland

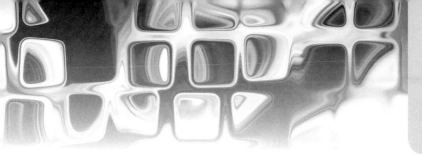

About the Editors

Both of us have unique backgrounds. For one, we are both men in nursing. When we entered the field of nursing, only around 2% of men were nurses. We both have clinical backgrounds in nursing, and then we both migrated to the world of administrative nursing. Later in our careers, we got postmaster degrees as nurse practitioners. Dr. Rundio had an extensive acute care background and initial certification as an acute care nurse practitioner followed by certification as an adult primary care nurse practitioner. Dr. Lorman achieved certification as a psychiatric mental health nurse practitioner.

Interestingly, both of our careers turned to where we were practicing in facilities serving patients with substance use disorders. Dr. Rundio practices at a residential addictions treatment facility in southern New Jersey. Dr. Lorman practices at a residential addictions treatment facility in southeastern Pennsylvania. We both teach at Drexel University, College of Nursing and Health Professions.

We both have developed and taught for several years certification review courses for both the American Nurses Credentialing Center (ANCC) and the American Nurses Association (ANA). Dr. Rundio developed and taught the Nurse Executive Review Certification Review Courses and the Adult Primary Care Nurse Practitioner Certification Review Courses. Dr. Lorman developed and taught the Psychiatric Mental Health Nurse Practitioner Review Courses.

Both of us are passionate about helping nurses to be successful as they pursue certification, and as the logical next step, went on to develop our first review manual in the primary care area focusing on Adult-Gerontology Nurse Practitioners and Family Nurse Practitioners.

We hope that you enjoy this review manual and find it a valuable part of your arsenal as you prepare for these certification examinations.

Sincerely,
Al Rundio
William J. Lorman
Coeditors

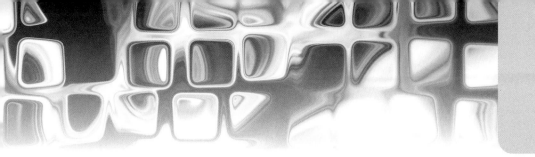

Preface

Much has happened to advance the practice of nurse practitioners since the role was first created by Dr. Loretta Ford in 1965.

Originally conceived as a primary care role, over the years there have been many specialty areas of practice identified for the nurse practitioner, such as the acute care nurse practitioner.

The Consensus Model for Advanced Practice has had a profound impact on the standardization of education for Advanced Practice Nursing. This model has clearly delineated the four roles of Advanced Practice Nursing: (1) the Clinical Nurse Specialist, (2) the Nurse Midwife, (3) the Nurse Anesthetist, and (4) the Nurse Practitioner. This model has also identified specific population foci for advanced practice nurses. It has also called for all programs to be accredited in order for advanced practice nurses to be eligible for the certification examinations. The model has also mandated that all advanced practice nurses achieve certification in their respective areas of practice. Gerontology has now become a major practice area with the adult primary and acute care nurse practitioner. Psychiatric Mental Health Nurse Practitioners now care for the entire family. This model has also helped to advance the independent practice of nurse practitioners. As of the writing of this review manual, approximately 50% of states have now achieved independent practice for nurse practitioners. This model also addresses the titling of Advanced Practice Nurses. The title of APRN (Advanced Practice Registered Nurse) has been recommended. Titling, certification, and independent practice are dependent upon each state making legislative changes as states are the bodies that actually license the advanced practice nurse. It will be some time before all states adopt some of these recommendations. A vast majority of nurses most likely remember the ANA (American Nurses Association) recommendation that the BSN degree be the entry-level degree to practice as a Registered Professional Nurse (RN). This recommendation was made in 1965, but is yet to be implemented in most states.

As many more nurses in many more states are getting certified in their respective areas of practice, this review manual has been written to help prepare adult-gerontology primary care and family nurse practitioners to be successful on these certification examinations.

This book has been a collaborative effort and has been written by individuals who specialize in the content of the chapters that have been written.

We hope that you find this manual a useful tool that enables your success on the certification examinations.

Sincerely,
Al Rundio, PhD, DNP, RN, APRN, ACNP-BC, ANP-BC, CARN-AP, NEA-BC, FNAP, FIAAN, FAAN
William J. Lorman, JD, PhD, RN, MSN, APRN, PMHNP-BC, CARN-AP, FIAAN
Coeditors

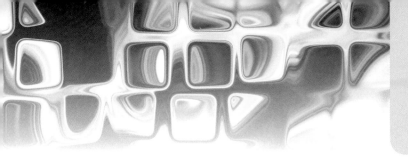

Acknowledgments

We would like to acknowledge all the authors of and contributors to this book. Without their willingness to share their expertise, this book would not be possible. They were also very timely with their submissions.

We would also like to acknowledge all nurse practitioners. Your expertise and care has positively impacted the provision of health care to many individuals. Many people would not have any health care if it were not for you.

We would also like to acknowledge the editorial staff of Wolters Kluwer for all their assistance and support through this process. A special thank-you to Julie Vitale and Maria McAvey for their diligent work on this book. We would not have met the production schedule without their expertise and assistance.

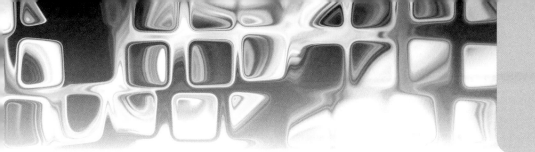

Contents

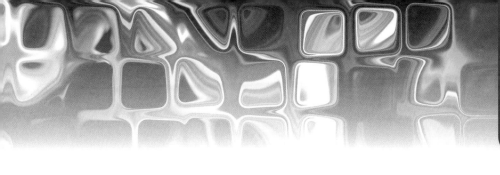

Chapter 1

Health Promotion

Brenda L. Douglass

Case Presentation

Directions: Carefully review the case study presented below. At the end of the chapter, answer the review questions. Compare your answers to the correct answers listed in the Review Section.

Source/Reliability: Patient, reliable.

Chief Complaint: "I want to get connected with a primary care doctor. I need to get some lab work done."

History of Present Illness: A 52-year-old female presents to the primary care office to establish care. For the past 4 years she has been uninsured and recently obtained health insurance through the health reform. During the time when she was without insurance, the patient reports obtaining care in the emergency department twice for bronchitis. Once she was seen at the local community health clinic about 2 years ago. Recommendations at that time were to complete blood work and preventive screenings. Due to not having health insurance coverage, the patient states she did not follow through with any of the recommendations. She reports following with a gynecologist, but stopped when she had no health insurance. She requests to have laboratory work ordered stating, "I know I am getting older. My father died of heart disease and diabetes and I want to get checked." She reports smoking 1 pack of cigarettes a day and has tried several times to quit smoking cold turkey. Relapses are attributed to weight gain when quitting smoking. "I tried to quit smoking because I know it's bad for my health and I can't afford cigarettes anymore. I don't make a lot of money."

Past Medical History:

Medical: Bronchitis, obesity, tobacco use. No hospitalizations.

Surgical: Cesarean section 1985.

Obstetric/Gynecologic: Gravida III, para II, abortion I. First birth at age 27, Caesarean section (secondary to dystocia); second, vaginal delivery. Last gynecologic examination with cervical screening about 5 years ago, reported as normal. Mammogram 5 years ago reported as normal. Sexually active with one partner. Denies history of sexually transmitted diseases. Sexual preference: men.

Psychiatric: Depressed mood about 3 days a week.

Health Maintenance: Last dental care about 10 years ago.

Screening Tests: Colonoscopy: never. Laboratory tests: about 8 years ago. Bone density study: never.

Immunizations: Tetanus >20 years ago; never had a flu or pneumonia vaccination.

Lifestyle: Physically active, no formal exercise regime. Nutrition/diet includes three 12 ounces of caffeinated coffee a day, 1 to 2 caffeinated soft drinks a day, 12 to 16 ounces of sweet ice tea a day. Limited plant-based foods, vegetables, fiber, or fruits.

Home Safety: Wears seatbelts when driving. No guns in household.

Allergies: Codeine. No latex allergy.

Medications: None.

Social: *Tobacco*: Smokes mentholated cigarettes, 1 pack/day, 31 pack-year-history. *Alcohol*: Two glasses of red wine 4 to 5 days a week with dinner. *Drug use:* Denies use of illegal drugs.

Personal History: *Education*: High school diploma. *Occupation*: Works as a cashier at a grocery store. *Marital Status:* Divorced, lives with her boyfriend. Children: 1 son age 25, 1 daughter age 23. *Financial*: Constraints. *Religion*: Christian. *Support person:* Boyfriend.

Family History: *Mother*: Living, age 72, colon cancer with partial bowel resection at age 48; osteoporosis, mild dementia. *Father*: Deceased, age 66, coronary artery disease, diabetes type II, hyperlipidemia, tobacco use, alcohol abuse. *Siblings*: 1 Brother, age 54, diabetes, hyperlipidemia, hypertension. 1 Sister, age 50, obese. *Maternal Grandfather*: Deceased, age 92, "old age." *Maternal Grandmother*: Deceased, age 84, colon cancer. *Paternal Grandfather*: Deceased, age 58, heart disease. *Paternal Grandmother:* Deceased, age 81, lung cancer, tobacco use.

Review of Systems/Health Promotion:
Constitutional/General Survey: Denies fever, chills, weight loss, or weakness. Denies fatigue. + Weight gain 10 pounds over past 2 years.
Skin: Denies rashes, lesions, itching, changes in hair or nails.
Head, Eyes, Ears, Nose, Throat (HEENT): **Head:** Denies head trauma, headache, lightheadedness, or dizziness. **Eye:** Denies eye pain, eye drainage, eye redness, spots, flashing lights, excessive tearing, double vision, glaucoma, or cataract. C/o visual changes (blurred) with reading and working on the computer. Last eye examination 8 years ago. No prescription contacts or glasses. + Use of nonprescription reading glasses. *Ears:* Denies hearing impairment, tinnitus, vertigo, earaches, infection, or discharge. **Nose/Sinus:** Denies nasal congestion, discharge, or itchiness. Denies nosebleeds or sinus problems. + Frequent colds. **Throat:** Denies sore throat, difficulty swallowing, sore tongue, dry mouth, postnasal drip or hoarse voice. **Mouth:** Denies bleeding gums. +Dental carries, last dental examination 8 years ago.
Neck: Denies swollen glands, lumps, pain, stiffness, or goiter.
Breast: Denies lumps, pain, discomfort, nipple discharge. Denies self breast examinations.
Lymph Nodes: Denies swollen lymph nodes.
Respiratory: (+)Dyspnea with exertion (walking up full flight of stairs or walking in windy weather). + Chronic productive cough, clear sputum. Denies hemoptysis. +History of bronchitis; denies chronic obstructive pulmonary disease (COPD), emphysema. Denies recent wheezing, history of associated upper respiratory infections. Chest X-ray in 2012 when treated for bronchitis.
Cardiovascular: Denies chest pain or discomfort. Denies heart palpitations, orthopnea, paroxysmal nocturnal dyspnea, or edema. No past cardiovascular testing.
Abdomen: Denies abdominal pain or discomfort. Denies heartburn, excessive belching, or flatulence. Denies appetite changes, nausea, vomiting, diarrhea, constipation, or change in bowel habits. Denies rectal bleeding, black or tarry stools, hemorrhoids. Denies jaundice, liver or gallbladder problems. EGD or colonoscopy, never.
Peripheral Vascular: Denies varicose veins, history of blood clots in legs, or swelling. Denies change in fingertip or toe color with cold weather. + Leg cramps and pain with walking long distances.
Urinary: Denies urinary frequency, urgency, nocturia, incontinence, odor, hematuria, burning or pain on urination. Denies kidney stones, urinary or kidney infections.
Genitalia: Denies vaginal discharge, itching, lesions/sores, or lumps. Menarche age 14. Denies menstrual irregularities until 3 years ago; menopause at age 50. +Hot flashes occasionally. Gravida III, para II, abortion I. 1 Caesarean section (nonprogressive delivery), 1 uncomplicated vaginal delivery, (1) induced abortion. Denies history of sexually transmitted diseases or abnormal cervical testing/PAP test.
Musculoskeletal: Denies muscle or joint pain, back pain, arthritis, joint stiffness, or neck pain. Denies trauma.
Psychiatric: Denies nervousness, anxiety, memory change, suicidal thoughts/attempt. +Depressed mood. +Moodiness. + Snoring. + Sleep difficulties with nighttime awakenings.
Neurologic: Denies numbness, seizures, headache, dizziness, vertigo, tremors, paralysis, or change in mental status. Denies changes in speech.
Hematologic: Denies anemia, fatigue, blood transfusions, easy bruising, or bleeding.
Endocrine: Denies thyroid problems, heat or cold intolerance, excessive sweating or hunger, or excessive thirst.

Physical Examination:

Vital Signs: T = 98.7°F   BP = 138/80 (right); 136/78 (left)   HR = 88 bpm   RR = 18/min Po_2 = 95% on room air *Height* = 5 feet 4 inches   *Weight* = 205 lbs.   BMI = 35.2   LMP: 2 years ago

General/Neuro/Psych: Pleasant, cooperative but mildly anxious. Well-groomed, dress appropriately for the season. Obese female.

Skin: Warm, normal turgor. Color pink. Nails without clubbing or cyanosis.

HEENT: **Head:** Scalp without lesions. Normocephalic/atraumatic. Hair dry. **Eyes:** Visual acuity 20/40 uncorrected each eye, 20/30 uncorrected both eyes. Conjunctiva pink, sclera. Pupils 3 mm, equally reactive to light. Extraocular movements intact. **Ears:** Tympanic membranes with dullness, no erythema, or discharge. No pain on movement with external tragus, normal pinna, no external abnormalities. **Nose:** Nasal mucosa pink, septum midline, no sinus pain, or tenderness. **Throat:** Oral mucosa pink, dentition good, no obvious caries, pharynx without exudates.

Neck: Trachea midline, neck supple, thyroid lobes palpable with fullness noted, no nodules.

Lymph nodes: No cervical, axillary, submandible, or inguinal adenopathy.

Thoracic/Lungs: Increased AP diameter, prolonged expiratory phase. Scattered rhonchi bilaterally, no wheezing.

Cardiovascular: Regular S1, S2 without heart murmurs. No jugular vein distention or carotid bruits.

Breasts: Pendulous, symmetric. No masses, nipple discharge, or dimpling.

Abdomen: Obese, soft, nontender with normal bowel sounds all quadrants. No masses. No costovertebral angle tenderness (CVAT).

Genitalia: Deferred

Rectal: Deferred

Extremities: Warm without edema. No varicosities or stasis changes. No ulcerations. All pulses +2 and symmetric. Lower extremities with loss of hair.

Musculoskeletal: No joint deformities. Gait steady. Full range of motion in all joints of the upper and lower extremities. Muscle strength +5/5 all four extremities.

Neurologic: **Mental Status:** Oriented to person, time, and place.

Assessment and Plan (with Rationale)

Well examination, age 52-year-old female

Plan: Clinical preventive health screenings and laboratory testing

- Mammogram screening.
  - Women aged 50 to 74: Baseline screening mammogram starting at 50 years of age and then every 2 years (biennial).
- Gynecologic examination with cervical screening, Papanicolaou (PAP) cytology testing.
  - Women aged 21 to 65: Pap smear (cytology) every 3 years until age 65 *or* for women aged 30 to 65 who want to extend the screening interval, screening with combined cytology, and HPV testing every 5 years.
- Colorectal screening, colonoscopy. Risk factors include age, family history of colon cancer, cigarette smoking, obesity, low dietary consumption of fruits and vegetables.
- Laboratory testing:
  - Complete blood count (CBC)
  - Comprehensive metabolic panel (CMP)
  - Lipid screening (at high risk for coronary heart disease [CHD]; family history of heart disease, tobacco use, obesity)
  - Hepatitis C virus (HCV)
    - Screening recommendations (USPSTF): Individuals born between 1945 and 1965, offer a one-time screening for HCV
- Self breast examinations
- Immunization according to adult immunization recommendations:
  - Influenza (inactivated) vaccination
    - Annual influenza vaccination recommended for all adults without contraindications
    - Pneumococcal vaccination
      - At high risk for pneumonia secondary to cigarette smoking
  - Tetanus, diphtheria, pertussis (Tdap)
    - One lifetime dose of Tdap followed by tetanus/diphtheria (Td) booster recommended every 10 years
- Follow-up in 2 to 3 weeks after completion of health screenings and serum laboratory testing

Dyspnea on exertion

Plan: Symptomatology of dyspnea with risk factor of tobacco use.

- Considerations: Cardiac and respiratory etiology. Increased AP diameter, prolonged expiratory phase are suggestive of COPD.
- Differential diagnoses: COPD, asthma, lung disorders such as pulmonary fibrosis, coronary artery disease, lung cancer, viral/bacterial infection.
- Risk factors: Cigarette smoking, age, family history of coronary artery disease, and cancer.
- Diagnostic studies: Complete electrocardiogram. Obtain chest X-ray. Spirometry to assess lung function.

Tobacco use disorder

Plan: Counsel on actual health symptoms (dyspnea on exertion) and health risks of tobacco use and benefits of quitting; strong recommendation to quit smoking.

- Differential diagnoses: Tobacco use disorder, nicotine withdrawal
- Risk factors: Family history of tobacco use (consideration to genetic tendency)
- Interventions:
  - Utilization of the five As (ask, advise, assess, assist, arrange). Assess readiness to make a quit attempt. Assist with a quit plan to include setting a target quit date (TQD)
    - Schedule a follow-up office visit within 1 week of TQD.
- Screen for lung cancer, 31-pack-year-history of smoking cigarettes.
  - Adults age 55 to 80 with a history of smoking: Annual screening for lung cancer with low-dose computed tomography (LDCT) in individuals with a 30-pack-year history

Obesity (BMI 35.2)/weight gain

Plan: Counsel on potential health risks of obesity such as with chronic health conditions (i.e., type 2 diabetes mellitus, hypertension, hyperlipidemia, obstructive sleep apnea).

- Differential diagnoses: Obesity, endocrine disorder
- Risk factors: Chronic diseases, elevated BMI 35.2 consistent with obesity, recent weight gain, sedentary lifestyle, dietary/nutritional intake, and family history of diabetes. Abnormal weight gain over the past 2 years of 10 pounds.
- Intervention: Health education recommendations including lifestyle modifications:
  - Obesity is a modifiable risk factor.
  - Healthful nutritional intake; educate on MyPlate recommendations.
  - Exercise three times a week with target of 150 minutes/week (dyspnea etiology must be considered initially).

Alcohol in excess

Plan: Two glasses of wine with dinner 4 to 5 times a week exceeds recommended guidelines.

- Differential diagnoses: Alcohol abuse, depression
- Guidelines recommend alcohol consumption in women no more than 1 drink/day.
- Risk factors: Depressed mood, financial constraints, family history of alcohol abuse (father)
- Intervention: counsel on potential health risks associated with alcohol misuse.

Depression

Plan: Screen for depression.

- Differential diagnoses: Major depressive disorder, metabolic disorders, thyroid disorder, depression attributed to menopausal state
- Risk factors: Alcohol use in excess of recommended guidelines, life stressors (financial), lower socioeconomic status
- Intervention: Further assessment warranted. Screening tool such as the PHQ-9 assessment tool for depression.

Menopausal state/symptoms

Plan: Menopausal symptoms, mild

- Differential diagnoses: Menopause, hypo- or hyperthyroidism
- Risk factors: Menopausal state, endocrine disorders
- Intervention: Educate on conservative measures such as lowering the room temperature, fans, dressing in light clothing, avoidance of triggers (spicy foods, stressful situations).

Sleep disturbances/snoring

Plan: Sleep disturbances with reported snoring.

- Differential diagnoses: Obstructive sleep apnea syndrome; insomnia related to stress reaction, depression, menopausal symptoms, nicotine withdrawal
- Risk factors: Obesity, central obesity, snoring, thicker neck circumference, tobacco use
- Intervention: Consider polysomnography (sleep study).

Family history of osteoporosis

Plan: Counsel on potential risk for osteoporosis

- Differential diagnoses: Osteopenia, osteoporosis
- Risk factors: Family history of osteoporosis, tobacco use, menopausal state
- Intervention: Counsel on risk of osteoporosis with tobacco use (smoking cigarettes decreasing bone density).
- Diagnostic: Complete bone density test. Weight bearing exercises. Calcium intake of 1,200 mg daily (dietary with calcium supplementation if needed to meet daily requirements)

Visual changes, (r/o) presbyopia

Plan: Visual changes

- Differential diagnoses: presbyopia, cataract, glaucoma, retinal disorders
- Risks: Reported visual changes in this case are suggestive of presbyopia, frequently apparent with advancing age due to loss of elasticity of the eye lens.
- Intervention: Refer to an ophthalmologist for a complete eye evaluation.

Note: The case presentation is a real-world scenario, although consideration should be given to addressing the needs of the patient in subsequent visits (prioritization).

Health Promotion

Introduction

Health promotion is defined by the World Health Organization (WHO) as a process enabling individuals to increase control over and to improve their health. Expanding beyond the focus on individual behavior by encapsulating a broad range of environmental and social interventions describes health promotion. Global health goals are intended to support individuals across the continuum of life to remain healthy, to promote healthy environments in which to live, and, in the presence of disability or chronic disease, to optimize health. Health promotion has application to all individuals with or without health problems. Individuals with health conditions (without the ability to prevent or cure) can benefit from health promotion strategies by slowing the functional decline and improving quality-of-life issues such as living independently, daily activities, and community life. The nation's public infrastructure provides resources to deliver essential public health services in communities.

United States Preventive Services Task Force

Based upon rigorous scientific evidence, the United States Preventive Services Task Force (USPSTF) develops preventive services recommendations for health professional and consumer information. The USPSTF is an "independent group of national experts in prevention and evidence-based medicine that works to improve the health of all Americans by making evidence-based recommendations about Clinical Preventive Services (CPS) such as screenings counseling services, or preventive medications." The Agency for Healthcare Research and Quality (AHRQ) provides administrative, research, technical, and communication support to the USPSTF in developing and dissemination of CPS.

CPS such as immunizations, screening tests, health behavioral intervention, and preventive medications can save lives and promote health and well-being. CPS can be critically important in disease detection, delaying the onset, or identification of disease processes in early, treatable stages, lending to a longer, quality life for adults.

Despite the widespread endorsement of benefits and raised awareness through media campaigns, it is estimated that only 50% of Americans receive recommended care. The Centers for Disease Control and Prevention (CDC) support the effectiveness of CPS as "potentially life-saving preventive services; regardless, statistics reveal only 25% of adults aged 50 to 64 years are current on preventive services and less than 50% of adults aged 65 years or older are up to date. A more pronounced gap exists among low-income Americans, minority groups (ethic and racial), and the older-adult population. Closing the 'prevention gap' could significantly reduce morbidity and mortality."

Chronic Disease

A national shift placing emphasis on health prevention and promotion correlates with underlying unhealthy lifestyles and environments lending to the staggering statistics on chronic disease. Promoting and preserving health can minimize the occurrence and consequences of disease and injury. Chronic diseases are preventable, have an enormous economic cost burden to the US health care system, and contribute considerably to morbidity and mortality. An estimated 86% of health care costs are spent on the treatment of chronic conditions and are the nation's leading causes of death and disability. The most common chronic diseases contributing to leading causes of death and disability in the United States are heart disease, cancer, stroke, diabetes, obesity, and arthritis. The top 10 leading causes of death ranked in order of prevalence account for nearly 75% of all deaths annually in the United States as listed below:

Leading Causes of Death in the United States (Top 10)[1]

- Heart disease
- Cancer
- COPD
- Stroke (cerebrovascular disease)
- Unintentional injuries
- Alzheimer disease
- Diabetes
- Influenza/pneumonia
- Kidney disease (nephritis, nephrotic syndrome, nephrosis)
- Intentional self-harm (suicide)

Of the leading causes of mortality, 7 of the 10 are related to chronic diseases (excludes unintentional injuries, intentional injuries, influenza/pneumonia) with heart disease and cancer accountable for close to 48% of all deaths. Contributing to chronic disease is the serious public health issue concerning the prevalence of obesity. More than one-third (34.9%) of adults and 17% of the youth in the United States are obese. Escalating rates of obesity contributes to rising chronic disease, escalated medical expenditures, and economical burden on the health care system. To become a healthy nation, a transformation of the health system embracing health prevention is critical.

Healthy People 2020

Healthy People 2020, under the umbrella of the United States Department of Health and Human Services (USDHHS), is a science-based national health promotion and disease prevention initiative, designed to improve the health of the nation. The 10-year national health objectives are based on identification of a wide-range of public health priorities with measureable objectives aimed at reducing the health threats. Overarching goals include increasing the quality and longevity of healthy life and elimination of health disparities by eliminating preventable disease, disability, injury, and premature death. Increasing public awareness and understanding of determinants concerning health, disease, and disability are integrated into the Healthy People 2020 mission. Engagement of various health sectors to capitalize by taking action supported by the "best available evidence and knowledge" together with identification of crucial research and data collection needs are added goals of Healthy People 2020.

Twenty-six Healthy People 2020 objectives are outlined under 12 Leading Health Indicator topics with illustrative targets of each to include as shown in Table 1-1.

---

[1]CDC (2014v).

Table 1-1: Healthy People 2020 Leading Health Indicators (LHI) Topics

Leading Indicator	Targeted Examples
1. Access to health services	Health coverage and accessible health service access for all Americans
2. Clinical preventive services	Increasing the number of individuals who have access to and take advantage of recommended CPS
3. Environmental quality	Improvement in air quality index and secondhand smoke exposure
4. Injury and violence	Reduce unintentional and intentional fatal injuries and violence-related injuries such as motor vehicle crashes, acts of violence, suicide, homicide, unintentional drug overdoses, domestic and school violence
5. Maternal (infant/child health)	Reduce all infant deaths and total preterm births.
6. Mental health	Reduce suicide rate. Reduce adolescent (added 12–17) major depressive episodes.
7. Nutrition, physical activity, and obesity	Increase fitness (aerobic and muscle-strengthening exercise). Reduce obesity. Increase dietary intake of fruits and vegetables. Decreased caloric intake of solid fats and added sugars.
8. Oral health	Increase utilization of dental care/dental health.
9. Reproductive and sexual health	Prevent unintended pregnancies, early detection and treatment of sexually transmitted diseases, decrease transmission of human immunodeficiency virus (HIV).
10. Social detriments	Improvement in social and physical environment detriments
11. Substance abuse	Reducing the number of individuals who abuse drugs and alcohol
12. Tobacco	Reduction in tobacco use and exposure to secondhand smoke

From United States Department of Health and Human Services (USDHHS). (2014a). *Healthy people 2020: About healthy people.* Retrieved from https://www.healthypeople.gov/2020/About-Healthy-People

Levels of Health Prevention

Three levels of health prevention are identified: *primary, secondary, and tertiary prevention. Primary prevention* measures are aimed at preventing the onset of disease. The purpose is to protect healthy individuals from developing a disease or experiencing an injury. An example includes immunizations for protection against an infectious disease.

Secondary prevention is for early screening and detection of disease. Secondary prevention includes strategies to identify and treat asymptomatic persons who have already developed risk factors or preclinical disease but in whom the disease or condition is not clinically evident (USPSTF, 1996). The goal is to slow or halt the progress of disease in its earliest stages. Obtaining a Papanicolaou smear to detect cervical dysplasia before the development of cancer and screening for high blood pressure are forms of secondary prevention.

Tertiary prevention activities are the restoration of health or involvement of care with an established disease (USPSTF, 1996). The aim is to limit the negative effects of the disease, restore to the highest function, and prevent disease-related complications (USPSTF, 1996). Prevent morbidity and mortality once disease has been established. An illustration includes treatment of hyperlipidemia in a patient with coronary artery disease or preventing complications of diabetes.

Primary Prevention—*"Prevention of disease"*[2]
- Immunization against infectious disease
- Health education

---

[2]Adapted from Dunphy, Winland-Brown, Porter, and Thomas (2011).

- Weight control, exercise
- Nutritional counseling
- Stress reduction
- Skin cancer prevention
- Seatbelt use, airbags in vehicles
- Avoidance of environmental hazards
- Elimination of allergen exposure
- Protective equipment (i.e., safety helmets, goggles, masks)
- Education on dangers of tobacco use, alcohol, or drug use
- Violence and bullying prevention
- Controlling potential hazards in the home or workplace environment

Secondary Prevention—*"Early screening and detection of the disease"*[2]

- Early screening and detection of disease to monitor risk factors for illness
- Cancer screenings—diabetes, skin, oral, lung, breast, testicular, prostate, ovarian, cervical, fecal occult blood
- Diabetes, hypertension, cardiovascular disease
- Laboratory tests to screen for disease (i.e., anemia, TSH for thyroid)
- Screening for high-risk behaviors (number of sex partners, suicide risk)
- Sexually transmitted disease
- Lead screening
- Anemia screening
- Height, weight, body mass index (BMI) screening
- Low-dose aspirin to prevent heart disease or stroke

Tertiary Prevention—*"Restoration of health or disease after illness has occurred"*[2]

- Restoration of health or disease after illness has occurred.
- Interventions to prevent further sequelae of disease processes (i.e., cardiovascular, respiratory, GI/GU, endocrine, immunodeficiency, infectious, dermatologic, gynecologic, neurologic, psychiatric, reproductive, oncology)
- Rehabilitation (cardiac rehabilitation, physical therapy, occupational therapy, speech therapy, addiction/drug rehabilitation)
- Support groups (i.e., breast cancer patients, Alcoholics Anonymous for alcohol)
- Hospice care
- Management of existing conditions (i.e., individual with diabetes who maintains good glycemic control)

Assessment of Health Risk Factors

A vital component of health promotion and disease prevention is to identify risk factors relative to disease. Health promotion differs from disease or illness prevention on the basis of motivation for the behavior. *Health promotion* is described as behavior motivated by the interest of a person to improve well-being and actualize individual health potential (Pender, 2011, Chapter 1). *Disease prevention* is behavior motivated by a desire to actively avoid illness and for early detection and intervention (Pender, 2011, Chapter 1). For health promotion and disease prevention to be effective, screening individuals with potential health-related risk factors presents an opportunity for behavioral modification to reduce the potential of disease, and early disease detection and intervention.

Nonmodifiable and Modifiable Risk Factors

Risk factors that increase one's risk of developing disease or infection are divided into two categories: *nonmodifiable and modifiable. Nonmodifiable* risk factors are those in which an individual cannot be changed and contribute to health conditions such as sex, age, race, ethnicity, and heredity. Awareness aimed toward health-promoting lifestyle modifications relative to modifiable risk factors can aid in prevention of disease and are key to improving health outcomes. *Modifiable* risk factors can be eliminated, controlled, or altered through behavioral change resulting in risk reduction of a health risk for a particular disease. Some examples of modifiable risk factors include weight, exercise/physical activity, nutrition, alcohol intake, or tobacco use. *Modifiable* risk factors contribute to an individual's likelihood of developing a particular disease or condition.

Identification risk factors
Nonmodifiable
- Age
- Ethnicity
- Genetic/family history
- Race
- Sex

Modifiable
- Lifestyle choices with diet/nutrition
- Sedentary lifestyle/lack of exercise or physical activity
- Social habits, alcohol consumption, tobacco use
- Stress reduction

Screening Test Statistical Measurements

"Screening is the presumptive identification of unrecognized disease or defects by means of tests, examinations, or other procedures that can be applied rapidly" as defined by the WHO. The goal of a screening test is to ensure the best possible detection of disease (high sensitivity) and as few as possible without a disease are overlooked or subjected to further diagnostic testing (high specificity). Factors to consider with screening tests include *specificity, sensitivity, positive predictive value,* and *negative predictive value.*

Specificity

Specificity refers to a measurement in the proportion of individuals without a disease correlating with a true negative result.

Sensitivity

Sensitivity is the ability of a test to accurately detecting those with a disease. A screening test with poor sensitivity may omit identification of an individual with the disease or condition resulting in a false-negative test results. The individual may have the disease but inaccurately are advised disease free or negative results. This refers to "false-positives," which is often a result of a highly sensitive test.

Positive Predictive Value

A *positive predictive value* correlates with the extent in which individuals have the disease in those who have a positive test result.

Negative Predictive Value

A *negative predictive value* correlates with the extent in which individuals are free of the disease in those who have a negative test result.

United States Preventive Service Task Force

National movements to include the Patient Protection and Affordable Care Act are placing a richer emphasis on health promotion and CPS. The United States Preventive Service Task Force (USPSTF), also known as the Task Force, was developed in 1984, is supported by the Department of Health and Human Services (HHS), and is an integral framework for evidence-based CPS recommendations (AHRQ, 2014). Subsequently to its inception, the USPSTF was moved under the umbrella of the Agency Healthcare Research and Quality (AHRQ) with enactment of the 1998 Public Health Service Act (AHRQ). Congressional mandates require the USPSTF to conduct rigorous scientific reviews of evidence leading to the development of evidence-based preventive services recommendations (AHRQ, 2014).

The recommendations are considered by many as "definitive standards for preventive services" (AHRQ), and the USPSTF work is recognized by the Patient Protection and Affordable Care Act, also known as the Affordable Care Act (ACA). A grade defines the strength of evidence and potential net benefit for the recommendation CPS. Aligned with the law, preventive services grade A or B must be covered without cost sharing (copayment or deductible) under guidelines of new health insurance plans or policies (AHRQ). An overview of the most common screening recommendations is provided in the next section.

USPSTF Screening Recommendations

Alcohol Misuse Screening (2013)

The consumption of alcoholic beverages in excess is detrimental to health and wellness. Alcohol misuse encompasses a spectrum of behaviors to include "risky or hazardous" alcohol use to including harmful alcohol ingestion, alcohol abuse, or dependence. Risky or hazardous alcohol consumption is consistent with drinking in excess of the recommended daily, weekly, or per-occasion amounts of alcohol with increased risk for health consequences. Alcohol is a central nervous system depressant rapidly absorbed into the bloodstream resulting in impairment. Alcohol is metabolized by the liver and reactions are individualized. Excess alcohol remains circulating in the body system and the effects of alcohol are directly linked to the amount of alcohol consumed. Alcohol misuse is associated with considerable morbidity and mortality.

Epidemiology:
- In 2012, 87.6% of adults aged 18 and older reported use of alcohol at a point in their lives.
  - 71% reported alcohol intake in the past year.
  - 56.3% reported alcohol intake in the prior month.
- In 2012, 24.6% of adults aged 18 or older reported binge drinking in the past month; 7.1% heaving alcohol drinking in the past month
- About 30% or an estimated 17 million adults aged 18 and above are reported to have alcohol use disorders (men 11.2 million; women 5.7 million) and "most engage in risky behaviors."
  - Approximately 1.4 million received treatment at a specialized facility.
- Over 85,000 deaths annually are attributed to alcohol-related causes, consistent with the third leading preventable cause of death in the US.
- In adults aged 20 to 64, excessive alcohol consumption has been attributable to 1 in 10 deaths.
- Adolescents aged 12 to 17 in 2012 an approximate 855,000 had alcohol use disorders (male 411,000 or 3.2%; females 444,000 or 3.6%).
  - Nearly 76,000 adolescents received treatment at a specialized facility.
- Economic burdens from excessive alcohol consumption in the US was estimated at 223.5 billion.

Risk Factors:
- Excessive alcohol consumption is defined as follows:
  - Heavy drinking is defined as 15 drinks or more per week for men; 8 drinks or more for women.
    - Standard drink equates to 14.0 g (0.6 ounces) of pure alcohol (such as 12 ounces of beer, 8 ounces of malt liquor, 5 ounces of wine, or 1.5 ounces or a "shot" of 80 proof/40% liquor).
  - Any alcohol ingestion by a pregnant women or those younger than age 21
  - Binge drinking
    - Defined as a BAC of 0.08% or above, commonly associated with alcohol consumption in about 2 hours of five drinks or more in men or four drinks or more in women
    - Binge drinking is more common in young adults aged 18 to 34 and aged 65 years and older.
    - Associated with alcohol poisoning along with other alcohol-related risk factors
- Behavioral changes (effects linked to exposure)
  - Cognitive impairment, altered judgment, lowered inhibitions
  - Slowed reaction time, slurred speech, blurred vision, ataxia
- Dependence on alcohol
- Risky or violent behavior
  - Intimate partner violence, unprotected sexual activity
- Depression and/or anxiety
- Suicide or homicide
- Motor vehicle crashes, alcohol-related driving arrests, trauma, injuries, drowning, fires

- Serious health problems:
  - Damaging effects on the brain (effects linked to exposure)
    - Blackouts and memory lapses
    - Chronic alcoholism can lead to alcoholic cerebellar degeneration/chronic cerebellar syndrome
      - Gait disturbances/ataxia, blurred vision, slowed reaction times, memory impairment
    - Hepatic encephalopathy
  - Malnutrition
    - Thiamine deficiency
      - Found in nearly 80% of adults with chronic alcohol use
      - Wernicke–Korsakoff syndrome (encephalopathy/psychosis)
        - Wernicke encephalopathy is characterized by the triad of oculomotor abnormalities, delirium, and ataxia and occurs secondary to thiamine deficiency.
        - Untreated Wernicke encephalopathy can progress to Korsakoff syndrome
  - Heart (cardiomyopathy, arrhythmias, stroke, hypertension)
  - Alcoholic hepatitis
  - Fibrosis
  - Severe liver disease/cirrhosis
  - Pancreatitis
  - Cancers (oropharyngeal, esophageal, liver, breast)
- Alcohol use in pregnancy is linked to fetal alcohol syndrome (FAS)
  - Underage drinking is associated with school problems, social issues, legal ramifications, changes in brain development, physical/sexual assault, unplanned pregnancy, and other alcohol-related risk factors
- Risks influential for alcohol misuse include the person's age, gender, level of education, genetic disposition, prenatal alcohol exposure, and family history of alcoholism.

Factors Decreasing Risk:
- Avoidance of alcohol use or alcohol use in moderation
  - Moderate alcohol consumption is defined as up to 2 drinks/day for men and 1 drink/day for women.
- Behavioral counseling interventions

Epidemiology/Risk Factors Sources: CDC (2014c, 2014i, 2014y) and National Institute on Alcohol Abuse and Alcoholism (NIH) (n.d., 2004, 2014).

Screening Test:
- Three screening instruments are considered by the USPSTF:
  - The alcohol use disorders identification test (AUDIT)
    - Most widely used
  - The abbreviated ADUTI consumption (AUDIT-C)
  - Single-question screening
    - For example, "How many times in the past year have you had five (for men) or four (for women and adults >65 years of age) or more drinks in a day?"
- Various other screening instruments are available for use such as follows:
  - Eye opener questionnaire—CAGE, cutdown, annoyed, guilt

Recommendation:
- Adults aged 18 and older: Screen for alcohol misuse and provide individuals "engaged in risky or hazardous drinking with brief behavioral counseling" aimed at alcohol reduction.
- Adolescents under age 18: Insufficient evidence for balancing benefits and harms of screening and intervention with behavioral counseling.

Source: USPSTF (2015).

Blood Pressure Screening (Adults 2015; Adolescents 2013)

Screening for hypertension is vital for detection and early intervention, particularly considering most individuals are asymptomatic. Goals include prevention of target organ damage (TOD) and comorbid conditions such as cardiovascular (i.e., myocardial infraction, stroke, heart failure), end-stage renal disease, and mortality. Accuracy with blood pressure measurement, integration of the most current evidence-based guidelines (JNC 8) for the management of hypertension, and clinical decision-making aimed at improving health outcomes.

Epidemiology:
- Prevalence of high blood pressure in American adults is estimated at 67 million (31%) equating to one in three adults.
- About one in three American adults have blood pressure readings that are above the recommended range.
- Less than half (47%) with hypertension are controlled.
- High blood pressure was a "primary or contributing cause of death for over 348,000 Americans" equating to about 1,000 deaths daily.
- The economic burden costs are over $47.5 billion annually including health-care services, lost productivity/work days, medications to treat hypertension.
- Hypertension in children/adolescents is reported between 1% and 5%.
  - BMI is the strongest correlating factor to hypertension in children/adolescents attributable to childhood overweight and obesity.
  - Youth with hypertension are at increased risk of hypertension during adulthood.
- Hypertension is the most common condition presenting in primary care.

Risk Factors:
- Age
  - Advancing age is a risk factor; in the older adult/elderly population, systolic blood pressure tends to be elevated as a result of stiffening of the large arteries.
- Obesity and weight gain
- Smoking tobacco
- Race (hypertension tends to be more prevalent, more severe, earlier onset in life, and with greater TOD in the African American population)
- High-sodium diet
- Excessive alcohol consumption
- Physical inactivity
- Diabetes mellitus
- Dyslipidemia
- Family history
- Risk factors for secondary hypertension (due to an underlying cause, consider secondary identifiable causes in severe or resistant hypertension refractory to treatment modalities):
  - Medication use
    - Nonsteroidal anti-inflammatory medications, oral contraceptives, antidepressants (selective serotonin reuptake inhibitors), glucocorticoids, decongestants containing pseudoephedrine, stimulants (methylphenidate, amphetamines), illegal drug use (methamphetamines, cocaine)
  - Endocrine
    - Hyperthyroidism, hypothyroidism, hyperparathyroid disease, primary aldosteronism, Cushing syndrome, pheochromocytoma
  - Renal
    - Renal artery stenosis, chronic kidney disease (CKD), polycystic kidney disease
  - Other
    - Coarctation of the aorta, obstructive sleep apnea

Factors Decreasing Risk:
- Maintain a healthy weight.
- Healthy dietary intake
- Reduction of dietary sodium intake
- Physical activity aligned with recommended guidelines
- Stress management
- Alcohol intake in moderation
- Avoidance of tobacco use

Epidemiology/Risk Factors Sources: CDC (2014p); American Heart Association (AHA) (2015); James et al. (2014); and Kaplan, Thomas, and Pohl (2014).

Screening Test:
- Sphygmomanometer (blood pressure cuff)
  - Two or more elevated readings on at least two visits over a period of one or more weeks are recommended for a diagnosis of hypertension.

- Accuracy in obtaining correct blood pressure measurement:
  - Patient:
    - Avoid strenuous exercise, food intake, smoking, or caffeine 30 minutes prior to measurement.
    - Avoid restrictive clothing (i.e., tight sleeve).
  - Clinician:
    - Proper cuff size/placement
      - Blood pressure cuff should cover 80% of upper arm and width at least 40% of the circumference of the upper arm.
      - Bladder of cuff should be over the midline over the brachial artery pulsation.
    - Proper position/preparation of the patient
      - Patient should be seated with the back supported and legs uncrossed.
      - Patient's arm at the level of the heart
      - Resting in a quiet environment for 5 minutes prior to measurement

Recommendation:
- Adults aged 18 and older: Screen for blood pressure every 2 years aligned with the seventh report of the Joint National Committee on Prevention Detection, Evaluation, and Treatment of High Blood Pressure (JNC 7). Screen for high blood pressure and obtain measurements outside of the clinical setting for diagnostic confirmation before initiating treatment.
- Children/Adolescents: Recommends against routine screening due to insufficient evidence assessing benefit and harms

Sources: USPSTF (2015) and Kaplan, Thomas, and Pohl (2014).

Breast Cancer Screening (2009)

Breast cancer is a group of cancer cells (malignant tumor) that begins in the breast cells. Breast cancer begins in the breast cells with the potential of spreading (metastasis) to other areas of the body. Strong supporting evidence exists that screening with film mammogram reduces breast cancer mortality. Mammography screening is the only method proven to be effective as a screening tool.

Epidemiology:
- Breast cancer is the most common cancer among American Women (all races/ethnicities).
- The most common cause of cancer-related deaths among Hispanic women
- The second most common cause of death from cancer among White, Black, American Indian/Alaska Native women, and Asian/Pacific Islander
- White women are more likely to develop breast cancer, whereas, African-American women are more likely to die secondary to breast cancer.

Risk Factors:
- Risk factors that influence the risk of breast cancer include the following:
- Gender: Female
- Age: 55 and older
- Cigarette smoking
- A personal history of breast cancer or noncancerous breast diseases
- Family history of breast cancer (maternal or paternal):
  - First-degree relative (mother, sister, or daughter) doubles the risk.
  - Most common hereditary breast cancer is the inherited mutation in the *BRCA1* and *BRACA2* genes.
- Long-term hormone replacement therapy (HRT)
- Radiation therapy to the breast or chest
- Exposure to diethylstilbestrol (DES) such as during pregnancy or when in the womb
- Dense breasts/fibrocystic breast disease
- Women with onset of menstrual periods before the age of 12 or menopause after the age of 55 (may be related to longer lifetime hormonal exposure with estrogen and progesterone).
- Drinking alcohol
- Night-shift work (linked to circadian rhythm disruption, reduced melatonin levels, exposure to light at night, fatigue)

Epidemiology/Risk Factors Sources: American Cancer Society (ACS) (2015a); CDC (2014j); International Agency for Research on Cancer [IARC] (2007); WHO (2014b).

Factors Decreasing Risk:

- Breastfeeding
- Physical activity
- Multiparity
- Exercise/physical activity
- Avoid smoking
- Maintain a healthy weight

Screening Test:

- Mammography (film)

Recommendation:

- Women aged 50 to 74: Baseline screening mammogram starting at 50 years of age and then every 2 years (biennial)
- Women before age 50: Decision based on individual case to include patient's values on specific benefits and harm
- Women aged 75 and older: Insufficient evidence for routine mammogram screening in women 75 years of age and older

Source: USPSTF (2015).

Cervical Cancer Screening (2012)

Cervical cancer is found in the lining of the cervix (the lower part of the uterus), also known as uterine cancer. Cancer prevention and early detection with a screening Papanicolaou (PAP) smear are vital to improving health outcomes. The most common types of cervical cancers are squamous cell carcinoma and adenocarcinoma. Most all cervical cancers are a result of human papillomavirus (HPV).

Epidemiology:

- All women are at risk for cervical cancer.
- Cervical cancer occurs most commonly after the age of 30.
- Hispanic women have the highest risk.
- American Indians and Alaskan natives have the lowest risk.

Risk Factors:

- HPV infection
  - >150 related viruses exist, some of which result in growths called papillomas (also known as warts).
- DES exposure (women with in utero exposure)
- Cigarette smoking
- Immunosuppression (such as with HIV/AIDS)
- Chlamydia infection
- Diet low in fruits and vegetables
- Overweight/obesity
- Multiple sexual partners (defined as more than four lifetime partners)
- Long-term use of oral contraceptives pills (5 years or more)
- Intrauterine device use
- Multiparity (three or more full-term pregnancies)
- Women younger than age 17 with first full-term pregnancy
- Poverty (secondary to inadequate access for screening)
- Family history of cervical cancer (mother, sister highest risk)

Factors Decreasing Risk:

- Recommended PAP and HPV screenings
- HPV vaccination
- Avoid smoking.
- Maintain a healthy weight.
- Limit number of sexual partners.

Epidemiology/Risk Factors Sources: CDC (2014k); ACS (2015b); and National Cancer Institute [NCI] (2015a, b).

Screening Test:
- PAP smear with cytology
- HPV testing with cytology

Recommendation:
- Women aged 21 to 65: Pap smear (cytology) every 3 years until age 65 or for women aged 30 to 65 who want to extend the screening interval, screening with combined cytology, and HPV testing every 5 years.
- Women older than age 65: No routine screening recommended (if adequate prior screening and who are not at high risk for cervical cancer).
- Women without a cervix (hysterectomy): Recommends against screening for cervical cancer in women without a cervix (hysterectomy) without a history of high-grade precancerous lesion (cervical intraepithelial neoplasia [CIN] grade 2 or 3) or cervical cancer.
- Women aged <21: Recommendations against routine screening

Note: The recommendations apply to women with a cervix, despite sexual history. The recommendation does not apply to women who are immunocompromised (such as with HIV positive individuals), women with in utero DES, or women with a diagnosis of high-grade precancerous cervical lesion or cervical cancer.

Source: USPSTF (2015).

Cholesterol/Lipid Disorder Screening (Adults 2008; Children/Adolescents 2007)

CHD is the leading cause of death in the US, and lipid abnormalities (dyslipidemia) is an important predictor of CHD. Primary objectives of screening for dyslipidemia are aimed at identification of individuals at risk for CHD and early intervention, with an end goal of lowering cardiovascular risk.

Epidemiology:
- Prevalence of dyslipidemia is estimated at 71 million (33.5%) of American adults.
- About one in three adults with dyslipidemia are controlled.
- Risk of CHD doubles with suboptimal levels of dyslipidemia.
- Less than half of adults with elevated LDL cholesterol are treated.

Risk Factors:
- Advanced age
- High cholesterol diet
- Obesity (BMI ≥ 30)
- Physical inactivity/sedentary lifestyle
- Familial hypercholesterolemia
- Diabetes mellitus
- History of previous CHD or atherosclerosis
- Family history of cardiovascular disease
- Tobacco use
- Hypertension

Factors Decreasing Risk:
- Healthy lifestyle modification focused on modifiable risk factors
  - Healthy dietary intake
    - Low in saturated fats, trans fats, and dietary cholesterol
    - High fiber and whole grains
    - Rich in vegetables and fruits
    - Portion control
- Physical activity/exercise aligned with recommended guidelines
  - For adults:
    - Target of 150 minutes (2 hours and 30 minutes) of moderate-intensity aerobic activity (i.e., brisk walking) every week and muscle-strengthening activities 2 or more days a week

      or

    - 75 minutes (1 hour and 15 minutes) of vigorous-intensity aerobic activity (i.e., jogging or running) every week and muscle-strengthening exercises

- Maintain a healthy weight (BMI in normal range).
- Avoid tobacco use.
- Limit alcohol.
- Pharmacologic treatment modalities for dyslipidemia (statin therapy mainstay of treatment)

Epidemiology/Risk Factors Sources: CDC (2012, 2014f); and Eckel et al. (2014)

Screening Test:
- Serum lipid (total cholesterol, high-density and low-density lipoprotein cholesterol), fasting state
  - Abnormal screening laboratory values should be repeated by a repeat test on another occasion for confirmation.
  - Insufficient evidence exists to include *triglycerides* in routine screening for dyslipidemia.

Recommendation:
- Men aged 35 and older: Strong recommendation to screen for lipid disorders
- Men aged 20 to 35 at increased risk for CHD[3]: Screen for lipid disorders.
- Women aged 45 and older: Strong recommendation to screen for lipid disorders
- Women aged 20 to 35 at increased risk for CHD[3]: Screen for lipid disorders.
- Men/women aged 20 to 35: not at increased CHD risk: No recommendation for or against screening for lipid disorders
- Youth aged 1 to 20: No recommendation for or against screening for lipid disorders

Source: USPSTF (2015).

Colorectal Screening (2008)

Colorectal cancer, also known as colon cancer, is a disease that develops in the tissues of the colon (the longest portion of the intestine). Adenocarcinomas (cancers that begin in cells that make and release mucus and other fluids) are the most common form of colon cancer. Rectal cancer develops in the tissues of the rectum (the last several inches of the large intestines, closest in proximity to the anus).

Epidemiology:
- Cancer is the second leading cause of death in the US, exceeded only by heart disease.
- Of all cancers, colorectal cancer is second leading cause of cancer-related deaths affecting both men and women in the US.
- In men and women, colorectal cancer is the third most common cancer.
- In 2014, an estimated 136,830 new cases of colon and rectal cancer were diagnosed (men and women combined).
- Deaths from colon and rectum cancer in the US account for 50,310 in 2014.
- A higher mortality rate of colorectal cancer is present in the African American population.

Risk Factors:
- Age
  - Greatest risk factor after 50 years of age for most individuals; 90% of all colorectal cancers are diagnosed after age 50.
- First-degree relative (risk doubles if relative was diagnosed before age 55)
- Personal history of colorectal cancer
- High-risk adenomas
- History of ovarian cancer
- Inflammatory bowel disease, Crohn disease, or ulcerative colitis
- Genetic predisposition (such as with familial adenomatous polyposis and hereditary nonpolyposis colorectal cancer [Lynch syndrome])
- Lack of exercise
- Diet low in fruit and vegetable intake
- Excessive alcohol consumption

---

[3]Note: Increased risk is defined by USPSTF as diabetes, past medical history of CHD or noncoronary atherosclerosis (i.e., abdominal aortic aneurysm, peripheral artery disease, carotid artery stenosis), family history of cardiovascular disease before age 50 in male relatives or age 60 in female relatives, tobacco use, hypertension, and/or obesity (BMI ≥ 30).

- Cigarette smoking
- Overweight/obesity

Factors Decreasing Risk:
- Routine screenings for colorectal cancer
  - Vast majority of colorectal cancers begin as precancerous polyps (abnormal growths) in the colon or rectum
  - Recommended CPS can aid in early detection of precancerous polyps with subsequent removal before turning to cancer (polypectomy)
- Physical activity
- Use of nonsteroidal anti-inflammatory drugs
- Daily use of aspirin (5 years or more)
- Removal of adenomatous polyps (large, >1.0 cm)
- Diet high in fruits and vegetables; low in fat and meat

Epidemiology/Risk Factors Sources: CDC (2014r, 2014ad); NCI (2014a, e, f, 2015a).

Screening Test:

There are three recommended screening tests for colorectal cancer (screening of the colon and rectum):
- High-sensitivity fecal occult blood test (FOBT)
  - Three consecutive stool samples annually. The test looks for the presence of microscopic blood in the stool.
- Sigmoidoscopy
  - Flexible, lighted tube passed through at the interior walls of the rectum and a portion of the colon.
- Colonoscopy
  - Flexible, lighted tube to examine the interior walls of the rectum and entire colon. Biopsies and polypectomy (removal of colonic polyps) may be completed.

Recommendation:
- Adults aged 50 to 75: The recommended screening includes high-sensitivity FOBT, sigmoidoscopy, or colonoscopy.
  - FOBT recommended annually
  - Sigmoidoscopy is recommended every 5 years.
  - Colonoscopy is recommended every 10 years.
  - Individuals at high risk should begin screening at a younger age and may need to test more frequently.
- Adults aged 76 to 85: Recommends against screening for colorectal screening. Beyond age 76, the decision to screen should be on an individual basis. There "may be considerations that support colorectal cancer screening in an individual patient."
- Adults aged 85 or older: Recommends against screening in this age group

Source: USPSTF (2015).

Depression Screening (Adults 2009; Adolescents 2009)

Depression, a state of mental health, is a mood disorder also referred to as major depressive disorder. According to the *Diagnostic and Statistical Manual of Mental Disorders* (DSM-IV-TR), depression is characterized by feelings of depressed mood or loss of interest in daily activities present in the same 2-week time period and represent a change from previous function. In addition to depressed mood or loss of interest in daily activities, at least five of the following symptoms must be present: (1) marked loss of interest or pleasure in most activities almost every day; (2) change in appetite/weight changes; (3) changes in sleep pattern (insomnia/hypersomnia); (4) changes in activity (psychomotor agitation/retardation); (5) fatigue or loss of energy; (6) guilt/worthlessness; (7) difficulty concentrating or more indecisiveness; and/or (8) suicidal thoughts or has a plan.

Epidemiology:
- Depression is the most common type of mental illness.
- Approximately 26% of the US population have clinical depression.
  - Depression can lead to suicide, which results in about 1 million deaths annually.
- Projections estimate by the year 2020 depression will be the second leading cause of disability throughout the world (second to ischemic heart disease).
- Major lifetime depression has been reported in women (11.7%) than in men (5.6%).

- Ethnic differences of major lifetime depression reveals 6.52% among Whites, 4.57% among Blacks, and 5.17% among Hispanic populations.
- Estimated prevalence of youth aged 13 to 18 years is 5.6% with a higher prevalence in girls (5.9%) as compared to boys (4.6%).
  - The majority of depressed youth are undiagnosed and untreated.
  - Among adolescents, lifetime prevalence may be as high as 20%.

Risk Factors:
- Individuals with comorbid mental health/psychiatric disorders
- Persons with substance abuse disorders
- Personal history of depression
  - Chronic disorder, at risk for relapse
- Family history of depression
- Associated chronic health disorders
- Unemployed individuals or low socioeconomic status
- Women are more at risk than men.
- Childbirth (i.e., postpartum depression)
- Stressful life events
- Poor social support
- Older adults with common life events (such as medical illness, bereavement, cognitive decline, institutional placement in residential, or inpatient settings)
- Adverse health behaviors associated with depression include smoking, alcohol consumption, physical inactivity, sleep disturbance.
- Adolescent risk factors include parental depression, comorbid chronic medical conditions or mental health disorders, or a major adverse life event.
  - Increased risk of suicide in youth aged 15 to 24; third leading cause of death in age group

Factors Decreasing Risk:
- Screening and treatment for individuals (adults/older adults) diagnosed with depression with psychotherapy, antidepressants, or both reduce morbidity.

Epidemiology/Risk Factors/Definition Sources: American Psychiatric Association (2013); CDC (2013); USPSTF (2015); WHO (2015a).

Screening Test:
- Formal instructions (various available) or informal screening such as two simple questions:
  - Eliciting information about mood and anhedonia
    - "Over the past 2 weeks, have you felt down, depressed, or hopeless?"
    - "Over the past 2 weeks have had felt little interest or pleasure in doing things?"
- Screening instruments include Patient Health Questionnaire [PHQ-9] (most widely used for adults and youth), Beck Depression Inventory for Primary Care, WHO-5.

Recommendation:
- Adults aged 18 and over: Screen for depression when staff-assisted depression care supports are available to accurately diagnose, provide effective treatment, and for follow-up.
- Adults aged 18 and over: The USPSTF recommends against routinely screening for depression when staff-assisted depression care supports are not in place.
  - Considerations may be given for screening patients on an individualized basis.

Source: USPSTF (2015).

Diabetes Mellitus, Type 2 Screening (2015)

Diabetes mellitus type 2 is a metabolic disorder characterized by insulin resistance that results in hyperglycemia (elevated blood glucose levels above the normal range) and/or relative insulin deficiency from insufficient production from the pancreas (American Diabetes Association [ADA], 2015a; CDC, 2011). Diabetes type 2 develops gradually over time and may take a decade or longer to progress from a normal blood sugar to the progression of impaired fasting glucose (IFG) to eventually diabetes (USPSTF, 2014, November 3).

Table 1-2: Test Values for Normal Glucose Metabolism, IFG or IGT, and Type 2 Diabetes

Test	Normal	IFG or IGT	Type 2 Diabetes
Hemoglobin A1c (%)	<5.7	5.7–6.4	>6.5 (on two separate tests)
Random plasma glucose (mg/dL)	<140	140–199	>200 (suggestive)
Fasting plasma glucose (mg/dL)	<100	100–125	>126
2-hour OTT (mg/dL)	<140	140–199	>200

From USPSTF (2014).

Insulin is the hormone allowing glucose (sugar) to enter into body cells for energy conversion (CDC, 2011). Hypertension and hyperlipidemia are associated with diabetes mellitus type 2 (Table 1-2).

Epidemiology:
- 9.3% or 29.1 million of US population have diabetes type 2
  - 21 million are diagnosed.
  - 8.1 million are undiagnosed.
- Type 2 diabetes accounts for 90% to 95% of the US population.
- 37% or 86 million of the US population aged 20 years or older had prediabetes (based on fasting glucose or hemoglobin A1C).
  - 51% were aged 65 years or older.

Risk Factors:
- Overweight or obesity
- Sedentary lifestyle
- Age 45 years or older
- Family history (first-degree relative)
- Genetic predisposition
- IFG
- Waist circumference:
  - Men >40 inches
  - Women >35 inches (nonpregnant women)
- Gestational diabetes (35% to 60% chance of developing diabetes type 2 in 10 years)
- Macrosomia (delivery of baby >9 pounds)
- Women with polycystic ovarian syndrome (PCOS)
- Hypertension
- Ethnicity/racial groups: African Americans, Hispanic/Latino Americans, American Indians, and some Pacific Islanders and Asian Americans

Factors Decreasing Risk:
- Lifestyle changes
  - Regular, physical activity/exercise
  - Healthy nutritional intake
- Maintaining healthy weight
- Moderate weight loss in high-risk individuals (5% to 10% of total body weight)

Epidemiology/Risk Sources: CDC (2011, June 11, 2014); and ADA (2015a).

Screening Tests:
- Fasting plasma glucose (FPG)
  - Requires a fasting state
  - Diabetes defined as FPG ≥ 126
  - Confirmatory FPG screening test recommended on a separate day

- Oral glucose tolerance test (OGTT)
  - Requires a fasting state
  - Blood glucose concentration is measured at 2 hours after ingestion of a 75-g glucose load.
- Hemoglobin A1C
  - Fasting state is not required; more convenient than FPG or OGTT
  - Measures long-term blood glucose concentration
  - Unaffected by acute changes in glucose levels (i.e., stress, illness)
- Random blood glucose levels: Not recommended for screening purposes
  - Affected by prandial state
  - Reflective of a single point-in-time blood glucose level

Note: A diagnosis of IFG, impaired oral glucose tolerance (IOGT), and type 2 diabetes mellitus requires repeat testing utilizing the same test on a different day as the preferred method for confirming. If the diagnosis is unable to be confirmed by findings of the two tests, but at one test is consist with high risk, the patient may be closely monitored by the clinician with a retest in 3 to 6 months.

Recommendation:
- Adults aged 40 to 70 years: Screen for abnormal blood glucose as a part of cardiovascular risk assessment in adults who are obese or overweight.
  - For patients with abnormal blood glucose, recommendations are to offer or refer patients to intensive behavioral counseling interventions promoting a healthful diet and physical activity.
  - In primary care settings, screen for abnormal blood glucose and type 2 diabetes mellitus in individuals who are at increased risk for diabetes.
- Screen for abnormal blood glucose and type 2 diabetes mellitus in those who are at increased risk for diabetes
  - Low risk with abnormal blood glucose levels: Screen every 3 years for adults with normal blood glucose levels.
  - High risk with near abnormal test values: Annual screening may be necessary.

Source: USPSTF (2015).

Hepatitis B Virus Infection (Adults/Adolescents 2013; Pregnant Women 2009)

Viral hepatitis is the leading cause of hepatocellular carcinoma (liver cancer) and the most common etiology for liver transplantation. Hepatitis B virus (HBV) infection is a serious illness that occurs as an acute infection (first 6 months of exposure) or lead to chronic infection. Chronic hepatitis B may result in potential long-term sequelae of cirrhosis, hepatic failure, and death. Hepatitis B, an infectious and contagious disease, is transmitted through blood, bodily fluids, or semen (percutaneous mucous membrane exposure to infectious blood or bodily fluids containing blood). The incubation period is 6 weeks to 6 months from the time of exposure to the onset of symptoms.

Epidemiology:
- Newly acquired HBV infection are estimated at 38,000 annually.
  - About half of new HBV infection cases are symptomatic (increases the risk of transmission to other persons)
  - Acute hepatitis B may be underreported due to some individuals being without symptoms.
  - An estimated 1% of acute cases of hepatitis B result in acute liver failure and death.
- Prevalence of chronic HBV infection in the US is estimated at 800,000 to 2.2 million individuals.
- About 3,000 individuals in the US die annually as a result of HBV-related illness.
- In infants infected with HBV during the first year of life, 80% to 90% will develop lifelong chronic hepatitis B (without immunoprophylaxis).
- In unimmunized persons, chronic HBV infection occurs in
  - >90% of infants
  - 25% to 50% of children aged 1 to 5 years
  - 6% to 10% of older children and adults
- In adults chronically infected during childhood, approximately 15% to 25% will die from prematurely from cirrhosis or hepatocellular carcinoma.

Risk Factors:
- Injection drug users, current or former (most important risk factor)
- Unprotected sex with an infected partner
- Perinatal transmission of infants born to an infected mother
- Unprotected sex with more than one partner
- Men who have sex with other men
- History of sexually transmitted infections (STIs)
- Persons who are HIV positive
- Household contacts of persons with chronic HBV infection
- Health-care and public safety workers at risk for occupational exposure to blood or blood-contaminated body fluids
  - Percutaneous needlestick injury
- Persons who are incarcerated or in correctional facilities
- Hemodialysis patients or immunosuppressive therapy (i.e., chemotherapy or immunosuppression due to organ transplantation)
- Persons with developmental disabilities or staff of facilities where persons with developmental disabilities reside
- Travelers to countries with intermediate or high risk of HBV and foreign-born persons in the US from high-risk countries
  - High prevalence: Sub-Saharan Africa, central and southeast Asia, and China
  - Intermediate prevalence: Mediterranean countries, Japan, Central Asia, Middle East, Latin and South America

Factors Decreasing Risk:
- Limiting exposure to blood and bodily fluids
- Hepatitis B vaccination
  - Routine vaccination of all infants with hepatitis B series (first dose administered at birth)
  - Adolescents and high-risk adults (i.e., injection drug users and household contacts of patients with HBV infection)
- Prevention of perinatal infection through recommended screening of all pregnant women
  - At birth, recommended immunoprophylaxis to provide hepatitis B immune globulin and hepatitis B vaccine within 12 hours of birth to the neonate

Epidemiology/Risk Factors Sources: CDC (2014g); WHO (2015b); and USPSTF (2015).

Screening Test:
- Laboratory testing with serology markers
  - Immunoassays for detecting hepatitis B surface antigen (HBsAg)
    - Test for hepatitis B surface antibodies to HBsAg (anti-HBs) and hepatitis B core antigen (anti-HBc) to distinguish between infection and immunity
      - HBsAg in acute and chronic infection
      - IgM anti-HBc is positive in acute infection only.

Recommendation:
- Adults/adolescents: Screen individuals at high risk[4] for HBV.
- Pregnant women: Screen all pregnant women at the initial prenatal visit.

Source: USPSTF (2015).

Hepatitis C Virus Infection (2013)

HCV infection is the most common chronic blood-borne infection in the US. HCV infection can cause both acute (first 6 months of exposure) and chronic infection, most commonly though progressing to a chronic condition. Chronic HCV is a leading indication for liver transplantation in the US. Serious health consequences secondary to chronic HCV infection include cirrhosis, hepatocellular carcinoma, hepatic failure, and death. HCV infection is transmitted via blood and bodily fluids, most commonly through large or repeated

---

[4]In the US, persons at high risk for HBV infection include persons who are HIV-positive, injection drug users, men who have sex with men, household contacts of persons with HBV infection, and persons from countries with a high prevalence of HBV infection.

percutaneous exposure to infected blood (i.e., blood transfusions from unscreened donors or injection drug use). Less commonly HCV infection is transmitted through sexual, occupational, perinatal exposure, although transmission of HCV infection has occurred. Detection of HCV RNA is within 1 to 3 weeks after exposure; antibody seroconversion occurs at 8 to 9 weeks. Unlike hepatitis B, no vaccine is available to prevent HCV infection, and therefore, primary prevention is of significant importance.

Epidemiology:
- Newly acquired HCV were estimated 16,000 in 2009; estimated deaths related to HCV infection in 2007 were about 15,000.
  - Only 849 cases were confirmed in 2007, although estimated to be significantly higher attributed to asymptomatic infection and underreporting (newly infected persons with HCV are typically asymptomatic).
  - Of the newly infected cases, an estimated 75% to 85% of persons develop chronic HCV, and 60% to 70% chronically infected individuals have evidence of active liver disease.
- Approximately 60% to 70% of newly infected individuals with HCV are asymptomatic or have a mild clinical presentation (increases the risk of transmission to other persons).
- An estimated 3.2 million persons have chronic HCV.
- A disproportionate percentage of the US population between 1999 and 2008 (estimated 75% of persons) born between 1945 and 1965 were chronically infected with HCV.
  - Between the 1970s and 1980s HCV was most prevalent.
    - About 200,000 cases in the 1908s; by 2001 decreased to 25,000 cases
- Injection drug use is the most important risk factor for HCV accounting for about 50% of cases on average.
  - Approximately one-third of persons aged 18 to 30 years are infected with HCV.
  - An estimated 70% to 90% of older persons and those with a history of injection drug use have HCV.
- HCV infection incidence has been attributed to a three-fold increase of hepatocellular carcinoma related to HCV infection 2 to 4 decades prior.

Risk Factors:
- Injection drug users (current or former)
- Recipients of clotting factor concentrates before to 1987
  - Risk reduced since more advanced methods for manufacturing/screening have been instituted.
- Recipients of blood transfusions or donated organs before July 1992
  - Risk of transfusion-associated hepatitis C has decreased since the advancement screening donated blood supply for HCV.
- Health-care and public safety workers at risk for occupational exposure to blood or blood-contaminated body fluids.
  - Percutaneous needlestick injury
- Perinatal transmission of infants born to an infected mother
- Persons who are HIV positive persons
- Persons who are incarcerated or in correctional facilities
- Hemodialysis patients
- Unregulated tattooing or piercing

Factors Decreasing Risk:
- Avoidance of high-risk behaviors (i.e., injection drug use)
- Screening and testing of blood, plasma, organ, tissue, and semen donors
- Limiting exposure to blood and bodily fluids

Epidemiology/Risk Factors Sources: CDC (2014, July 17); CDC (2015, January 5); and USPSTF (2015).

Screening Test:
- Immunoassays for detecting anti-HCV antibody testing
  - HCV antibody nonreactive (no HCV antibody detected)
  - HCV antibody reactive (presumptive HCV infection)
  - HCV antibody reactive, HCV RNA detected (current HCV infection)
  - HCV antibody reactive, HCV RNA not detected (no current HCV infection)

Recommendation:
- Adults: Screen individuals at high risk for HCV.
- Individuals born between 1945 and 1965: Offer a one-time screening for HCV.

Source: USPSTF (2015).

Human Immunodeficiency Virus Infection Screening (2013)

Human Immunodeficiency Virus (HIV) attacks the immune system by destroying CD4+ T cells and over time leaves the host susceptible to opportunistic infections. HIV can result in acquired immunodeficiency syndrome (AIDS). There is no cure presently and HIV remains a serious health issue. However, advances in screening, early detection, and treatment intervention has brought about the management of HIV as a chronic disease with a near-to-normal life expectancy. HIV is transmitted through blood and bodily fluids (blood, semen, preseminal fluid, vaginal fluids, rectal fluids, or breast milk from an infected person), predominantly through sharing of drug, anal or vaginal sex or by sharing injection drug use equipment with an HIV infected person. The highest risk of newly acquired infections was among men who have sex with men and among the African American population. HIV is not detectable until approximately 10 to 15 days after infected, although diagnostic immunoassays may be falsely negative. If high clinical suspicion for HIV exposure exists, repeat testing in 1 to 2 weeks is recommended. Antiretroviral therapy aimed at viral suppression is the mainstay of treatment.

Epidemiology:
- Prevalence of newly acquired HIV infection is estimated at 50,000 annually (incidence relatively stable since the mid-1990s).
  - In 2010, 47,500 newly acquired infections were reported.
  - African Americans are the most HIV affected racial/ethnic group.
    - An approximate 44% of newly acquired HIV infections in 2010 were African Americans.
  - Men who had sex with men accounted for 63% of all newly acquired HIV infections in 2010.
- Nearly 50% of HIV-infected persons in the US are unaware of their infection (increases the risk of transmission to other persons).
- An approximate of 1.2 million individuals in the US were living with HIV in 2011.
  - Of the 1.2 million, about 14% were unaware of being infected.
  - Only 4 out of 10 individuals living with HIV were in HIV medical care.
- The highest risk group of new HIV infections are among men who have sex with men.

Risk Factors:
- Gay, bisexual men, and men who have sex with other men
  - More affected than any other group in the US
  - Among all gay and bisexual men, about 36% were African American/black men.
- Engaging in anal, vaginal, or oral sex with men who have sex with men, multiple partners, or anonymous partners without using a condom
  - CDC recommends testing every 3 to 6 months for all sexually active males who have sex with other men.
- Injection drug use or sharing of drug injection equipment
- Sex partners of persons who are HIV-infected, bisexual, or use injection drug use.
- Persons who exchange sex for money or drugs
- Personal history of hepatitis, tuberculosis, or malaria
- Recipients of clotting factor concentrates from 1978 to 1985
  - Risk reduced since more advanced methods for manufacturing/screening have been instituted.
- Recipients of blood transfusions from 1978 to 1985
  - Risk of transfusion-associated HIV has decreased since the advancement screening donated blood supply for HIV.
- Health-care and public safety workers at risk for occupational exposure to blood or blood-contaminated body fluids
  - Percutaneous needlestick injury
- Perinatal transmission of infants born to an infected mother
- Persons who are incarcerated or in correctional facilities
- Hemodialysis patients
- Unregulated tattooing or piercing

Factors Decreasing Risk:
- Abstinence, limiting sexual partners, less risky sexual behaviors (oral sex is much less risky than anal or vaginal sex)
- Avoidance of injection drug use or sharing of drug use equipment
- Protection with consistent use of latex condoms
- Test for HIV status
- With known exposure, prompt treatment with postexposure prophylaxis
- Screening if planning pregnancy or early in pregnancy

Epidemiology/Risk Factors Sources: CDC (2014aa, 2015b); National Institute of Health (NIH) (2015); and USPSTF (2015).

Screening Test:
- Immunoassays for detecting HIV p24 antigen and HIV antibody testing
  - If positive, follow by a confirmatory HIV-1/HIV-2 antibody differentiation immunoassay.

Recommendation:
- Adolescents/adults aged 15 to 65: Screen for HIV.
  - Additionally, younger adolescents and older adults at increased risk should be screened.
- Pregnant women: Screen all pregnant women including untested women who present in labor and whose HIV status is unknown.

Source: UPSTF (2015).

Lung Cancer Screening (2013)

Lung cancer develops in the lung tissues, typically in the cells lining the air passages. The most common type is non–small cell accounting for an estimated 85% of all lung cancer cases. Subtypes of non–small cell lung cancer include squamous cell carcinoma, adenocarcinoma, and large cell carcinoma. Small cell lung cancer, also known as oat cell cancer, is responsible for about 10% to 15% of lung cancers and tends to spread quickly. Lung carcinoid tumors, referred to as neuroendocrine tumors, account for less than 5% of lung cancers and typically are characterized by slow growth. Metastases (spreading to lymph nodes or other organs of the body) are uncommon with lung carcinoid tumors. Slow growth and rarely (metastases) are typical of lung carcinoid tumors. Lung cancer is associated with a poor prognosis, and 90% of individuals with lung cancer die of the disease and therefore prevention is key.

Epidemiology:
- Lung cancer is the most preventable type of cancer in the world.
- Lung cancer is a leading cause of cancer death in both men and women in the US.
- Lung cancer is the third most common cancer in the US.
- Estimated 224, 210 new lung cancer cases (morbidity) from non–small cell and small cell combined in 2014 (males 116,000; females 108,210)
- Estimated 159,260 deaths (mortality) from non–small cell and small cell in the US in 2014 (males 86,930; females 72,330)
- Lung cancer accounts for an approximate 27% of all cancer deaths in the US (men and women combined) and each year more individuals die of lung cancer than colon, breast, and prostate cancers combined.
- Black males have a highest incidence of developing lung cancer (about 20% more likely than white males), followed by white, American Indian/Alaska Native, Asian/Pacific Islander, and Hispanic men.
- In women, White women have the highest incidence, followed by Black, American Indian/Alaska Native, Asian/Pacific Islander, and Hispanic women.
- Incidence of lung cancer increases with age occurring most often in individuals aged 55 and older.
- Approximately 37% of the US adults are current or former smokers.
- Average 5-year survival rate for lung cancer is low (17%); higher when diagnosed at an early stage (52%)
  - Only 15% of lung cancers are diagnosed at an early stage.
    - Prevention and early detection are vital to improving health outcomes.

Risk Factors:
- Cigarette smoking
  - Most important risk factor
  - Smoking is a modifiable risk factor
- Age
  - Increasing age and cumulative tobacco smoke exposure are the two most common risk factors for lung cancer.
- Occupational exposures to carcinogens
- Radon exposure
- Family history of lung cancer, pulmonary fibrosis, or chronic obstructive pulmonary disease
- Secondhand smoke exposure
- Air pollution

Factors Decreasing Risk:
- Smoking cessation (quitting)
  - Significantly reduces a person's risk of developing and dying of lung cancer
- Less than 50 years of age
- Years since quitting (longer abstinence decreases lung cancer risk)
- Avoidance of secondhand smoke exposure
- Reducing or eliminating radon exposure
  - Radon testing for home environment
- Reducing or eliminating occupational carcinogen exposures

Epidemiology/Risk Factors Sources: CDC (2014x); ACS (2015); and NCI (2014c).

Screening Test:
- LDCT

Recommendation:
- Adults aged 55 to 80 with a history of smoking: Annual screening for lung cancer with LDCT in individuals with a 30-pack-year-history and currently smoke or have quit within the past 15 years
  - Screening should be discontinued once an individual has not smoked for 15 years or develops a health condition that substantially limits life expectancy or has curative lung surgery.

Source: USPSTF (2015).

Obesity (Adults 2012; Children/Adolescents 2010)

Obesity in the past two decades has been drastically increased and is a serious public health issue. Chronic health conditions are associated with obesity, some of which correspond with disability and leading causes of preventable death. Promoting healthy lifestyles with integration good nutrition, physical activity/exercise, and maintaining a healthy weight are endeavors to improve health outcomes.

Epidemiology:
- Prevalence of obesity in adults is estimated at 78.6 million or more than one-third (34.9%) of adults in the US.
- Obesity is attributed to morbidity and disability resulting from preventable health diseases.
- Increased mortality is associated with obesity, particularly in adults <65 years of age.
- Economic burden of obesity in the US estimated at 147 billion in 2008.
- Childhood obesity reflects an estimated 12.7 million (17%) among the nation's youth aged 2 to 19 years.
  - Nearly one in five youth aged 2 to 19 are obese.
  - Obesity is more prevalent among Hispanics (22.4%) and non-Hispanic Black (20.2%) youth than White youth (14.1%) and Asian youth (8.6%).

Risk Factors:
- Sedentary lifestyle/lack of physical exercise
- Unhealthy diet and eating habits
- Advancing age
  - Decreased metabolism
  - Menopause in women
- Socioeconomic factors
  - Lifelong-learned patterns from family environments
  - Lack of education
  - Cost barriers
- Quitting smoking (related to weight gain)
- Abdominal obesity increases risk of obesity-related diseases.
  - Male: Waist circumference >40 inches
  - Female: Waist circumference >35 increases
- Eating disorders
- Mental health disorders
  - Depression, anxiety
- Hypothyroidism

- Genetics
  - Family history of obesity including disorders such as Prader–Willi syndrome and Bardet–Biedi syndrome
- Associated comorbid and chronic health conditions
  - Type 2 diabetes mellitus (adult/youth), metabolic syndrome, CHD, heart failure, stroke, dyslipidemia, hypertension
  - Restrictive lung disease and asthma
  - Gastroesophageal reflux disease
  - Various cancers (endometrial, breast, colon)
  - Liver and gallbladder disease
  - Sleep apnea and respiratory issues
  - Osteoarthritis
  - Gynecological problems (abnormal menses, infertility)

Factors Decreasing Risk:
- Comprehensive lifestyle intervention and behavior modification
  - Lifelong changes
    - Counseling on nutrition, exercise/physical activity, healthy weight
- Healthy weight
  - Caloric restriction/setting weight loss goals
  - Weight reduction
    - 5% can reduce the incidence of type II diabetes mellitus
    - Lower incidence of health-related conditions
    - Mortality all-cause reduction
- Healthy dietary intake
  - Diet rich in fruits and vegetables
  - Low in saturated fats, trans fats, and dietary cholesterol
  - High fiber and whole grains
  - Rich in vegetables and fruits
  - Portion control
- Physical activity/exercise aligned with recommended guidelines.
  - For adults:
    - Target of 150 minutes (2 hours and 30 minutes) of moderate-intensity aerobic activity (i.e., brisk walking) every week and muscle-strengthening activities 2 or more days a week

      or

    - 75 minutes (1 hour and 15 minutes) of vigorous-intensity aerobic activity (i.e., jogging or running) every week and muscle-strengthening exercises
  - For youth:
    - Target of 60 minutes (1 hour) or more each day
- Bariatric surgery
  - Recommended for individuals who have failed lifestyle changes with dietary modification, exercise, and pharmacologic intervention
  - BMI 40 or 35 with comorbidities (hypertension, dyslipidemia, IFG, diabetes mellitus, obstructive sleep apnea)
- Self-monitoring
  - Monitoring weight on a regular basis

Epidemiology/Risk Factors Sources: CDC (2011, 2014f, 2014l, 2014o, 2014, August 25, 2014s); and Dunphy, Winland-Brown, Porter, and Thomas (2011).

Screening Test:
- Weight and height to determine a BMI
  - BMI <18.5 → Underweight
  - BMI = 18.5 to 24.9 → Normal weight
  - BMI = 25 to 29.9 → Overweight
  - BMI > 30 → Obese
  - BMI >40 (or 35 in presence of comorbid conditions) → Severe obesity

Recommendation:
- All adults: Screen for obesity. Recommended offering or referring patients with a body mass index (BMI ≥ 30) to intensive, multicomponent behavioral intervention such as follows:
  - Individual or group sessions, weight loss setting goals, improvement of diet/nutrition, physical activity/ exercise sessions, addressing barriers preventing behavior change, strategies for maintenance of lifestyle modification changes
- Children/adolescents aged 6 and older: Screen for obesity. Offer or refer for comprehensive intervention with promoting behavioral changes toward weight reduction.

Source: USPSTF (2015).

Prostate Cancer Screening (2012)

Carcinoma of the prostate forms in the tissues of the prostate and predominantly occurs in older men. The median age for prostate cancer is 72 years. Most prostate cancers grow slowly, but some may have rapid growth and spread quickly. More than 95% of primary prostate cancers are adenocarcinomas. When localized, prostate cancer may be cured and typically responds to treatment when widespread. Although prostate cancer is a serious health problem, most do not die from the disease.

Epidemiology:
- Prostate cancer is the most common cancer among men in the US.
- Prostate cancer is the second leading cause of cancer-related death in American men (lung cancer is first).
- About 1 in 38 men will die from prostate cancer.
- Estimated 233,000 in 2014 died from new prostate cancer cases (morbidity).
- Estimated 29,480 deaths (mortality) in 2014 attributed to prostate cancer.
- Black men have the highest rate of developing prostate cancer followed by White, Hispanic, Asian/Pacific Islander, and American Indian/Alaska Native men.

Risk Factors:
- Risk of prostate cancer increases with age.
  - Risk rapidly increases after age 50.
  - Approximately 6 out of 10 cases are diagnosed in men aged 65 or older.
  - Rare before age 40
- Family history (greater risk two- to threefold with first-degree relative of father, brother, or son)
- One in seven men will be diagnosed during a person's lifetime.
- Dietary intake:
  - High in red meat or high-fat dairy products; low in fruits and vegetables may slightly increase the risk of developing prostate cancer
- Genetic mutations
  - Inherited mutations of the *BRCA1* or *BRCA2* genes (raises risk of breast/ovarian cancers) may increase the risk in some men for prostate cancer.
  - Men with hereditary nonpolyposis colorectal cancer (Lynch syndrome) may have an increased risk for prostate cancer.

Factors Decreasing Risk:
- Some medications used to treat benign prostatic hypertrophy (BPH), a noncancerous condition.
  - Finasteride and dutasteride have shown a reduction in the diagnosis of prostate cancer.

Epidemiology/Risk Factors Sources: ACS (2015d); CDC (2014h); NCI (2014d); and Prostate Cancer Foundation (2015).

Screening Test:
- Digital rectal examination (DRE)
- Prostate-specific antigen (PSA) test
  - An organ-specific marker, often used as a tumor marker (not precise)
  - Increased PSA levels may be suggestive of disease progression or metastatic disease.

Recommendation:
- The USPSTF recommends against PSA screening for prostate cancer.

Source: USPSTF (2015).

Skin Cancer Screening (2009)

The most common cancer in the US is skin cancer and includes three primary types of skin cancer: melanoma, basal cell carcinoma, and squamous cell carcinoma. Of these, melanoma is the most serious and responsibility for morbidity and mortality. The two most common types of skin cancer, basal cell and squamous cell carcinomas, are highly curable. A causative factor in all three types of skin cancers are exposure to ultraviolet (UV) light and therefore, an emphasis on prevention is key to risk reduction.

Epidemiology:
- Melanoma accounts for an estimated 5% to 6% of skin cancer diagnoses; attributed to 75% of mortality-related skin cancer.
- Prevalence of melanoma[5] (diagnosed) in 2011 was estimated at 70,853 in the US (41,573 men; 29,280 women).
- Mortality (deaths) in 2011 attributable to melanomas of the skin was estimated at 12,212 in the US (8,241 men; 3,971 women).
- Over 3.5 million cases of basal cell and squamous cell carcinomas are diagnosed every year in the US.

Risk Factors:
- Unprotected and/or excessive exposure to UV radiation (sunlight or tanning booths or sun lamps)
- Fair-skinned individuals (more sensitive and at greater risk for UV effects)
  - Pale skin, natural red, or blonde hair
- Severe sunburns
- Personal history of skin cancer
- Personal history of certain types of pigmented lesions (dysplastic or atypical nevi), several large nondysplastic nevi, many small nevi, or with a moderate amount of freckling—two- to threefold risk of developing melanoma
- Family history of skin cancer
  - First-degree relative (parent, sibling, or child) at greater risk
  - Familial dysplastic nevus syndrome or with several dysplastic or atypical nevi are at high risk of melanoma (greater than fivefold risk)
- Excessive exposure
  - High-intensity, chronic exposure greater risk
- Melanoma risk increases after age 20 years.
- Organ transplantation individuals receiving immunosuppressive drug therapy (in particularly increased risk of squamous cell carcinomas)
- Workplace exposure to coal tar, creosote, pitch, arsenic compounds, or radium exposure

Factors Decreasing Risk:
- Avoid exposure to the sun at the most intense time of the day, midday between 10 AM and 4 PM.
  - Seek shade.
  - Wear a wide-brim hat; sunglasses.
- Broad spectrum sunscreen containing a sun protector factor (SPF) of 30 or higher
  - Reapply every 2 hours and after swimming, towel drying, or sweating.
- Prevent sunburn.
- Avoid tanning beds or sun lamps.

Epidemiology/Risk Factors Sources: ACS (2014b); CDC (2015c); NCI (2014b).

Screening Test:
- Visual examination of the skin including self-examination and clinical examination

Recommendation:
- All adults without a history of premalignant or malignant lesions: The USPSTF recommends against screening for skin cancer with a whole-skin examination by a primary care clinician or self-examination of the skin by the patient for early detection of cutaneous melanoma, squamous cell, or basal cell cancer in the general adult population.[6]

---

[5]Melanoma is a reportable cancer in the US cancer registries. More reliable statistics are available for melanoma compared to basal cell and squamous cell carcinomas, which uncommonly result in metastasis or death.

[6]Surveillance in high-risk populations such as individuals with familial syndromes (i.e., familial atypical mole and melanoma syndrome) were not examined by the USPSTF.

- Adults, adolescents, and children aged 10 to 24; fair-skinned individuals: Counseling is recommended to minimize exposure of UV radiation to reduce skin cancer risk.

Source: USPSTF (2015).

Sexually Transmitted Diseases Screening (2014)

STIs are spread by sexual contact and are a major health problem in the nation. Often individuals may be asymptomatic, thereby increasing the risk of transmission. Serious health-related consequences of STIs include pelvic inflammatory disease (PID), cancer, infertility, ectopic pregnancy, and chronic pelvic pain. Some complications secondary to untreated STIs include cervical cancer, genital tract infections, infertility, hepatitis viruses, HIV, and PID. In pregnancy or during delivery, untreated STIs may result may result in perinatal infection, serious physical and mental disabilities, and death.

Epidemiology:
- Approximately 20 million new cases of STIs occur annually in the US.
  - About half of the cases are individuals aged 15 to 24 years.
- Bacterial vaginosis (BV):
  - Most common infection in women aged 15 to 44 years
    - Not considered an STI
    - Greater risk of contracting an STI with BV present
  - Prevalence is estimated at 21.2 million (29.2%) among women in the US.
  - Non-White women at a higher risk (African American 51%; Mexican Americans 32%) as compared to White women (23%)
- Chlamydia (*Chlamydia trachomatis*):
  - Most common reported bacterial STI in the US, affecting both men and women
  - Prevalence in 2013 was estimated at 1,401,906 cases in the US.
    - Often underreported due to individuals being asymptomatic; including unreported cases, prevalence is estimated at 2.86 million cases
  - Prevalence among young persons aged 14 to 24 is about threefold that of persons aged 25 to 39.
  - About 1 in 15 sexually active females aged 14 to 19 are infected with chlamydia.
- Gonorrhea (*Neisseria gonorrhoeae bacterium*):
  - In 2013, an approximate 333,004 cases of gonorrhea were reported.
    - Highest reported rates of infection are among sexually active teenagers, young adults, and African Americans
  - Approximately 820,000 individuals contract new gonorrheal infections annually.
    - Less than half of the cases are detected or reported.
    - Among the 820,000 cases, about 570,000 were among persons aged 15 to 24 years.
  - Congenital gonorrhea (gonorrhea that may be transmitted to an infant during childbirth) can result in fetal death or physical and mental developmental disabilities.
- Hepatitis (A, B, and C)
  - Mode of transmission via sexual contact
  - Viral hepatitis is the leading cause of liver cancer and most frequent etiology necessitating for a liver transplant.
  - An estimated 4.4 million have chronic hepatitis and the majority are unaware of being infected with hepatitis.
  - Hepatitis A virus (HAV):
    - Occurs during sexual activity secondary to fecal–oral contact or contamination
    - HAV is a self-limiting disease and not chronic in nature; however, about 10% to 15% of individuals experience a relapse of symptoms in the first 6 months following the acute illness.
  - HBV:
    - In individuals seeking treatment in sexually transmitted diseases (STD) clinics, about 10% to 40% have evidence of prior or current HBV infection.
    - In persons infected with HBV, 39% had previous screening for an STD or sought care before becoming infected with HBV.
      - Suggestive of many missed opportunities to vaccinate at-risk individuals

- HCV:
  - ○ Approximately 15% to 20% of HCV infected cases have no risk factors except a history of sexual exposure.
- Herpes (herpes simplex viruses type I [HSV-1] or type 2 [HSV-2]):
  - An approximate 15.5% of individuals aged 14 to 49 have genital herpes in the US.
    - ○ Overall prevalence is thought to be higher than 15.5% as HSV-1 is attributed to an increasing number of cases.
  - Prevalence in the US was estimated at 776,000 new genital herpes infection annually.
  - HSV-2 is more common among women (20.3%) than men (10.6%) in aged 14 to 49.
  - Predominantly, HSV-2 is transmitted from men to women, as compared to women to men.
  - Higher prevalence of HSV-2 exists in non-Hispanic Blacks (41.8%) than among non-Hispanic Whites (11.3%).
  - Majority of individuals with HSV-2 are unaware of their STI.
    - ○ Approximately 87.4% of 14- to 49-year-old persons infected with HSV-2 have not been diagnosed clinically.
  - Genital ulcerative disease resulting from genital herpes increases the risk of transmitting and acquiring HIV.
    - ○ Two- to fourfold greater risk of contracting HIV if exposed to HIV when genital herpes is present (genital herpes comprises the integrity of the skin secondary to ulcerations)
- Human immunodeficiency virus (HIV)
  - Individuals with an STI are at greater risk of contracting HIV or are more likely to acquire in the future.
  - Syphilis and HIV have been closely linked in men who have sex with men.
    - ○ In 2012, about 75% of reported syphilis cases in the US were men who had sex with men.
    - ○ Men who have syphilis are at higher risk for being diagnosed with HIV.
    - ○ HIV is more closely linked with gonorrhea than chlamydia.
    - ○ Herpes is commonly found in association with HIV.
      - ○ Individuals with HSV-2 are at about a threefold risk for contracting HIV infection.
  - HIV and syphilis have been closely linked in men who have sexual relations with men.
- HPV:
  - Most common STI in the US
    - ○ So common that most sexually active men and women will contract at least one type of HPV (over 100 types) in their lifetime
  - Prevalence of Americans has been estimated at 79 million.
  - Estimated about 14 million newly infected HPV cases occur annually.
  - Genital warts, a complication of HPV, is responsible for about 360,000 cases; cervical cancer accounts for about 10,000 cases in females annually.
    - ○ Prevention of about 21,000 HPV-related cancers are possible with the HPV vaccination.
- Syphilis (*Treponema pallidum*):
  - In 2013, 56,471 new cases of syphilis were reported.
    - ○ Of these, 17,535 were primary and secondary syphilis, the earliest and most transmissible states of syphilis.
    - ○ Highest incidence was found among men aged 20 to 29.
    - ○ The majority were among Black, Hispanic, and other racial/ethnic minorities.
  - 350 cases of congenital syphilis were reported in 2013.
    - ○ Incidence was 10.4 times higher among infants born to Black or 3.5 times Hispanic mothers as compared to White mothers.
- Trichomoniasis (*Trichomonas vaginalis*):
  - Most common curable STI
  - Prevalence of trichomoniasis has been estimated at 3.7 million in the US.
    - ○ Of the 3.7 million cases, about 70% are asymptomatic.
  - Trichomoniasis is more common among women than men.
    - ○ Older women are more commonly infected.

Risk Factors:
- More than one sexual partner; multiple sexual partners
- Adolescents are at higher risk of STIs than adults.

- Sexual relations initiated at an early onset of age
- Men who have sex with men
- Women who have sex with women
- Sexual relations with an individual who has an STI
- New partner in the past 60 days
- History of prior STIs
- Illicit drug use
  - Intravenous drug use or sexual partner with use of intravenous drug use
- African American race
- Unmarried status
- Homelessness
- Individuals with mental illness or a disability
- Persons with a history of sexual abuse
- Patients at public STI clinics
- Low income persons in urban settings
- Persons in correctional facilities

Factors Decreasing Risk:
- Abstinence from sexual relations
- Less risky sexual behaviors
- Latex condom protection (vaginal, anal, or oral sex)
- Preexposure vaccination
  - HPV
    - Vaccination (Gardasil/Cervarix) is recommended for the following:
      - All adolescents (male/female) aged 11 or 12 years
      - Gay and bisexual men (or any man who has sex with a man) through age 26
      - Immunosuppressed men and women including persons living with HIV/AIDS through age 26 (if not fully vaccinated during youth)
  - Hepatitis A and B
    - Vaccination is the most effective means of reducing HAV and HBV.
    - HAV prevention vaccine is recommended for persons aged $\geq$ 12 months and at risk populations:
      - Unvaccinated individuals at risk for HAV should be vaccinated (men who have sex with men; persons with illicit drug use; chronic liver disease; individuals in direct contact with persons infected with HAV) and all adults seeking protection from HBV
      - Postexposure: For individuals not vaccinated and exposed to HAV, recommendation is to administer a single vaccine.
    - HBV prevention vaccine is recommended for persons aged $\geq$ 12 months and at-risk populations:
      - Unvaccinated adolescents, all unvaccinated adults at risk for HBV infection (multiple sex partners, persons not in a monogamous relationship, current or recent injection drug use, men who have sex with men, household or sexual contact with HBV surface antigen–positive contact), and all adults seeking protection from HBV
- Monogamous relationship
- Limit number of sexual partners.
- Personal screening for STIs and limiting transmission
- Knowledge of the partner's sexual history and negative STI status
- Immunization for HPV, HAV, and HBV

Epidemiology/Risk Factors Sources: CDC (2011a, 2014d, 2014t, 2014u, 2014af, 2015d); USPSTF (2015).

Screening Test:
- Identification of adolescents and adults who are at increased risk for STIs and implementing intensive behavioral counseling
- For specific STI diagnostic considerations and treatment modalities, refer to the women's health chapter.

Recommendation:
- Sexually active adults and adolescents: Recommendation for intensive behavioral counseling who are at risk for STIs

Source: USPSTF (2015).

Tobacco Use Counseling and Interventions (Adults 2015; Children/Adolescents 2013)

Tobacco use, primarily cigarette smoking, is the leading cause of preventable disease, disability, and death in the US. Nearly every system of the body is harmed by smoking cigarettes. Health risks are associated with smokeless tobacco (tobacco products not burned) such as chewing tobacco, oral tobacco, spitting tobacco, dip, chew, and snuff). Secondhand smoke contains toxic chemicals and carcinogens (cancer-causing agents) that are health detriments.

Epidemiology:
- Cigarette smoking remains the leading cause of preventable death in the US.
- An estimated 18.1% or 42.1 million adults aged 18 or older smoke cigarettes in the US.
- In 2012 an estimated 6.7% of middle school and 23.3% of high school youth used tobacco products (cigarettes, cigars, hookahs, snus, smokeless tobacco, bidis, pipes, dissolvable tobacco, Keteks, and electronic cigarettes).
- Tobacco-related deaths are estimated for more than 480,000 deaths annually (or one in every five deaths) including deaths from secondhand smoke (men 278,544; women 201,773).
    - Death attributed to secondhand smoke is estimated at 42,000 each year in the US.
    - Of the tobacco-related deaths, an estimated 161,000 are attributable to cancer, 128,000 from cardiovascular disease, and 103,000 related to respiratory diseases.
        - Approximately 80% of all deaths from COPD are a result of smoking.
- Cigarette smoking is more common among men (20.5%) than women (15.8%).
- Lung cancer is the leading cause of death in men and women in the US.
    - Smoking causes about 90% of all lung cancer deaths in men and women.
- Costs attributed to tobacco use are estimated at $193 billion annually.
    - Direct medical expenses $96 billion a year
    - Lost productivity $97 billion a year

Risk Factors:
- Smoking cigarettes is known to cause the following:
    - Cardiovascular disease, stroke, peripheral arterial disease (PAD)
    - Lung diseases such as chronic bronchitis, chronic obstructive pulmonary disease, emphysema
    - Various cancers such as lung, bladder, blood, cervical, colorectal, esophageal, gastric, renal, larynx, liver, or oropharynx
    - Premature death
    - Fertility issues in both men and women
    - Preterm delivery, stillbirth, low birth weight, and ectopic pregnancy in women; SIDS; and fertility issues in both men and women
    - Osteoporosis
    - Oral disease
    - Cataract development
    - Chronic inflammation and adverse effects on immune function
- Cigarette use is associated with premature death.
    - On average, life expectancy is about 10 years shorter for individuals who smoke than for nonsmokers.
- An approximate 600 ingredients are found in cigarettes and when burned create over 7,000 toxic chemicals, of which 69 are known carcinogens.
- Smokeless tobacco is associated with oropharyngeal cancers, esophageal, and pancreatic along with cardiovascular disease.
- Secondhand smoke in adults has been linked to cardiovascular disease, lung cancer and various cancers; respiratory diseases and infections; and death.
- Secondhand smoke in youth has been associated with ear infections, asthma exacerbations, respiratory symptoms and infections, and an increased risk of sudden infant death syndrome (SIDS).

- Risks influential for tobacco use are various to include race/ethnicity, education, age, socioeconomic status. Disparities exist in geographical areas, particularly relative to smoke-free protective states and tobacco prevention funding endeavors.

Factors Decreasing Risk:

- Quitting tobacco use reduces risk of health diseases such as cardiovascular, lung disorders, cancers, premature death, and other various health conditions linked to smoking. There are immediate and long-term benefits to quitting smoking to include the risk of cardiovascular, pulmonary diseases, and cancers.
- Smoking cessation prior to the age of 40 reduces the risk of dying from smoking-related diseases by an estimated 90%.
- Quitting smoking can reduce a women's risk of preterm delivery, stillbirth, low birth weight, and ectopic pregnancy, SIDS, along with fertility issues in both men and women.
- Smoking cessation can reduce the risk of osteoporosis, oral disease, and cataract development.
- Quitting the use of smoke-less tobacco reduces the risk of oropharyngeal cancer and oral disease.
- No safe level of secondhand exposure exists; smoke-free environments are critical to health.

Epidemiology/Risk Factors Sources: ACS (2014a); AHRQ (2012); American Lung Association (2015); CDC (2014w, 2014ae, 2014ah); USDHHS (2014c); and WHO (2014d).

Screening Test:

- Recognition of the five *As* behavioral framework aimed at a strategic approach for intervention.
  - Five *As* behavioral counseling framework encompasses five major steps:
    - **Ask** every patient at every visit about tobacco use status.
    - **Advise** with a strong, clear, and personalized message to quit tobacco use.
    - **Assess** the individual's willingness to make a quit attempt.
    - **Assist** those interested in making a quit attempt with counseling and pharmacotherapy.
    - **Arrange** a follow-up office visit (in person or by phone) in the first week after the quit date preferably.

Recommendation:

- Adults who are not pregnant: Recommended to ask all adults about tobacco use, advise to stop using tobacco, and provide behavioral interventions and US Food and Drug Administration (FDA)-approved pharmacotherapy for cessation of tobacco.
  - The five As is a recommended framework to utilize as a common approach for recognition and counseling of tobacco use behaviors.
  - All adults: Ask all adults about tobacco use and provide cessation interventions for those who use tobacco products (utilizing the five As behavioral counseling framework).
- Pregnant women: Ask all pregnant women about tobacco use, advise to stop using tobacco, and provide behavioral interventions for cessation of tobacco use in pregnant women and provide "augmented, pregnancy-tailored counseling for those who smoke."
- School-aged children/adolescents: Recommended for primary care clinicians to provide interventions with education or brief counseling to prevent the initiation of tobacco use

Source: USPSTF (2015).

Nutrition

United States Department of Agriculture 2010 Dietary Guidelines for Americans and *ChooseMyPlate*

Promotion of healthy nutritional intake and maintenance of healthy body weights are among the national goals. The prevalence of obesity has escalated tremendously over the past several decades, with rates doubling for adults and tripling for children. In 2011, over one-third of US adults (more than 72 million) and about 17% of youth were obese. Childhood and adult obesity has considerable health consequences such as chronic diseases and the economic burden on the US health-care system. Type 2 diabetes mellitus, heart disease, stroke, hypertension, dyslipidemia, sleep apnea, and cancers are among some of the potential health risks linked to obesity.

RECOMMENDATIONS

The health and nutrition of adults and youth are among national priorities with endeavors at the community, state, and national level. The national *2010 Dietary Guidelines for Americans for a Healthier Life* are a joint endeavor by the US Department of Agriculture (USDA) and the US Department of Health and Human Services (USDHHS). Guidelines are released every 5 years with the next release slated for 2015. Three overarching concepts of the 2010 Dietary Guidelines for Americans for a Healthier Life include the following:

- Balance of caloric intake with physical activity to achieve and sustain a healthy weight
- Consumption of nutrient-dense foods such as vegetables, fruits, whole grains, low-fat and fat-free dairy products, and seafood
- A reduction of foods with sodium, saturated fats, trans fat, cholesterol, refined grains, and added sugars

Promoting health, reduction of chronic diseases, and decreasing the prevalence of obesity describes the overall aim of the US dietary guidelines.

In June 2011, the USDA replaced MyPyramid with the *MyPlate* nutritional initiative, which can be found on the website ChooseMyPlate.gov. Developed by the First Lady Michelle Obama and USDA secretary, *MyPlate* was released as the USDA's new food icon. *MyPlate*, a communication initiative, serves as a visual reminder promoting Americans to select healthful food choices and build healthy plates at mealtimes. Specific recommendations on the *MyPlate* food groups correlate with the 2010 Dietary Guidelines and each of the five USDA food groups (fruits, vegetables, grains, protein foods, and dairy). For healthy nutrition, *MyPlate* recommends a diet:

- Rich in a variety of vegetables (dark-green vegetables, red and yellow vegetables, raw, cooked, fresh, or frozen)
- Focused on fruits (fruits, berries, melons, 100% fruit juice)
- High in foods containing fiber
- Low in refined grains (white flour, white bread, white rice, pasta)
- High in whole grains (whole wheat, bran, brown rice, oatmeal, barley, whole wheat pasta)—at least half of grains should be whole grains.
- Protein foods (lean meats or poultry, seafood, beans, eggs, soy products, nuts, peanut butter)
  - At least 8 ounces of seafood per week for adults
- Fat-free or low-fat dairy products (low-fat or reduced-fat milk, yogurt, cheese, frozen yogurt)
- Avoid saturated and trans fat products (hydrogenated or partially hydrogenated products, butter, stick margarine, baked goods, pastries, fried foods, meats with visible fat).
- Avoid food and beverages with added sugars (soda, energy drinks, desserts, dairy desserts such as ice cream); drink plenty of water.
- Limit sodium intake to as follows:
  - Adults/youth: 2,300 mg of sodium a day (about one teaspoon of salt)
  - Adults aged 51 and older, individuals with hypertension, African Americans of any age, diabetes, or CKD: 1,500 mg of sodium a day

Objectives of the 2010 Dietary Guidelines for Americans and *MyPlate* are aimed at eating a "healthful diet, promotion of health, and prevention of disease."

Sources: CDC (2012b, 2014s); United States Department of Agriculture (USDA) (n.d.); USDHHS (2015b, 2015c).

Physical Activity/Exercise

National Physical Activity Guidelines

In 2008, the Physical Activity Guidelines for Americans (PAG), the first national guidelines for physical activity ever developed, was prepared. Over 80% of adults do not meet the required guidelines for aerobic and muscle-strengthening activities, and greater than 80% of youth do not meet aerobic physical activity guidelines. Regular physical activity is vital to health and wellness, achieving and maintenance of a healthy weight, and reducing the risk of chronic diseases or disability. Regular physical activity includes active participation in moderate or vigorous physical activities together with muscle-strengthening exercises.

Recommendation:

Adults (Aged 18 to 64 years)
- Avoidance of physical activity/sedentary lifestyle.
  - Some physical activity has benefits over physical inactivity.
- At least 150 minutes (2 hours and 30 minutes) a week of moderate-intensity or 75 minutes (1 hour and 15 minutes) of vigorous-intensity aerobic physical activity, or an equivalent combination of both moderate- and vigorous-intensity aerobic activity. Exercises preferred spread throughout a week.
  - Moderate-intensity examples: Brisk walking, water aerobics, bicycling, tennis, dancing, general gardening, golfing, walking a dog
  - Vigorous-intensity examples: Race walking, jogging, running, swimming laps, aerobic dancing, bicycling 10 miles/hour or faster, jumping rope, heavy gardening, hiking uphill or with a heavy backpack
  - Muscle-strengthening examples:
    o Defined as exercises that increases the skeletal muscle strength, power, endurance, and mass
    o Examples: Lifting weights, push-ups, sit-ups, heavy gardening (digging, shoveling), yoga, working with resistance bands

Older Adults (Aged 65 years and Older)
- When chronic conditions impede the ability to meet physical activity guidelines of 150 minutes of moderate-intensity aerobic activity, recommendations are to be as physically activity as abilities and conditions permit.
- To maintain or improve balance if at risk of falling, recommendations are for older adults to perform exercises.
- Older adults should determine their level of effort for physical activity as it correlates to their level of fitness.
- Older adults with chronic health conditions should understand whether or how their health conditions may affect their ability to perform regular physical activity safely.

Guidelines for Safe Physical Activity
- Understand risks; know that physical activity is safe for almost all individuals.
- Select types of physical activity that align with current fitness level and health goals.
- Increase length and duration of physical activity over time; "start low and go slow."
- Wear protective gear, choose safe environments, and make sensible choices about when, where, and how to be physically active.
- Consult a health-care provider when chronic disorders or symptoms are present about the type and amount of physical activity.

Guidelines for Women during Pregnancy and the Postpartum Period
- Healthy women, not already active or performing vigorous-intensity activity, should have at least 150 minutes of moderate-intensity aerobic activity a week during pregnancy and in the postpartum period.

Youth (Aged 2 years to 17)
- Aerobic exercises 60 or more minutes a day
  - Examples: Running, brisk walking
- Muscle-strengthening activities at least 3 days a week for 60 minutes or more
  - Examples: Playing on a jungle gym, gymnastics, push-ups
- Bone-strengthening activities at least 3 days a week for 60 minutes or more
  - Examples: Jumping rope, running

Sources: CDC (2014ab) and USDHHS (2015d, 2015e).

Immunizations

Vaccinations/Immunity

Immunizations provide immunity (protection from an infectious disease) and are examples of primary prevention. Vaccinations are a strategy to reduce infectious diseases across the nation and "among the most cost-effective preventative services." Immunizations have contributed to longer life expectancy in the 20th century. Reductions in mortality rates attributed to infectious diseases are largely a result of immunizations, predominantly apparent in improved child survival. Programs central to childhood immunizations provide an illustration. For every birth cohort vaccinated according the recommended immunization schedule, 33,000 lives are saved, 14 million cases of disease is prevented, and health-care costs are reduced by $9.9 billion of direct costs and $33.4 billion in indirect costs.

Despite immunization recommendations in the US targeting 17 vaccine-preventable diseases across the lifespan, infectious diseases "remain a major cause of illness, disability and death." In the US,

- Preventable diseases to include tuberculosis (TB), influenza, and viral hepatitis account for the leading causes of morbidity and mortality.
- An estimated 42,000 adults and 300 children die annually as a result of vaccine-preventable diseases.
- Nearly 226,000 people are hospitalized annually as a result of influenza, and between 3,000 and 49,000 die from influenza complications—most are adults.
- An estimated 32,000 cases of invasive pneumococcal disease occurred in 2012 resulting in 3,300 deaths.
- Annual cases of herpes zoster (shingles) are estimated at 1 million individuals and of those many continue to experience long-term complications related to postherpetic neuralgia.
- HPV in the US results in about 17,000 cancers in women, 9,000 cancers in men annually, and an approximate 4,000 women who die from cervical cancer each year.

Although there are only a few of the staggering statistics, opportunity exists to immunize the youth, adults, and the older adult as a strategy to limit or eradicate infectious diseases.

Immunity occurs through the development of antibodies to a disease within a person. Two basic types of immunity exist: active and passive. *Active immunity* occurs "when exposure to a disease organism triggers the immune system to produce antibodies to that disease." This transpires in one of two ways: through *natural immunity* or *vaccine-induced immunity*. In *natural immunity*, the person develops antibodies as a result of being infected with the actual disease. In *vaccine-induced immunity*, "a killed or weakened form of the disease organism through vaccination" triggers the development of disease specific antibodies. Active immunity offers long-term protection and some life-long. Passive immunity is achieved when an individual receives antibodies to a disease, thus developing immunity to that disease. Two methodologies provide examples: when transferred from a mother to fetus through the placenta or administration through a vaccination (artificially) such as with immune globulin (IG), antibody containing blood products. A benefit to passive immunity is immediate protection, as compared to active immunity that takes time to develop (often several weeks). Passive immunity lasts for a short time (a few weeks or months), whereas active immunity is longer lasting and the preferred method.

Herd immunity, also known as community immunity, is when a considerable portion of a community is immunized against a contagious disease. Herd immunity significantly reduces the risk across a community for an infectious disease outbreak, relative to the infectious disease for which persons were protected against. In this type of community immunity, even susceptible individuals who are not candidates for the vaccination are afforded some protection by disease containment and minimizing transmission of the disease. Some illustrations within a community include influenza, measles, mumps, and pneumococcal disease.

Sources: CDC (2014n, 2014t) and USDHHS (2013, 2015a).

Vaccinations

Recommended Adult Immunization Schedules for the United States, 2015 (Figs. 1-1 to 1-4).

Recommended Adult Immunization Schedule—United States - 2016
Note: These recommendations must be read with the footnotes that follow
containing number of doses, intervals between doses, and other important information.

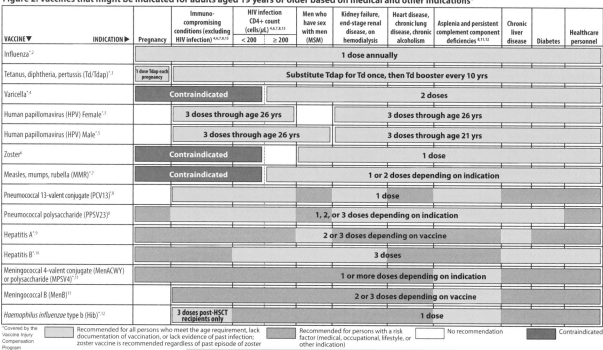

Figure 1. Recommended immunization schedule for adults aged 19 years or older, by vaccine and age group[1]

VACCINE▼ AGE GROUP►	19-21 years	22-26 years	27-49 years	50-59 years	60-64 years	≥ 65 years
Influenza[*,2]	1 dose annually					
Tetanus, diphtheria, pertussis (Td/Tdap)[*,3]	Substitute Tdap for Td once, then Td booster every 10 yrs					
Varicella[*,4]	2 doses					
Human papillomavirus (HPV) Female[*,5]	3 doses					
Human papillomavirus (HPV) Male[*,5]	3 doses					
Zoster[6]					1 dose	
Measles, mumps, rubella (MMR)[*,7]	1 or 2 doses depending on indication					
Pneumococcal 13-valent conjugate (PCV13)[*,8]					1 dose	
Pneumococcal 23-valent polysaccharide (PPSV23)[8]	1 or 2 doses depending on indication					1 dose
Hepatitis A[*,9]	2 or 3 doses depending on vaccine					
Hepatitis B[*,10]	3 doses					
Meningococcal 4-valent conjugate (MenACWY) or polysaccharide (MPSV4)[*,11]	1 or more doses depending on indication					
Meningococcal B (MenB)[11]	2 or 3 doses depending on vaccine					
Haemophilus influenzae type b (Hib)[*,12]	1 or 3 doses depending on indication					

*Covered by the Vaccine Injury Compensation Program

☐ Recommended for all persons who meet the age requirement, lack documentation of vaccination, or lack evidence of past infection; zoster vaccine is recommended regardless of past episode of zoster

☐ Recommended for persons with a risk factor (medical, occupational, lifestyle, or other indication)

☐ No recommendation

Report all clinically significant postvaccination reactions to the Vaccine Adverse Event Reporting System (VAERS). Reporting forms and instructions on filing a VAERS report are available at www.vaers.hhs.gov or by telephone, 800-822-7967.

Information on how to file a Vaccine Injury Compensation Program claim is available at www.hrsa.gov/vaccinecompensation or by telephone, 800-338-2382. To file a claim for vaccine injury, contact the U.S. Court of Federal Claims, 717 Madison Place, N.W., Washington, D.C. 20005; telephone, 202-357-6400.

Additional information about the vaccines in this schedule, extent of available data, and contraindications for vaccination is also available at www.cdc.gov/vaccines or from the CDC-INFO Contact Center at 800-CDC-INFO (800-232-4636) in English and Spanish, 8:00 a.m. - 8:00 p.m. Eastern Time, Monday - Friday, excluding holidays.

Use of trade names and commercial sources is for identification only and does not imply endorsement by the U.S. Department of Health and Human Services.

The recommendations in this schedule were approved by the Centers for Disease Control and Prevention's (CDC) Advisory Committee on Immunization Practices (ACIP), the American Academy of Family Physicians (AAFP), the America College of Physicians (ACP), the American College of Obstetricians and Gynecologists (ACOG) and the American College of Nurse-Midwives (ACNM).

Figure 2. Vaccines that might be indicated for adults aged 19 years or older based on medical and other indications[1]

VACCINE▼ INDICATION►	Pregnancy	Immuno-compromising conditions (excluding HIV infection)[4,6,7,8,13]	HIV infection CD4+ count (cells/µL)[4,6,7,8,13] < 200	≥ 200	Men who have sex with men (MSM)	Kidney failure, end-stage renal disease, on hemodialysis	Heart disease, chronic lung disease, chronic alcoholism	Asplenia and persistent complement component deficiencies[8,11,12]	Chronic liver disease	Diabetes	Healthcare personnel
Influenza[*,2]	1 dose annually										
Tetanus, diphtheria, pertussis (Td/Tdap)[*,3]	1 dose Tdap each pregnancy	Substitute Tdap for Td once, then Td booster every 10 yrs									
Varicella[*,4]	Contraindicated			2 doses							
Human papillomavirus (HPV) Female[*,5]	3 doses through age 26 yrs			3 doses through age 26 yrs							
Human papillomavirus (HPV) Male[*,5]	3 doses through age 26 yrs			3 doses through age 21 yrs							
Zoster[6]	Contraindicated			1 dose							
Measles, mumps, rubella (MMR)[*,7]	Contraindicated			1 or 2 doses depending on indication							
Pneumococcal 13-valent conjugate (PCV13)[*,8]		1 dose									
Pneumococcal polysaccharide (PPSV23)[8]	1, 2, or 3 doses depending on indication										
Hepatitis A[*,9]	2 or 3 doses depending on vaccine										
Hepatitis B[*,10]	3 doses										
Meningococcal 4-valent conjugate (MenACWY) or polysaccharide (MPSV4)[*,11]	1 or more doses depending on indication										
Meningococcal B (MenB)[11]	2 or 3 doses depending on vaccine										
Haemophilus influenzae type b (Hib)[*,12]	3 doses post-HSCT recipients only	1 dose									

*Covered by the Vaccine Injury Compensation Program

☐ Recommended for all persons who meet the age requirement, lack documentation of vaccination, or lack evidence of past infection; zoster vaccine is recommended regardless of past episode of zoster

☐ Recommended for persons with a risk factor (medical, occupational, lifestyle, or other indication)

☐ No recommendation

☐ Contraindicated

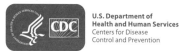 **U.S. Department of Health and Human Services** Centers for Disease Control and Prevention

These schedules indicate the recommended age groups and medical indications for which administration of currently licensed vaccines is commonly recommended for adults aged ≥19 years, as of February 2016. For all vaccines being recommended on the Adult Immunization Schedule: a vaccine series does not need to be restarted, regardless of the time that has elapsed between doses. Licensed combination vaccines may be used whenever any components of the combination are indicated and when the vaccine's other components are not contraindicated. For detailed recommendations on all vaccines, including those used primarily for travelers or that are issued during the year, consult the manufacturers' package inserts and the complete statements from the Advisory Committee on Immunization Practices (www.cdc.gov/vaccines/hcp/acip-recs/index.html). Use of trade names and commercial sources is for identification only and does not imply endorsement by the U.S. Department of Health and Human Services.

Figure 1-1: Recommended adult immunization schedules, United States, 2016.

Footnotes—recommended immunization schedule for adults aged 19 years or older: United States, 2016 may be accessed at www.cdc.gov/vaccines/schedules/downloads/adult/adult-schedule.pdf

*Note: The recommendations must be read with the footnotes that follow containing number of doses, intervals between doses, and other important information.

Source: Centers for Disease Control and Prevention. (2015, April 6). *Immunization schedules: Adult immunization schedules*. Retrieved from www.cdc.gov/vaccines/schedules/downloads/adult/adult-schedule.pdf

Footnotes—Recommended Immunization Schedule for Adults Aged 19 Years or Older: United States, 2016

1. Additional information
- Additional guidance for the use of the vaccines described in this supplement is available at www.cdc.gov/vaccines/hcp/acip-recs/index.html.
- Information on vaccination recommendations when vaccination status is unknown and other general immunization information can be found in the General Recommendations on Immunization at www.cdc.gov/mmwr/preview/mmwrhtml/rr6002a1.htm.
- Information on travel vaccine requirements and recommendations (e.g., for hepatitis A and B, meningococcal, and other vaccines) is available at wwwnc.cdc.gov/travel/destinations/list.
- Additional information and resources regarding vaccination of pregnant women can be found at www.cdc.gov/vaccines/adults/rec-vac/pregnant.html.

2. Influenza vaccination
- Annual vaccination against influenza is recommended for all persons aged ≥6 months. A list of currently available influenza vaccines can be found at http://www.cdc.gov/flu/protect/vaccine/vaccines.htm.
- Persons aged ≥6 months, including pregnant women, can receive the inactivated influenza vaccine (IIV). An age-appropriate IIV formulation should be used.
- Intradermal IIV is an option for persons aged 18 through 64 years.
- High-dose IIV is an option for persons aged ≥65 years.
- Live attenuated influenza vaccine (LAIV [FluMist]) is an option for healthy, non-pregnant persons aged 2 through 49 years.
- Recombinant influenza vaccine (RIV [Flublok]) is approved for persons aged ≥18 years.
- RIV, which does not contain any egg protein, may be administered to persons aged ≥18 years with egg allergy of any severity; IIV may be used with additional safety measures for persons with hives-only allergy to eggs.
- Health care personnel who care for severely immunocompromised persons who require care in a protected environment should receive IIV or RIV; health care personnel who receive LAIV should avoid providing care for severely immunosuppressed persons for 7 days after vaccination.

3. Tetanus, diphtheria, and acellular pertussis (Td/Tdap) vaccination
- Administer 1 dose of Tdap vaccine to pregnant women during each pregnancy (preferably during 27–36 weeks' gestation) regardless of interval since prior Td or Tdap vaccination.
- Persons aged ≥11 years who have not received Tdap vaccine or for whom vaccine status is unknown should receive a dose of Tdap followed by tetanus and diphtheria toxoids (Td) booster doses every 10 years thereafter. Tdap can be administered regardless of interval since the most recent tetanus or diphtheria-toxoid-containing vaccine.
- Adults with an unknown or incomplete history of completing a 3-dose primary vaccination series with Td-containing vaccines should begin or complete a primary vaccination series including a Tdap dose.
- For unvaccinated adults, administer the first 2 doses at least 4 weeks apart and the third dose 6–12 months after the second.
- For incompletely vaccinated (i.e., less than 3 doses) adults, administer remaining doses.
- Refer to the ACIP statement for recommendations for administering Td/Tdap as prophylaxis in wound management (see footnote 1).

4. Varicella vaccination
- All adults without evidence of immunity to varicella (as defined below) should receive 2 doses of single-antigen varicella vaccine or a second dose if they have received only 1 dose.
- Vaccination should be emphasized for those who have close contact with persons at high risk for severe disease (e.g., health care personnel and family contacts of persons with immunocompromising conditions) or are at high risk for exposure or transmission (e.g., teachers; child care employees; residents and staff members of institutional settings, including correctional institutions; college students; military personnel; adolescents and adults living in households with children; nonpregnant women of childbearing age; and international travelers).
- Pregnant women should be assessed for evidence of varicella immunity. Women who do not have evidence of immunity should receive the first dose of varicella vaccine upon completion or termination of pregnancy and before discharge from the health care facility. The second dose should be administered 4–8 weeks after the first dose.
- Evidence of immunity to varicella in adults includes any of the following:
  — documentation of 2 doses of varicella vaccine at least 4 weeks apart;
  — U.S.-born before 1980, except health care personnel and pregnant women;
  — history of varicella based on diagnosis or verification of varicella disease by a health care provider;
  — history of herpes zoster based on diagnosis or verification of herpes zoster disease by a health care provider; or
  — laboratory evidence of immunity or laboratory confirmation of disease.

5. Human papillomavirus (HPV) vaccination
- Three HPV vaccines are licensed for use in females (bivalent HPV vaccine [2vHPV], quadrivalent HPV vaccine [4vHPV], and 9-valent HPV vaccine [9vHPV]) and two HPV vaccines are licensed for use in males (4vHPV and 9vHPV).
- For females, 2vHPV, 4vHPV, or 9vHPV is recommended in a 3-dose series for routine vaccination at age 11 or 12 years and for those aged 13 through 26 years, if not previously vaccinated.
- For males, 4vHPV or 9vHPV is recommended in a 3-dose series for routine vaccination at age 11 or 12 years and for those aged 13 through 21 years, if not previously vaccinated. Males aged 22 through 26 years may be vaccinated.
- HPV vaccination is recommended for men who have sex with men through age 26 years who did not get any or all doses when they were younger.
- Vaccination is recommended for immunocompromised persons (including those with HIV infection) through age 26 years who did not get any or all doses when they were younger.
- A complete HPV vaccination series consists of 3 doses. The second dose should be administered 4–8 weeks (minimum interval of 4 weeks) after the first dose; the third dose should be administered 24 weeks after the first dose and 16 weeks after the second dose (minimum interval of 12 weeks).

- HPV vaccines are not recommended for use in pregnant women. However, pregnancy testing is not needed before vaccination. If a woman is found to be pregnant after initiating the vaccination series, no intervention is needed; the remainder of the 3-dose series should be delayed until completion or termination of pregnancy.

6. Zoster vaccination
- A single dose of zoster vaccine is recommended for adults aged ≥60 years regardless of whether they report a prior episode of herpes zoster. Although the vaccine is licensed by the U.S. Food and Drug Administration for use among and can be administered to persons aged ≥50 years, ACIP recommends that vaccination begin at age 60 years.
- Persons aged ≥60 years with chronic medical conditions may be vaccinated unless their condition constitutes a contraindication, such as pregnancy or severe immunodeficiency.

7. Measles, mumps, rubella (MMR) vaccination
- Adults born before 1957 are generally considered immune to measles and mumps. All adults born in 1957 or later should have documentation of 1 or more doses of MMR vaccine unless they have a medical contraindication to the vaccine or laboratory evidence of immunity to each of the three diseases. Documentation of provider-diagnosed disease is not considered acceptable evidence of immunity for measles, mumps, or rubella.
Measles component:
- A routine second dose of MMR vaccine, administered a minimum of 28 days after the first dose, is recommended for adults who:
  — are students in postsecondary educational institutions,
  — work in a health care facility, or
  — plan to travel internationally.
- Persons who received inactivated (killed) measles vaccine or measles vaccine of unknown type during 1963–1967 should be revaccinated with 2 doses of MMR vaccine.
Mumps component:
- A routine second dose of MMR vaccine, administered a minimum of 28 days after the first dose, is recommended for adults who:
  — are students in a postsecondary educational institution,
  — work in a health care facility, or
  — plan to travel internationally.
- Persons vaccinated before 1979 with either killed mumps vaccine or mumps vaccine of unknown type who are at high risk for mumps infection (e.g., persons who are working in a health care facility) should be considered for revaccination with 2 doses of MMR vaccine.
Rubella component:
- For women of childbearing age, regardless of birth year, rubella immunity should be determined. If there is no evidence of immunity, women who are not pregnant should be vaccinated. Pregnant women who do not have evidence of immunity should receive MMR vaccine upon completion or termination of pregnancy and before discharge from the health care facility.
Health care personnel born before 1957:
- For unvaccinated health care personnel born before 1957 who lack laboratory evidence of measles, mumps, and/or rubella immunity or laboratory confirmation of disease, health care facilities should consider vaccinating personnel with 2 doses of MMR vaccine at the appropriate interval for measles and mumps or 1 dose of MMR vaccine for rubella.

8. Pneumococcal vaccination
- General information
  — Adults are recommended to receive 1 dose of 13-valent pneumococcal conjugate vaccine (PCV13) and 1, 2, or 3 doses (depending on indication) of 23-valent pneumococcal polysaccharide vaccine (PPSV23).
  — PCV13 should be administered at least 1 year after PPSV23.
  — PPSV23 should be administered at least 1 year after PCV13, except among adults with immunocompromising conditions, anatomical or functional asplenia, cerebrospinal fluid leak, or cochlear implant, for whom the interval should be at least 8 weeks; the interval between PPSV23 doses should be at least 5 years.
  — No additional dose of PPSV23 is indicated for adults vaccinated with PPSV23 at age ≥65 years.
  — When both PCV13 and PPSV23 are indicated, PCV13 should be administered first; PCV13 and PPSV23 should not be administered during the same visit.
  — When indicated, PCV13 and PPSV23 should be administered to adults whose pneumococcal vaccination history is incomplete or unknown.
- Adults aged ≥65 years (immunocompetent) who:
  — have not received PCV13 or PPSV23: administer PCV13 followed by PPSV23 at least 1 year after PCV13.
  — have not received PCV13 but have received a dose of PPSV23 at age ≥65 years: administer PCV13 at least 1 year after PPSV23.
  — have not received PCV13 but have received 1 or more doses of PPSV23 at age <65 years: administer PCV13 at least 1 year after the most recent dose of PPSV23. Administer a dose of PPSV23 at least 1 year after PCV13 and at least 5 years after the most recent dose of PPSV23.
  — have received PCV13 but not PPSV23 at age <65 years: administer PPSV23 at least 1 year after PCV13.
  — have received PCV13 and 1 or more doses of PPSV23 at age <65 years: administer PPSV23 at least 1 year after PCV13 and at least 5 years after the most recent dose of PPSV23.
- Adults aged ≥19 years with immunocompromising conditions or anatomical or functional asplenia (defined below) who:
  — have not received PCV13 or PPSV23: administer PCV13 followed by PPSV23 at least 8 weeks after PCV13. Administer a second dose of PPSV23 at least 5 years after the first dose of PPSV23.
  — have not received PCV13 but have received 1 dose of PPSV23: administer PCV13 at least 1 year after the PPSV23. Administer a second dose of PPSV23 at least 8 weeks after PCV13 and at least 5 years after the first dose of PPSV23.

(Continued on next page)

Figure 1-1: (*continued*)

Footnotes—Recommended Immunization Schedule for Adults Aged 19 Years or Older: United States, 2016

- have not received PCV13 but have received 2 doses of PPSV23: administer PCV13 at least 1 year after the most recent dose of PPSV23.
  - have received PCV13 but not PPSV23: administer PPSV23 at least 8 weeks after PCV13. Administer a second dose of PPSV23 at least 5 years after the first dose of PPSV23.
  - have received PCV13 and 1 dose of PPSV23: administer a second dose of PPSV23 at least 8 weeks after PCV13 and at least 5 years after the first dose of PPSV23.
  - If the most recent dose of PPSV23 was administered at age <65 years, at age ≥65 years, administer a dose of PPSV23 at least 8 weeks after PCV13 and at least 5 years after the last dose of PPSV23.
  - Immunocompromising conditions that are indications for pneumococcal vaccination are: congenital or acquired immunodeficiency (including B- or T-lymphocyte deficiency, complement deficiencies, and phagocytic disorders excluding chronic granulomatous disease), HIV infection, chronic renal failure, nephrotic syndrome, leukemia, lymphoma, Hodgkin disease, generalized malignancy, multiple myeloma, solid organ transplant, and iatrogenic immunosuppression (including long-term systemic corticosteroids and radiation therapy).
  - Anatomical or functional asplenia that are indications for pneumococcal vaccination are: sickle cell disease and other hemoglobinopathies, congenital or acquired asplenia, splenic dysfunction, and splenectomy. Administer pneumococcal vaccines at least 2 weeks before immunosuppressive therapy or an elective splenectomy, and as soon as possible to adults who are newly diagnosed with asymptomatic or symptomatic HIV infection.
- Adults aged ≥19 years with cerebrospinal fluid leaks or cochlear implants: administer PCV13 followed by PPSV23 at least 8 weeks after PCV13; no additional dose of PPSV23 is indicated if aged <65 years. If PPSV23 was administered at age <65 years, at age ≥65 years, administer another dose of PPSV23 at least 5 years after the last dose PPSV23.
- Adults aged 19 through 64 years with chronic heart disease (including congestive heart failure and cardiomyopathies, excluding hypertension), chronic lung disease (including chronic obstructive lung disease, emphysema, and asthma), chronic liver disease (including cirrhosis), alcoholism, or diabetes mellitus, or who smoke cigarettes: administer PPSV23. At age ≥65 years, administer PCV13 at least 1 year after PPSV23, followed by another dose of PPSV23 at least 1 year after PCV13 and at least 5 years after the last dose of PPSV23.
- Routine pneumococcal vaccination is not recommended for American Indian/Alaska Native or other adults unless they have an indication as above; however, public health authorities may consider recommending the use of pneumococcal vaccines for American Indians/Alaska Natives or other adults who live in areas with increased risk for invasive pneumococcal disease.

9. Hepatitis A vaccination
- Vaccinate any person seeking protection from hepatitis A virus (HAV) infection and persons with any of the following indications:
  - men who have sex with men;
  - persons who use injection or noninjection illicit drugs;
  - persons working with HAV-infected primates or with HAV in a research laboratory setting;
  - persons with chronic liver disease and persons who receive clotting factor concentrates;
  - persons traveling to or working in countries that have high or intermediate endemicity of hepatitis A (see footnote 1); and
  - unvaccinated persons who anticipate close personal contact (e.g., household or regular babysitting) with an international adoptee during the first 60 days after arrival in the United States from a country with high or intermediate endemicity of hepatitis A (see footnote 1). The first dose of the 2-dose hepatitis A vaccine series should be administered as soon as adoption is planned, ideally 2 or more weeks before the arrival of the adoptee.
- Single-antigen vaccine formulations should be administered in a 2-dose schedule at either 0 and 6–12 months (Havrix), or 0 and 6–18 months (Vaqta). If the combined hepatitis A and hepatitis B vaccine (Twinrix) is used, administer 3 doses at 0, 1, and 6 months; alternatively, a 4-dose schedule may be used, administered on days 0, 7, and 21–30 followed by a booster dose at 12 months.

10. Hepatitis B vaccination
- Vaccinate any person seeking protection from hepatitis B virus (HBV) infection and persons with any of the following indications:
  - sexually active persons who are not in a long-term, mutually monogamous relationship (e.g., persons with more than 1 sex partner during the previous 6 months); persons seeking evaluation or treatment for a sexually transmitted disease (STD); current or recent injection drug users; and men who have sex with men;
  - health care personnel and public safety workers who are potentially exposed to blood or other infectious body fluids;
  - persons who are aged <60 years with diabetes as soon as feasible after diagnosis; persons with diabetes who are aged ≥60 years at the discretion of the treating clinician based on the likelihood of acquiring HBV infection, including the risk posed by an increased need for assisted blood glucose monitoring in long-term care facilities, the likelihood of experiencing chronic sequelae if infected with HBV, and the likelihood of immune response to vaccination;
  - persons with end-stage renal disease (including patients receiving hemodialysis), persons with HIV infection, and persons with chronic liver disease;
  - household contacts and sex partners of hepatitis B surface antigen–positive persons, clients and staff members of institutions for persons with developmental disabilities, and international travelers to regions with high or intermediate levels of endemic HBV infection (see footnote 1); and
  - all adults in the following settings: STD treatment facilities, HIV testing and treatment facilities, facilities providing drug abuse treatment and prevention services, health care settings targeting services to injection drug users or men who have sex with men, correctional facilities, end-stage renal disease

programs and facilities for chronic hemodialysis patients, and institutions and nonresidential day care facilities for persons with developmental disabilities.
- Administer missing doses to complete a 3-dose series of hepatitis B vaccine to those persons not vaccinated or not completely vaccinated. The second dose should be administered at least 1 month after the first dose; the third dose should be administered at least 2 months after the second dose (and at least 4 months after the first dose). If the combined hepatitis A and hepatitis B vaccine (Twinrix) is used, give 3 doses at 0, 1, and 6 months; alternatively, a 4-dose Twinrix schedule may be used, administered on days 0, 7, and 21–30, followed by a booster dose at 12 months.
- Adult patients receiving hemodialysis or with other immunocompromising conditions should receive 1 dose of 40 mcg/mL (Recombivax HB) administered on a 3-dose schedule at 0, 1, and 6 months or 2 doses of 20 mcg/mL (Engerix-B) administered simultaneously on a 4-dose schedule at 0, 1, 2, and 6 months.

11. Meningococcal vaccination
- General information
  - Serogroup A, C, W, and Y meningococcal vaccine is available as a conjugate (MenACWY [Menactra, Menveo]) or a polysaccharide (MPSV4 [Menomune]) vaccine.
  - Serogroup B meningococcal (MenB) vaccine is available as a 2-dose series of MenB-4C vaccine (Bexsero) administered at least 1 month apart or a 3-dose series of MenB-FHbp (Trumenba) vaccine administered at 0, 2, and 6 months; the two MenB vaccines are not interchangeable, i.e., the same MenB vaccine product must be used for all doses.
  - MenACWY vaccine is preferred for adults with serogroup A, C, W, and Y meningococcal vaccine indications who are aged ≤55 years, and for adults aged ≥56 years: 1) who were vaccinated previously with MenACWY vaccine and are recommended for revaccination or 2) for whom multiple doses of vaccine are anticipated; MPSV4 vaccine is preferred for adults aged ≥56 years who have not received MenACWY vaccine previously and who require a single dose only (e.g., persons at risk because of an outbreak).
  - Revaccination with MenACWY vaccine every 5 years is recommended for adults previously vaccinated with MenACWY or MPSV4 vaccine who remain at increased risk for infection (e.g., adults with anatomical or functional asplenia or persistent complement component deficiencies, or microbiologists who are routinely exposed to isolates of *Neisseria meningitidis*).
  - MenB vaccine is approved for use in persons aged 10 through 25 years; however, because there is no theoretical difference in safety for persons aged >25 years compared to those aged 10 through 25 years, MenB vaccine is recommended for routine use in persons aged ≥10 years who are at increased risk for serogroup B meningococcal disease.
  - There is no recommendation for MenB revaccination at this time.
  - MenB vaccine may be administered concomitantly with MenACWY vaccine but at a different anatomic site, if feasible.
  - HIV infection is not an indication for routine vaccination with MenACWY or MenB vaccine; if an HIV-infected person of any age is to be vaccinated, administer 2 doses of MenACWY vaccine at least 2 months apart.
- Adults with anatomical or functional asplenia or persistent complement component deficiencies: administer 2 doses of MenACWY vaccine at least 2 months apart and revaccinate every 5 years. Also administer a series of MenB vaccine.
- Microbiologists who are routinely exposed to isolates of *Neisseria meningitidis*: administer a single dose of MenACWY vaccine; revaccinate with MenACWY vaccine every 5 years if remain at increased risk for infection. Also administer a series of MenB vaccine.
- Persons at risk because of a meningococcal disease outbreak: if the outbreak is attributable to serogroup A, C, W, or Y, administer a single dose of MenACWY vaccine; if the outbreak is attributable to serogroup B, administer a series of MenB vaccine.
- Persons who travel to or live in countries in which meningococcal disease is hyperendemic or epidemic: administer a single dose of MenACWY vaccine and revaccinate with MenACWY vaccine every 5 years if the increased risk for infection remains (see footnote 1); MenB vaccine is not recommended because meningococcal disease in these countries is generally not caused by serogroup B.
- Military recruits: administer a single dose of MenACWY vaccine.
- First-year college students aged ≤21 years who live in residence halls: administer a single dose of MenACWY vaccine if they have not received a dose on or after their 16th birthday.
- Young adults aged 16 through 23 years (preferred age range is 16 through 18 years): may be vaccinated with a series of MenB vaccine to provide short-term protection against most strains of serogroup B meningococcal disease.

12. *Haemophilus influenzae* type b (Hib) vaccination
- One dose of Hib vaccine should be administered to persons who have anatomical or functional asplenia or sickle cell disease or are undergoing elective splenectomy if they have not previously received Hib vaccine. Hib vaccination 14 or more days before splenectomy is suggested.
- Recipients of a hematopoietic stem cell transplant (HSCT) should be vaccinated with a 3-dose regimen 6–12 months after a successful transplant, regardless of vaccination history; at least 4 weeks should separate doses.
- Hib vaccine is not recommended for adults with HIV infection since their risk for Hib infection is low.

13. Immunocompromising conditions
- Inactivated vaccines (e.g., pneumococcal, meningococcal, and inactivated influenza vaccines) generally are acceptable and live vaccines generally should be avoided in persons with immune deficiencies or immunocompromising conditions. Information on specific conditions is available at www.cdc.gov/vaccines/hcp/acip-recs/index.html.

Figure 1-1: (*continued*)

TABLE. Contraindications and precautions to commonly used vaccines in adults [1*†]

Vaccine	Contraindications	Precautions
Influenza, inactivated (IIV)[2]	• Severe allergic reaction (e.g., anaphylaxis) after previous dose of any influenza vaccine; or to a vaccine component, including egg protein	• Moderate or severe acute illness with or without fever • History of Guillain-Barré Syndrome within 6 weeks of previous influenza vaccination • Adults with egg allergy of any severity may receive RIV; adults with hives-only allergy to eggs may receive IIV with additional safety measures[2]
Influenza, recombinant (RIV)	• Severe allergic reaction (e.g., anaphylaxis) after previous dose of RIV or to a vaccine component. RIV does not contain any egg protein[2]	• Moderate or severe acute illness with or without fever • History of Guillain-Barré Syndrome within 6 weeks of previous influenza vaccination

Influenza, live attenuated (LAIV)[2,3]	• Severe allergic reaction (e.g., anaphylaxis) to any component of the vaccine, or to a previous dose of any influenza vaccine
	• In addition, ACIP recommends that LAIV not be used in the following populations:
	  — pregnant women
	  — immunosuppressed adults
	  — adults with egg allergy of any severity
	  — adults who have taken influenza antiviral medications (amantadine, rimantadine, zanamivir, or oseltamivir) within the previous 48 hours; avoid use of these antiviral drugs for 14 days after vaccination
		• Moderate or severe acute illness with or without fever.
		• History of Guillain-Barré Syndrome within 6 weeks of previous influenza vaccination
		• Asthma in persons aged 5 years and older
		• Other chronic medical conditions, e.g., other chronic lung diseases, chronic cardiovascular disease (excluding isolated hypertension), diabetes, chronic renal or hepatic disease, hematologic disease, neurologic disease, and metabolic disorders

Tetanus, diphtheria, pertussis (Tdap); tetanus, diphtheria (Td)	• Severe allergic reaction (e.g., anaphylaxis) after a previous dose or to a vaccine component • For pertussis-containing vaccines: encephalopathy (e.g., coma, decreased level of consciousness, or prolonged seizures) not attributable to another identifiable cause within 7 days of administration of a previous dose of Tdap, diphtheria and tetanus toxoids and pertussis (DTP), or diphtheria and tetanus toxoids and acellular pertussis (DTaP) vaccine	• Moderate or severe acute illness with or without fever • Guillain-Barré Syndrome within 6 weeks after a previous dose of tetanus toxoid-containing vaccine • History of Arthus-type hypersensitivity reactions after a previous dose of tetanus or diphtheria toxoid-containing vaccine; defer vaccination until at least 10 years have elapsed since the last tetanus toxoid-containing vaccine • For pertussis-containing vaccines: progressive or unstable neurologic disorder, uncontrolled seizures, or progressive encephalopathy until a treatment regimen has been established and the condition has stabilized
Varicella[3]	• Severe allergic reaction (e.g., anaphylaxis) after a previous dose or to a vaccine component • Known severe immunodeficiency (e.g., from hematologic and solid tumors, receipt of chemotherapy, congenital immunodeficiency, or long-term immunosuppressive therapy,[4] or patients with human immunodeficiency virus [HIV] infection who are severely immunocompromised) • Pregnancy	• Recent (within 11 months) receipt of antibody-containing blood product (specific interval depends on product)[5] • Moderate or severe acute illness with or without fever • Receipt of specific antivirals (i.e., acyclovir, famciclovir, or valacyclovir) 24 hours before vaccination; avoid use of these antiviral drugs for 14 days after vaccination
Human papillomavirus (HPV)	• Severe allergic reaction (e.g., anaphylaxis) after a previous dose or to a vaccine component	• Moderate or severe acute illness with or without fever • Pregnancy
Zoster[3]	• Severe allergic reaction (e.g., anaphylaxis) to a vaccine component • Known severe immunodeficiency (e.g., from hematologic and solid tumors, receipt of chemotherapy, or long-term immunosuppressive therapy,4 or patients with HIV infection who are severely immunocompromised) • Pregnancy	• Moderate or severe acute illness with or without fever • Receipt of specific antivirals (i.e., acyclovir, famciclovir, or valacyclovir) 24 hours before vaccination; avoid use of these antiviral drugs for 14 days after vaccination
Measles, mumps, rubella (MMR)[3]	• Severe allergic reaction (e.g., anaphylaxis) after a previous dose or to a vaccine component • Known severe immunodeficiency (e.g., from hematologic and solid tumors, receipt of chemotherapy, congenital immunodeficiency, or long-term immunosuppressive therapy,[4] or patients with HIV infection who are severely immunocompromised) • Pregnancy	• Moderate or severe acute illness with or without fever • Recent (within 11 months) receipt of antibody-containing blood product (specific interval depends on product)[5] • History of thrombocytopenia or thrombocytopenic purpura • Need for tuberculin skin testing[6]
Pneumococcal conjugate (PCV13)	• Severe allergic reaction (e.g., anaphylaxis) after a previous dose or to a vaccine component, including to any vaccine containing diphtheria toxoid	• Moderate or severe acute illness with or without fever
Pneumococcal polysaccharide (PPSV23)	• Severe allergic reaction (e.g., anaphylaxis) after a previous dose or to a vaccine component	• Moderate or severe acute illness with or without fever
Hepatitis A	• Severe allergic reaction (e.g., anaphylaxis) after a previous dose or to a vaccine component	• Moderate or severe acute illness with or without fever
Hepatitis B	• Severe allergic reaction (e.g., anaphylaxis) after a previous dose or to a vaccine component	• Moderate or severe acute illness with or without fever
Meningococcal, conjugate (MenACWY); meningococcal, polysaccharide (MPSV4)	• Severe allergic reaction (e.g., anaphylaxis) after a previous dose or to a vaccine component	• Moderate or severe acute illness with or without fever
Meningococcal serogroup B (MenB)	• Severe allergic reaction (e.g., anaphylaxis) after a previous dose or to a vaccine component	• Moderate or severe acute illness with or without fever
Haemophilus influenzae Type b (Hib)	• Severe allergic reaction (e.g., anaphylaxis) after a previous dose or to a vaccine component	• Moderate or severe acute illness with or without fever

1. Vaccine package inserts and the full ACIP recommendations for these vaccines should be consulted for additional information on vaccine-related contraindications and precautions and for more information on vaccine excipients. Events or conditions listed as precautions should be reviewed carefully. Benefits of and risks for administering a specific vaccine to a person under these circumstances should be considered. If the risk from the vaccine is believed to outweigh the benefit, the vaccine should not be administered. If the benefit of vaccination is believed to outweigh the risk, the vaccine should be administered. A contraindication is a condition in a recipient that increases the chance of a serious adverse reaction. Therefore, a vaccine should not be administered when a contraindication is present.

2. For more information on use of influenza vaccines among persons with egg allergies and a complete list of conditions that CDC considers to be reasons to avoid receiving LAIV, see CDC. Prevention and control of seasonal influenza with vaccines: recommendations of the Advisory Committee on Immunization Practices (ACIP) — United States, 2015–16 Influenza Season. *MMWR* 2015;64(30):818-25.

3. LAIV, MMR, varicella, or zoster vaccines can be administered on the same day. If not administered on the same day, live vaccines should be separated by at least 28 days.

4. Immunosuppressive steroid dose is considered to be ≥2 weeks of daily receipt of 20 mg of prednisone or the equivalent. Vaccination should be deferred for at least 1 month after discontinuation of such therapy. Providers should consult ACIP recommendations for complete information on the use of specific live vaccines among persons on immune-suppressing medications or with immune suppression because of other reasons.

5. Vaccine should be deferred for the appropriate interval if replacement immune globulin products are being administered. See CDC. General recommendations on immunization: recommendations of the Advisory Committee on Immunization Practices (ACIP). *MMWR* 2011;60(No. RR-2). Available at www.cdc.gov/vaccines/pubs/pinkbook/index.html.

6. Measles vaccination might suppress tuberculin reactivity temporarily. Measles-containing vaccine may be administered on the same day as tuberculin skin testing. If testing cannot be performed until after the day of MMR vaccination, the test should be postponed for at least 4 weeks after the vaccination. If an urgent need exists to skin test, do so with the understanding that reactivity might be reduced by the vaccine.

* Adapted from CDC. Table 6. Contraindications and precautions to commonly used vaccines. General recommendations on immunization: recommendations of the Advisory Committee on Immunization Practices. MMWR 2011;60(No. RR-2):40–41 and from Hamborsky J, Kroger A, Wolfe C, eds. Appendix A. Epidemiology and prevention of vaccine preventable diseases. 13th ed. Washington, DC: Public Health Foundation, 2015. Available at www.cdc.gov/vaccines/pubs/pinkbook/index.html.

† Regarding latex allergy, consult the package insert for any vaccine administered.

CS260933-D

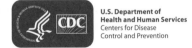

U.S. Department of Health and Human Services
Centers for Disease Control and Prevention

Figure 1-2: Contraindications and precautions to commonly used vaccines in adults, United States, 2015.
Source: Centers for Disease Control and Prevention. (2015, January 15). *Sexually transmitted diseases (STDs)*. Retrieved from www.cdc.gov/std/

Recommended Immunization Schedules for Persons Aged 0 Through 18 Years
UNITED STATES, 2016

This schedule includes recommendations in effect as of January 1, 2016. Any dose not administered at the recommended age should be administered at a subsequent visit, when indicated and feasible. The use of a combination vaccine generally is preferred over separate injections of its equivalent component vaccines. Vaccination providers should consult the relevant Advisory Committee on Immunization Practices (ACIP) statement for detailed recommendations, available online at http://www.cdc.gov/vaccines/hcp/acip-recs/index.html. Clinically significant adverse events that follow vaccination should be reported to the Vaccine Adverse Event Reporting System (VAERS) online (http://www.vaers.hhs.gov) or by telephone (800-822-7967).

The Recommended Immunization Schedules for Persons Aged 0 Through 18 Years are approved by the

Advisory Committee on Immunization Practices
(http://www.cdc.gov/vaccines/acip)

American Academy of Pediatrics
(http://www.aap.org)

American Academy of Family Physicians
(http://www.aafp.org)

American College of Obstetricians and Gynecologists
(http://www.acog.org)

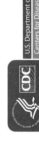

U.S. Department of Health and Human Services
Centers for Disease Control and Prevention

Figure 1-3: Recommended immunizations for persons aged 0 through 18 years, United States, 2016
Footnotes—recommended immunization schedule for persons aged 0 through 18 years or older: United States, 2016 may be accessed at www.cdc.gov/vaccines/schedules/hcp/imz/child-adolescent.html
*Note: The recommendations must be read with the footnotes that follow.
Source: Centers for Disease Control and Prevention. (2015, April 6). *Immunization schedules: Child and adolescent schedule.* Retrieved from www.cdc.gov/vaccines/schedules/hcp/imz/child-adolescent.html

Figure 1. Recommended immunization schedule for persons aged 0 through 18 years – United States, 2016.

(FOR THOSE WHO FALL BEHIND OR START LATE, SEE THE CATCH-UP SCHEDULE [FIGURE 2]).

These recommendations must be read with the footnotes that follow. For those who fall behind or start late, provide catch-up vaccination at the earliest opportunity as indicated by the green bars in Figure 1. To determine minimum intervals between doses, see the catch-up schedule (Figure 2). School entry and adolescent vaccine age groups are shaded.

Vaccine	Birth	1 mo	2 mos	4 mos	6 mos	9 mos	12 mos	15 mos	18 mos	19–23 mos	2–3 yrs	4–6 yrs	7–10 yrs	11–12 yrs	13–15 yrs	16–18 yrs
Hepatitis B[1] (HepB)	1st dose	←2nd dose→			←————— 3rd dose —————→											
Rotavirus[2] (RV) RV1 (2-dose series); RV5 (3-dose series)			1st dose	2nd dose	See footnote 2											
Diphtheria, tetanus, & acellular pertussis[3] (DTaP: <7 yrs)			1st dose	2nd dose	3rd dose		←———— 4th dose ————→					5th dose				
Haemophilus influenzae type b[4] (Hib)			1st dose	2nd dose	See footnote 4		3rd or 4th dose, See footnote 4									
Pneumococcal conjugate[5] (PCV13)			1st dose	2nd dose	3rd dose		←— 4th dose —→									
Inactivated poliovirus[6] (IPV: <18 yrs)			1st dose	2nd dose	←————— 3rd dose —————→							4th dose				
Influenza[7] (IIV; LAIV)					Annual vaccination (IIV only) 1 or 2 doses						Annual vaccination (LAIV or IIV) 1 or 2 doses			Annual vaccination (LAIV or IIV) 1 dose only		
Measles, mumps, rubella[8] (MMR)							←— 1st dose —→					2nd dose				
Varicella[9] (VAR)							←— 1st dose —→					2nd dose				
Hepatitis A[10] (HepA)							2-dose series, See footnote 10									
Meningococcal[11] (Hib-MenCY ≥ 6 weeks; MenACWY-D ≥ 9 mos; MenACWY-CRM ≥ 2 mos)						See footnote 11								1st dose		Booster
Tetanus, diphtheria, & acellular pertussis[12] (Tdap: ≥ 7 yrs)														(Tdap)		
Human papillomavirus[13] (2vHPV: females only; 4vHPV, 9vHPV: males and females)														(3-dose series)		
Meningococcal B[11]														See footnote 11		
Pneumococcal polysaccharide[5] (PPSV23)												See footnote 5				

Legend:
- Range of recommended ages for all children
- Range of recommended ages for catch-up immunization
- Range of recommended ages for certain high-risk groups
- Range of recommended ages for non-high-risk groups that may receive vaccine, subject to individual clinical decision making
- No recommendation

This schedule includes recommendations in effect as of January 1, 2016. Any dose not administered at the recommended age should be administered at a subsequent visit, when indicated and feasible. The use of a combination vaccine generally is preferred over separate injections of its equivalent component vaccines. Vaccination providers should consult the relevant Advisory Committee on Immunization Practices (ACIP) statement for detailed recommendations, available online at http://www.cdc.gov/vaccines/hcp/acip-recs/index.html. Clinically significant adverse events that follow vaccination should be reported to the Vaccine Adverse Event Reporting System (VAERS) online (http://www.vaers.hhs.gov) or by telephone (800-822-7967). Suspected cases of vaccine-preventable diseases should be reported to the state or local health department. Additional information, including precautions and contraindications for vaccination, is available from CDC online (http://www.cdc.gov/vaccines/recs/vac-admin/contraindications.htm) or by telephone (800-CDC-INFO [800-232-4636]).

This schedule is approved by the Advisory Committee on Immunization Practices (http://www.cdc.gov/vaccines/acip), the American Academy of Pediatrics (http://www.aap.org), the American Academy of Family Physicians (http://www.aafp.org), and the American College of Obstetricians and Gynecologists (http://www.acog.org).

NOTE: The above recommendations must be read along with the footnotes of this schedule.

Figure 1-3: (*continued*)

FIGURE 2. Catch-up immunization schedule for persons aged 4 months through 18 years who start late or who are more than 1 month behind —United States, 2016.

The figure below provides catch-up schedules and minimum intervals between doses for children whose vaccinations have been delayed. A vaccine series does not need to be restarted, regardless of the time that has elapsed between doses. Use the section appropriate for the child's age. Always use this table in conjunction with Figure 1 and the footnotes that follow.

Vaccine	Minimum Age for Dose 1	Minimum Interval Between Doses			
		Dose 1 to Dose 2	Dose 2 to Dose 3	Dose 3 to Dose 4	Dose 4 to Dose 5
Children age 4 months through 6 years					
Hepatitis B[1]	Birth	4 weeks	8 weeks *and* at least 16 weeks after first dose. Minimum age for the final dose is 24 weeks.		
Rotavirus[2]	6 weeks	4 weeks	4 weeks[2]		
Diphtheria, tetanus, and acellular pertussis[3]	6 weeks	4 weeks	4 weeks	6 months	6 months[3]
Haemophilus influenzae type b[4]	6 weeks	4 weeks if first dose was administered before the 1st birthday. 8 weeks (as final dose) if first dose was administered at 12 through 14 months. No further doses needed if first dose was administered at age 15 months or older.	4 weeks[4] if current age is younger than 12 months **and** first dose was administered at younger than age 7 months, **and** at least 1 previous dose was PRP-T (ActHIB, Pentacel) or unknown. **OR** 8 weeks (as final dose)[4] if current age is younger than 12 months **and** first dose was administered at age 7 through 11 months (wait until at least 12 months old); **OR** if current age is 12 through 59 months **and** first dose was administered before the 1st birthday, **and** second dose administered at younger than 15 months; **OR** if both doses were PRP-OMP (PedvaxHIB, Comvax) **and** were administered before the 1st birthday (wait until at least 12 months old). No further doses needed if previous dose was administered at age 15 months or older.	8 weeks (as final dose) This dose only necessary for children age 12 through 59 months who received 3 doses before the 1st birthday.	
Pneumococcal[5]	6 weeks	4 weeks if first dose administered before the 1st birthday. 8 weeks (as final dose for healthy children) if first dose was administered at the 1st birthday or after. No further doses needed for healthy children if first dose administered at age 24 months or older.	4 weeks if current age is younger than 12 months and previous dose given at <7months old. 8 weeks (as final dose for healthy children) if previous dose given between 7–11 months (wait until at least 12 months old); **OR** if current age is 12 months or older and at least 1 dose was given before age 12 months. No further doses needed for healthy children if previous dose administered at age 24 months or older.	8 weeks (as final dose) This dose only necessary for children aged 12 through 59 months who received 3 doses before age 12 months or for children at high risk who received 3 doses at any age.	
Inactivated poliovirus[6]	6 weeks	4 weeks[6]	4 weeks[6]	6 months[6] (minimum age 4 years for final dose).	
Measles, mumps, rubella[8]	12 months	4 weeks			
Varicella[9]	12 months	3 months			
Hepatitis A[10]	12 months	6 months			
Meningococcal[11] (Hib-MenCY ≥ 6 weeks; MenACWY-D ≥9 mos; MenACWY-CRM ≥ 2 mos)	6 weeks	8 weeks[11]	See footnote 11	See footnote 11	
Children and adolescents age 7 through 18 years					
Meningococcal[11] (Hib-MenCY ≥ 6 weeks; MenACWY-D ≥9 mos; MenACWY-CRM ≥ 2 mos)	Not Applicable (N/A)	8 weeks[11]			
Tetanus, diphtheria; tetanus, diphtheria, and acellular pertussis[12]	7 years[12]	4 weeks	4 weeks if first dose of DTaP/DT was administered before the 1st birthday. 6 months (as final dose) if first dose of DTaP/DT or Tdap/Td was administered at or after the 1st birthday.	6 months if first dose of DTaP/DT was administered before the 1st birthday.	
Human papillomavirus[13]	9 years	Routine dosing intervals are recommended.[13]			
Hepatitis A[10]	N/A	6 months			
Hepatitis B[1]	N/A	4 weeks	8 weeks **and** at least 16 weeks after first dose.		
Inactivated poliovirus[6]	N/A	4 weeks	4 weeks[6]	6 months[6]	
Measles, mumps, rubella[8]	N/A	4 weeks			
Varicella[9]	N/A	3 months if younger than age 13 years. 4 weeks if age 13 years or older.			

NOTE: The above recommendations must be read along with the footnotes of this schedule.

Figure 1-3: (*continued*)

43

Footnotes — Recommended immunization schedule for persons aged 0 through 18 years—United States, 2016

For further guidance on the use of the vaccines mentioned below, see: http://www.cdc.gov/vaccines/hcp/acip-recs/index.html.
For vaccine recommendations for persons 19 years of age and older, see the Adult Immunization Schedule.

Additional information

- For contraindications and precautions to use of a vaccine and for additional information regarding that vaccine, vaccination providers should consult the relevant ACIP statement available online at http://www.cdc.gov/vaccines/hcp/acip-recs/index.html.
- For purposes of calculating intervals between doses, 4 weeks = 28 days. Intervals of 4 months or greater are determined by calendar months.
- Vaccine doses administered ≤4 days or less before the minimum interval are considered valid. Doses of any vaccine administered ≥5 days earlier than the minimum interval or minimum age should not be counted as valid doses and should be repeated as age-appropriate. The repeat dose should be spaced after the invalid dose by the recommended minimum interval. For further details, see *MMWR, General Recommendations on Immunization and Reports* / Vol. 60 / No. 2; Table 1. *Recommended and minimum ages and intervals between vaccine doses* available online at http://www.cdc.gov/mmwr/pdf/rr/rr6002.pdf.
- Information on travel vaccine requirements and recommendations is available at http://wwwnc.cdc.gov/travel/destinations/list.
- For vaccination of persons with primary and secondary immunodeficiencies, see Table 13, "Vaccination of persons with primary and secondary immunodeficiencies," in *General Recommendations on Immunization* (ACIP), available at http://www.cdc.gov/mmwr/pdf/rr/rr6002.pdf; and American Academy of Pediatrics. "Immunization in Special Clinical Circumstances," in Kimberlin DW, Brady MT, Jackson MA, Long SS eds. *Red Book: 2015 report of the Committee on Infectious Diseases. 30th ed.* Elk Grove Village, IL: American Academy of Pediatrics.

1. Hepatitis B (HepB) vaccine. (Minimum age: birth)

Routine vaccination:

At birth:

- Administer monovalent HepB vaccine to all newborns before hospital discharge.
- For infants born to hepatitis B surface antigen (HBsAg)-positive mothers, administer HepB vaccine and 0.5 mL of hepatitis B immune globulin (HBIg) within 12 hours of birth. These infants should be tested for HBsAg and antibody to HBsAg (anti-HBs) at age 9 through 18 months (preferably at the next well-child visit) or 1 to 2 months after completion of the HepB series if the series was delayed; CDC recently recommended testing occur at age 9 through 12 months (see http://www.cdc.gov/mmwr/preview/mmwrhtml/mm6439a6.htm.
- If mother's HBsAg status is unknown, within 12 hours of birth administer HepB vaccine regardless of birth weight. For infants weighing less than 2,000 grams, administer HBIG in addition to HepB vaccine within 12 hours of birth. Determine mother's HBsAg status as soon as possible and, if mother is HBsAg-positive, also administer HBIG for infants weighing 2,000 grams or more as soon as possible, but no later than age 7 days.

Doses following the birth dose:

- The second dose should be administered at age 1 or 2 months. Monovalent HepB vaccine should be used for doses administered before age 6 weeks.
- Infants who did not receive a birth dose should receive 3 doses of a HepB-containing vaccine on a schedule of 0, 1 to 2 months, and 6 months starting as soon as feasible. See Figure 2.
- Administer the second dose 1 to 2 months after the first dose (minimum interval of 4 weeks), administer the third dose at least 8 weeks after the second dose AND at least 16 weeks after the first dose. The final (third or fourth) dose in the HepB vaccine series should be administered **no earlier than age 24 weeks.**
- Administration of a total of 4 doses of HepB vaccine is permitted when a combination vaccine containing HepB is administered after the birth dose.

Catch-up vaccination:

- Unvaccinated persons should complete a 3-dose series.
- A 2-dose series (doses separated by at least 4 months) of adult formulation Recombivax HB is licensed for use in children aged 11 through 15 years.
- For other catch-up guidance, see Figure 2.

2. Rotavirus (RV) vaccines. (Minimum age: 6 weeks for both RV1 [Rotarix] and RV5 [RotaTeq])

Routine vaccination:

Administer a series of RV vaccine to all infants as follows:
1. If Rotarix is used, administer a 2-dose series at 2 and 4 months of age.
2. If RotaTeq is used, administer a 3-dose series at ages 2, 4, and 6 months.
3. If any dose in the series was RotaTeq or vaccine product is unknown for any dose in the series, a total of 3 doses of RV vaccine should be administered.

Catch-up vaccination:

- The maximum age for the first dose in the series is 14 weeks, 6 days; vaccination should not be initiated for infants aged 15 weeks, 0 days or older.
- The maximum age for the final dose in the series is 8 months, 0 days.
- For other catch-up guidance, see Figure 2.

3. Diphtheria and tetanus toxoids and acellular pertussis (DTaP) vaccine. (Minimum age: 6 weeks. Exception: DTaP-IPV [Kinrix, Quadracel]: 4 years)

Routine vaccination:

- Administer a 5-dose series of DTaP vaccine at ages 2, 4, 6, 15 through 18 months, and 4 through 6 years. The fourth dose may be administered as early as age 12 months, provided at least 6 months have elapsed since the third dose.
- Inadvertent administration of 4th DTaP dose early: If the fourth dose of DTaP was administered at least 4 months, but less than 6 months, after the third dose of DTaP, it need not be repeated.

3. Diphtheria and tetanus toxoids and acellular pertussis (DTaP) vaccine (cont'd)

Catch-up vaccination:

- The fifth dose of DTaP vaccine is not necessary if the fourth dose was administered at age 4 years or older.
- For other catch-up guidance, see Figure 2.

4. Haemophilus influenzae type b (Hib) conjugate vaccine. (Minimum age: 6 weeks for PRP-T [ActHIB, DTaP-IPV/Hib (Pentacel) and Hib-MenCY (MenHibrix)], PRP-OMP [PedvaxHIB or COMVAX], 12 months for PRP-T [Hiberix])

Routine vaccination:

- Administer a 2- or 3-dose Hib vaccine primary series and a booster dose (dose 3 or 4 depending on vaccine used in primary series) at age 12 through 15 months to complete a full Hib vaccine series.
- The primary series with ActHIB, MenHibrix, or Pentacel consists of 3 doses and should be administered at 2, 4, and 6 months of age. The primary series with PedvaxHIB or COMVAX consists of 2 doses and should be administered at 2 and 4 months of age; a dose at age 6 months is not indicated.
- One booster dose (dose 3 or 4 depending on vaccine used in primary series) of any Hib vaccine should be administered at age 12 through 15 months. An exception is Hiberix vaccine. Hiberix should only be used for the booster (final) dose in children aged 12 months through 4 years who have received at least 1 prior dose of Hib-containing vaccine.
- For recommendations on the use of MenHibrix in patients at increased risk for meningococcal disease, please refer to the meningococcal vaccine footnotes and also to *MMWR* February 28, 2014 / 63(RR01):1-13, available at http://www.cdc.gov/mmwr/PDF/rr/rr6301.pdf.

Catch-up vaccination:

- If dose 1 was administered at ages 12 through 14 months, administer a second (final) dose at least 8 weeks after dose 1, regardless of Hib vaccine used in the primary series.
- If both doses were PRP-OMP (PedvaxHIB or COMVAX), and were administered before the first birthday, the third (and final) dose should be administered at age 12 through 59 months and at least 8 weeks after the second dose.
- If the first dose was administered at age 7 through 11 months, administer the second dose at least 4 weeks later and a third (and final) dose at age 12 through 15 months or 8 weeks after second dose, whichever is later.
- If first dose is administered before the first birthday and second dose administered at younger than 15 months, a third (and final) dose should be administered 8 weeks later.
- For unvaccinated children aged 15 months or older, administer only 1 dose.
- For other catch-up guidance related to MenHibrix, please see the meningococcal vaccine footnotes and also *MMWR* February 28, 2014 / 63(RR01);1-13, available at http://www.cdc.gov/mmwr/PDF/rr/rr6301.pdf.

Vaccination of persons with high-risk conditions:

- Children aged 12 through 59 months who are at increased risk for Hib disease, including chemotherapy recipients and those with anatomic or functional asplenia (including sickle cell disease), human immunodeficiency virus (HIV) infection, immunoglobulin deficiency, or early component complement deficiency, who have received either no doses or only 1 dose of Hib vaccine before 12 months of age, should receive 2 additional doses of Hib vaccine 8 weeks apart; children who received 2 or more doses of Hib vaccine before 12 months of age should receive 1 additional dose.
- For patients younger than 5 years of age undergoing chemotherapy or radiation treatment who received a Hib vaccine dose(s) within 14 days of starting therapy or during therapy, repeat the dose(s) at least 3 months following therapy completion.
- Recipients of hematopoietic stem cell transplant (HSCT) should be revaccinated with a 3-dose regimen of Hib vaccine starting 6 to 12 months after successful transplant, regardless of vaccination history; doses should be administered at least 4 weeks apart.
- A single dose of any Hib-containing vaccine should be administered to unimmunized* children and adolescents 15 months of age and older undergoing an elective splenectomy; if possible, vaccine should be administered at least 14 days before procedure.

Figure 1-3: *(continued)*

For further guidance on the use of the vaccines mentioned below, see: http://www.cdc.gov/vaccines/hcp/acip-recs/index.html.

4. **Haemophilus influenzae type b (Hib) conjugate vaccine (cont'd)**
- Hib vaccine is not routinely recommended for patients 5 years or older. However, 1 dose of Hib vaccine should be administered to unimmunized* persons aged 5 years or older who have anatomic or functional asplenia (including sickle cell disease) and unvaccinated persons 5 through 18 years of age with HIV infection.

  Patients who have not received a primary series and booster dose or at least 1 dose of Hib vaccine after 14 months of age are considered unimmunized.

5. **Pneumococcal vaccines. (Minimum age: 6 weeks for PCV13, 2 years for PPSV23)**

   Routine vaccination with PCV13:
   - Administer a 4-dose series of PCV13 vaccine at ages 2, 4, and 6 months and at age 12 through 15 months.
   - For children aged 14 through 59 months who have received an age-appropriate series of 7-valent PCV (PCV7), administer a single supplemental dose of 13-valent PCV (PCV13).

   Catch-up vaccination with PCV13:
   - Administer 1 dose of PCV13 to all healthy children aged 24 through 59 months who are not completely vaccinated for their age.
   - For other catch-up guidance, see Figure 2.

   Vaccination of persons with high-risk conditions with PCV13 and PPSV23:
   All recommended PCV13 doses should be administered prior to PPSV23 vaccination if possible.
   1. For children 2 through 5 years of age with any of the following conditions: chronic heart disease (particularly cyanotic congenital heart disease and cardiac failure); chronic lung disease (including asthma if treated with high-dose oral corticosteroid therapy); diabetes mellitus; cerebrospinal fluid leak; cochlear implant; sickle cell disease and other hemoglobinopathies; anatomic or functional asplenia; HIV infection; chronic renal failure; nephrotic syndrome; diseases associated with treatment with immunosuppressive drugs or radiation therapy, including malignant neoplasms, leukemias, lymphomas, and Hodgkin disease; solid organ transplantation; or congenital immunodeficiency:
       1. Administer 1 dose of PCV13 if any incomplete schedule of 3 doses of PCV (PCV7 and/or PCV13) were received previously.
       2. Administer 2 doses of PCV13 at least 8 weeks apart if unvaccinated or any incomplete schedule of fewer than 3 doses of PCV (PCV7 and/or PCV13) were received previously.
       3. Administer 1 supplemental dose of PCV13 if 4 doses of PCV7 or other age-appropriate complete PCV7 series was received previously.
       4. The minimum interval between doses of PCV (PCV7 or PCV13) is 8 weeks.
       5. For children with no history of PPSV23 vaccination, administer PPSV23 at least 8 weeks after the most recent dose of PCV13.
   2. For children aged 6 through 18 years who have cerebrospinal fluid leak; cochlear implant; sickle cell disease and other hemoglobinopathies; anatomic or functional asplenia; congenital or acquired immunodeficiencies; HIV infection; chronic renal failure; nephrotic syndrome; diseases associated with treatment with immunosuppressive drugs or radiation therapy, including malignant neoplasms, leukemias, lymphomas, and Hodgkin disease; generalized malignancy; solid organ transplantation; or multiple myeloma:
       1. If neither PCV13 nor PPSV23 has been received previously, administer 1 dose of PCV13 now and 1 dose of PPSV23 at least 8 weeks later.
       2. If PCV13 has been received previously but PPSV23 has not, administer 1 dose of PPSV23 at least 8 weeks after the most recent dose of PCV13.
       3. If PPSV23 has been received but PCV13 has not, administer 1 dose of PCV13 at least 8 weeks after the most recent dose of PPSV23.
   - For children aged 6 through 18 years with chronic heart disease (particularly cyanotic congenital heart disease and cardiac failure), chronic lung disease (including asthma if treated with high-dose oral corticosteroid therapy), diabetes mellitus, alcoholism, or chronic liver disease, who have not received PPSV23, administer 1 dose of PPSV23. If PCV13 has been received previously, then PPSV23 should be administered at least 8 weeks after any prior PCV13 dose.
   - A single revaccination with PPSV23 should be administered 5 years after the first dose to children with sickle cell disease or other hemoglobinopathies; anatomic or functional asplenia; congenital or acquired immunodeficiencies; HIV infection; chronic renal failure; nephrotic syndrome; diseases associated with treatment with immunosuppressive drugs or radiation therapy, including malignant neoplasms, leukemias, lymphomas, and Hodgkin disease; generalized malignancy; solid organ transplantation; or multiple myeloma.

6. **Inactivated poliovirus vaccine (IPV). (Minimum age: 6 weeks)**

   Routine vaccination:
   - Administer a 4-dose series of IPV at ages 2, 4, 6 through 18 months, and 4 through 6 years. The final dose in the series should be administered on or after the fourth birthday and at least 6 months after the previous dose.

   Catch-up vaccination:
   - In the first 6 months of life, minimum age and minimum intervals are only recommended if the person is at risk of imminent exposure to circulating poliovirus (i.e., travel to a polio-endemic region or during an outbreak).
   - If 4 or more doses are administered before age 4 years, an additional dose should be administered at age 4 through 6 years and at least 6 months after the previous dose.
   - A fourth dose is not necessary if the third dose was administered at age 4 years or older and at least 6 months after the previous dose.

6. **Inactivated poliovirus vaccine (IPV). (Minimum age: 6 weeks) (cont'd)**
- If both OPV and IPV were administered as part of a series, a total of 4 doses should be administered, regardless of the child's current age. If only OPV were administered, and all doses were given prior to 4 years of age, one dose of IPV should be given at 4 years or older, at least 4 weeks after the last OPV dose.
- IPV is not routinely recommended for U.S. residents aged 18 years or older.
- For other catch-up guidance, see Figure 2.

7. **Influenza vaccines. (Minimum age: 6 months for inactivated influenza vaccine [IIV], 2 years for live, attenuated influenza vaccine [LAIV])**

   Routine vaccination:
   - Administer influenza vaccine annually to all children beginning at age 6 months. For most healthy, nonpregnant persons aged 2 through 49 years, either LAIV or IIV may be used. However, LAIV should NOT be administered to some persons, including 1) persons who have experienced severe allergic reactions to LAIV, any of its components, or to a previous dose of any other influenza vaccine; 2) children 2 through 17 years receiving aspirin or aspirin-containing products; 3) persons who are allergic to eggs; 4) pregnant women; 5) immunosuppressed persons; 6) children 2 through 4 years of age with asthma or who had wheezing in the past 12 months; or 7) persons who have taken influenza antiviral medications in the previous 48 hours. For all other contraindications and precautions to use of LAIV, see MMWR August 7, 2015 / 64(30):818-25 available at http://www.cdc.gov/mmwr/pdf/wk/mm6430.pdf.

   For children aged 6 months through 8 years:
   - For the 2015-16 season, administer 2 doses (separated by at least 4 weeks) to children who are receiving influenza vaccine for the first time. Some children in this age group who have been vaccinated previously will also need 2 doses. For additional guidance, follow dosing guidelines in the 2015-16 ACIP influenza vaccine recommendations, MMWR August 7, 2015 / 64(30):818-25, available at http://www.cdc.gov/mmwr/pdf/wk/mm6430.pdf.
   - For the 2016-17 season, follow dosing guidelines in the 2016 ACIP influenza vaccine recommendations.

   For persons aged 9 years and older:
   - Administer 1 dose.

8. **Measles, mumps, and rubella (MMR) vaccine. (Minimum age: 12 months for routine vaccination)**

   Routine vaccination:
   - Administer a 2-dose series of MMR vaccine at ages 12 through 15 months and 4 through 6 years. The second dose may be administered before age 4 years, provided at least 4 weeks have elapsed since the first dose.
   - Administer 1 dose of MMR vaccine to infants aged 6 through 11 months before departure from the United States for international travel. These children should be revaccinated with 2 doses of MMR vaccine, the first at age 12 through 15 months (12 months if the child remains in an area where disease risk is high), and the second dose at least 4 weeks later.
   - Administer 2 doses of MMR vaccine to children aged 12 months and older before departure from the United States for international travel. The first dose should be administered on or after age 12 months and the second dose at least 4 weeks later.

   Catch-up vaccination:
   - Ensure that all school-aged children and adolescents have had 2 doses of MMR vaccine; the minimum interval between the 2 doses is 4 weeks.

9. **Varicella (VAR) vaccine. (Minimum age: 12 months)**

   Routine vaccination:
   - Administer a 2-dose series of VAR vaccine at ages 12 through 15 months and 4 through 6 years. The second dose may be administered before age 4 years, provided at least 3 months have elapsed since the first dose. If the second dose was administered at least 4 weeks after the first dose, it can be accepted as valid.

   Catch-up vaccination:
   - Ensure that all persons aged 7 through 18 years without evidence of immunity (see MMWR 2007 / 56 [No. RR-4], available at http://www.cdc.gov/mmwr/pdf/rr/rr5604.pdf) have 2 doses of varicella vaccine. For children aged 7 through 12 years, the recommended minimum interval between doses is 3 months (if the second dose was administered at least 4 weeks after the first dose, it can be accepted as valid); for persons aged 13 years and older, the minimum interval between doses is 4 weeks.

10. **Hepatitis A (HepA) vaccine. (Minimum age: 12 months)**

    Routine vaccination:
    - Initiate the 2-dose HepA vaccine series at 12 through 23 months; separate the 2 doses by 6 to 18 months.
    - Children who have received 1 dose of HepA vaccine before age 24 months should receive a second dose 6 to 18 months after the first dose.
    - For any person aged 2 years and older who has not already received the HepA vaccine series, 2 doses of HepA vaccine separated by 6 to 18 months may be administered if immunity against hepatitis A virus infection is desired.

    Catch-up vaccination:
    - The minimum interval between the 2 doses is 6 months.

Figure 1-3: *(continued)*

For further guidance on the use of the vaccines mentioned below, see: http://www.cdc.gov/vaccines/hcp/acip-recs/index.html.

10. **Hepatitis A (HepA) vaccine (cont'd)**

Special populations:
- Administer 2 doses of HepA vaccine at least 6 months apart to previously unvaccinated persons who live in areas where vaccination programs target older children, or who are at increased risk for infection. This includes persons traveling to or working in countries that have high or intermediate endemicity of infection; men having sex with men; users of injection and non-injection illicit drugs; persons who work with HAV-infected primates or with HAV in a research laboratory; persons with clotting-factor disorders; persons with chronic liver disease; and persons who anticipate close personal contact (e.g., household or regular babysitting) with an international adoptee during the first 60 days after arrival in the United States from a country with high or intermediate endemicity. The first dose should be administered as soon as the adoption is planned, ideally 2 or more weeks before the arrival of the adoptee.

11. **Meningococcal vaccines. (Minimum age: 6 weeks for Hib-MenCY [MenHibrix], 9 months for MenACWY-D [Menactra], 2 months for MenACWY-CRM [Menveo], 10 years for serogroup B meningococcal [MenB] vaccines: MenB-4C [Bexsero] and MenB-FHbp [Trumenba])**

Routine vaccination:
- Administer a single dose of Menactra or Menveo vaccine at age 11 through 12 years, with a booster dose at age 16 years.
- Adolescents aged 11 through 18 years with human immunodeficiency virus (HIV) infection should receive a 2-dose primary series of Menactra or Menveo with at least 8 weeks between doses.
- For children aged 2 months through 18 years with high-risk conditions, see below.

Catch-up vaccination:
- Administer Menactra or Menveo vaccine at age 13 through 18 years if not previously vaccinated.
- If the first dose is administered at age 13 through 15 years, a booster dose should be administered at age 16 through 18 years with a minimum interval of at least 8 weeks between doses.
- If the first dose is administered at age 16 years or older, a booster dose is not needed.
- For other catch-up guidance, see Figure 2.

Clinical discretion:
- Young adults aged 16 through 23 years (preferred age range is 16 through 18 years) may be vaccinated with either a 2-dose series of Bexsero or a 3-dose series of Trumenba vaccine to provide short-term protection against most strains of serogroup B meningococcal disease. The two MenB vaccines are not interchangeable; the same vaccine product must be used for all doses.

Vaccination of persons with high-risk conditions and other persons at increased risk of disease:

Children with anatomic or functional asplenia (including sickle cell disease):

Meningococcal conjugate ACWY vaccines:
1. Menveo
   o *Children who initiate vaccination at 8 weeks:* Administer doses at 2, 4, 6, and 12 months of age.
   o *Unvaccinated children who initiate vaccination at 7 through 23 months:* Administer 2 doses, with the second dose at least 12 weeks after the first dose AND after the first birthday.
   o *Children 24 months and older who have not received a complete series:* Administer 2 primary doses at least 8 weeks apart.
2. MenHibrix
   o *Children who initiate vaccination at 6 weeks:* Administer doses at 2, 4, 6, and 12 through 15 months of age.
   o If the first dose of MenHibrix is given at or after 12 months of age, a total of 2 doses should be given at least 8 weeks apart to ensure protection against serogroups C and Y meningococcal disease.
3. Menactra
   o *Children 24 months and older who have not received a complete series:* Administer 2 primary doses at least 8 weeks apart. If Menactra is administered to a child with asplenia (including sickle cell disease), do not administer Menactra until 2 years of age and at least 4 weeks after the completion of all PCV13 doses.

Meningococcal B vaccines:
1. Bexsero or Trumenba

Children with persistent complement component deficiency (includes persons with inherited or chronic deficiencies in C3, C5-9, properdin, factor D, factor H, or taking eculizumab [Soliris®]):

Meningococcal conjugate ACWY vaccines:
1. Menveo
   o *Children who initiate vaccination at 8 weeks:* Administer doses at 2, 4, 6, and 12 months of age.
   o *Unvaccinated children who initiate vaccination at 7 through 23 months:* Administer 2 doses, with the second dose at least 12 weeks after the first dose AND after the first birthday.
   o *Children 24 months and older who have not received a complete series:* Administer 2 primary doses at least 8 weeks apart.
2. MenHibrix
   o *Children who initiate vaccination at 6 weeks:* Administer doses at 2, 4, 6, and 12 through 15 months of age.
   o If the first dose of MenHibrix is given at or after 12 months of age, a total of 2 doses should be given at least 8 weeks apart to ensure protection against serogroups C and Y meningococcal disease.

3. Menactra
   o *Children 9 through 23 months:* Administer 2 primary doses at least 12 weeks apart.
   o *Children 24 months and older who have not received a complete series:* Administer 2 primary doses at least 8 weeks apart.

Meningococcal B vaccines:
1. Bexsero or Trumenba
   o *Persons 10 years or older who have not received a complete series.* Administer a 2-dose series of Bexsero, at least 1 month apart. Or a 3-dose series of Trumenba, with the second dose at least 2 months after the first and the third dose at least 6 months after the first. The two MenB vaccines are not interchangeable; the same vaccine product must be used for all doses.

For children who travel to or reside in countries in which meningococcal disease is hyperendemic or epidemic, including countries in the African meningitis belt or the Hajj
- administer an age-appropriate formulation and series of Menactra or Menveo for protection against serogroups A and W meningococcal disease. Prior receipt of MenHibrix is not sufficient for children traveling to the meningitis belt or the Hajj because it does not contain serogroups A or W.

For children at risk during a community outbreak attributable to a vaccine serogroup
- administer or complete an age- and formulation-appropriate series of MenHibrix, Menactra, or Menveo, Bexsero or Trumenba.

For booster doses among persons with high-risk conditions, refer to *MMWR* 2013 / 62(RR02);1-22, available at http://www.cdc.gov/mmwr/preview/mmwrhtml/rr6202a1.htm.

For other catch-up recommendations for these persons, and complete information on use of meningococcal vaccines, including guidance related to vaccination of persons at increased risk of infection, see *MMWR* March 22, 2013 / 62(RR02);1-22, and *MMWR* October 23, 2015 / 64(41); 1171-1176 available at http://www.cdc.gov/mmwr/pdf/rr/rr6202.pdf, and http://www.cdc.gov/mmwr/pdf/wk/mm6441.pdf.

12. **Tetanus and diphtheria toxoids and acellular pertussis (Tdap) vaccine. (Minimum age: 10 years for both Boostrix and Adacel)**

Routine vaccination:
- Administer 1 dose of Tdap vaccine to all adolescents aged 11 through 12 years.
- Tdap may be administered regardless of the interval since the last tetanus and diphtheria toxoid-containing vaccine.
- Administer 1 dose of Tdap vaccine to pregnant adolescents during each pregnancy (preferred during 27 through 36 weeks gestation) regardless of time since prior Td or Tdap vaccination.

Catch-up vaccination:
- Persons aged 7 years and older who are not fully immunized with DTaP vaccine should receive Tdap vaccine as 1 (preferably the first) dose in the catch-up series; if additional doses are needed, use Td vaccine. For children 7 through 10 years who receive a dose of Tdap as part of the catch-up series, an adolescent Tdap vaccine dose at age 11 through 12 years should NOT be administered. Td should be administered instead 10 years after the Tdap dose.
- Persons aged 11 through 18 years who have not received Tdap vaccine should receive a dose followed by tetanus and diphtheria toxoids (Td) booster doses every 10 years thereafter.
- Inadvertent doses of DTaP vaccine:
  - If administered inadvertently to a child aged 7 through 10 years may count as part of the catch-up series. This dose may count as the adolescent Tdap dose, or the child can later receive a Tdap booster dose at age 11 through 12 years.
  - If administered inadvertently to an adolescent aged 11 through 18 years, the dose should be counted as the adolescent Tdap booster.
- For other catch-up guidance, see Figure 2.

13. **Human papillomavirus (HPV) vaccines. (Minimum age: 9 years for 2vHPV [Cervarix], 4vHPV [Gardasil] and 9vHPV [Gardasil 9])**

Routine vaccination:
- Administer a 3-dose series of HPV vaccine on a schedule of 0, 1-2, and 6 months to children aged 11 through 12 years. 9vHPV, 4vHPV or 2vHPV may be used for females, and only 9vHPV or 4vHPV may be used for males.
- The vaccine series may be started at age 9 years.
- Administer the second dose 1 to 2 months after the first dose (minimum interval of 4 weeks); administer the third dose 16 weeks after the second dose (minimum interval of 12 weeks) and 24 weeks after the first dose.

Catch-up vaccination:
- Administer the vaccine series to females (2vHPV or 4vHPV or 9vHPV) and males (4vHPV or 9vHPV) at age 13 through 18 years if not previously vaccinated.
- Administer HPV vaccine beginning at age 9 years to children and youth with any history of sexual abuse or assault who have not initiated or completed the 3-dose series.
- Use recommended routine dosing intervals (see Routine vaccination above) for vaccine series catch-up.

Figure 1-3: (*continued*)

CS260933-A

Vaccine-Preventable Diseases and the Vaccines that Prevent Them

Diphtheria (Can be prevented by Tdap vaccine)

Diphtheria is a very contagious bacterial disease that affects the respiratory system, including the lungs. Diphtheria bacteria can be passed from person to person by direct contact with droplets from an infected person's cough or sneeze. When people are infected, the diptheria bacteria produce a toxin (poison) in the body that can cause weakness, sore throat, low-grade fever, and swollen glands in the neck. Effects from this toxin can also lead to swelling of the heart muscle and, in some cases, heart failure. In severe cases, the illness can cause coma, paralysis, and even death.

Hepatitis A (Can be prevented by HepA vaccine)

Hepatitis A is an infection in the liver caused by hepatitis A virus. The virus is spread primarily person-to-person through the fecal-oral route. In other words, the virus is taken in by mouth from contact with objects, food, or drinks contaminated by the feces (stool) of an infected person. Symptoms include fever, tiredness, loss of appetite, nausea, abdominal discomfort, dark urine, and jaundice (yellowing of the skin and eyes). An infected person may have no symptoms, may have mild illness for a week or two, or may have severe illness for several months that requires hospitalization. In the U.S., about 100 people a year die from hepatitis A.

Hepatitis B (Can be prevented by HepB vaccine)

Hepatitis B is an infection of the liver caused by hepatits B virus. The virus spreads through exchange of blood or other body fluids, for example, from sharing personal items, such as razors or during sex. Hepatitis B causes a flu-like illness with loss of appetite, nausea, vomiting, rashes, joint pain, and jaundice. The virus stays in the liver of some people for the rest of their lives and can result in severe liver diseases, including fatal cancer.

Human Papillomavirus (Can be prevented by HPV vaccine)

Human papillomavirus is a common virus. HPV is most common in people in their teens and early 20s. It is the major cause of cervical cancer in women and genital warts in women and men. The strains of HPV that cause cervical cancer and genital warts are spread during sex.

Influenza (Can be prevented by annual flu vaccine)

Influenza is a highly contagious viral infection of the nose, throat, and lungs. The virus spreads easily through droplets when an infected person coughs or sneezes and can cause mild to severe illness. Typical symptoms include a sudden high fever, chills, a dry cough, headache, runny nose, sore throat, and muscle and joint pain. Extreme fatigue can last from several days to weeks. Influenza may lead to hospitalization or even death, even among previously healthy children.

Measles (Can be prevented by MMR vaccine)

Measles is one of the most contagious viral diseases. Measles virus is spread by direct contact with the airborne respiratory droplets of an infected person. Measles is so contagious that just being in the same room after a person who has measles has already left can result in infection. Symptoms usually include a rash, fever, cough, and red, watery eyes. Fever can persist, rash can last for up to a week, and coughing can last about 10 days. Measles can also cause pneumonia, seizures, brain damage, or death.

Meningococcal Disease (Can be prevented by MCV vaccine)

Meningococcal disease is caused by bacteria and is a leading cause of bacterial meningitis (infection around the brain and spinal cord) in children. The bacteria are spread through the exchange of nose and throat droplets, such as when coughing, sneezing or kissing. Symptoms include nausea, vomiting, sensitivity to light, confusion and sleepiness. Meningococcal disease also causes blood infections. About one of every ten people who get the disease dies from it. Survivors of meningococcal disease may lose their arms or legs, become deaf, have problems with their nervous systems, become developmentally disabled, or suffer seizures or strokes.

Mumps (Can be prevented by MMR vaccine)

Mumps is an infectious disease caused by the mumps virus, which is spread in the air by a cough or sneeze from an infected person. A child can also get infected with mumps by coming in contact with a contaminated object, like a toy. The mumps virus causes fever, headaches, painful swelling of the salivary glands under the jaw, fever, muscle aches, tiredness, and loss of appetite. Severe complications for children who get mumps are uncommon, but can include meningitis (infection of the covering of the brain and spinal cord), encephalitis (inflammation of the brain), permanent hearing loss, or swelling of the testes, which rarely can lead to sterility in men.

Pertussis (Whooping Cough) (Can be prevented by Tdap vaccine)

Pertussis is caused by bacteria spread through direct contact with respiratory droplets when an infected person coughs or sneezes. In the beginning, symptoms of pertussis are similar to the common cold, including runny nose, sneezing, and cough. After 1-2 weeks, pertussis can cause spells of violent coughing and choking, making it hard to breathe, drink, or eat. This cough can last for weeks. Pertussis is most serious for babies, who can get pneumonia, have seizures, become brain damaged, or even die. About two-thirds of children under 1 year of age who get pertussis must be hospitalized.

Pneumococcal Disease
(Can be prevented by Pneumococcal vaccine)

Pneumonia is an infection of the lungs that can be caused by the bacteria called pneumococcus. This bacteria can cause other types of infections too, such as ear infections, sinus infections, meningitis (infection of the covering around the brain and spinal cord), bacteremia and sepsis (blood stream infection). Sinus and ear infections are usually mild and are much more common than the more severe forms of pneumococcal disease. However, in some cases pneumococcal disease can be fatal or result in long-term problems, like brain damage, hearing loss and limb loss. Pneumococcal disease spreads when people cough or sneeze. Many people have the bacteria in their nose or throat at one time or another without being ill—this is known as being a carrier.

Polio (Can be prevented by IPV vaccine)

Polio is caused by a virus that lives in an infected person's throat and intestines. It spreads through contact with the feces (stool) of an infected person and through droplets from a sneeze or cough. Symptoms typically include sudden fever, sore throat, headache, muscle weakness, and pain. In about 1% of cases, polio can cause paralysis. Among those who are paralyzed, up to 5% of children may die because they become unable to breathe.

Rubella (German Measles) (Can be prevented by MMR vaccine)

Rubella is caused by a virus that is spread through coughing and sneezing. In children rubella usually causes a mild illness with fever, swollen glands, and a rash that lasts about 3 days. Rubella rarely causes serious illness or complications in children, but can be very serious to a baby in the womb. If a pregnant woman is infected, the result to the baby can be devastating, including miscarriage, serious heart defects, mental retardation and loss of hearing and eye sight.

Tetanus (Lockjaw) (Can be prevented by Tdap vaccine)

Tetanus is caused by bacteria found in soil. The bacteria enters the body through a wound, such as a deep cut. When people are infected, the bacteria produce a toxin (poison) in the body that causes serious, painful spasms and stiffness of all muscles in the body. This can lead to "locking" of the jaw so a person cannot open his or her mouth, swallow, or breathe. Complete recovery from tetanus can take months. Three of ten people who get tetanus die from the disease.

Varicella (Chickenpox) (Can be prevented by varicella vaccine)

Chickenpox is caused by the varicella zoster virus. Chickenpox is very contagious and spreads very easily from infected people. The virus can spread from either a cough, sneeze. It can also spread from the blisters on the skin, either by touching them or by breathing in these viral particles. Typical symptoms of chickenpox include an itchy rash with blisters, tiredness, headache and fever. Chickenpox is usually mild, but it can lead to severe skin infections, pneumonia, encephalitis (brain swelling), or even death.

> If you have any questions about your child's vaccines, talk to your healthcare provider.

Last updated on 02/02/2015 - CS254242-A

Figure 1-4: Vaccine-preventable diseases and the vaccines that prevent them, United States, 2015. Source: Centers for Disease Control and Prevention [CDC]. (2015, January 26). *Immunization schedules for preteens and teens in easy-to-read formats.* Retrieved from www.cdc.gov/vaccines/schedules/easy-to-read/preteen-teen.html#print

Review Section

Review Questions

1. By ordering a serum fasting glucose level for a patient with obesity and risk factors for diabetes, a nurse practitioner exemplifies what level of prevention?

   a. Primary
   b. Secondary
   c. Tertiary
   d. Intermediary

2. A 45-year-old male patient presents to the primary care office for a follow-up visit to review his laboratory results: a body mass index (BMI) of 34.2 and an elevated fasting glucose level of 106 mg/dL. The patient has reported a family history of coronary heart disease. When counseling the patient about his risk for developing type 2 diabetes mellitus, the nurse practitioner identifies which of the following as a modifiable risk factor?

   a. Obesity
   b. Age
   c. Sex
   d. Ethnicity

3. Lydia, a 53-year-old female patient, arrives for her annual wellness visit. During her visit 1 year ago, she completed a colorectal screening with a colonoscopy and a mammogram. Her last cervical PAP smear, which was completed 2 years ago, was reported as normal. The patient reports being sexually active in

a monogamous relationship. Which health screening does the nurse practitioner now recommend?

a. Mammogram
b. Cervical PAP smear
c. Complete blood count
d. Fecal occult blood test

4. Sam, a 68-year-old male patient and former postal worker who retired 2 years ago, reports participating in minimal physical activity: mostly, he sits on the sofa and watches "old-time" movies or uses his computer. Since retiring, the patient has gained 26 pounds and his BMI is 31. The nurse practitioner advises the patient that his BMI is:

a. within normal limits.
b. at the optimum target.
c. above the normal range.
d. below normal limits.

5. The nurse practitioner is precepting a newly graduated nurse. The preceptee requires further instruction about the 2010 Dietary Guidelines for Americans (DGA), and the *MyPlate* recommendations for nutrition when stating that patients should be:

a. "eat a diet rich in vegetables and fruits."
b. "choose lean meats for protein."
c. "avoid foods and beverages with added sugars."
d. "limit sodium intake to 2,500 mg a day."

6. A healthy, 25-year-old patient seeks to improve his or her health through exercise. The nurse practitioner counsels that the guidelines recommend a minimum of:

a. 150 minutes a week of moderate-intensity or 75 minutes of vigorous-intensity aerobic physical activity, or an equivalent combination of both moderate- and vigorous-intensity aerobic activity.
b. 120 minutes a week of moderate-intensity or 60 minutes of vigorous-intensity aerobic physical activity, or an equivalent combination of both moderate- and vigorous-intensity aerobic activity.
c. 100 minutes a week of moderate-intensity or 45 minutes of vigorous-intensity aerobic physical activity, or an equivalent combination of both moderate- and vigorous-intensity aerobic activity.
d. 60 minutes a week of moderate-intensity or 60 minutes of vigorous-intensity aerobic physical activity, or an equivalent combination of both moderate- and vigorous-intensity aerobic activity.

7. Which of the following immunizations is appropriate to administer?

a. Hepatitis B vaccine to a 32-year-old female patient who has an anaphylactic reaction to baker's yeast
b. Pneumococcal vaccine (PCV23) to a 61-year-old male patient who smokes cigarettes
c. Shingles vaccine (Zostavax) to a 71-year-old-male patient undergoing chemotherapy
d. Influenza vaccine to a 24-year-old female patient with a severe allergic reaction to eggs

8. Which screening test, if any, is indicated for a 67-year-old patient with a 35-pack-year-history of smoking cigarettes?

a. Chest X-ray
b. Low-dose computed tomography (LDCT)
c. Chest X-ray followed by a LDCT
d. No screening tests are recommended.

9. Comprehensive health screening in a 56-year-old male patient who has a history of injection drug use includes:

a. immunoassays for hepatitis A.
b. hepatitis B surface antigen (HBsAg).
c. HIV p24 antigen and HIV antibody testing.
d. All of the above

10. Strategies to assist an individual in quitting smoking include:

a. offer FDA-approved pharmacotherapy for tobacco use disorders.
b. counseling on the potential health risks of smoking cigarettes.
c. brief intervention for treating tobacco use disorders with the five As: Ask, Advise, Assess, Assist, Arrange
d. All of the above

Answers with Rationales

1. (b) Primary Prevention

   Rationale: *Secondary prevention* is for early screening and detection of disease. Secondary prevention includes strategies to identify and treat asymptomatic persons who have already developed risk factors or preclinical disease but in whom the disease or condition is not clinically evident.

2. (a) Obesity

   Rationale: *Nonmodifiable* risk factors are those that an individual cannot change and that contribute to health conditions (e.g., sex, age, race, ethnicity, and heredity). Awareness aimed toward health-promoting lifestyle modifications relative to modifiable risk factors can aid in prevention of disease and are key to improving health outcomes. *Modifiable* risk factors (e.g., obesity) can be eliminated, controlled, or altered through behavioral change resulting in risk reduction of a health risk for a particular disease.

3. (d) Fecal occult blood test

   Rationale: Guideline recommendations for women aged 50 to 74 include a baseline screening mammogram starting at 50 years of age and then every 2 years (biennial). For women aged 21 to 65, a Pap smear (cytology) is recommended every 3 years until age 65. For women aged 45 and older, guidelines assert a strong recommendation to screen for lipid disorders, but not a complete blood count. In adult women aged 50 to 75, recommendations for colorectal screening includes a high-sensitivity fecal occult blood test (FOBT) annually, colonoscopy every 10 years, or sigmoidoscopy every 5 years. Since the patient had a colonoscopy 2 years ago, FOBT is indicated at this visit.

4. (c) BMI is above the normal range, placing him at risk for chronic health conditions, such as type 2 diabetes mellitus. The nurse practitioner should counsel the patient regarding physical activity.

   Rationale: BMI of 31 is consistent with obesity. Recommendations for obesity include offering or referring patients with a body mass index (BMI $\geq$ 30) to intensive, multicomponent behavioral intervention, such as individual or group sessions; weight-loss-setting goals; improvement of diet/nutrition; physical activity/exercise sessions; addressing barriers that prevent behavior change; and strategies for maintenance of lifestyle modification changes.

   (d) Limit sodium intake to 2,500 mg a day.

   Rationale: The 2010 Dietary Guidelines for Americans and *MyPlate* recommend limiting sodium to 2,300 mg of sodium a day (about 1 teaspoon of salt) for adults/adolescents and 1,500 mg of sodium a day for adults aged 51 years and older, individuals with hypertension, African Americans of any age, and those with diabetes or CKD. The 2010 Dietary Guidelines for Americans and *MyPlate* recommendations include eating a diet rich in a variety vegetables (dark-green vegetables, red and yellow vegetables, raw, cooked, fresh, or frozen), focused on fruits (fruits, berries, melons, 100% fruit juice), and choosing protein foods, such as lean meats.

5. (a) At least 150 minutes a week of moderate-intensity or 75 minutes of vigorous-intensity aerobic physical activity, or an equivalent combination of both moderate- and vigorous-intensity aerobic activity is recommended.

   Rationale: Guidelines recommend at least 150 minutes (2 hours and 30 minutes) a week of moderate-intensity or 75 minutes (1 hour and 15 minutes) of vigorous-intensity aerobic physical activity, or an equivalent combination of both moderate- and vigorous-intensity aerobic activity. Exercises are preferably spread throughout a week.
   1. Moderate-intensity examples: brisk walking, water aerobics, bicycling, tennis, dancing, general gardening, golfing, walking a dog
   2. Vigorous-intensity examples: race walking, jogging, running, swimming laps, aerobic dancing, bicycling 10 miles/hour or faster, jumping rope, heavy gardening, hiking uphill or with a heavy backpack
   3. Muscle-strengthening examples: lifting weights, push-ups, sit-ups, heavy gardening (digging, shoveling), yoga, working with resistance bands

6. (b) Pneumococcal vaccine (PCV23) to a 61-year-old male patient who smokes cigarettes

   Rationale: Patients with tobacco use disorders are at risk for pneumonia, and therefore, pneumococcal vaccine is indicated. Hepatitis B vaccine is contraindicated with a history of anaphylactic reaction to baker's yeast. Shingles (zoster) vaccine is contraindicated in patients who are on immunosuppressive therapy or on chemotherapy. In patients with severe allergic reactions (i.e., anaphylaxis) to egg protein, influenza vaccine is contraindicated.

7. (b) Low-dose computed tomography (LDCT)

    Rationale: Guidelines recommend screening for lung cancer for adults aged 55 to 80 with a history of smoking. The recommendation is an annual LDCT in individuals with a 30 pack-year-history who currently smoke or have quit within the past 15 years.

8. (d) All of the above

    Rationale: In adults, recommendations include screening individuals at high risk for HBV, including injection drug users who are HIV positive, men who have sex with men, household contacts of persons with HBV infection, and persons from countries with a high prevalence of HBV infection. All adults at high risk for HCV should be screened. Individuals born between 1945 and 1965 should be offered a one-time screening for HCV. Adolescents and adults aged 15 to 65 years should be screened for HIV. The patient is at high risk for HBV, HCV, and HIV; the nurse practitioner should recommend screening for all.

9. (d) All of the above

    Rationale: Guidelines recommend asking all adults about tobacco use and providing cessation interventions for those who use tobacco products (utilizing the five As behavioral counseling framework). The five As behavioral framework, when aimed at a strategic approach for intervention, can aid in an individual quitting tobacco use. Effective tobacco intervention combining the five As, counseling, and pharmacotherapy can enhance the chances of successfully quitting tobacco.

Suggested Readings

Agency for Healthcare Research and Quality. (2012, December). *Five major steps to intervention (The 5As)*. Rockville, MD: AHRQ. Retrieved from http://www.ahrq.gov/professionals/clinicians-providers/guidelines-recommendations/tobacco/5steps.html

Agency for Healthcare Research and Quality. (2014, June). *Preface: Guide to clinical preventive services*. Rockville, MD: AHRQ. Retrieved from http://www.ahrq.gov/professionals/clinicians-providers/guidelines-recommendations/guide/preface.html

American Cancer Society. (2014a.) *Healthy risks of secondhand smoke*. Retrieved from http://www.cancer.org/cancer/cancercauses/tobaccocancer/secondhand-smoke

American Cancer Society. (2014b.). *Skin cancer facts*. Retrieved from http://www.cancer.org/cancer/cancercauses/sunanduvexposure/skin-cancer-facts

American Cancer Society. (2015a). *Breast cancer*. Retrieved from http://www.cancer.org/cancer/breastcancer/index

American Cancer Society. (2015b). *Cervical cancer*. Retrieved from http://www.cancer.org/cancer/cervicalcancer/

American Cancer Society. (2015c). *Lung cancer*. Retrieved from http://www.cancer.org/cancer/lungcancer/index

American Cancer Society. (2015d). *Prostate cancer*. Retrieved from http://www.cancer.org/cancer/prostatecancer/index

American Diabetes Association. (2015). *Diabetes type 2*. Retrieved from http://www.diabetes.org/diabetes-basics/type-2/facts-about-type-2.html

American Heart Association. (2015). *High blood pressure*. Retrieved from http://www.heart.org/HEARTORG/Conditions/HighBloodPressure/High-Blood-Pressure-or-Hypertension_UCM_002020_SubHomePage.jsp

American Lung Association. (2015). *What's in a cigarette*. Retrieved from http://www.lung.org/stop-smoking/about-smoking/facts-figures/whats-in-a-cigarette.html

American Psychiatric Association. (2013). Depressive disorders. In *Diagnostic and statistical manual of mental disorders* (DSM-V-TR) (5th ed.). Washington, DC: APA. Retrieved from http://dsm.psychiatryonline.org/doi/book/10.1176/appi.books.9780890425596

Centers for Disease Control and Prevention. (2010, December 21). *Viral hepatitis populations: STDs and viral hepatitis*. Retrieved from http://www.cdc.gov/hepatitis/Populations/STDs.htm

Centers for Disease Control and Prevention. (2011, January 28). *2010 STD treatment guidelines*. Retrieved from http://www.cdc.gov/std/treatment/2010/toc.htm

Centers for Disease Control and Prevention. (2011, March 14). *CDC features: Clinical preventive services for older adults*. Retrieved from http://www.cdc.gov/features/preventiveservices/index.html

Centers for Disease Control and Prevention. (2011, August 11). *Diabetes*. Retrieved from http://www.cdc.gov/chronicdisease/resources/publications/AAG/ddt.htm

Centers for Disease Control and Prevention. (2011, November 9). *Physical activity: How much physical exercise do children need?* Retrieved from http://www.cdc.gov/physicalactivity/everyone/guidelines/children.html

Centers for Disease Control and Prevention. (2012a, October 16). *Cholesterol: Fast facts*. Retrieved from http://www.cdc.gov/cholesterol/facts.htm

Centers for Disease Control and Prevention. (2012b, October 29). *Nutrition for everyone*. Retrieved from http://www.cdc.gov/nutrition/everyone/index.html

Centers for Disease Control and Prevention. (2013, October 4). *Mental health: Burden of mental illness*. Retrieved from http://www.cdc.gov/mentalhealth/basics/burden.htm

Centers for Disease Control and Prevention. (2014a). *National diabetes statistics report: Estimates of diabetes and its burden in* the United States, 2014. Retrieved from http://www.cdc.gov/diabetes/pubs/statsreport14/national-diabetes-report-web.pdf

Centers for Disease Control and Prevention. (2014b January 16). *Healthy aging: Clinical preventive services*. Retrieved from http://www.cdc.gov/aging/services/

Centers for Disease Control and Prevention. (2014c, January 16). *Alcohol and public health: Facts sheets—Binge drinking*. Retrieved from http://www.cdc.gov/alcohol/fact-sheets/binge-drinking.htm

Centers for Disease Control and Prevention. (2014d, January 31). *Recommended immunization schedule for persons age 0 through 18: United States, 2014*. Retrieved from http://www.cdc.gov/vaccines/schedules/hcp/imz/child-adolescent.html

Centers for Disease Control and Prevention. (2014e, January 31b). *Contraindications and precautions to commonly used vaccines in adults: United States, 2014*. Retrieved from http://www.cdc.gov/vaccines/schedules/hcp/imz/adult-contraindications.html

Centers for Disease Control and Prevention. (2014f, March 3). *Physical activity: How much physical activity do you need?* Retrieved from http://www.cdc.gov/physicalactivity/everyone/guidelines/index.html

Centers for Disease Control and Prevention. (2014g, March 21). *Hepatitis B information for health professionals*. Retrieved from http://www.cdc.gov/hepatitis/HBV/HBVfaq.htm#overview

Centers for Disease Control and Prevention. (2014h, April 9). *Prostate cancer*. Retrieved from http://www.cdc.gov/cancer/prostate/

Centers for Disease Control and Prevention. (2014i, April 17). *CDC features: Data & statistics, excessive drinking*. Retrieved from http://www.cdc.gov/features/alcoholconsumption/

Centers for Disease Control and Prevention. (2014j, May 6). *What are the risk factors for breast cancer*. Retrieved from http://www.cdc.gov/cancer/breast/basic_info/risk_factors.htm

Centers for Disease Control and Prevention. (2014k, May 6). *What are the risk factors for cervical cancer*. Retrieved from http://www.cdc.gov/cancer/cervical/basic_info/risk_factors.htm

Centers for Disease Control and Prevention. (2014l, May 9). *Chronic disease prevention and health promotion*. Retrieved from http://www.cdc.gov/chronicdisease/overview/index.htm

Centers for Disease Control and Prevention. (2014m, May 9). *Overweight and obesity: Adult obesity facts*. Retrieved from http://www.cdc.gov/obesity/data/adult.html

Centers for Disease Control and Prevention. (2014n, May 19). *Vaccines and immunizations: Immunity types*. Retrieved from http://www.cdc.gov/vaccines/vac-gen/immunity-types.htm

Centers for Disease Control and Prevention. (2014o, July 1). *Healthy weight: Assessing your weight*. Retrieved from http://www.cdc.gov/healthyweight/assessing/index.html

Centers for Disease Control and Prevention. (2014p, July 7). *High blood pressure*. Retrieved from http://www.cdc.gov/bloodpressure/index.htm

Centers for Disease Control and Prevention. (2014q, July 17). *Hepatitis C information for health professionals*. Retrieved from http://www.cdc.gov/hepatitis/HCV/

Centers for Disease Control and Prevention. (2014r, September 2). *Colorectal (colon) cancer: Colorectal cancer statistics*. Retrieved from http://www.cdc.gov/cancer/colorectal/statistics/

Centers for Disease Control and Prevention. (2014s, September 10). *Physical activity and health*. Retrieved from http://www.cdc.gov/obesity/index.html

Centers for Disease Control and Prevention. (2014t, September 18a). *Recommended adult immunization schedule by vaccine and age group: United States, 2014*. Retrieved from http://www.cdc.gov/vaccines/schedules/hcp/imz/adult.html

Centers for Disease Control and Prevention. (2014u, September 18b). *Vaccine information for adults: Vaccine-preventable adult diseases*. Retrieved from http://www.cdc.gov/vaccines/adults/vpd.html

Centers for Disease Control and Prevention. (2014v, October 31a). *Morbidity and Mortality Weekly Report (MMWR). CDC National Health Report: Leading causes of morbidity and mortality and associated behavioral risk and protective factors-United States, 2005–2013*. Retrieved from http://www.cdc.gov/mmwr/preview/mmwrhtml/su6304a2.htm?s_cid=su6304a2_w

Centers for Disease Control and Prevention. (2014w, October 31b). *Smokeless tobacco: Health effects*. Retrieved from http://www.cdc.gov/tobacco/data_statistics/fact_sheets/smokeless/health_effects/index.htm

Centers for Disease Control and Prevention. (2014x, November 6). *Lung cancer*. Retrieved from http://www.cdc.gov/cancer/lung/index.htm

Centers for Disease Control and Prevention. (2014y, November 7). *Alcohol and public health: Frequently asked questions*. Retrieved from http://www.cdc.gov/alcohol/faqs.htm

Centers for Disease Control and Prevention. (2014z, November 13). *Tobacco use: Secondhand smoke*. Retrieved from http://www.cdc.gov/tobacco/basic_information/secondhand_smoke/

Centers for Disease Control and Prevention. (2014aa, November 25a). *Vital signs: HIV care saves lives*. Retrieved from http://www.cdc.gov/VitalSigns/hiv-aids-medical-care/index.html

Centers for Disease Control and Prevention. (2014ab, November 25b). *Physical activity*. Retrieved from http://www.cdc.gov/physicalactivity/

Centers for Disease Control and Prevention. (2014ac, November 26). *Immunization schedules: Adult immunization schedules United States, 2014*. Retrieved from http://www.cdc.gov/vaccines/schedules/hcp/adult.html

Centers for Disease Control and Prevention. (2014ad, December 1). *Colorectal (colon) screening*. Retrieved from http://www.cdc.gov/cancer/colorectal/basic_info/risk_factors.htm

Centers for Disease Control and Prevention. (2014ae, December 11). *Youth and tobacco use*. Retrieved from http://www.cdc.gov/tobacco/data_statistics/fact_sheets/youth_data/tobacco_use/

Centers for Disease Control and Prevention. (2014af, December 16). *2013 Sexually transmitted diseases surveillance: STDs in women and infants*. Retrieved from http://www.cdc.gov/std/stats13/womenandinf.htm

Centers for Disease Control and Prevention. (2014ag, December 29). *Chronic disease prevention and health promotion*. Retrieved from http://www.cdc.gov/chronicdisease/

Centers for Disease Control and Prevention. (2014ah, December 31). *Smoking & tobacco use*. Retrieved from http://www.cdc.gov/tobacco/index.htm

Centers for Disease Control and Prevention. (2015a, January 5). *Viral hepatitis statistics & surveillance: Surveillance for viral hepatitis—United States, 2012*. Retrieved from http://www.cdc.gov/hepatitis/Statistics/2012Surveillance/Commentary.htm

Centers for Disease Control and Prevention. (2015b, January 12). *HIV/AIDS*. Retrieved from http://www.cdc.gov/hiv/

Centers for Disease Control and Prevention. (2015c, January 13). *Skin cancer*. Retrieved from http://www.cdc.gov/cancer/skin/

Centers for Disease Control and Prevention. (2015d, January 15). *Sexually transmitted diseases (STDs)*. Retrieved from http://www.cdc.gov/std/

Centers for Disease Control and Prevention. (2015e, January 26). *Immunization schedules for preteens and teens in easy-to-read formats*. Retrieved from http://www.cdc.gov/vaccines/schedules/easy-to-read/preteen-teen.html#print

Centers for Disease Control and Prevention. (2015f, April 6). *Immunization schedules: Adult immunization schedules*. Retrieved from http://www.cdc.gov/vaccines/schedules/hcp/adult.html

Centers for Disease Control and Prevention. (2015g, April 6). *Immunization schedules: Child and adolescent schedule*. Retrieved from http://www.cdc.gov/vaccines/schedules/hcp/imz/child-adolescent.html

Dunphy, L., Winland-Brown, J., Porter, B., & Thomas, D. (2011). *Primary care: The art and science of advanced practice nursing* (3rd ed.). Philadelphia, PA: F.A. Davis Company.

Eckel, R., Jakicic, J., Ard, J., DeJesus, J., Houston-Miller, N., Hubbard, V.,. . .Yanovski, S. (2014). 2013 AHA/ACC Guideline on lifestyle management to reduce cardiovascular risk: A report of the American College of Cardiology/American Heart Association Task Force on Practice Guidelines. *Journal of the American College of Cardiology*, 63(25), 2960–2984. doi:10.1016/j.jacc2013.11.003

International Agency for Research on Cancer. (2007). IARC Monographs Programme finds cancer hazards associated with shiftwork, painting, and firefighting. Retrieved from http://www.iarc.fr/en/media-centre/pr/2007/pr180.html

James, P., Oparil, S., Carter, B., Cushman, W., Dennison-Himmelfarb, C., Handler, J., Lackland, D. (2014). 2014 Evidence-based guidelines for the management of high blood pressure in adults: Report from the panel members appointed to the eighth Joint National Committee (JNC 8). *Journal of the American Medical Association*, 311(5), 507–520. doi:10.1001/jama.2013.284427

Kaplan, N., Thomas, G., & Pohl, M. (2014, December 17). Blood pressure measurement in the diagnosis and management of hypertension in adults. In G. Bakris & J. Forman (Eds.), *UpToDate*. Waltham, MA: UpToDate. Retrieved from http://www.uptodate.com/contents/blood-pressure-measurement-in-the-diagnosis-and-management-of-hypertension-in-adults

Kristi, A. H., Shenson, D., Woolf, S. H., Bradley, C., Liaw, W.R., Rothemich, S. F.,. . . Slonim, A. (2013). Clinical and community delivery systems for preventive care: an integration framework. *American Journal of Preventive Medicine*, 45(4), 508–516. doi:10.1016/j.amepre.2013.06.008

Lok, A. S. F. (2014, December). Diagnosis of Hepatitis B. In R. Esteban & J. Mitty (Eds.), *UpToDate*. Waltham, MA: UpToDate. Retrieved from http://www.uptodate.com/contents/diagnosis-of-hepatitis-b-virus-infection

National Breast Cancer Foundation. (2012). *What is breast cancer?* Retrieved from http://www.nationalbreastcancer.org/what-is-cancer

National Cancer Institute. (2014a). *Colon and rectal cancer*. Retrieved from http://www.cancer.gov/cancertopics/types/colon-and-rectal

National Cancer Institute. (2014b). *Skin cancer*. Retrieved from http://www.cancer.gov/cancertopics/types/skin

National Cancer Institute. (2014c). *Lung cancer: Lung cancer prevention*. Retrieved from http://www.cancer.gov/cancertopics/pdq/prevention/lung/HealthProfessional

National Cancer Institute. (2014d). *Prostate cancer: General information about prostate cancer*. Retrieved from http://www.cancer.gov/cancertopics/types/prostate

National Cancer Institute. (2014e). *Colorectal cancer prevention: Overview*. Retrieved from http://www.cancer.gov/cancertopics/pdq/prevention/colorectal/HealthProfessional/page2#_150_toc

National Cancer Institute. (2014f). *Colorectal cancer prevention: Who is at risk?* Retrieved from http://www.cancer.gov/cancertopics/pdq/prevention/colorectal/HealthProfessional

National Cancer Institute. (2015a). *Cervical cancer*. Retrieved from http://www.cancer.gov/cancertopics/pdq/treatment/cervical/HealthProfessional/page1

National Cancer Institute. (2015b). *SEER cancer statistics factsheets: Colon and rectum cancer*. Retrieved from http://seer.cancer.gov/statfacts/html/colorect.html

National Institute on Alcohol Abuse and Alcoholism. (n.d.). *Alcohol & Your health: Alcohol facts and statistics*. Retrieved from http://www.niaaa.nih.gov/alcohol-health/alcohols-effects-body

National Institute on Alcohol Abuse and Alcoholism. (2004). *Alcohol alert: Alcohol's damaging effects on the brain*. Retrieved from http://pubs.niaaa.nih.gov/publications/aa63/aa63.htm

National Institute on Alcohol Abuse and Alcoholism. (2014, July). *Alcohol & your health: Alcohol facts and statistics*. Retrieved from http://www.niaaa.nih.gov/alcohol-health/overview-alcohol-consumption/alcohol-facts-and-statistics

Pender, N., Murdaugh, C., & Parsons, M. A. (2011). Global Health Promotion: Challenges of the 21st Century. In N. Pender, C. Murdaugh, & M. A. Parsons (eds.), *Health promotion in nursing practice* (6th ed., p. 203). Upper Saddle River, NJ: Pearson Education, Inc.

Prostate Cancer Foundation. (2015). *Understanding prostate cancer: Prevention*. Retrieved from http://www.pcf.org/site/c.leJRIROrEpH/b.5802029/k.31EA/Prevention.htm

United States Department of Agriculture. (n.d.). *ChooseMyPlate*. Retrieved from http://www.choosemyplate.gov/index.html

United States Department of Health and Human Services. (2008). *Developing healthy people 2020: Recommendations for the framework and format of healthy people 2020*. Retrieved from https://www.healthypeople.gov/sites/default/files/PhaseI_0.pdf

United States Department of Health and Human Services. (2013). *Community immunity: Herd immunity*. Retrieved from http://www.vaccines.gov/basics/protection/

United States Department of Health and Human Services. (2014a). *Healthy people 2020: About healthy people*. Retrieved from https://www.healthypeople.gov/2020/About-Healthy-People

United States Department of Health and Human Services. (2014b). *Healthy people 2020: About healthy people*. Retrieved from https://www.healthypeople.gov/2020/leading-health-indicators/2020-LHI-Topics

United States Department of Health and Human Services. (2014c). *Healthy people 2020: About healthy people*. Retrieved from https://www.healthypeople.gov/2020/topics-objectives/topic/tobacco-use

United States Department of Health and Human Services. (2015a). *Healthy people 2020: Immunizations and infectious diseases.* Retrieved from https://www.healthypeople.gov/2020/topics-objectives/topic/immunization-and-infectious-diseases

United States Department of Health and Human Services. (2015b). *Office of Disease Prevention and Health Promotion: Dietary guidelines for Americans, 2010.* Retrieved from http://www.health.gov/dietaryguidelines/2010.asp

United States Department of Health and Human Services. (2015c). *Healthy people 2020: Nutrition and weight status.* Retrieved from https://www.healthypeople.gov/2020/topics-objectives/topic/nutrition-and-weight-status

United States Department of Health and Human Services. (2015d). *Healthy people 2020: Physical activity.* Retrieved from https://www.healthypeople.gov/2020/topics-objectives/topic/physical-activity

United States Department of Health and Human Services. (2015e, February 1). *Office of Disease Prevention and Health Promotion: 2008 Physical activities guidelines for Americans.* Retrieved from http://www.health.gov/paguidelines/

United States Preventative Services Task Force. (1996). Guide to clinical preventive services (2nd ed.). Baltimore, MD: Williams & Wilkins. Retrieved from http://odphp.osophs.dhhs.gov/pubs/GUIDECPS/PDF/Frontmtr.PDF

United States Preventative Services Task Force. (2014a). *Published Recommendations.* Retrieved from http://www.ahrq.gov/professionals/clinicians-providers/guidelines-recommendations/guide/section2.html

United States Preventative Services Task Force. (2014b, June). *Published recommendations, Section 2: Recommendations for adults.* Retrieved from http://www.uspreventiveservicestaskforce.org/uspstopics.htm

United States Preventative Services Task Force. (2015). *Published recommendations.* Retrieved from http://www.uspreventiveservicestaskforce.org/BrowseRec/Index/browse-recommendations

World Health Organization. (2014a). *Health promotion.* Retrieved from http://www.who.int/topics/health_promotion/en/

World Health Organization. (2014b). *Breast cancer: Prevention and control.* Retrieved from http://www.who.int/cancer/detection/breastcancer/en/

World Health Organization. (2014c). *Cancer: Screening for various cancers.* Retrieved from http://www.who.int/cancer/detection/variouscancer/en/

World Health Organization. (2014d). *Tobacco.* Retrieved from http://www.who.int/mediacentre/factsheets/fs339/en/

World Health Organization. (2015a). *Depression.* Retrieved from http://www.who.int/mediacentre/factsheets/fs369/en/

World Health Organization. (2015b). *Hepatitis B.* Retrieved from http://www.who.int/mediacentre/factsheets/fs204/en/

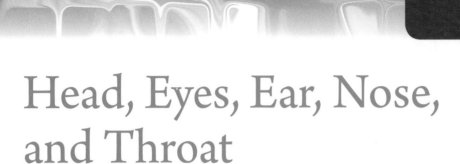

Chapter 2

Head, Eyes, Ear, Nose, and Throat

Ellen D. Feld ● Ann McDonough Madden ● Megan E. Schneider ● Diana D. Smith ● and Patrick C. Auth

Case Presentation

Directions: Review the case study below carefully. At the end of the chapter, answer the questions. Proceed then to the Review Section. Compare your answers to what you find in the review section along with the rationales.

History of Present Illness: This is a 77-year-old female widow who resides in an assisted living facility (ALF) who presents to her nurse practitioner with a 3-year history of progressive hearing loss. Patient states her friends noticed her hearing loss is more noticeable and suggested she be evaluated. Patient states she is able to manage hearing a one-to-one conversation; however, she has difficulty hearing when there is more than one person speaking at the same time. She had no family history of hearing loss. She denied pain, numbness, or weakness. The patient's Past Medical History (PMH) is significant for Degenerative Joint Disease (DJD) hips and knees, hypertension, macular degeneration, diabetes mellitus type 2, urinary urgency, and rare incontinence. Denies history of head or neck malignancies.

Past Medical History:
Degenerative joint disease bilaterally in knees with chronic pain × 15 years
Hypertension × 22 years
Macular degeneration × 2 months
Diabetes 2 × 12 years
Urinary urgency and rare incontinence × 3 years

Family and Social History:
Mother had hypertension; no family history of depression, hearing loss, dementia, head or neck cancer. There is no history of tobacco or alcohol use.

Medications:
Verapamil SR 360 mg daily
Ranitidine 150 mg at bedtime
Hydrochlorothiazide 12.5 mg daily
Enteric-coated aspirin 81 mg daily
Acetaminophen 650 mg p.o. every 6 hours p.r.n. pain
Multivitamin adult, daily

Medical Allergies:
Penicillin (PCN) (hives)

Physical Examination:

Vital signs: T = 99°F   Height = 63 inches in shoes   Weight = 120 lbs (54 kg)
PR = 70/min, regularly, regular   RR = 12/min, regular, shallow

BP:	Right Arm	Left Arm
Supine		
Sitting	160/80	160/82
Standing	164/92	

General Survey: Well developed well nourished (WDWN) Caucasian female in No Apparent Distress (NAD) appears stated age of 77 years. Speech clear and goal directed. Answers questions quickly and accurately. Clean and neatly groomed. Ambulates with assistance.

Skin: Olive complexion, warm, smooth, moist with rapid turgor, freely mobile. Well-healed 5-cm scar over the dorsum of the right hand. Vellus hair evenly distributed to finger to toes. **Nails curved:** Nail beds pink with capillary refill <1 second. No erythema, cyanosis, jaundice, petechiae, ecchymosis, or clubbing.

Head, Eyes, Ears, Nose, Throat (HEENT): **Head:** Symmetrical and proportionate to body habitus. Nontender to palpation. No deformities or lesions. Face is symmetrical at rest and upon movements. Thin black hair is evenly distributed over scalp. **Eyes:** Visual acuity; uncorrected OS-20/50 OD-20/50 OU = 20/50. Cornea and lenses are clear and colorless without opacities and scares. Fundi are pinkish-yellow, A:V ration = 2:3; disc: cup 1:2. Disc margins are distinct bilaterally; macula shows yellowish-colored retinal deposits (drusen bodies). No AV nicking, narrowing, banking, copper/silver wiring, hemorrhages, exudates, neovascularization. **Ears:** Symmetrical in alignment and position, auricles are nontender without edema, deformities, or erythema. Auditory acuity equal bilaterally to finger rubbing. Weber: Without lateralization, Rinne: AC>BC bilaterally. Auditory canals are patent with excess cerumen. TMs are pearly gray. Landmarks: Cone of light, umbo, malleolar processes, pars flaccida, and pars tensa all distinct and in normal anatomic positions. No erythema, edema, injection, exudates, perforation, air/fluid levels, air bubbles, bulging, or retraction. **Nose:** Symmetrical positioning, and alignment, without deformity. Nares are patent bilaterally. Mucosa and turbinates are pinkish-red, moist and without erythema, edema, polyps, exudate, discoloration, bogginess, bleeding.

Nodes: No visible masses, nodules, or enlargement. Nontender and nonpalpable cervical, supraclavicular, infraclavicular, axillary, epitrochlear, and inguinal nodes.

Mouth: **Lips:** Pink, moist, and symmetrical without lesions, cracking, or fissures. **Gums:** Full, pink, moist without edema. **Uvula:** Symmetrical at rest and upon phonation. **Posterior pharynx:** Pink and moist without exudates, erythema, injection, or discharge.

Chest (Respirations): Shallow and unlabored, regular rhythm at 12/min. **Chest wall:** Nontender. **Breath sounds:** Vesicular in distal airways; bronchovesicular over larger airways. No wheezes, rhonchi, crackles, egophony

Heart: **Rate and rhythm:** Regular at 70/min. PMI palpable 9 cm lateral to the MSL in the left, fifth ICS; approx. 1 cm diameter; strong and lasting approx. two-third of systole, S1>S2 at apex, no murmurs, gallops, rubs, or splitting heart sounds.

Abdomen: Normal (active) BS × 4 quads. Soft, nontender without masses, rebound tenderness, tenderness, guarding, or fluid wave.

Neurologic: CN I–CN XII grossly intact bilaterally. Romberg normal. **Gait:** Antalgic secondary to bilateral knee pain. **Get-up-and-go test:** 18 seconds. Uses arms to arise from chair. DTR's +2/+4 UE and LE extremities bilaterally.

Laboratory: Sodium = 140 mEq/L; Potassium = 4.2 mEq/L; Chloride = 100 mEq/L; BUN = 24 mg/dL; Creatinine = 1.4 mg/dL; Glucose = 88 mg/dL; Hemoglobin = 14.9 g/dL; Hematocrit = 44%; Audiogram showed bilateral symmetrical sensorineural hearing loss; ECG NSR

Diagnosis (Age-related): Presbycusis

Eye Disorders

Entropion

Description of the Disease: An entropion is an inward turning of the lid margin, and it may be classified as involutional, cicatricial, spastic, or congenital.

Etiology:
- Involutional entropion is the most common type and occurs during normal aging when the preseptal orbicularis muscle migrates upward, the lower lid retractors disinsert, and the eyelid becomes more lax.

Epidemiology:
- Older population
- May be congenital

Risk Factors:
- Extensive scarring of the conjunctiva and tarsus
- Scarring, infection, or spastic conditions

Signs and Symptoms:
- Eye irritation, which may result in blepharospasm
- Redness
- Light sensitivity
- Dryness
- Increased lacrimation
- Foreign-body sensation
- Scratching of the cornea by ashes

Differential Diagnosis:
- Epiblepharon
- Trichiasis
- Distichiasis

Diagnostic Studies:
- None

Treatment:
- Surgery is an effective treatment for all types of entropion.
- Temporary treatments include taping the lower lid to the cheek and injection of botulinum toxin.

Ectropion

Description of the Disease: An ectropion is an outward turning of the lid margin, and it may be classified as involutional, paralytic, cicatricial, mechanical, or congenital.

Etiology:
- Involutional ectropion results from horizontal lid laxity associated with aging.

Epidemiology:
- Common in the elderly
- Following a seventh nerve palsy
- Orbicularis oculi muscle relaxation

Risk Factors:
- Can be congenital or have cicatricial causes

Signs and Symptoms:
- Eye tearing and irritation and possibly exposure keratitis
- Drooping of the eyelid
- Redness
- Light sensitivity
- Dryness
- Foreign-body sensation

Differential Diagnosis:
- Eyelid malignancy
- Eyelid retraction caused by proptosis

Diagnostic Studies:
- None

Treatment:
- Surgery that shortens the lid horizontally is an effective treatment.

Dacryocystitis

Description of the Disease: Dacryocystitis is an inflammation of the lacrimal drainage system.

Etiology:
- It typically occurs in postmenopausal women as a result of chronic inflammation that produces fibrosis in the nasolacrimal duct, which can lead to stasis of tears and secondary infections.

Epidemiology:
- Usually presents in people over 40, peak age is 60 to 70, postmenopausal women and infants
- In acute cases, *Staphylococcus aureus* and B-hemolytic strep
- In chronic cases: *S. epidermidis*, anaerobic strep, *Candida albicans*

Risk Factors:
- Congenital: Both sexes are at equal risk.

Signs and Symptoms:
- Eye tearing and discharge
- In acute dacryocystitis there is also pain, inflammation, swelling, and tenderness in the area of the lacrimal sac.
- Purulent material can sometimes be expressed through the lacrimal puncta.
- In chronic dacryocystitis tearing, matting of lashes and expressible mucoid material are the only symptoms.

Differential Diagnosis:
- Infected sebaceous cyst
- Acute ethmoid sinusitis
- Cellulitis
- Allergic rhinitis.

Diagnostic Studies:
- Usually none
- Consider computed tomography (CT) scan or magnetic resonance imaging (MRI) when etiology is in question.
- Complete blood count (CBC) to check for leukocytosis

Treatment:
- Acute dacryocystitis is treated with systemic antibiotics; occasionally incision and drainage is needed.
- Antibiotic drops are used in the chronic form.
- In both forms, surgical correction, usually by dacryocystorhinostomy (where a permanent fistula is formed between the lacrimal sac and the nose), is a definitive treatment.

Retinal Detachment

Description of the Disease: A condition in which the retina peels away from its supporting tissues

Etiology:
- Most cases begin with a hole or tear in the peripheral retina—patients with peripheral retinal thinning are at particular risk for this.

Epidemiology:
- Occurs between 40 and 70
- Most common in patients with myopia >6 diopters

Risk Factors:
- Myopia
- Trauma
- Prior cataract extraction

- Leukemia
- Diabetes
- Angiomatosis
- Eclampsia
- Breast cancer
- Melanoma
- Sickle cell disease

Signs and Symptoms:
- Scotomata
- Flashing lights
- Floaters
- There may be an afferent pupillary defect and decreased visual acuity if the area of detachment includes the fovea.

Differential Diagnosis:
- Posterior vitreous detachment
- Retinal vein or artery occlusion
- Optic neuritis
- CVA
- Migraine

Diagnostic Studies:
- Slit lamp
- No laboratory tests are usually needed unless a cause for the detachment is unknown.
- CT or MRI is used only if a tumor or foreign body is suspected.

Treatment:
- Urgent surgery is indicated.
- Surgical techniques include cryosurgery, laser, and pneumatic retinopexy.

Retinal Vein Occlusion

Description of the Disease: A condition in which thrombosis produces occlusion of either the central retinal vein or one of its branches.

Epidemiology:
- More than 50% of patients have associated cardiovascular disease.

Etiology:
- Depending on the area of retinal venous drainage effectively occluded it is broadly classified as central retinal vein occlusion, hemispheric retinal vein occlusion, or branch retinal vein occlusion.

Risk Factors:
- Other risk factors include diabetes, hypertension, dyslipidemia, hypercoagulability, vasculitis, glaucoma, and vein compression from thyroid disease or orbital tumors.

Signs and Symptoms:
- Variable, painless loss of vision
- Optic disc edema
- Cotton wool spots
- Diffuse retinal hemorrhages ("blood-and-thunder fundus")
- A normal contralateral fundus helps distinguish this from papilledema.

Differential Diagnosis:
- Papilledema
- Optic neuritis
- Retinal artery occlusion
- Diabetic retinopathy

Diagnostic Studies:
- Fluorescein angiography may be used to determine the degree of retinal ischemia and diagnose macular edema. Optical coherence tomography may be used to diagnose macular edema and gauge response to treatment.

Treatment:
- There is no specific treatment for retinal vein occlusion.
- The resultant macular edema may sometimes be treated with argon laser photocoagulation or intravitreal injections of steroids or anti-VEGF (vascular endothelial growth factor) agents.

Retinal Artery Occlusion

Description of the Disease: A condition in which either the central retinal artery or one of its branches is acutely occluded resulting in sudden, painless visual loss.

Etiology:
- A condition in which either the central retinal artery or one of its branches is acutely occluded resulting in sudden, painless visual loss.

Epidemiology:
- Usually occurs in patients between the ages of 50 and 80

Risk Factors:
- Geriatric patients who have concurrent hypertension, cardiac arrhythmia, diabetes, or atherosclerosis

Signs and Symptoms:
- Partial or total monocular
- Painless loss of vision is the hallmark.
- Prior transient loss of vision (amaurosis fugax) may have occurred.
- Retina appears pale and opaque with a characteristic "cherry red spot" at the macula.

Differential Diagnosis:
- Retinal vein occlusion
- Optic neuritis
- CVA
- Migraine

Diagnostic Studies:
- Electrocardiogram (ECG)
- Fasting blood sugar
- Lipid profile
- Partial thromboplastin time (PTT)
- Erythrocyte sedimentation rate (ESR)

Treatment:
- Giant cell arteritis must be immediately ruled out in older patients; if present, immediate high-dose systemic steroids are indicated.
- In embolic central retinal artery occlusion, anterior chamber paracentesis and IV acetazolamide may reduce intraocular pressure.
- Inhaled oxygen–carbon dioxide mixture may increase retinal Po_2 via retinal vasodilatation.
- Rarely, thrombolytic therapy is used.

Presbyopia

Description of the Disease: Presbyopia is the loss of accommodation that results from aging.

Etiology:
- It is caused by progressive stiffening of the lens with aging and occurs in all people beginning around age 45. Symptoms worsen until around age 55 when they stabilize but persist.

Epidemiology:
- Occurs in all people beginning around age 45

Risk Factors:
- Can be congenital

Signs and Symptoms:
- Individuals are unable to read small print or discriminate fine, close objects.
- Symptoms are worse in dim light or with fatigue.

Differential Diagnosis:
- Cataracts
- Macular degeneration
- Diabetic retinopathy
- Hyperopia (if refractive history is unknown)

Diagnostic Studies:
- Thorough eye examination by ophthalmologist or optometrist

Treatment:
- Use of a "plus" lens via reading glasses, multifocal lenses, or contact lenses

Cataract

Description of the Disease: A cataract is an opacification of the lens that results in loss of vision.

Etiology:
- Aging is the most common cause; 50% of individuals 65 to 74 are affected, as are 70% of those over 75.

Epidemiology:
- Usually occurs >60 years of age

Risk Factors:
- Other risk factors include trauma, diabetes, heredity, and radiation therapy and glucocorticoid treatment.

Signs and Symptoms:
- Progressive loss of vision
- Impaired red reflex on funduscopic examination.

Differential Diagnosis:
- Macular degeneration
- Presbyopia
- Retinal disease

Diagnostic Studies:
- Through eye examination by ophthalmologist or optometrist

Treatment:
- Surgical removal of the lens with implantation of a plastic or silicone replacement lens.

Glaucoma

Description of the Disease: Glaucoma is an acquired optic neuropathy characterized by optic disc cupping and visual field loss and usually associated with increased intraocular pressure. There are multiple types of glaucoma, with primary open-angle glaucoma being the most common.

Etiology:
- The mechanism of increased intraocular pressure is impairment in the outflow of the aqueous humor due to abnormalities in the drainage system. The increased pressure causes retinal ganglion cell death and axonal loss; the optic nerve then atrophies.

Epidemiology:
- It is more common in Black than in White patients and is the leading cause of blindness in African Americans.

Risk Factors:
- African American heritage
- Individuals with vascular disease such as hypertension, those with migraine, diabetes, or cardiovascular disease
- Individuals with family history of glaucoma

Signs and Symptoms:
- Open-angle glaucoma may be initially asymptomatic and is often not detected until extensive bilateral visual field loss has occurred.
- Acute narrow-angle glaucoma is characterized by a sudden onset of pain and ocular inflammation.
- On funduscopic examination the physiologic cup appears enlarged ("cupping"), and the cup–disc ratio is increased. Intraocular pressure measurements are elevated.

Differential Diagnosis:
- Iris cysts
- Melanocytoma
- Fuchs' adenoma
- Uveal melanoma

Diagnostic Studies:
- Thorough eye examination by ophthalmologist including tonometry
- Central field testing
- Pachymetry

Treatment:
- Topical adrenergic agonists, prostaglandin analogs, carbonic anhydrase inhibitors, or cholinergic agonists
- Laser trabeculoplasty and surgical intervention are also sometimes used.

Age-Related Macular Degeneration

Description of the Disease: Age-related macular degeneration is a disorder that causes progressive destruction of the macula, leading to loss of central vision; there are two types: "wet" (exudative) and "dry" (nonexudative).

Etiology:
- It affects people over age 55 and is the leading cause of irreversible blindness in the developed world.

Epidemiology:
- It is a multifactorial disease involving genetic susceptibility and risk factors listed below.

Risk Factors:
- Increasing age
- White race
- Smoke

Signs and Symptoms:
- Gradual, painless, bilateral central vision loss
- Drusen (yellow deposits) are visible on funduscopic examination in the dry form. In the wet form, neovascularization, hemorrhages, and scarring may be evident.

Differential Diagnosis:
- Angioid streaks
- Toxic lesions
- Cuticular drusen
- Sarcoidosis
- Ocular histoplasmosis

Diagnostic Studies:
- Amsler grid
- Angiography
- Electroretinogram

Treatment:
- Smoking cessation is recommended, and oral vitamins may reduce the risk of progression in certain subgroups of patients.
- Intravitreal injections of anti-VEGF antibodies are the preferred treatment for macular degeneration with neovascularization.

Presbycusis

Description of the Disease: Multifactorial age-related hearing impairment with predisposition for high-frequency hearing loss

Epidemiology:
- One-third of adults aged 61 to 70, 80% of adults older than 85
- Greater hearing loss and earlier onset in men

Etiology:
- Genetic predisposition and environmental insults result in decreased cochlear sensitivity.
- Cochlear hair cell degeneration and loss of auditory neurons in the organ of Corti result in high-frequency sound loss, making human speech difficult to understand. Decreased cochlear blood supply and loss of cortical auditory neurons cause hearing loss in all frequencies, making sound localization difficult.

Risk Factors:
- Genetic and environmental influence
- Excessive noise exposure
- Ototoxic medications (e.g., aminoglycosides, salicylates, NSAIDs, diuretics)
- Chronic disease that impairs cochlear vascular supply (e.g., diabetes mellitus and cardiovascular disease)
- Smoking

Signs and Symptoms:
- Gradual onset with exacerbation in noisy environments and selective high-frequency sound loss
- Physical examination unremarkable

Differential Diagnosis:
- Acoustic neuroma
- TM perforation
- Cerumen impaction
- Trauma

Diagnostic Studies:
- Audiometric testing

Treatment:
- Hearing aids
- Cochlear implants

Acoustic Neuroma

Description of the Disease: Benign tumor of the Schwann cells of the vestibular nerve. Also called acoustic schwannoma

Epidemiology:
- Fourth to sixth decade is most common.

Etiology:
- Proliferation of Schwann cells

Risk Factors:
- Unilateral disease (most common) usually idiopathic
- Bilateral disease associated with neurofibromatosis type 2

Signs and Symptoms:
- Unilateral sensorineural hearing impairment with poor speech discrimination, often progressive but may be sudden
- Tinnitus
- Continuous vertigo or disequilibrium
- Headache
- Facial numbness or palsy
- Horizontal nystagmus

Differential Diagnosis:
- Neurofibromatosis type 2
- Meningioma
- Meniere disease
- Multiple sclerosis
- Other intracranial or facial tumors

Diagnostic Studies:
- Audiometric testing
- MRI with contrast is the gold standard.

Treatment:
- Surgical excision
- Radiation therapy

Tinnitus

Description of the Disease: Perception of noise in the absence of an external acoustic stimulus

Epidemiology:
- Prevalence increases with age
- Slightly more common in men

Etiology:
- Any disease that damages the auditory system may cause tinnitus (e.g., noise-induced hearing impairment, otitis, cerumen impaction, Meniere disease, cholesteatoma, acoustic neuroma, ototoxic medications)
- Neurogenic causes (e.g., brain injury, multiple sclerosis, migraine, meningitis)

Risk Factors:
- Excessive noise exposure
- Ototoxic medications (e.g., aminoglycosides, salicylates, NSAIDs)
- Chronic autoimmune, endocrine, and vascular disease
- Emotional distress, anxiety, depression

Signs and Symptoms:
- Ringing, buzzing, clicking, or roaring in unilateral or bilateral ears
- May occur with ear pain or fullness
- Meniere disease suggested by low-pitched roaring tinnitus, fluctuating sensorineural hearing loss, and vertigo

Differential Diagnosis:
- See Etiology

Diagnostic Studies:
- Audiometric testing
- Tympanometry
- Asymmetric tinnitus or audiometric testing or neurologic symptoms are indications for MRI.

Treatment:
- Treat any found pathologic causes
- Relaxation or cognitive–behavioral therapy for patients significantly distressed by symptoms

Cerumen Impaction

Description of the Disease: Accumulation of cerumen that causes symptoms, prevents examination, or both

Epidemiology:
- Prevalence increases with age.

Etiology:
- Cerumen, composed of glandular secretions, sloughed epithelial cells, and hair, is a normal finding in the external ear canal that migrates laterally. An impaction can partially or completely obstruct the canal.

Risk Factors:
- Narrow or deformed ear canals
- Dense hair growth
- Production of drier harder wax due to atrophy of cerumen glands

Signs and Symptoms:
- Hearing loss
- Ear pain, discomfort, or sensation of fullness
- Tinnitus
- Dizziness
- Partial or complete cerumen obstruction of the ear canal on examination; after removal, look for signs of canal or tympanic membrane trauma.

Differential Diagnosis:
- Foreign body
- Otitis externa

Diagnostic Studies:
- None

Treatment:
- Cerumenolytic agents
- Ear canal irrigation
- Manual removal (curette, forceps, suction)

Nose Disorders

Epistaxis

Description of the Disease: Epistaxis is identified as hemorrhaging from the nostril, nasal cavity, or nasopharynx.

Epidemiology:
- Epistaxis is a relatively common event that is typically self-limiting. It is estimated that approximately 60% of the population will experience a nosebleed, with less than 10% of those individuals requiring medical attention.
- Age distribution is bimodal, with increased incidence in children aged 2 to 10 years and in older adults aged 50 to 80 years. The spike occurring in older patients may be accounted for by the physiologic changes that occur in the nasal mucosa with aging. These changes, including mucosal epithelium atrophy and changes in the nasal vasculature, promote drying of the nasal mucous membranes in the elderly.

Etiology:
- Ninety percent of nose bleeds are categorized as anterior nosebleeds and occur on the anteroinferior septum where a highly vascularized area, the Kiesselbach plexus, is located.
- This area is susceptible to trauma and excessive drying. Posterior nasal cavity epistaxis is less common. These types of bleeds are more frequently associated with arteriosclerotic disease and hypertension.

Risk Factors:
- In any patient presenting with epistaxis, it is important to assess the patient for underlying causes of bleeding.
- Risk factor assessment should include asking about dry climate, nose picking, nasal/facial injury, use of supplemental oxygen, anticoagulant/antiplatelet/ASA/NSAID medication use, and substance inhalation.
- A thorough PMH should be obtained to identify any history of significant disease processes including bleeding disorders, liver disease, or hypertension.

Signs and Symptoms:
- Patients may present complaining of unilateral or bilateral epistaxis.
- Most nose bleeds are painless. However, patients may experience dizziness, anxiety, difficulty breathing, sore throat, nausea, and/or vomiting (usually secondary to swallowing blood).
- If the nose bleed is secondary to facial trauma, the patient may complain of facial bruising, pain, or deformity.

Differential Diagnosis:
- Trauma
- Mucosal dryness
- Inflammatory process—rhinitis, infection (sinusitis, URI)
- Drug-induced causes—nasal sprays, NSAID, inhaled substances (cocaine)
- Structural abnormalities—deviated nasal septum, septal perforation, nasal surgery
- Neoplasms (benign or malignant)
- Hematologic causes—thrombocytopenia, von Willibrand disease, hemophilia
- Vascular abnormalities—arteriosclerosis, hereditary hemorrhagic telangiectasia (HHT or Osler–Weber–Rendu syndrome), endometriosis
- Idiopathic causes

Diagnostic Studies:
- Routine diagnostic or laboratory studies are typically not required for single or infrequent episodes of epistaxis with identifiable causes.

- If recurrent or severe bleeding occurs, then a hematocrit and type and crossmatch should be obtained.
- If a bleeding disorder is suspected, bleeding time may be used as a screening tool.
- In cases of anticoagulant use or suspected liver disease, the international normalized ratio (INR)/ prothrombin time (PT) may be obtained.
- Other hematologic studies may be required as necessary.
- A CT scan may be ordered to help evaluate or diagnose suspected foreign bodies, neoplasms, or infections.

Treatment:
Anterior Epistaxis:
- Most bleeding can be controlled using direct pressure. The patient should sit upright, leaning forward slightly to prevent blood from entering the oropharynx which may help reduce the swallowing of blood. The patient should pinch nostrils firmly for approximately 10 to 15 minutes.
- If manual compression does not stop the bleeding, then a cotton pledget impregnated with a vasoconstrictor (e.g., oxymetazoline or phenylephrine 0.25%) and anesthetic (2% lidocaine) may be inserted with light pressure applied for another 10 minutes to help control bleeding. If continued oozing occurs, chemical cauterization with silver nitrate or electrocautery may be considered. Should epistaxis continue after failed manual compression and cauterization attempts, nasal packing using tampons, balloons, or gauze impregnated with thrombogenic agents or petroleum should be utilized.

Posterior Epistaxis:
- Posterior bleeding is difficult to manage and control because the site of bleeding cannot be visualized. Posterior epistaxis may be initially managed through posterior packing with petroleum-impregnated gauze or a posterior balloon. Patients should be hospitalized as IV sedation and analgesia are often necessary.
- Hospitalization also allows for close monitoring of patients for vasovagal syncope, and close monitoring of the packing to prevent displacement and possible recurrent bleed.
- Surgical management for posterior epistaxis including ligation of the internal maxillary artery and the ethmoid arteries may be considered when posterior packing fails. Endovascular embolization of the facial artery or the internal maxillary artery is also utilized in some circumstances to obtain hemorrhagic control.
- Inspection of the oropharynx for persistent bleeding should occur in patients who have been treated or packed. Should bleeding continue after packing, patients should be referred to the emergency department. For patients who have received packing and achieved good control, packing should remain in place for 3 to 5 days with follow-up to an otolaryngologist.
- Patients are typically placed on antistaphylococcal antibiotics (cephalexin 500 mg q.i.d. or clindamycin 150 mg q.i.d.) to prevent significant complications such as toxic shock syndrome while packing is in place. Other nonpharmacologic management includes the following:
  - Avoidance of vigorous exercise, bending, or straining for several days
  - Avoidance of nose blowing for 7 to 10 days after the nosebleed
  - Saline nasal spray on packing or in nares several times per day to keep moist
  - Application of petroleum jelly or bacitracin ointment in the nares twice daily
  - Use of home humidifier/vaporizer
  - Avoidance of trauma/nose picking
  - Humidified face tent/mask if utilizing supplemental oxygen (avoid nasal cannula except at meal times)

Allergic Rhinitis

Description of the Disease: Allergic rhinitis is an inflammation of the mucous membranes in the eyes, Eustachian tubes, middle ear, nose, and pharynx, and is characterized by a combination of symptoms including rhinorrhea, sneezing, nasal itching, and nasal congestion.

Epidemiology:
- It is estimated that approximately 20% of the population is affected by allergic rhinitis. Allergic rhinitis can occur at any age, but the onset of allergic rhinitis is typically during childhood, adolescence, and young adulthood. The incidence and severity of allergic rhinitis typically decrease with age.

Etiology:
- Allergic rhinitis is a complex immunoglobulin E (IgE)-mediated response to environmental triggers. The most common environmental allergens include dust, pollens, molds, and animal dander.

Risk Factors:
- Asthma or allergies
- Living or working in an environment with continual exposure to allergens
- Family members with asthma or allergies (as there is a genetic component)

Signs and Symptoms:
- Nasal congestion
- Runny nose
- Itching of nose, ears, eyes, or roof of mouth, tearing
- Postnasal drip
- Sneezing
- Earache
- Sinus pressure or pain
- Fatigue, or lack of energy
- In the geriatric population, patients may also complain of crusting in the nose, loss of smell, nasal dryness, or cough. A thorough history should be obtained noting the timing, duration, and severity of symptoms as well as any response to any medication. Particular attention should be paid to any cyclical or seasonal nature to the symptoms, and possible environmental or occupational exposures.
- Physical examination should primarily focus on the HEENT. Classically, allergic rhinitis exhibits pale, boggy, blue–gray turbinates. However, hyperemia may also be present. The mucus of a patient with allergic rhinitis is typically thin and watery. However, nonallergic rhinitis mucus may also be of that consistency.
- Eye examination: Lacrimation, injection, or swelling of the palpebral conjunctiva, "allergic shiners," Dennie–Morgan lines
- Ear examination: Retraction of the tympanic membrane, air/fluid levels, bubbles, and decreased mobility of the tympanic membrane with pneumatic insufflation
- Oropharynx: Cobblestoning of posterior pharynx
- Lung examination should be performed to assess for signs of asthma.
- A skin examination should be performed to assess for signs of atopic dermatitis.

Differential Diagnosis:
- Allergic rhinitis
- Nonallergic rhinitis: Vasomotor rhinitis, atrophic rhinitis, gustatory rhinitis, medication induced rhinitis, and viral rhinitis
- Sinusitis

Diagnostic Studies:
- Utilization of allergy skin testing is helpful in identifying specific hypersensitivity-producing allergens. In older patients, skin testing responses may be decreased due to aging and photo damage. Therefore, testing should occur on sun-protected areas such as the low back. Alternatively, in vitro testing or radioallergosorbent testing (RAST) may be utilized.
- Total serum IgE and total blood eosinophil count are neither sensitive nor specific for the diagnosis of allergic rhinitis, but may help support the diagnosis when considered with the patient's entire clinical presentation.
- Imaging studies such as radiography and CT scans may be helpful in identifying structural abnormalities, or comorbid conditions and complications.
- Rhinolaryngoscopy is not routinely performed but may be utilized to assess structural abnormalities such as polyps, deviated septum, masses, adenoid hypertrophy, etc.

Treatment:
- First consideration in the management of allergic rhinitis should be avoidance of environmental triggers. Depending on the allergen, this may include shutting windows during peak seasonal blooms of pollens and molds, or regular vacuuming, washing of bed linens, covering of mattresses and pillows with plastic covers, removal of carpets, or removal of pets. This might be significant for older patients who spend more time indoors.
- Antihistamines: First-generation antihistamines (e.g., chlorpheniramine, diphenhydramine) are not recommended in the elderly due to their potential interactions with other drugs and adverse effects on the central nervous system. Second-generation antihistamines (e.g., loratadine, cetirizine, fexofenadine, desloratadine, and levocetirizine) are used in treating mild allergic rhinitis and are tolerated much better

as they have little sedating or anticholinergic effects. Topical antihistamines, such as azelastine, are a good alternative to oral antihistamines and may be used as monotherapy or in conjunction with intranasal steroids.

- Intranasal steroids are first-line treatment for moderate to severe allergic rhinitis, and are generally well tolerated by the older patient. However, they may aggravate nasal drying and crusting, so patient education regarding humidification and maintaining moisture in the nares is particularly important.
- Decongestants should be used cautiously in the elderly due to their α-adrenergic and central nervous system effects, and should be avoided in patients with hypertension, coronary artery disease, cerebral vascular disease, and bladder neck obstruction.
- Leukotriene inhibitors (e.g., montelukast, zileuton) are approved for use in the treatment of allergic rhinitis. They are not as effective as intranasal steroids, but are well tolerated. They are often used in combination with antihistamines or intranasal steroids to help reduce the inflammation of allergic rhinitis.
- Immunotherapy is generally considered a last-line therapy for patients with refractory allergic rhinitis and with moderate to severe symptoms.

Granulomatosis with Polyangiitis (Wegener Granulomatosis)

Description of the Disease: Granulomatosis with polyangiitis (GPA), known previously as Wegener granulomatosis, is a systemic vasculitis of the small and medium veins and arteries with characteristic necrotizing granulomatous inflammation.

Epidemiology:
- GPA is a relatively rare disorder estimated to affect 1 in 25,000 people. Although GPA may be diagnosed at any age, it is rare in childhood and most commonly diagnosed in the fourth and fifth decades of life. Approximately 90% of patients diagnosed with GPA are Caucasian; it is much less frequently diagnosed in other ethnic groups. The male-to-female ratio is approximately the same.

Etiology:
- Although the etiology of GPA is unknown, immunologic processes are thought to play a role. It is a multisystem disease most commonly manifesting in the upper respiratory, pulmonary, and renal systems. However, any organ may be affected.

Risk Factors:
- No known risk factors

Signs and Symptoms:
- As GPA is a multisystem condition, signs and symptoms are dependent upon which organs are affected. Onset of symptoms may be insidious or acute. Constitutional symptoms may include fever, night sweats, fatigue, loss of appetite, and weight loss. Other possible signs and symptoms may include the following:
  - Upper respiratory tract: Sinusitis is the most common presentation of GPA. GPA should be considered in patients with recurrent sinus infections refractory to multiple antibiotic treatments. Other upper respiratory tract symptoms may include rhinorrhea, epistaxis, nasal ulcers, crusting, septal perforation, nasal chondritis with pain, and potential collapse of the nasal structure resulting in "saddle nose" deformity. Laryngeal stenosis may occur, causing symptoms of hoarseness, stridor, or wheezing. Otic manifestations include ear infections, sensorineural hearing loss, vertigo.
  - Eye: Signs and symptoms of conjunctivitis, episcleritis, uveitis, nasolacrimal duct occlusion, proptosis
  - Lower respiratory tract: Cough, chest pain, hemoptysis, shortness of breath
  - Kidneys: Hematuria (typically later in the disease)
  - Musculoskeletal: Myalgia, joint pain
  - Skin: Palpable purpura
  - Nerves: Sensorimotor neuropathies, cranial nerve palsies, mononeuropathy complex

Differential Diagnosis:
- The differential diagnosis is dependent upon the clinical presentation of this disease, as GPA may involve different organs and present with a different constellations of symptoms.
- Should GPA present only with upper respiratory symptoms, typically the differential diagnosis will include the consideration of infectious and neoplastic disease processes (including nasal neoplastic killer/T-cell lymphoma or lethal midline granuloma [LMG]), cocaine use, and ruling out other forms of vasculitis.
- Should pulmonary and renal symptomology occur, consideration of various pneumonias (bacterial, fungal), autoimmune disorders (Goodpasture syndrome, systemic lupus erythematosus, sarcoidosis),

various forms of glomerulonephritis, malignancy, and various forms of vasculitis (polyarteritis nodosa, microscopic polyangiitis, Churg–Strauss syndrome) would be considered.

Diagnostic Studies:
- Routine tests that may be ordered are CBC with differential, serum albumin and total protein, urinalysis, serum creatinine, ESR, and C-reactive protein (CRP). These are nonspecific but supporting tests for GPA.
- CBC may reveal mild normochromic normocytic anemia typical of chronic disease. ESR and CRP are typically elevated; serum albumin and total protein may be decreased.
- If glomerular involvement is present, urinalysis may reveal red blood cells (RBCs) and RBC casts, and proteinuria; serum creatinine may be elevated.
- Chest radiology or CT scans may be helpful if suspecting GPA. Most patients have abnormal findings such as nodules (with or without cavitation), masses, infiltrates, opacities of alveolar hemorrhage, or atelectasis.
- Serologic testing antineutrophil cytoplasmic autoantibodies (ANCAs) with confirmatory enzyme-linked immunosorbent assay (ELISA) for antibodies are performed when a high suspicion of GPA exists. Positive c-ANCA directed against PR-3 is highly suggestive for GPA.
- Confirmatory tissue biopsy from a site of active disease is conclusive.

Treatment:
- The mainstay of treatment for GPA is a combination of corticosteroids and other immunosuppressant agents such as cyclophosphamide, rituximab, or methotrexate (typically used in less severe cases of GPA).
- Initial treatment is typically 1.5 to 2 mg/kg/day of oral cyclophosphamide and 1 mg/kg/day of prednisone for 3 to 6 months or until remission occurs. Fifty percent of patients will have at least one relapse of the disease. Remission maintenance therapy is important and involves continued corticosteroids, but replacing cyclophosphamide and rituximab with azathioprine, methotrexate, or leflunomide.
- Typical maintenance therapy lasts at least 18 months. Relapse is usually treated with cyclophosphamide and steroids.

Lethal Midline Granuloma (Natural Killer/T-Cell Lymphoma)

Description of the Disease: Most LMGs are caused by natural killer/T-cell lymphoma (NKTL), a form of non-Hodgkin lymphoma, primarily found in the nasal cavity, paranasal sinuses, and nasopharynx.

Epidemiology:
- LMG-NKTL is a rare disease comprising approximately 0.17% to 1.5% of all non-Hodgkin lymphomas.
- It is most commonly found in people of Asian, Central or South American, or Mexican descent. Any age group may be affected; however, it is most commonly diagnosed in the sixth decade of life.
- Males are three times more likely than females to be diagnosed.

Etiology:
- Most non-Hodgkin lymphomas are of B-cell origin. Only about 10% of non-Hodgkin lymphomas are of non–B-cell classification.
- It is still uncertain whether NKTL represents the presence of natural killer cells or simply a T-cell with unusual cell markers. NKTL is found primarily in the nasal cavity. Occurrence is associated with Epstein–Barr virus (EBV) >95% of identified cases.

Risk Factors:
- Risk factors for non-Hodgkin lymphoma and NKTL include the following: gender (male predominance); age (increased incidence with age); race/ethnicity (Asians have greater incidence); immunosuppression—both inherited conditions (e.g., Klinefelter syndrome, Chédiak–Higashi syndrome, ataxia telangiectasia syndrome) and acquired conditions (e.g., HIV, immunodeficiency secondary to mediations/drugs); associated infections (e.g., EBV); external/environmental exposures (phenoxy herbicides, insecticides, irradiation, and prior chemotherapy or radiotherapy); autoimmune disorders (e.g., celiac sprue, systemic lupus erythematosus , Sjögren syndrome, rheumatoid arthritis).

Signs and Symptoms:
- Nasal LMG-NKTL is characterized by midline facial destruction, but may patients initially present with generalized symptoms such as fever, fatigue, or weight loss. More specific symptomology may include

nasal congestion, facial swelling, epistaxis, pain, septal perforation, purulent nasal discharge, halitosis, changes in vision or hearing, ulcerations on the palate, or dysphagia. Should LMG-NKTL occur in the pulmonary system or GI tract, symptoms related to those systems may arise. The physical examination should focus on the HEENT examination, but also include the lung examination and abdominal examination to help identify other extranodal manifestations of NKTL.

Differential Diagnosis:
- The differential diagnosis for LMG-NKTL includes B-cell/non-Hodgkin lymphoma and granulomatosis with polyangiitis (Wegener's granuloma). Depending on the initial presentation, cocaine abuse, infections, trauma, malignancies, autoimmune/inflammatory disease processes such as sarcoidosis, systemic lupus erythematosus, or polyarteritis nodosa may be considered

Diagnostic Studies:
- Laboratory tests including a CBC, liver function tests, renal function tests, uric acid, and calcium levels are obtained. Patients with elevated lactic dehydrogenase have been noted to have poorer outcomes. EBV titers should also be obtained. Flexible nasopharyngoscopy and direct laryngoscopy should be performed to assess the scope of the lesion. CT scans and MRIs may be obtained to evaluate the extent of the disease, structural destruction involved, and for staging purposes. Primary site biopsy and histologic evaluation, including immunophenotyping for CD54 especially, are of particular diagnostic importance.

Treatment:
- Clinical outcomes for patients diagnosed with LMG-NKTL are poor. The 5-year survival rate is approximately 20%. Due to the rarity of LMG-NKTL, management protocols are unclear. Most treatment guidelines recommend a combination of chemotherapy and moderate-dose radiation therapy. CHOP (cyclophosphamide, doxorubicin, vincristine, prednisone) chemotherapy regimens are utilized. However, nasal LMG-NKTL is particularly resistant to this standard therapy and high rates of relapse occur. Experimental regimens using the SMILE protocol (dexamethasone, methotrexate, ifosfamide, l-asparaginase, and etoposide) have shown potential, but significant myelotoxicity utilizing this regimen indicates further study is required.

Mouth

Xerostomia

Description of the Disease: Sensation of dry mouth secondary to decreased salivary production

Epidemiology:
- 29% to 58% of older Americans
- M = F

Etiology:
- Decreased salivary flow
- Medication side effect
- Chronic illness

Risk Factors:
- Head or neck radiation
- Human immunodeficiency virus
- Medication use (antidepressants and antipsychotics, antihypertensives, antihistamines, and anticholinergics)
- Salivary gland aplasia
- Sjögren syndrome
- Smoking
- Sustained caffeine use
- Sustained ETOH use

Signs and Symptoms:
- Dry mouth
- Burning sensation

- Changes in taste
- Dysphagia

Differential Diagnoses:
- None

Diagnostic Studies:
- None

Treatment:
- Consider medication change, if possible.
- Increase water; avoid alcohol and caffeine
- OTC: Salivary substitutes, mouthwashes and rinses
- RX: Pilocarpine (Salagen) and cevimeline (Evoxac).

Leukoplakia and Erythroplakia

Description of the Disease: Precancerous lesions of the oral cavity

Epidemiology:
- Sex: Men > women; male-to-female ratio is 3:1.
- Age: 80% of patients are older than 40 years. Most common in the fifth to seventh decades of life.

Etiology:
- Idiopathic/unknown. May have a viral connection

Risk Factors:
- Tobacco use
- ETOH consumption
- Immunosuppressed conditions
- Nutritional deficiencies

Signs and Symptoms:
- Often asymptomatic
- Homogenous leukoplakia: Uniformly white patch in buccal mucosa
- Verrucous leukoplakia: White flecks or fine nodules on an atrophic erythematous base
- Erythroplakia: Red macule or patch with velvety texture

Differential Diagnoses:
- Oral candidiasis
- Squamous cell carcinoma

Diagnostic Studies:
- Biopsy

Treatment:
- Surgical excision
- Cryotherapy and laser ablation also used
- Discontinue tobacco and alcohol use
- Close follow-up as it is a precursor to squamous cell CA

Oral Candidiasis

Description of the Disease: Fungal infection caused by yeasts from the genus *Candida*.

Epidemiology:
- Sex: M = F
- Age: Middle aged–older adults

Etiology:
- *Candida albicans* is the most common cause.

Risk Factors:
- Diabetes
- Medications: Antibiotics and corticosteroids

- Ill-fitting dentures
- Smoking
- Decreased salivation—see Xerostomia
- Immunodeficient diseases: HIV, cancer

Signs and Symptoms:
- White patches on the surface of the oral mucosa and tongue
- Can be wiped off to reveal an erythematous base. Bleeding may occur.

Differential Diagnose:
- Oral leukoplakia

Diagnostic Studies:
- KOH stain reveals hyphae.

Treatment:
- Consider medication change.
- Smoking cessation
- Antifungals—topical and oral as needed, for example, nystatin troches

Cancer of the Oral Mucosa

Description of the Disease: Cancer of the oral cavity. Often with precancerous lesions present.

Epidemiology:
- Sex: M > F
- Age: middle aged–older adults
- Race: African American > White
- In developed countries: Eighth most common form of cancer overall

Etiology:
- Squamous cell carcinoma—90% of oral cancer

Risk Factors:
- ETOH use
- Tobacco use
- Betel use
- Poor oral hygiene
- Immunosuppressive states
- Sunlight exposure
- Human papilloma virus

Signs and Symptoms:
- Leukoplakia, erythroplakia, granular ulcer, nonhealing lesions, and cervical adenopathy
- On examination, pay close attention to lateroventral surface of tongue, floor of the mouth, and lips.

Differential Diagnoses:
- Oral leukoplakia
- Oral candidiasis
- Oral lichen planus

Diagnostic Studies:
- Biopsy and staging

Treatment:
- Refer to surgery and oncology.
- Eliminate tobacco and ETOH use.

Cancer of the Larynx

Description of the Disease: Laryngeal cancer includes tumors of the supraglottis, glottis, or subglottis.

Epidemiology:
- Sex: M > F

Etiology:
- Squamous cell carcinoma–96% of laryngeal carcinomas

Risk Factors:
- ETOH use
- Tobacco use
- Human papilloma virus

Signs and Symptoms:
- Dysphagia, dysphonia, neck mass, pain, weight loss, fatigue
- Oral lesions in oropharynx examination
- Adenopathy and masses in neck examination

Differential Diagnoses:
- Laryngitis
- Fungal laryngitis
- Sarcoidosis
- Tuberculosis
- Wegener's granulomatosis

Diagnostic Studies:
- CT Scan
- CXR
- PET scan

Treatment:
- Refer to surgery and oncology

Dental Abscess

Description of the Disease: Collection of pus around tooth structures

Epidemiology:
- None

Etiology:
- Normal host bacteria such as *Bacteroides, Fusobacterium, Actinomyces,* and *Streptococcus viridans.*

Risk Factors:
- Poor oral hygiene

Signs and Symptoms:
- Fever, pain, swelling, and gingival bleeding

Differential Diagnoses:
- Peritonsillar abscess
- Advanced gingivitis

Diagnostic Studies:
- Simple abscess: None
- Complicated abscess: CBC, blood cultures, and needle aspirate

Treatment:
- Hydration, antibiotics, and analgesic as needed
- Refer to oral–maxillofacial specialist p.r.n.

Review Section

Review Questions

1. A 65-year-old man with a history of smoking presents with difficulty reading and seeing faces for several months. Examination of the retina reveals drusen. Which of the following is the most likely diagnosis?

   a. Presbyopia
   b. Bilateral retinal artery occlusion
   c. Bilateral cataracts
   d. Age-related macular degeneration

2. A 70-year-old woman presents to the Emergency Department with an acute onset of a painful, red, left eye. Tonometry reveals increased intraocular pressure. Which of the following is the most likely diagnosis?

   a. Acute retinal vein occlusion
   b. Narrow-angle glaucoma
   c. Open-angle glaucoma
   d. Dacryocystitis

3. Which of the following is used in the treatment of age-related macular degeneration?

   a. Anti-VEGF agents
   b. Topical prostaglandin analogs
   c. Laser trabeculoplasty
   d. Intravenous acetazolamide

4. A 68-year-old man presents with decreased vision. Below is the patient's funduscopic examination result.

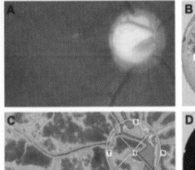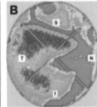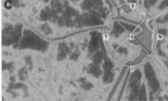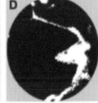

Source: **A.** National Institutes of Health (NIH). https://openi.nlm.nih.gov/detailedresult.php?img=PMC3218163_opth-5-1549f2&req=4

Which of the following is a likely concurrent finding?

   a. Increased intraocular pressure
   b. Drusen
   c. Neovascularization
   d. Impaired red reflex

5. The majority of oral cancers are characterized as:

   a. basal cell carcinoma.
   b. human papillomavirus.
   c. squamous cell carcinoma.
   d. human herpes virus.

6. Where is the most common site for oral cancers to present?

   a. Lateroventral surface of the tongue
   b. Lips
   c. Floor of the mouth
   d. Buccal mucosa

7. Which of the following is the most common etiologic agent of oral candidiasis?

   a. *Staphylococcus aureus*
   b. *Streptococcus pneumonia*
   c. *Candida tropicalis*
   d. *Candida albicans*

8. A 65-year-old man presents to your clinic complaining of clear nasal discharge accompanied by "itchy eyes" for 2 weeks. He states that these symptoms "usually happen every autumn." He is able to perform his daily activities, but finds the symptoms "bothersome." Patient denies fever, ear pain, epistaxis, cough, changes in vision. Past medical history of this patient is significant for hypertension for 5 years, which is well controlled by quinapril 10 mg i tab p.o. b.i.d. Initial management of this patient would include:

   a. diphenhydramine HCl 25 mg i–ii tabs q.i.d.
   b. cetirizine HCl 10 mg i tab q.d.
   c. immunotherapy to determine allergen.
   d. supportive care including fluids, over the counter ocular antihistamines, and oral decongestants.

9. Which of the following statements are *true* regarding granulomatosis with polyangiitis (GPA)?

   a. Positive c-ANCA directed against PR-3 is highly suggestive for GPA.
   b. GPA is one of the more common causes of epistaxis in the elderly aged >80.
   c. GPA is a systemic vasculitis affecting medium-to-large blood vessels.
   d. Those at higher risk for GPA include persons of Southeast Asian descent.

10. Which of the following drug classifications is ototoxic medication?

   a. Proton pump inhibitors
   b. Serotonin–norepinephrine reuptake inhibitors
   c. Glucocorticoids
   d. Aminoglycosides

Answers with Rationales

1. (d) Age-related macular degeneration

   Rationale: Difficulty reading and seeing faces suggests central vision loss, which is characteristic of age-related macular degeneration. Drusen are a frequent finding on funduscopic examination of patients with macular degeneration. Neither presbyopia, retinal artery occlusion, nor cataracts are associated with drusen or a preferential loss of central vision.

2. (b) Narrow-angle glaucoma

   Rationale: Increased intraocular pressure defines glaucoma. Open-angle glaucoma usually presents insidiously, while closed-angle (acute) glaucoma presents acutely with a painful red eye.

3. (a) Anti-VEGF agents

   Rationale: Intravitreal injections of anti-VEGF antibodies are the preferred treatment for macular degeneration with neovascularization. Topical prostaglandin analogs and laser trabeculoplasty may be used to treat glaucoma. Intravenous acetazolamide may be used in cases of embolic central retinal artery occlusion to reduce intraocular pressure.

4. (a) Increased intraocular pressure

   Rationale: The photograph shows an enlarged physiologic cup and increased cup-to-disc ratio, which, along with increased intraocular pressure, are characteristic of glaucoma. Drusen and neovascularization may be found in macular degeneration. Dense cataracts may result in an impaired red reflex.

5. (c) squamous cell carcinoma.

   Rationale: Over 95% of oral cavity cancers are squamous cell carcinomas, and these cancers are further subdivided by how closely they resemble normal lining cells: well differentiated, moderately differentiated, and poorly differentiated. Other types of cancers of the oral cavity include cancers of the salivary glands such as mucoepidermoid carcinoma and adenoid cystic carcinoma, sarcomas (tumors arising from bone, cartilage, fat, fibrous tissue, or muscle), and melanomas. Tobacco and alcohol use are the major risk factors for most cancers of the head and neck including the oral cavity.

6. (a) Lateroventral surface of the tongue

   Rationale: Oral or mouth cancer most commonly involves the tongue, and most common site for oral cancers presents along the lateral–ventral surface of the tongue. It may also occur on the floor of the mouth, cheek lining, gingiva (gums), lips, or palate (roof of the mouth).

7. (d) *Candida albicans*

   Rationale: *Candida albicans* is the most commonly implicated organism in oral candidiasis. *C. albicans* is carried in the mouths as a normal component of the oral microbiota. This candidal carriage state is not considered a disease, but when *Candida* species become pathogenic and invade host tissues, oral candidiasis can occur. This change usually constitutes an opportunistic infection of normally harmless microorganisms because of local (i.e., mucosal) or systemic factors altering host immunity.

8. (b) cetirizine HCl 10 mg i tab q.d.

   Rationale: Diagnosis is allergic rhinitis. Patient's symptoms are mild. Second-generation antihistamines are first drug of choice. Diphenhydramine (first-generation antihistamine) has significant side effects particularly in the elderly population. Immunotherapy is considered a last-line treatment. Oral decongestants should not be used in elderly patient with hypertension.

9. (a) Positive c-ANCA directed against PR-3 is highly suggestive for GPA.

Rationale: Serologic testing antineutrophil cytoplasmic autoantibodies (ANCAs) with confirmatory enzyme-linked immunosorbent assay (ELISA) for antibodies are performed when a high suspicion of GPA exists. Positive c-ANCA directed against PR-3 pattern correlates highly with the diagnosis of GPA. Sinusitis is the most common presentation in patients with GPA. Epistaxis in the elderly is most commonly caused by dry mucous membranes. GPA is a systemic vasculitis affecting small to medium vessels. Ninety percent of patients with GPA are Caucasian. (Southeast Asians have a higher incidence of *LMG-NKTL*.)

10. (d) Aminoglycosides

Rationale: Aminoglycosides are commonly prescribed antibiotics with deleterious side effects to the inner ear. Antibiotics in the aminoglycosides class, such as gentamicin and tobramycin, may produce cochieotoxicity. This ototoxicity may occur from antibiotic binding to NMDA receptors in the cochlea and damaging neurons through excitotoxicity. Aminoglycoside-induced production of reactive oxygen species may also damage cells of the cochlea.

Suggested Readings

Baguley, D., McFerran, D., & Hall, D. Tinnitus. *The Lancet, 382*(9904), 1600–1607. Retrieved from https://www-clinicalkey-com.ezproxy2.library.drexel.edu/#!/content/journal/1-s2.0-S0140673613601427?scrollTo=%23hl0000288

Chakravarthy, U., Evans, J., & Rosenfeld, P. J. (2010). Age-related macular degeneration. *BMJ, 340*, c981.

D'amico, D. J. Clinical practice: Primary retinal detachment. *The New England Journal of Medicine, 359*, 2346.

Gonsalves, W. C., Wrightson, A. S., & Henry, R. C. (2008). Common oral conditions in older persons. *American Family Physician, 78*(7), 845–852. Retrieved from http://www.aafp.org/afp/2008/1001/p845.html#abstract

Kakizaki, H., Malhotra, R., Madge, S. N., & Selva, D. (2009). Lower eyelid anatomy: an update. *Annals of Plastic Surgery, 63*, 344.

McCance, K. L., & Heuther, S. E. (Eds.). (2014). *Pathophysiology: The biologic basis for disease in adults and children* (7th ed.). St. Louis, MO: Elsevier.

Onerci, M. (2002). Dacryocystorhinostomy. Diagnosis and treatment of nasolacrimal canal obstructions. *Rhinology, 40*, 49.

Pinto, J. M., & Jeswani, S. (2010). Rhinitis in the geriatric population. *Allergy, Asthma, and Clinical Immunology, 6*(1), 10. doi:10.1186/1710-1492-6-10

Roland, P. S., Smith, T. L., Schwartz, S. R., Rosenfeld, R. M., Ballachanda, B., Earll, J. M., . . . Wetmore S. (2008). Clinical practice guideline: Cerumen impaction. *Otolaryngology Head and Neck Surgery, 139*(3 Suppl 2):S1–S21. Retrieved from https://www-clinicalkey-com.ezproxy2.library.drexel.edu/#!/content/practice_guide_summary/31-s2.0-13402

Rudkin, A. K., Lee, A. W., & Chen, C. S. (2009). Central retinal artery occlusion: Timing and mode of presentation. *European Journal of Neurology, 16*, 674.

Sha S-H., Talaska, A. E., & Schacht, J. (2009). Age-related changes in the auditory system. In J. B. Halter, J. G. Ouslander, M. E. Tinetti, S. Studenski, K. P. High, & S. Asthana (Eds.). *Hazzard's geriatric medicine and gerontology* (6th ed.). Retrieved from http://accessmedicine.mhmedical.com/book.aspx?bookid=371

Slavin, R. G. (2009). Treating rhinitis in the older population: special considerations. *Allergy, Asthma, and Clinical Immunology, 6*(1), 10. doi:10.1186/1710-1492-6-10

Walling, A. D., & Dickson, G. M. (2012). Hearing loss in older adults. *American Family Physician, 85*(12), 1150–1156. Retrieved from http://www.aafp.org/afp/2012/0615/p1150.html

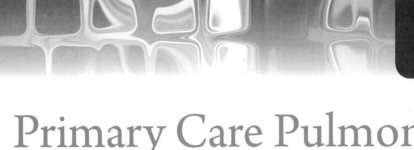

Chapter 3

Primary Care Pulmonary Disorders

Kathleen Bradbury-Golas

Case Presentation

Directions: Carefully review the case study presented below. At the end of the chapter, answer the review questions. Compare your answers with the correct answers listed in the Review Section.

History of Present Illness (HPI): A 72-year-old white woman presents to the office with her full chart, stating that she is changing medical practices because of a new location. She presents with mild dyspnea on exertion, with a respiratory rate of 26, but claims she is not really "too short of breath." However, she states that her feet and ankles have been "swelling up" over the past few weeks and that she has been coughing more and more, sometimes very severely. The cough has been productive with the mucous changing from clear to thick white to a thick yellow-green mucous. She presents to the office as a new patient. She says that she was diagnosed with a "smoker's cough" by her last health care provider.

As you review the chart, you note the following information:

Past Medical History:
Chronic bronchitis from 50-pack-year smoking history
Osteoarthritis
Pneumonia two times, with hospitalization
Seasonal allergies

Medications:
Prednisone 5 mg p.o. daily maintenance
Singular 10 mg daily
Advair 250/50 one puff b.i.d.
Albuterol metered dose inhaler (MDI) two puffs every 4 to 6 hours prn during exacerbations
Albuterol nebulizer prn during exacerbations
Oxygen 2 L via nasal cannula prn for SOB

Allergy: PCN, Bactrim

Social: Quit smoking 5 years ago; drinks 1 Manhattan daily. No illegal drugs

Immunizations: Flu and Pneumovax up to date; unsure of tetanus

Previous Diagnostic Data:
Pulmonary function tests (PFTs): Forced expiratory volume in 1 second (FEV_1) 45% predicted; does not change with inhaled bronchodilator
Pulse oximetry decreases to 90% with moderate activity

Echocardiogram from 6 months ago: EF 50%

Laboratory data from 6 months ago: Electrolytes and profiles all without deviations except the following: Hgb = 14.5; Hct = 45%.

Review of Systems/Health Promotion:

Constitutional: Denies fever at this time, but had a fever 2 days ago (maximum 100.5°F), denies weight loss, chills.

Head, Eyes, Ears, Nose, Throat (HEENT): **Head:** Denies headache, head trauma or injury, dizziness, lightheadedness. Denies head lesions or bumps. **Eyes:** Patient denies eye pain, drainage, dryness, excessive tearing, blurred vision or visual changes; spots, specks, flashing lights, glaucoma, or cataracts. Reports use of corrective lenses for reading. *Last vision exam was 1 year ago.* **Ears:** Denies ear pain, hearing loss, tinnitus, drainage, or use of hearing device. **Nose/Sinus:** Denies nasal congestion, nosebleeds, pain, and nasal drainage/dryness/itching. **Throat:** Denies sore throat, difficulty swallowing, bleeding gums, dry mouth, and hoarseness.

Dental: Last exam was 3 months ago.

Respiratory: See History of Present Illness (HPI). Dyspnea rated 3/10 in severity at present but has intermittent episodes where it is 9/10, at which she uses her oxygen. + history COPD. Denies wheezing at present. Positive SOB, especially on exertion (walking into examination room); productive cough of white to green sputum; increased use of albuterol MDI on daily basis (at least every 4 hours).

Cardiovascular: Denies chest pain, murmur, paroxysmal nocturnal dyspnea or palpitations; positive swollen feet and ankles; one-pillow orthopnea.

Gastrointestinal: Denies loss of appetite, heartburn, pain, diarrhea, constipation, bloating, incontinence, nausea, vomiting, hemorrhoids, or rectal bleeding. She reports moving her bowels normally daily. *Last colonoscopy 5 years ago without any polyps.*

Urinary: Patient reports voiding normally, and reports clear and yellow urine. Denies incontinence, burning, pain, odor, hematuria, polyuria, urgency, retention, nocturia, urinary infections, and kidney stones.

Neurologic: Denies numbness, seizures, headache, dizziness, vertigo, paralysis, or change in mental status.

Psychiatric: Patient states occasional nervousness, tension especially when SOB, denies feeling depressed or having recent mood changes.

Hematologic: Denies anemia, easy bruising or bleeding, fatigue, blood transfusions.

Endocrine: Denies heat or cold intolerance, weight gain or loss, excessive thirst or hunger.

Physical Examination:

Vital Signs: T = 98.2°F   BP = 148/94   HR = 98 bpm   RR = 24 to 28/min Po_2 = 93% on RA
Height = 5 ft 3 inches   Weight = 112 lb   BMI = 19.7

General/Neuro/Psych: AAO times three; appropriate and cleanly dressed; pleasant and cooperative. Good historian.

HEENT: **Head:** The skull is normocephalic/atraumatic (NC/AT). No lesions. Hair with average texture. **Eyes:** Sclera white, conjunctiva pink. **Ears:** Normal pinna, no external abnormalities. Acuity accurate to whispered voice. Tympanic membranes with correct cone of light. **Nose:** Nasal mucosa pink, septum midline, no sinus tenderness. **Throat:** Oral mucosa pink, dentition good, no obvious caries, pharynx without exudates.

Neck: Trachea midline, neck supple, thyroid isthmus palpable, lobes not felt.

Lymph nodes: No cervical, axillary, submandible adenopathy.

Thoracic/Lungs: Increased AP diameter. Diffuse expiratory wheezing and diffuse rhonchi bilaterally; crackles in lower right lobe. Prolonged expiratory phase; some pursed-lip breathing noted.

Cardiovascular: Regular $S_1 S_2$. The Point of Maximum Impulse (PMI) is tapping, 7 cm lateral to the midsternal line in the fifth intercostal space. Trace edema bilateral lower extremities. No signs of cyanosis.

Musculoskeletal: Gait steady. Full range of motion in all joints of the upper and lower extremities. Muscle strength 5/5 in all four extremities.

Case Study Review Questions and Answers

1. What is the most likely diagnosis for this patient at this time? Based on your diagnosis, what stage of the GOLD criteria would the patient be exhibiting?
   Acute exacerbation of chronic obstructive pulmonary disease (COPD)
   Severe COPD as per GOLD criteria

2. What are the differential diagnoses that could also be considered for this patient?
   Asthma, cystic fibrosis, pneumonia

3. What is the pathophysiology that has occurred with this disease process?
   Fifty-year history of cigarette smoking is major cause leading to mucous gland hypertrophy with hypersecretion, ciliary dysfunction, destruction of the lung parenchyma, and airway remodeling. The result of these changes over time includes narrowing of the airways, fixed airway obstruction, poor mucous clearance, cough, wheezing, dyspnea. In this case, emphysema is the major contributor to the COPD (probably had chronic bronchitis in 40s to 50s).

4. What diagnostics, with rationale, would you order at this time?
   CXR: PA/Lateral (look for possible pneumonia, lung hyperinflation, diaphragm flattening, heart size)
   CBC with differential (rule out infectious process and determine degree of polycythemia)
   Cultures as indicated
   Pulse Oximetry

5. Although spirometry through pulmonary function tests is the leading diagnostic test of lung function, what is the relationship/ratio of FVC and FEV_1 in this patient? How does that determine treatment?
   In COPD patients, both the forced vital capacity (FVC) and the forced expiratory volume after 1 second (FEV_1) are reduced, and the ratio of the FEV1 to the FVC is less than 0.7, indicating airway obstruction. Using a bronchodilator may result in some improvement of both the FVC and the FEV_1, but neither will return to normal (fixed obstruction). Determining severity helps to determine treatment. In this case, the ratio is 45% predicted, which is stage 3 (severe). As noted, this patient is already on an inhaled corticosteroids / long-acting β_2 agonist (ICS/LABA) combo, but was also started on maintenance oral steroids (no longer recommended at this time). She also has the SABA MDI for exacerbations.

6. What treatment modalities would you expect to use at this time with the symptomatology presented?
   Maintain current medications as prescribed
   Mucolytic agent
   Antibiotic (owing to change in sputum color and high risk for pneumonia)—either a macrolide or a quinolone is appropriate at this time.

7. What is the goal for this patient? What educational/counseling modalities/possible referrals are necessary to achieve the best outcome for this patient?
   Goals for treatment: Improve symptoms and functional status; prevent recurrence of exacerbation; improve quality of life by preserving optimal lung function.
   Teaching/counseling/potential referrals:
   1. Dietary: Low-carb diet because high-carb diets increase CO_2 production, increasing pulmonary workload. Check on malnourishment status.
   2. Medications being initiated, side effects, etc.; check on proper usage of current medications; take medications as prescribed.
   3. Eliminate irritants; pace activities; influenza vaccine yearly.
   4. Referrals:
      a. Pulmonary rehabilitation
      b. Pulmonologist (as indicated)
      c. Registered dietitian (as needed)

8. What is your plan for follow-up?
   1. For acute exacerbation: Evaluate within 1 to 2 days on status.
   2. For chronic COPD and those on oxygen, follow-up every 1 to 3 months depending on stability.
      a. Monitor weight (COPDers have a tendency to lose weight).
      b. Monitor for osteoporosis (higher tendency).
      c. If started on theophylline in future, monitor for therapeutic serum levels.

9. What diagnostic is now being recommended for cancer screening in the 30- to 74-year-old age group? What are the criteria for this screening?
   Low-dose CT scanning for those patients within the age group who have a $\geq$30-pack-year history of cigarette smoking.

Pulmonary Review

Introduction to Pulmonary Complaints

Pulmonary or respiratory complaints are among the most common reasons encountered in the primary care setting. Dyspnea and cough are vague symptoms, often nonspecific, and may stem from not only the pulmonary system but other systems as well, such as cardiac, neurological, ENT, or even gastrointestinal for cough.

Assessment: A very detailed history and physical examination along with a social history of tobacco use and an analysis of symptoms will help direct the health care provider toward potential causes of complaints. The full history and analysis of the chief complaint will assist in guiding the provider in the physical examination sequence. Note whether the patient can give a history without being short of breath or with audible wheezing.

- Inspect the rate, rhythm, depth, and use of accessory muscles. Note the chest movement, configuration, symmetry, and diameter.
- Palpate any area of pain or discomfort; note expansion and symmetry and quality of tactile fremitus.
- Percuss lung fields for areas of dullness or hyperresonance.
- Auscultate all lung fields with special attention to any area that had previous abnormalities detected. Note the qualities with each breath sound (tracheal, bronchial, vesicular) and the presence/location of any adventitious lung sounds (crackles, wheezes, rhonchi, rales).

Pulmonary disorders are often delineated as either upper or lower in nature. A thorough respiratory examination, including multiple diagnostics, may be necessary to differentiate the cause of the symptoms.

Upper Pulmonary Disorders

Cough

Description of the Disease: A defensive mechanism to clear the airway of secretions and any inhaled particles.

Epidemiology and Etiology/Risk Factors:
- Classified as acute (less than 3 weeks duration) and chronic (3 or more weeks in duration, classically around 8 weeks).
- Pertussis, always thought to be only a childhood illness, is increasing in adults secondary to lack of booster vaccination.
- Exposure to pharyngeal irritants; foreign body aspirations, cardiac disorders, respiratory disorders, gastroesophageal reflux disease (GERD), and medications are common causes of a cough.

Signs and Symptoms:
- **Subjective Complaints:**
  - Cough that interferes with activities of daily living (ADL) or decreasing quality of life (QoL).
  - Fatigue, rhinitis, tickle in throat, postnasal drainage, fever, sputum production, shortness of breath are all possible complaints that accompany a cough.
  - Need to get a thorough history of the cough, its onset, duration, course, sputum production, time of day, and other characteristics to assist in making a diagnosis of cause.
- **Physical Examination Findings:**
  - May be normal.
  - A complete ENT, cardiac, and respiratory assessment should be performed on any patient who complains of a cough.
- **Differential Diagnoses:**
  - Environmental irritant such as tobacco smoking, dust, pollutants.
  - Lower respiratory tract infections.
  - Upper respiratory tract infections.
  - Medication induced (ACE inhibitors).
  - GERD.

- **Diagnostic Studies**:
  - None indicated.
  - Depending on presentation, chest radiography (CXR) and spirometry studies would be the most likely indicated.
- **Treatment**: Supportive only
  - Pharmacological:
    - ○ Avoid antibiotics.
    - ○ Ascertain the cause of the cough and treat accordingly.
    - ○ Cough suppressants.
  - Nonpharmacological:
    - ○ Smoking cessation; secondhand smoke avoidance.
    - ○ Pertussis vaccination as indicated.
    - ○ Follow-up and referral:
      - ○ None indicated.
- **Geriatric Considerations**:
  - Certain cold medications (especially decongestants) produce adverse effects in the elder population.
  - Narcotic-based cough suppressants have a higher fall risk indication.

Upper Respiratory Infection/Common Cold

Description of the Disease: A self-limiting respiratory tract infection usually resulting from a viral infection of the respiratory tract. URI is the most frequent reason for a primary care office visit.

Epidemiology and Etiology/Risk Factors:
- Usually caused by the rhinovirus. Other viral causes include respiratory syncytial virus (RSV), adenovirus, and parainfluenza viruses.
- Incubation period is between 1 and 3 days; can last up to 14 days.
- Droplet or direct contact exposure to virus. Crowded environments increase risk.
- Affects all ages.
- Tobacco use increases risk by 50%.

Signs and Symptoms:
- **Subjective Complaints:**
  - Generalized malaise.
  - Body aches.
  - Low-grade fever.
  - Nasal congestion and discharge (starts clear, progresses to thick yellow, then returns to clear), Sneezing. If purulent nasal discharge lasts longer than 2 weeks, consider bacterial sinusitis.
  - Sore throat, postnasal drip, cough.
- **Physical Examination Findings:**
  - May be normal.
  - Inflamed nasal mucosa, rhinorrhea, postnasal drainage.
  - Erythema of the throat but no exudates.
  - Dull tympanic membranes.
  - Low-grade fever.
- **Differential Diagnoses:**
  - Influenza
  - Allergic rhinitis
  - Acute sinusitis
  - Strep pharyngitis
- **Diagnostic Studies:**
  - None indicated
- **Treatment:** Supportive only
  - Pharmacological: No antibiotics indicated. Topical and oral decongestants, antihistamines, NSAIDs and/or acetaminophen as needed, cough suppressants as indicated.

- Nonpharmacological:
  - ○ Smoking cessation; secondhand smoke avoidance.
  - ○ Vaccinations: Annual influenza immunization. Pneumococcal vaccine as indicated.
  - ○ Increase fluids, vaporizer/humidifier, saline nasal sprays/rinses.
  - ○ Vitamin C and probiotics have no proven preventive effects, but may help to reduce severity and duration of symptoms.
  - ○ Handwashing.
  - ○ Follow-up and referral:
    - ○ None indicated. Recovery takes approximately 7 to 10 days; smokers 3 to 4 days longer.
- **Geriatric Considerations:**
  - Certain cold medications (especially decongestants) produce adverse effects in the elder population.

Asthma

Description of the Disease: Asthma is a chronic, reversible inflammatory airway disease that has episodes of wheezing, breathlessness, chest tightness, and cough. There are four major classifications of asthma. Table 3-1 outlines the classification.

Epidemiology and Etiology:

- Asthma is one of the most chronic diseases of childhood, affecting more than 7 million children and over 25 million people overall in the United States.
- Its prevalence has been markedly increasing over the past two decades.
- A cycle of host and environmental factors that causes airway inflammation.
- Environmental factors include but are not limited to irritants (tobacco smoke being number one), animal dander, allergens, pollens, mold, cold air, and exercise.
- Results in airway hyperresponsiveness, bronchial constriction, airway edema, mucous formation, with possible plugs and airway remodeling.

Risk Factors:

- Genetic predisposition
- Environmental exposures

Table 3-1: Asthma Classification and Symptomatology

Classification	Symptoms[a]	Frequency of Occurrence
Intermittent	Normal forced expiratory volume between episodes. Peak expiratory flow rate (PEFR) greater than 80% predicted with variability less than 20%.	• Symptoms occur on fewer than 2 d/wk. • Do not interfere with normal activities. • Nighttime symptoms occur on fewer than 2 d/mo. • Uses short-acting β agonist no more than 2 d/wk.
Mild persistent	PEFR greater than or equal to 80% predicted with variability 20%–30%.	• Symptoms occur greater than 2 times/wk but less than 1/d. • Exacerbations affect activity somewhat. • Nighttime symptoms occur greater than 2 d/mo.
Moderate persistent	PEFR greater than 60% and greater than 80% predicted with variability greater than 30%.	• Daily symptoms. • Uses short-acting β_2 agonist daily. • Affects activity level. • Severe episodes greater than or equal to 2/wk. • Nighttime symptoms occur greater than 1/wk.
Severe persistent	PEFR less than or equal to 60% predicted with greater than 30% variability.	• Continuous symptoms. • Limited physical activity owing to symptoms. • Frequent exacerbations and nighttime symptoms.

[a]Difficulty breathing, wheezing, chest tightness, and coughing occur in all classifications, but worsen as indicated below.

- Obesity
- Food allergies, GERD, viral infections

Signs and Symptoms: Symptoms can be immediate or 4 to 6 hours after exposure (late response).
- **Subjective Complaints:**
  - Cough, usually worse at night, often unproductive. Paroxysms may be triggered by deep respiratory effort.
  - Wheezing.
  - Chest tightness and difficulty breathing, especially with activity.
- **Physical Examination Findings:**
  - At times may be normal
  - Signs of respiratory distress
  - Rhinitis, nasal polyps, swollen turbinates (asthmatics often have other allergies)—a complete ENT examination is essential
  - Wheezing, prolonged expiratory phase
  - Eczema
  - Allergic shiners and cobblestone conjunctiva
- **Differential Diagnoses:**
  - Chronic obstructive pulmonary disease (COPD)
  - GERD
  - CHF
  - Cough secondary to specific medications, such as ACE inhibitors
  - Pneumonia
  - Benign or malignant tumors
- **Diagnostic Studies:**
  - Spirometry is the gold standard. Evaluates forced vital capacity (FVC) and forced expiratory volume in 1 second (FEV_1) before and after the inhalation of a short-acting bronchodilator. Airflow obstruction is indicated by a reduced FEV_1/FVC ratio.
  - Peak flow meter measurements—used not for diagnostics but to monitor symptoms and determine response to therapy.
  - Bronchial provocation testing: Used when asthma is suspected but spirometry is nondiagnostic. When a patient inhales histamine or methacholine, there is a fall in the FEV_1.
  - CXR to exclude other causes and evaluate cardiac status.
  - Complete blood count (CBC) to rule out other causes.
  - Allergy testing, especially for persistent asthma.
  - Arterial blood gases (ABG) for patients in respiratory distress (respiratory alkalosis is common).
- **Treatment:**
  - Pharmacological: Medications are prescribed in a stepwise fashion based on severity and symptomatology. Table 3-2 summarizes the six steps for prescribing medications. (See Table 3-4 for commonly used medications.)
  - Nonpharmacological:
    - Evaluate patients after treatment begins. Determine whether well controlled or poorly controlled. All patients must have an asthma action plan for self-management and when to come into the office.
    - Avoid triggers by keeping windows closed, removing carpets, washing linens frequently, controlling dust, etc.
    - Smoking cessation; secondhand smoke avoidance.
    - Vaccinations: Annual influenza immunization. Pneumococcal vaccine as indicated.
    - Education: About all medications, side effects of medication and MDI use, how to use inhaler properly.
    - Follow-up and referral:
      - Follow-up within 24 hours for acute attacks to monitor for improvement.
      - For mild intermittent and persistent asthma: Follow-up every 3 to 6 months to monitor status.
      - Referrals: Pulmonologist and allergist as indicated.
- **Geriatric Considerations:**
  - Asthma is associated with many comorbid conditions.
  - Respiratory viruses are often the trigger.
  - If using steroids, monitor the patient for complications (such as hyperglycemia, increased intraocular pressure).

Table 3-2: Asthma Severity and Medication Options

Asthma Severity	Pharmacological Agents
Step 1: Mild intermittent asthma	• No long-term preventive medications necessary. • Short-acting β agonist prn via MDI. May be used up to 4 times/day for exacerbations.
Step 2: Mild persistent asthma	• Low-dose inhaled corticosteroids (ICS) daily. • Can alternate with mast cell stabilizers and leukotriene modifiers.
Step 3: Moderate persistent asthma	• Low-dose ICS plus a long-acting β₂ agonist (LABA).
Step 4: Severe persistent asthma	• Medium- to high-dose ICS plus either a leukotriene modifier or theophylline.
Step 5	• High-dose ICS with LABA or leukotriene modifier.
Step 6	• High-dose ICS with LABA and oral corticosteroid. Or • Consider omalizumab for patients with allergies.
Exercise-induced bronchospasm	• Short-acting inhaled β₂ agonist shortly before exercise (30 minutes). Works for approximately 2–3 h. • LABA before exercise (effective for approximately 10–12 h).

- Asthma medications have a greater adverse effect rate in the elderly, and there may be additional drug interactions owing to polypharmacy.
- Elder patients may not be able to inhale as deeply as necessary; consider nebulizer treatment instead.

Acute Bronchitis

Description of the Disease: Inflammation of the tracheobronchial smooth muscle, resulting in a respiratory tract infection (chest cold) or irritant. It is usually self-limiting in healthy people, but will last longer in those who smoke.

Epidemiology and Etiology:
- More common in fall and winter.
- Majority are viral if there is no underlying cardiopulmonary disease present. Adenoviral, Influenza A and B, RSV, and rhinovirus most common.
- A secondary bacterial infection can occur as part of an acute URI.
- Chemical irritants can also lead to the inflammatory effect.
- Occurs in all age groups.

Risk Factors:
- Very old and very young
- Tobacco smoke (primary and secondary)
- Air pollutants
- Sinusitis

Signs and Symptoms:
- **Subjective Complaints:**
  - Sudden onset of cough, no other signs of other respiratory infection.
  - Dry, nonproductive cough, which later becomes productive. If sputum becomes mucopurulent, secondary infection may be presenting.
  - Complaints of shortness of breath, wheezing, and malaise.
  - Droplet and direct contact exposure.
- **Physical Examination Findings:**
  - Dry hacking cough.
  - Crackles, rhonchi, and wheezing, which can be altered or clear with cough.
  - Erythema of the throat but no exudates.

- No evidence of consolidation on palpation and auscultation (no egophony; equal fremitus).
- Possible low-grade fever.
- **Differential Diagnoses:**
  - URI (common cold)
  - Influenza
  - Acute sinusitis
  - Bronchial pneumonia
  - CHF
  - Tuberculosis (TB)
- **Diagnostic Studies:**
  - None indicated in beginning.
  - If unresolved, CBC and chest radiography may be indicated.
  - Tuberculin skin test (TST [PPD]) if exposed to TB.
- **Treatment:** Supportive only
  - Pharmacological: No antibiotics indicated, unless a treatable pathogen has been identified.
    - Influenza cause: Amantadine or rimatadine therapy
    - Treatable pathogen identified:
      - Amoxicillin 500 mg every 8 hours
      - Trimethoprim-sulfamethoxazole DS every 12 hours.
      - PCN allergy: Clarithromycin 500 mg every 12 hours or azithromycin z pack, take as directed.
      - Quinolones should be used only for more serious infections, previous antibiotic failure, or in patients, especially elderly ones, with multiple comorbidities.
    - Inhaled short-acting β agonist alone or in combination with steroids (MDI or nebulizer).
    - Oral steroids for severe bronchospasm.
    - Decongestants, antipyretic analgesics as needed.
    - Expectorants such as guaifenesin with dextromethorphan.
    - Cough suppressant, with or without narcotic for cough interfering with ADLs or QoL.
  - Nonpharmacological:
    - Smoking cessation; secondhand smoke avoidance.
    - Vaccinations: Annual influenza immunization. Pneumococcal vaccine as indicated.
    - Increase fluids, vaporizer/humidifier/steam, saline nasal sprays/rinses.
    - Vitamin C and probiotics have no proven preventive effects, but may help to reduce severity and duration of symptoms.
    - Handwashing.
    - Follow-up and referral:
      - None usually indicated, but may need reassessment within 72 hours start of treatment. Recovery approximately 7 to 14 days; smokers 3 to 4 days longer.
      - Pulmonary referral for coughs lasting greater than 3 months.
- **Geriatric Considerations:**
  - Can be serious, especially if patient has underlying lung or heart disease or if part of influenza.

Lower Respiratory Disorders

Chronic Obstructive Pulmonary Disease

Description of the Disease: This is a progressive, chronic expiratory airway obstruction usually due to either chronic bronchitis or emphysema. There is airway flow limitation that is inflammatory in nature and not always reversible. Each disorder will be addressed separately in this section.

CHRONIC BRONCHITIS

Description of the Disease: Increased mucous production with recurrent cough over at least 3 months a year for two consecutive years, despite therapy.

Epidemiology and Etiology:
- Unable to determine the true incidence of this alone because there is a lack of diagnostic criteria that doesn't overlap with asthma and emphysema.
- More common in adults.
- Excessive mucous production due to enlarged bronchial mucous glands and loss of ciliated cells leads to a productive cough. Usually in response to acute airway injury or continuous exposure to noxious environmental irritants.
- Surface epithelium, edema, and inflammation thicken small airways, smooth muscle hyperplasia, mucous plugging; possible bacterial colonization of the airways.
- Not genetic in nature.

Risk Factors:
- Tobacco smoke (primary and secondary)
- Cannabis use
- Air or occupational pollutants
- Emphysema
- Chronic aspiration or GERD; severe pneumonia at earlier age

Signs and Symptoms:
- **Subjective Complaints:**
  - Cough and increasing sputum production.
  - Intermittent shortness of breath, wheezing.
- **Physical Examination Findings:**
  - Rarely diagnostic; lung sounds may be normal.
  - Wheezing, decreased breath sounds, scattered bilateral crackles/rhonchi. Noisy in nature.
  - Distant heart sounds, possible cyanosis.
  - Weight gain.
  - Peripheral edema.
  - Often referred to as the "blue bloater."
- **Differential Diagnoses:**
  - Acute bronchitis
  - Asthma
  - Cystic fibrosis
  - Lung cancer
  - GERD
  - TB
  - Normal aging process
- **Diagnostic Studies:**
  - Pulse oximetry and/or ABGs: May show increased Pco_2 or decreased Po_2/O_2 sat levels.
  - CBC: Hemoglobin level may be increased; ABGs: $Paco_2$ may be slightly elevated.
  - Sputum culture to identify any bacteria.
  - CXR: Exclude other disease processes; check heart enlargement. May show increased interstitial markings, especially at the bases; diaphragms not flattened (Fig. 3-1).
  - Pulmonary function tests (PFTs): Decreased FEV_1; poor/absent reversibility to bronchodilator.
  - Sweat test to rule out cystic fibrosis.
- **Treatment:** Supportive only.
  - Pharmacological: No antibiotics indicated, unless a treatable pathogen has been identified.
    - Bronchodilators/anticholinergics are first-line therapy:
      - Short-acting β_2 agonist via inhalation every 4 to 6 hours.
      - Anticholinergic inhalation daily.
      - Long-acting β_2 agonist via inhalation or nebulizer every 12 hours.
    - Steroid therapy is the second line of therapy:
      - Inhaled corticosteroid for moderate to severe disease. If no response, discontinue after 6 to 8 weeks' trial.
      - Systemic corticosteroids: Pulse dosing may be best for chronic bronchitis with reversibility (40 mg/day, tapering downward).

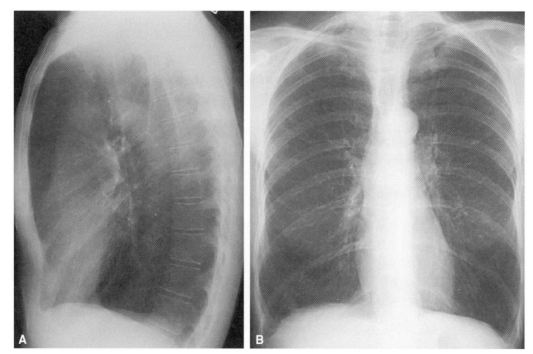

Figure 3-1: A. Enlarged AP diameter; **B.** Clear.

- ○ Other:
  - ○ Theophylline 400 mg/day; note serum level and therapeutic range and renal/liver function.
  - ○ Combination of inhaled corticosteroid, long-acting β agonist and anticholinergic.
  - ○ Mucolytic agents.
  - ○ Antipyretic analgesics as needed.
  - ○ Treatable pathogen identified:
    - ○ Low-dose macrolides such as erythromycin 250 to 500 every 6 hours, clarithromycin 500 mg every 12 hours, or azithromycin z pack; take as directed. Short course of antibiotics is more effective and safer than longer courses.
- ● Nonpharmacological:
  - ○ Smoking cessation; secondhand smoke avoidance.
  - ○ Vaccinations: Annual influenza immunization. Pneumococcal vaccine as indicated.
  - ○ Increase fluids, vaporizer/humidifier/steam.
  - ○ Home oxygenation, if O_2 sat is below 89%.
  - ○ Follow-up and referral:
    - ○ None usually indicated, but may need reassessment in 3 to 4 days after treatment for exacerbation started.
    - ○ Pulmonary rehabilitation as indicated.
    - ○ Pulmonary referral for coughs lasting longer than 3 months.
    - ○ Hospitalization may be required for acute exacerbation with respiratory distress.

EMPHYSEMA

Description of the Disease: Abnormal, permanent enlargement of the air sacs, with destruction of elastic recoil. Many patients have both chronic bronchitis and emphysema, which leads to the diagnosis of COPD. Emphysema involves both the lung parenchyma and the airways. COPD is staged according to the Global Initiative for COPD (GOLD) criteria. This staging system classifies patients with COPD according to their degree of airflow obstruction, which is measured during PFTs. See Table 3-3 for summary of staging criteria.

Epidemiology and Etiology:
- ● COPD is the fourth leading cause of death in the United States.
- ● More common in adults.

Table 3-3: GOLD Criteria/Clinical Findings/Treatment

Stage	Severity/Spirometry Findings	Treatment
0	At risk; normal PFTs	None
1	Mild; FEV_1 greater than 80% predicted; chronic cough; $FEV_1/FVC < 0.7$	First line: Short-acting anticholinergic (SAMA) or β adrenergic (SABA) as needed. Second line: Can use long-acting anticholinergic (LAMA) or β adrenergic (LABA) depending on symptoms.
2	Moderate; FEV_1 greater than 50% but less than 80% predicted; dyspnea on exertion; $FEV_1/FVC < 0.7$	First line: LAMA or LABA Second line: LAMA and LABA
3	Severe; FEV_1 greater than 30% but less than 50% predicted; increasing shortness of breath, lower exercise capacity, and many exacerbations; $FEV_1/FVC < 0.7$	First line: Inhaled corticosteroid (ICS) and LAMA *Or* ICS and LABA. Second line: LAMA and LABA.
4	Very severe; FEV_1 less than 30% predicted or less than 50% with chronic respiratory failure ($Pao_2 < 60$ mm Hg) or right-sided heart failure; $FEV_1/FVC < 0.7$	First line: Inhaled corticosteroid (ICS) and LAMA *Or* ICS and LABA. Second line: Combination of ICA with LAMA or LABA; can add a phosphodiesterase 4 inhibitor (PDE 4).

- One of the leading causes of readmissions to acute care facilities and one of the first diagnoses for readmission reduction in the Medicare Shared Saving Plan of the Affordable Care Act (2010).
- In emphysema, the entire lung is affected; the bronchi are usually clear of secretions, alveoli are enlarged, and there is atrophy and bullae formation.
- α_1-Antitrypsin screening for those patients who are under 45 years old and have COPD or with family member who has disease.

Risk Factors:
- Tobacco smoke (primary and secondary)—leading cause.
- Cannabis use.
- Air or occupational pollutants.
- Genetic factor: α_1-antitrypsin deficiency.
- Recurrent/chronic lower respiratory infections or disease.
- Age (usually occurs in fifth decade of life).

Signs and Symptoms:
- **Subjective Complaints:**
  - Minimal cough, scant sputum.
  - Shortness of breath/dyspnea, occasional respiratory infections.
  - Orthopnea.
- **Physical Examination Findings:**
  - Rarely diagnostic; lung sounds may be normal.
  - Minimal wheezing.
  - Decreased breath sounds; increased vocal fremitus and egophony (increased resonance and high-pitched quality).
  - Hyperresonance on percussion.
  - Distant heart sounds, slight/absent cyanosis.
  - Barrel chest; often referred to as the "pink puffer."
  - Use of accessory muscles, pursed-lip breathing.
  - Usually no peripheral edema.
  - Weight loss.
  - Jugular venous distention (JVD) with advanced disease.
  - Patient's heart is markedly lateral to normal placement in PMI, she has peripheral edema. She does not necessarily have full form of this but is heading toward it.

- **Differential Diagnoses:**
  - Asthma
  - Sleep apnea
  - Lung cancer
  - GERD
  - Reactive airway dysfunction process
  - Normal aging process
- **Diagnostic Studies:**
  - Pulse oximetry and/or ABGs: May show normal/elevated P_{CO_2} or slightly decreased P_{O_2}/O_2 sat levels.
  - CBC: Normal or polycythemia (increased RBC/Hg levels).
  - Desaturation on six-minute walking test.
  - Sputum culture as indicated.
  - CXR: Small heart, hyperinflation, flat diaphragms, possible bullae.
  - PFTs: Spirometry is the gold standard for diagnosing and determining progression/severity of the disease. Although the FVC and FEV_1 reduce over time, in normal patients the ratio of FEV_1 to FVC is greater than 0.7.
    - ○ Decreased FVC.
    - ○ Decreased FEV_1 determines airflow obstruction; poor/absent reversibility to bronchodilator; increased residual volume and functional residual capacity.
  - Perform a TST (PPD) if TB is suspected.
- **Treatment:** See Table 3-3 for treatment based on severity; Table 3-4 for commonly used medications.
  - Pharmacological: No antibiotics indicated, unless a treatable pathogen has been identified.
    - ○ Bronchodilators/anticholinergics are first-line therapy.
    - ○ Steroid therapy is the second line of therapy: Although long-term oral use is no longer recommended as maintenance therapy because of its extensive side effects.
    - ○ Other:
      - ○ Combination of inhaled corticosteroid, long-acting β agonist, and anticholinergic.
      - ○ Mucolytic Agents.
      - ○ Phosphodiesterase-4 inhibitor (PDE-4).
      - ○ α_1-antitrypsin to maintain level above 80 mg/dL.

Table 3-4: Examples of Commonly Used Medications for Asthma and COPD (List Is Not All-Inclusive)

Classification	Examples
Short-acting β agonists (SABA)	Albuterol (ProAir, Proventil, Ventolin) Levalbuterol (Xopenex)
Long-acting β agonists (LABA)	Salmeterol (Serevent)
Short-acting anticholinergics (SAMA)	Ipratropium bromide (Atrovent)
Long-acting anticholinergics (LAMA)	Tiotropium (Spiriva)
Combination SABA and anticholinergic	Albuterol/ipratropium (Combivent)
Methylxanthines	Aminophylline, theophylline
Inhaled corticosteroids (ICS)	Beclomethasone (Qvar), budesonide (Pulmicort), fluticasone (Flovent)
Combination LABA and ICS	Formoterol/budesonide (Symbicort), salmeterol/fluticasone (Advair)
Phosphodiesterase 4 (PDE4) inhibitor	Roflumilast
Leukotrine modifiers	Montelukast (Singular)

- ○ Treatable pathogen identified:
  - ○ Low-dose macrolides such as erythomycin 250 to 500 every 6 hours, clarithromycin 500 mg every 12 hours, or azithromycin z pack; take as directed. Short course of antibiotics is more effective and safer than longer courses.
- ● Nonpharmacological:
  - ○ Smoking cessation; secondhand smoke avoidance.
  - ○ Vaccinations: Annual influenza immunization. Pneumococcal vaccine as indicated.
  - ○ Increase fluids, vaporizer/humidifier/steam.
  - ○ Home oxygenation, if O_2 sat is below 88%.
  - ○ Follow-up and referral:
    - ○ Pulmonary rehabilitation as indicated.
    - ○ Pulmonary referral for coughs lasting longer than 3 months.
    - ○ Hospitalization may be required for acute exacerbation with respiratory distress.
    - ○ Hospice referral for uncompensated COPD.
- ● **Geriatric Considerations:**
  - ● Presentation may not be typical.
  - ● Patients may have difficulty with inhalers.
  - ● Side effects of medications may be exaggerated.

Pneumonia

Description of the Disease: Inflammation and consolidation of the lung tissue, including the alveoli and interstitial tissues. Usually categorized as either community acquired (outpatient or within 72 hours of hospitalization) or hospital acquired (greater than 72 hours of hospitalization).

Epidemiology and Etiology:
- ● Community acquired: Usually from a colonized infection of *Streptococcus pneumoniae* or the inhalation of another atypical pathogen (*M. pneumonia and C. pneumonia, Haemophilus influenza*).
- ● Viruses account for approximately one third of pneumonias, with influenza, parainfluenza, and adenovirus being the most common. They are more common in children than adults.
- ● Hospital acquired: In addition to *S. pneumonia* and *H. influenza*, other common organisms include but are not limited to *Staphylococcus aureus, Klebsiella pneumonia, and moraxella catarrhalis*.
- ● Bacterial pneumonia is the sixth leading cause of death in the United States.

Risk Factors:
- ● Very old, immunocompromised, asthma, COPD, DM, renal failure.
- ● Overuse of antibiotics has led to resistance.
- ● Tobacco smoke (primary and secondary).

Signs and Symptoms:
- ● **Subjective Complaints:**
  - ● Fatigue, headache, malaise, body aches, vague abdominal pain with nausea.
  - ● Fever, chills, rigor and shortness of breath.
  - ● Chest pain that worsens with inspiration.
  - ● Productive cough with purulent sputum (not in all patients).
- ● **Physical Examination Findings:**
  - ● Tachypnea (leading predictor).
  - ● Crackles (present in the majority of patients; do not clear with coughing), wheezes, and decreased breath sounds.
  - ● Positive whispered pectoriloquy (increased loudness); positive egophony ("e" sounds like "a") and positive bronchophony (voice sounds louder).
  - ● Increased fremitus.
  - ● Dullness on percussion.
  - ● Note any change in respiratory status such as use of accessory muscles, cyanosis.
  - ● Fever greater than 100.4°F.
- ● **Differential Diagnoses:**
  - ● Other types of pneumonia
  - ● Atelectasis

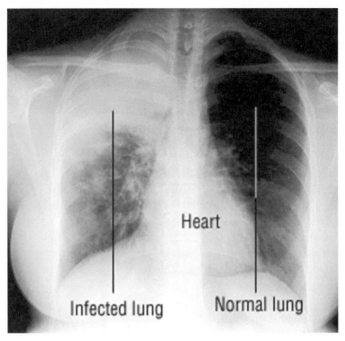

Figure 3-2: Pneumonia on chest X-ray. Source: Harvard Medical School (N.D.). Patient Education Center: Pneumonia. Retrieved from www.patienteducationcenter.org/articles/pneumonia/

- COPD
- Asthma
- Lung abscess
- CHF
- TB
- **Diagnostic Studies:**
  - Pulse oximetry.
  - CXR: Posteroanterior (PA) and lateral—infiltrates confirm the diagnosis. In the early part of the disease, the CXR may be negative because of dehydration. See Figure 3-2.
  - CBC with differential (elevated WBC with left shift if bacterial in nature).
  - Cultures: Blood and sputum, especially for the critically ill and to determine specific pathogen.
  - Electrolytes: To determine degree of dehydration.
  - Rapid viral testing for rule-out diagnoses.
  - TST (PPD) if exposed to TB.
- **Treatment:**
  - Pharmacological–bacterial:
    - Outpatient adult:
      - Healthy, no antibiotics in past 3 months: Macrolide such as azithromycin 500 mg day 1, 250 mg days 2 to 4; clarithromycin 500 mg b.i.d. times 10 days; erythromycin 500 mg b.i.d. for 10 days. Can substitute with doxycycline if allergic.
      - With comorbid conditions: Quinolone such as levofloxacin 750 mg for 5 days; moxifloxacin 400 mg daily for 10 days. Can use β-lactam penicillin (such as amoxicillin and amoxicillin–clavulanate) plus a macrolide.
    - Inpatient adult:
      - Non-ICU: IV antibiotics to start, then switch to oral compounds. β-Lactam (such as cefotaxime, ceftriaxone) plus a macrolide OR a quinolone for 14 days.
  - Pharmacological—viral:
    - Antiviral agents, such as zanamirvir MDI, combination of oseltamirvir and rimantadine.
    - Antipyretic analgesics as needed.
    - Expectorants such as guaifenesin with dextromethorphan.
    - Avoid cough suppressants.

- Nonpharmacological:
  - CURB-65 to determine whether patient requires hospitalization. Based on a patient having at least three of the following five criteria:
    - Confusion
    - Uremia (BUN greater than 19 mg/dL)
    - Respiratory rate greater than 30 bpm
    - Blood pressure less than 90 mm Hg SBP or 60 mm Hg DBP
    - 65 years of age
  - Smoking cessation; secondhand smoke avoidance.
  - Vaccinations: Annual influenza immunization. Pneumococcal vaccine as indicated.
  - Increase fluids, vaporizer/humidifier/steam, saline nasal sprays/rinses.
  - Follow-up and referral:
    - Pulmonary/infectious disease: Seriously ill, respiratory distress, suspected biological warfare agents.
    - Outpatient: Follow up by phone in 24 hours; schedule office visit for 2 weeks to evaluate treatment.
- **Geriatric Considerations:**
  - Can be serious, especially if patient has underlying lung or heart disease or if part of influenza.
  - Seen more in the elderly adult and those with multiple comorbidities.
  - May initially present with weakness or mental status change, and may not have a fever.

Pulmonary Tuberculosis

Description of the Disease: Acute or chronic bacterial infection caused by a mycobacterium. Usually affects the lungs, but other organs may be involved, such as lymph nodes, abdomen, and bones. TB occurs from inhalation of airborne bacilli, which multiply in alveoli and are then transported to other sites. The accumulation of activated T cells and macrophages creates a granuloma that limits replication of the organism. Eventually, a solid necrosis forms, establishing the latent disease. For those with ineffective immune systems, progressive TB develops.

Epidemiology and Etiology:
- Caused by *Mycobacterium tuberculosis* or *mycobacterium bovis*.
- For those individuals who are not immunocompromised, the infection is self-limited and often subclinical. Many are asymptomatic.
- Infection occurs when T cell status is compromised. Active disease occurs from either a primary infection or reactivation of latent infection.
- 85% of infections occur within the lungs, and are contagious.
- Found worldwide with approximately one third of the world's population infected with latent TB. Approximately 3.4 cases per 100,000 population in the United States.
- Drug-resistant TB is increasing and is about 5% to 10% in the United States.

Risk Factors:
- Homelessness, institutionalized settings, close contact with infected individuals.
- Immigrant populations (check states with highest immigrant workers); foreign-born people.
- Immunocompromised individuals.
- Smoking, alcoholism, drug abuse, and malnutrition.

Signs and Symptoms:
- **Subjective Complaints:**
  - Known exposure to TB.
  - Fever, night sweats, chills.
  - Weight loss, malaise.
  - Painless enlarged lymph nodes.
  - Pulmonary TB: Cough, hemoptysis, pleuritic chest pain.
  - May have other system complaints: Abdominal pain, mass, neurological complaints.
- **Physical Examination Findings:**
  - Often normal.
  - Crackles in upper chest.
  - Positive bronchophony, positive pectoriloquy.

Table 3-5: First-Line Treatment Options for TB

Regimen 1 (Preferred)	Regimen 2
Initial phase: Isoniazid (INH) 5 mg/kg Rifampin (RIF) 10 mg/kg Pyrazinamide (PZA) 15–30 mg/kg Ethambutol (EMB) 15–20 mg/kg All once daily for 8 wk	Initial phase INH/RIF/PZA/EMB daily for 2 wk, then twice weekly for 6 wk
Or	*Or*
INH/RIF/PZA/EMB 5 d/wk for 8 wk	INH/RIF/PZA/EMB 5 days/week for 2 weeks, then twice weekly for 6 weeks
Continuation phase INH/RIF daily for 18 wk *Or* INH/RIF 5 d/wk for 18 wk[a] *Or* INH/RIF 2–3 times/wk for 18 wks[a] *Or* INH/rifapentine once weekly for 18 wks[a]	**Continuation phase** INH/RIF 2–3 times/wk for 18 wk *Or* INH/rifapentine once weekly for 18 wk[a]
	Pregnant patients: INH/RIF/EMB supplement with pyridoxine 25 mg/d

[a] Dependent on HIV status and CD4 counts.

- Lymphadenopathy.
- Meningeal irritation signs.
- **Differential Diagnoses:**
  - Pneumonia
  - Malignancy
  - Fungal infections
- **Diagnostic Studies:**
  - TST—old PPD: Method is 0.1 mL intradermally into volar aspect of forearm. Results are as follows:
    - 5 mm or more: Determine whether the person has close contact with a person with TB or is immunocompromised or has an abnormal CXR—this could be consistent with active disease.
    - 10 mm or more: Ascertain whether the person is homeless, HIV infected, uses illicit drugs, nursing home resident, or living within an institutional setting. If positive, this could mean high risk for active TB.
    - 15 mm or more: Even without risk factors, this person is positive for possible TB.
    - False-positive purified protein derivative (PPD) results can occur from steroids or BCG. False negatives can occur with HIV, alcoholism, renal failure, and malnutrition.
  - Alternative to TST/PPD is QuantiFERON TB gold: Used to detect both TB and latent TB infections.
  - CXR: PA and lateral—infiltrates with or without effusion, atelectasis, or adenopathy. Cavitary lesions and upper lobe disease may be present.
  - Acid fast bacilli (AFB) Cultures: three different morning sputum samples. Treatment is based on culture and sensitivity.
  - Biopsy: Granuloma with central caseating necrosis.
  - Interferon gamma release assays (IGRAs) measure interferon release after stimulation by *M. tuberculosis* antigens. This is preferred in testing people who have had BCG.
- **Treatment:** Must have accurate body weight for the dosing of all TB medications.
  - Pharmacological: See Table 3-5 for initial and continuation phases
    - Ensure compliance with directly observed therapy (DOT)—mandatory for patients with coexistent HIV disease, multidrug resistant TB, and those who may be noncompliant with therapy.
    - Steroids can be used for those who have TB meningitis or pericarditis.
    - Antipyretic analgesics as needed.

- Nonpharmacological:
  - ○ Airborne isolation with personal sealed respirators.
  - ○ Baseline liver function tests and color vision test before starting therapy.
  - ○ Follow-up with contacts exposed to infected person.
  - ○ Report to state and local health departments.
  - ○ Ensure patient is aware of all medication side effects:
    - ○ Isoniazid (INH): Peripheral neuropathy (supplement with daily pyridoxine)
    - ○ Rifampin (RIF): Orange discoloration of urine, contact lenses, GI upset
    - ○ Pyrazinamde (PZA): Increased uricemia, hepatotoxicity
    - ○ Ethambutol (EMB): Fever, rash, and optic neuritis
    - ○ Streptomycin (SM): Ototoxicity
  - ○ Follow-up and referral:
    - ○ Regular follow-up every 4 to 8 weeks.
    - ○ Repeat CXR after 2 to 3 months of therapy. Monitor liver enzymes as indicated.
    - ○ Infectious disease: For inpatient and outpatient management.
  - ○ Bacille Calmette–Guérin (BCG) vaccine is a live vaccine that is available to prevent disseminated TB. It does not prevent against *M. tuberculosis*.

Other Pulmonary Disorders

Primary Lung Cancer

Description of the Disease: Primary pulmonary malignancies may occur anywhere from the tracheobronchial tree to peripheral lung tissue. It can be either small cell cancer or non–small cell cancer.

Epidemiology and Etiology:
- Leading cause of cancer-related deaths in the United States.
- Non–small cell cancer accounts for over 85% of all lung cancers.
  - Adenocarcinoma is the most common type in the United States. It metastasizes early, has a poor prognosis, and is the most common type in nonsmokers.
  - Squamous cell carcinoma is the dose-related effect with smoking. Much slower growing.
  - Large cell cancer is similar in prognosis to adenocarcinoma.
- Small cell cancer is usually centrally located, has early metastasis, and is very aggressive.
- Other types of lung cancer include mesothelioma, carcinoid tumor, and sarcoma.
- Can be staged using the NSCLC (0 to IV looking at the tumor, lymph node status, and presence of metastasis) or SCLS (looks at disease location and metastasis).
- Most tumors (60%) occur in upper lung lobes; only 30% in the lower lobes.
- Spread occurs usually to the lymph nodes and to other body organs or by local extension into the chest wall, diaphragm, pulmonary vessels, esophagus, and pericardium.

Risk Factors:
- Tobacco smoke (primary and secondary)—accounts for 95% of lung cancer in men and 85% lung cancer in women.
- Environmental/occupational exposures (such as asbestos, ionizing radiation, metals).
- Lung scarring from TB.
- Radiation therapy to breast or chest.

Signs and Symptoms:
- **Subjective Complaints:**
  - May be totally asymptomatic until condition is advanced.
  - Pulmonary: Cough (similar to "smoker's cough" of chronic bronchitis), dyspnea, hemoptysis, wheezing/stridor.
  - General: Fatigue, malaise, body aches, bone pain, weight loss, fever, chills, anemia.
  - Other: Pleuritic chest pain, shoulder pain, dysphagia, hoarseness, neurologic symptoms.

- **Physical Examination Findings:**
  - There may not be any significant changes on examination, depending on the degree of disease severity.
  - Unilateral wheezing, enlarged/palpable lymph nodes.
- **Differential Diagnoses:**
  - COPD
  - CHF
  - TB
  - Lung abscess
  - Bronchitis
- **Diagnostic Studies:**
  - CXR: PA and lateral—compare with old films when possible. Can show nodule/mass, persistent infiltrate, atelectasis, pleural effusion, hilar mass. CXR is the first step to further workup.
  - CT scan of chest with contrast: Nodule/mass and lymphadenopathy.
  - Brain MRI: To note metastasis. Additional CT scans to diagnose other metastatic disease.
  - CBC, liver function tests, and comprehensive metabolic profile to establish baseline data.
  - Electrolytes: To determine degree of dehydration.
  - Bronchoscopy with biopsy with pathology review.
- **Treatment:**
  - Pharmacological:
    - Chemotherapy
    - Pain management
  - Nonpharmacological:
    - Surgery: Only about 25% of patients are candidates for surgery.
    - Radiation therapy.
    - Smoking cessation.
    - Realistic assessment of condition and prognosis with patient and family.
    - Follow-up and referral:
      - Surgical consult
      - Oncology consult
      - Palliative care/hospice care
    - Screening: American Cancer Society, American College of Chest Physicians, and U.S. Preventive Services Task Force (USPSTF) have recommended that adults between the ages of 55 and 74 years of age with at least a 30-pack-year history of current/prior cigarette use receive annual low-dose CT scans of the chest to screen for lung cancer.
- **Geriatric Considerations:**
  - Cancer treatments are often very aggressive and may be more toxic in older patients.
  - Older patients experience more side effects from chemotherapy.
  - With non–small cell cancer that has metastasized, chemotherapy assists in palliating symptoms and improving QoL.

Obstructive Sleep Apnea

Description of the Disease: Repetitive episodes of reduction or cessation of breathing (apnea) due to narrowing or occlusion of the upper airway during sleep. The apnea episodes disrupt sleep, terminate with a gasp or snort, and lead to excessive daytime sleepiness.

Epidemiology and Etiology:
- Occurs in middle-aged men and women and with a higher incidence in obese or hypertensive patients.
- Increase incidence in those that smoke, have some form of nasal obstruction, or drink alcohol/take sedative prior to sleep.
- Naso- or oropharynx (enlarged tonsils or uvula, low soft palate, a large or posteriorly located tongue) collapses during inspiration causes the apnea episodes.

Risk Factors:
- Obesity (incidence between 38% and 88%)
- Hypertension
- Metabolic syndrome

Signs and Symptoms:
- **Subjective Complaints:** Screen all patients who complain of feeling tired. See Table 3-6 for screening tool.
  - Excessive daytime sleepiness or fatigue.
  - Tired on awakening, headache on awakening, sore throat/dry mouth.
  - Unable to concentrate; decrease in memory, irritable with frequent mood changes.
  - Loud snoring while sleeping (occurs in 60% of all patients).
  - Snort or gasp that awakens patient from sleep.
  - Significant other notes apneic episodes at night.
- **Physical Examination Findings:**
  - Most patients have a normal physical examination, with the exception of possible risk factors.
  - Head and neck: Concentrate on this area, and note any of the following: Short neck with large circumference, narrowing of the lateral airway, tonsillar hypertrophy, soft palate edema, enlarged tongue, deviated nasal septum, and poor nasal airflow.
- **Differential Diagnoses:**
  - Narcolepsy
  - Depression
  - Primary snoring
  - Restless leg syndrome
  - Sleep deprivation
- **Diagnostic Studies:**
  - Polysomnography (PSG), a nighttime sleep study, is the gold standard for diagnosis. Will assist in determining the following:
    - Severity of hypoxemia, sleep disruption, and any associated cardiac dysrhythmias
    - Number of apneic episodes
- **Treatment:**
  - Pharmacological—none
  - Nonpharmacological:
    - Weight loss and avoiding alcohol, smoking, and sedatives before bedtime.
    - Continuous positive airway pressure (CPAP) therapy is the mainstay treatment for moderate to severe obstructive sleep apnea (OSA). Bilevel positive airway pressure (BiPAP) therapy can also be used.
    - Possible surgical interventions: Tracheotomy, bariatric surgery, uvulopalatoplasty, and any other upper airway corrections.
    - Follow-up and referral:
      - Pulmonary Referral for sleep test and management of therapy.
      - Surgical Referral for any needed surgical intervention.

Table 3-6: STOP-BANG Screening Tool for Obstructive Sleep Apnea

S = **S**noring	**B** = **B**MI greater than 35
T = **T**iredness	**A** = **A**ge greater than 50
O = **O**bserved you stop breathing	**N** = **N**eck circumference greater than 40 cm (15.7 inches
P = Blood **P**ressure	**G** = **G**ender male

High risk equals the patient having equal to/greater than three positive items. If at high risk, refer for sleep testing.

Review Section

Review Questions

1. You, as the NP, are examining a 35-year-old woman who is complaining of severe wheezing for the past few days. She has a history of asthma and is using budesonide on a daily basis, and has been using her albuterol more frequently. However, it is not effective. Her peak expiratory flow measurement is only 55% of her personal best. You auscultate diffuse severe wheezing bilaterally and note a dry cough, with mild shortness of breath. Based on these findings, what medication should be added to her medication regimen?

   a. Salmeterol inhaler
   b. Montelukast by mouth
   c. Systemic oral corticosteroids, such as prednisone
   d. Oral theophylline

2. When teaching a patient about using inhalers, which of the following information should be included?

   a. Do not shake any of the inhalers
   b. Separate inhaler medications by 30 minutes
   c. Refrigerate all inhaler medications to maintain effectiveness
   d. Rinse mouth after using each inhaler

3. When teaching a patient how to use a home peak expiratory flow to measure changes and determine when treatment is required, which of the following zones would her expiratory compliance be at 50% to 80% of her personal best?

   a. Red zone
   b. Green zone
   c. White zone
   d. Yellow zone

4. When prescribing medications for COPD, which of the following drug classifications should be implemented FIRST?

   a. Inhaled β_2 agonist bronchodilator
   b. Xanthines, such as theophylline
   c. Oral Corticosteroids
   d. Inhaled anticholinergic bronchodilator

5. A patient presents at the local clinic after living in a homeless shelter for 2 months. He comes in complaining of an increase in a productive cough, weakness, general malaise, body aches. He thinks he is having night fevers because he complains of night sweats. Which of the following tests would you order first?

   a. Tuberculin skin test (TST or Mantoux)
   b. CBC
   c. Sputum culture
   d. Chest X-ray

6. A patient presents with complaints of fever, difficulty breathing, and cough for 4 days. On examination, the NP notes increased tactile fremitus and dullness on percussion on the left lung base. The NP diagnoses community-acquired pneumonia (CAP). These clinical manifestations likely indicate:

   a. Pulmonary embolus
   b. Cavitation
   c. Severe atelectasis
   d. Consolidation

7. You diagnose a 72-year-old patient with community-acquired pneumonia. He has a history of CHF and DM-2. Based on the American Thoracic Society Consensus Guidelines on the Management of CAP, which of the following antibiotics is recommended for use in this patient?

   a. Macrolide
   b. Cephalosporin
   c. β-Lactamase inhibitor amoxicillin
   d. Fluoroquinolone

8. According to the American Thoracic Society, when prescribing antibiotics for CAP in the outpatient setting, what is the usual length of time for antimicrobial therapy?

   a. 7 to 10 days
   b. 5 to 7 days
   c. 2 to 5 days
   d. 10 to 14 days

9. Which of the following is the definitive test for obstructive sleep apnea?

   a. 48-hour Holter monitor
   b. ENT specialist confirming enlarged abnormal uvula
   c. Overnight polysomnogram
   d. Subjective symptoms and history of apnea episodes

10. Which of the following is the *most common* mode of transmission of a viral upper respiratory infection?

   a. Air pollution
   b. Hand-to-hand transmission
   c. Persons coughing into the air
   d. Unclean silverware and plates

Answers with Rationales

1. (c) Systemic oral corticosteroids, such as prednisone

   Rationale: Systemic oral corticosteroids should be used in an acute attack. Prednisone should be used in short burst regimen and then tapered to the lowest dose, before being discontinued. This patient is already on a steroid MDI, which should be continued throughout and following oral treatment.

2. (d) Rinse mouth after using each inhaler

   Rationale: Rinsing the mouth after use of a steroid inhaler is essential to prevent oral candidiasis (thrush). A patient who has a bad taste should brush his/her teeth. Steroid MDIs should be used after β_2 agonist MDI.

3. (d) Yellow zone

   Rationale: An asthma patient should be instructed to record his or her personal best (80% to 100%) when feeling well, with no symptoms. This is considered the "green" zone. With the beginning symptoms and progression, a yellow zone (50% to 80% personal best) is cautionary. A red zone (less than 50%) indicates that an attack is occurring and rescue interventions should be started.

4. (a) Inhaled β_2 agonist bronchodilator

   Rationale: Although all medications are used in COPD, inhaled β_2 agonist bronchodilators are prescribed first during stage 1 of the GOLD criteria. Other medications are initiated as the disease progresses through the other stages.

5. (a) Tuberculin skin test (TST or Mantoux)

   Rationale: Because of the symptomatology and the patient's current living conditions, he is at high risk for contracting tuberculosis. Although any of the diagnostics is appropriate, a TST should be completed first, followed by the other diagnostics to confirm the diagnosis.

6. (d) Consolidation

   Rationale: Dullness on percussion and tactile fremitus are indications of consolidation, especially with CAP. Atelectasis and PE will have decreased breath sounds and complaints of dyspnea. Cavitation is seen on CXR, indicating possible TB.

7. (d) Fluoroquinolone

   Rationale: Patients with comorbidities should be started on a respiratory fluoroquinolone OR both a β-lactamase inhibitor amoxicillin and an advanced macrolide. Using one medication instead of two medications increases medication compliance.

8. (b) 5 to 7 days

   Rationale: Patients being treated in the outpatient setting should be on antibiotics for 5 to 7 days on average. Levofloxacin is usually 750 mg daily times 5 days; azithromycin or clarithromycin packs are usually for a 5-day course.

9. (c) Overnight polysomnogram

   Rationale: Although the subjective symptoms and history of apnea episodes will add to your suspicions of OSA, the definitive test is an overnight polysomnogram. It is an all-night recording of the patient's sleep and helps to identify the presence, type, and severity of the sleep apnea.

10. (b) Hand-to-hand transmission

   Rationale: Although viral URIs can also be contracted through inhaled particles from people sneezing and coughing, the common cold is most commonly transmitted through hand-to-hand transmission, making handwashing the best preventable method of decreasing new cases.

Suggested Readings

Blait, K., & Evelo, A. (2013). COPD: Overview and survey of NP knowledge. *The Nurse Practitioner, 38*(6), 18–26.

Cash, J., & Glass, C. (2014). *Family practice guidelines* (3rd ed.). Philadelphia, PA: Springer Publishing.

Chernecky, C. C., & Berger, B. J. (Eds.) (2012). *Laboratory tests and diagnostic procedures* (6th ed.). Philadelphia, PA: Saunders.

Kamanager, N. (2014). *Bacterial pneumonia.* Retrieved from http://emedicine.medscape.com/article/300157-overview

McPhee, S., Papadakis, M., & Rabow, M. (Eds.) (2015). *Current medical diagnosis and treatment* (54th ed.). New York, NY: McGraw Hill Medical.

Rance, K., & O'Laughlen, M. (2014). Managing asthma in older adults. *The Journal for Nurse Practitioners, 10*(1), 1–9.

U.S. Department of Health and Human Services. (2007). *Diagnosis and management of asthma.* Retrieved from www.nhlbi.nih.gov/health-pro/guidelines/current/asthma-guidelines

WebMD Medical Reference. (2012). *GOLD criteria for COPD.* Retrieved from www.webmd.com/lung/copd/gold-criteria-for-copd

Williams, B., & Chang, B. (2014). *Current diagnosis and treatment geriatrics* (2nd ed.). New York, NY: McGraw Hill Medical.

Yates, C. (2013). Assessing asthma control. *The Nurse Practitioner, 38*(6), 40–47.

Chapter 4

Cardiovascular System

Catherine J. Morse

Introduction: This chapter addresses the most common cardiac diagnoses that the Adult Primary Care Nurse Practitioner may see in practice. While the incidence of cardiac issues can increase with advancing age it can occur across the spectrum of adulthood. The chapter begins with a case study of a common cardiac problem.

Case Presentation

Directions: Carefully review the case study presented below. At the end of the chapter, answer the review questions. Compare your answers to the correct answers listed in the Review Section.

Chief Complaint: A 78-year-old male presents with pain in his lower left extremity while walking back and forth to the bathroom.

History of Present Illness: The pain has been occurring for the past month only while walking. He can make it to the bathroom (approximately 30 ft) but then while walking back he has been experiencing pain the in left calf. The pain is an "ache" or "cramp-like" and goes way after he sits down. When the pain is present, it is a 4–5/10 pain scale. He denies pain at rest, or any recent trauma. He does not have a history of deep vein thrombosis (DVT), baker's cyst, varicose veins, or peripheral arterial disease. He has tried a heating pad at home with no effect; no medications have been taken. He does have a history of heart failure with reduced ejection fraction, coronary artery disease, acute myocardial infarction, remote history of smoking (40 pack-year) quit 10 years ago, hypertension (HTN), and dyslipidemia.

Past Medical History: Heart failure with reduced ejection fraction (last echo 1 month ago), HTN, dyslipidemia, coronary heart disease (Drug Eluting Stent [DES] stent to Left anterior descending [LAD] in 2014, DES stent to Right Coronary Artery [RCA] in 2013), acute myocardial infarction (AMI) in 2013, obesity

Past Social History: Cholecystectomy in 2000

Social History: Lives alone, denies ETOH = alcohol or street drugs, + smoking history of 40 pack-years, quit 10 years ago

Current Medications:
Carvediol 12.5 mg p.o. b.i.d.
ASA 81 mg p.o. daily
Clopidogrel 75 mg p.o. daily
Enalapril 10 mg p.o. b.i.d.
Furosemide 20 mg p.o. b.i.d.
KCL 20 mEq p.o. daily
Atorvasatin 20 mg p.o. daily
Protonix 40 mg p.o. daily

Review of Systems:
Constitution: Denies trouble sleeping, recent unintended weight loss, fevers, or night sweats
Eyes: Denies visual changes, glaucoma, cataracts, and wears glasses. Last eye examination 1 month ago

Ears, Nose, Mouth, and Throat: Denies nasal stuffiness, nose bleeds, ear pain, tinnitus, throat pain, dry mouth, thrush, nonhealing ulcers

Cardiovascular: Denies chest pain (CP), chest tightness, or palpitations. + shortness of breath (SOB) with activity at his normal level. He can walk about 50 ft before becoming SOB, but this has been restricted lately due to pain in his left calf. 2 + pillow orthopnea (not changed), no paroxysmal nocturnal dyspnea (PND), + peripheral edema at his usual amount

Respiratory: Denies cough, hemoptysis, wheezing, or pain with breathing. SOB, see under cardiovascular (CV).

Gastrointestinal: Denies swallowing difficulties, + Gastroesophageal reflux disease (GERD) but symptoms under control with protonix. Denies nausea, changes in bowel habits, blood in stools, hematemesis, or bright red blood per rectum (BRBPR)

Genitourinary (GU): Gets up frequently to void but thinks it is due to his diuretics (no change from usual), denies pain with urination, blood in urine, or foul smelling urine

Integumentary: Denies rashes, new bruising, or skin breakdown

Neurologic: Denies cerebral vascular accident (CVA), Transient ischemic attack (TIA), amaurosis fugax, visual changes

Psychiatric: Denies depression, suicidal thoughts, anxiety, memory loss, or stress

Endocrine: Denies heat or cold intolerance, change in appetite, thyroid, or diabetes (DM)

Hematologic/Lymphatic: Denies easy bleeding, + bruising but no more than normal

Allergic/Immunologic: No known drug allergies (NKDA), flu, and pneumovax vaccine in 2014

Physical Assessment:

Vital Signs: HR = 78 and regular BP = 105/65 RR = 22 SPO_2 on room air 95% Temperature = 98.4°F orally

General: Pleasant gentleman in no acute distress

Head, Eyes, Ears, Nose, and Throat: Normocephalic atraumatic, no jugular venous distention (JVD) or hepatojuglar reflux (HJR), no carotid bruits, no lymphadenopathy

Chest: Symmetrical, nontender, bilateral excursion

Lungs: Scattered fine crackles in bases, no wheezing. Air entry decreased slightly bilaterally. No egophony

Heart: PMI displaced to left lateral position, S1, S2, and S3 audible. Soft systolic murmur II/VI best heard at apex without radiation

Abdomen: Soft nontender, without heptomegaly or splenomegaly. No bruits, + bowel sounds (BS)

GU: Deferred

Extremities: Lower extremities with + 1 edema bilaterally, pulses only present with Doppler on left (posterior tibialis [PT]/dorsalis pedis [DP]), on right + 1 DP/PT. Decreased hair distribution on the left

Differential Diagnosis: Peripheral arterial disease, baker's cyst, DVT, muscular injury or strain, popliteal entrapment syndrome, osteoarthritis, venous disease, chronic compartment syndrome

Diagnostics:

Ankle–Brachial Index (ABI): Left <0.5, right 0.5 to 0.79

Echo: 2D with M mode

    AV diameter: 2.1 cm

    EF biplane: 30%

    IVSd: 1.5 cm

    LA diameter: 5.7 cm

    LVESDs: 3.4 cm

    LEVDDs: 2.7 cm

    LVPWd: 1.6 cm

    RA area: 18.1 cm^2

    MV E/A ratio: 0.7

Cardiac Function:

Left Atrium: Moderately dilated left atrium (LA) chamber size

Right Atrium: Dilated RA chamber size

Left Ventricle: Normal LV size. Systolic function was moderately to markedly reduced. Ejection fraction was estimated in the range of 25% to 30%. Paradoxical septal motion. Moderate to severe septal hypokinesis. Mild hypokinesis of the lateral and inferior walls; otherwise global LV hypokinesis.

Right Ventricle: Normal RV chamber size. Systolic function was normal

Aorta: The root exhibited normal size

Aortic Valve: Anatomically normal. The valve was trileaflet. There was no aortic valve regurgitation.

Mitral Valve: There was mild to moderate annular calcification. There was diffuse thickening. There was no regurgitation.

Tricuspid Valve: Anatomically normal. There was trace regurgitation.

Summary:

Left Ventricle: Systolic function was moderately to markedly reduced. Ejection fraction was estimated to be 25% to 30%.

Diagnosis and Patient Goals:

Peripheral arterial disease—ABI less than 0.5 indicating significant disease. Invasive testing to further delineate anatomy and consult to vascular surgeon as the patient wishes to aggressively treat the disease. Continue with progressive, consistent exercise program. Already on antiplatelet therapy. Order basic metabolic panel (BMP) in anticipation of ordering pentoxifylline

Heart failure with reduced ejection fraction—Compensated, continue current therapy and lifestyle changes

HTN—Well controlled, continue current therapy and lifestyle changes

Dylipidemia—Reassess fasting lipids

Pharmacologic Interventions:

The patient is already on antiplatelet medications, ASA 81 to 325 mg is recommended for peripheral arterial disease (PAD). In order to increase walking distances, pentoxifylline (Trental) or cilostazol (Pletal) can be considered. In this patient cilostazol is contraindicated due to the history of heart failure and increased risk of death.

Treatment:

Refer for magnetic resonance angiogram (MRA) and surgical evaluation for PAD.
Refer to physical therapy for PAD walking program.
Lipids have not been evaluated in last 90 days—recheck.
Check BMP prior to ordering pentoxifylline to assess creatinine clearance.

Coronary Heart Disease

Description of the Disease: Coronary heart disease is the obstruction of blood flow, partial or complete, in the coronary arteries. This results in a mismatch between myocardial oxygen demand and supply resulting in the most common symptom, chest pain (angina).

Epidemiology:

- Coronary heart disease was responsible for 1 out of 7 deaths in the United States in 2011. This resulted in 375,295 Americans dying from coronary disease in 2011.
- Approximately every 34 seconds one American has a coronary event, and approximately every 1 minute 24 seconds, an American will die from a coronary event.

Etiology:

- It is most commonly due to atherosclerosis, but other causes include coronary spasm, myocardial bridges, tumors, congenital anomalies, vasculitides, granulomas, scarring from previous trauma or radiation, and aortic dissection. Transient coronary artery obstruction can be the result of vasospasm, embolus, or a thrombus.

Risk Factors:

- Risk factors can be divided into modifiable and nonmodifiable risk factors. See List 4-1 for a complete list. Most patients with coronary heart disease have some identifiable risk factor(s).

List 4-1: Risk Factors for Coronary Heart Disease

Modifiable	
- Risk	- Hypertension
- Factors	- Gender
Non—Modifiable	- Diabetes
- Risk	- Race
- Factors	- Obesity
- Smoking	- Heredity
- Age	- Increased Stress and Type A Personality
	- Use of Oral Contraceptives Hyperlipidemia

Signs and Symptoms:
- Patient presentation of coronary heart disease can be varied with gender differences in signs and symptoms. However, the most common signs and symptoms of heart disease include chest pain, shortness of breath, palpitations, syncope or near syncope, and fatigue.
- The severity of symptoms varies greatly. Angina pectoris is often described as a sensation of tightness, burning, squeezing, aching, "gas pains," or indigestion. Often the discomfort can be felt behind the sternum or just to the left.
- If radiation of the discomfort or pain occurs, it is typically to the jaw and left shoulder. However, there can be many different presentations and atypical chest pain or angina equivalents need to be in the forefront of the Nurse Practitioner's mind while assessing this population.

Different Types of Angina:
- Chronic Stable Angina
  - Predictable in terms of provoking factors and relieving factors
  - Typically lasts between 2 and 30 minutes
  - Cheat pain that lasts longer than 30 minutes is more consistent with myocardial infarction.
  - Often precipitated by stress or exertion and relieved with rest or nitrates
- Unstable Angina
  - A change in intensity, frequency, or character of the patient's typical angina pattern
  - For example, previously stable extertional angina that is now occurring at rest
- Variant Angina
  - This is angina that is not predictable and can occur at rest and with activity.
- Prinzmetal Angina
  - Occurs at rest, typically in the early morning hours, but is not associated with the usual precipitating factors
  - Tends to effect women less than 50 years of age
  - Often involves the right coronary artery
  - Can be associated with cocaine abuse, tobacco abuse, nitric oxide deficiency, stimulation of α receptors

Common Signs:
- Hypo or hypertension
- A gallop on cardiac assessment
- Transient apical systolic murmur from mitral regurgitation from papillary muscle dysfunction during acute ischemia
- New-onset dysrhythmias (atrial or ventricular)
- Secondary findings
  - Nicotine-stained fingers in smokers
  - Barrel chest secondary to COPD
  - Peripheral edema (evidence of heart failure)

Differential Diagnoses:
- The first critical step is to discern if this is a potentially life-threatening cause of chest pain and to differentiate between noncardiac and cardiac pain. List 4-2 lists the must-not-miss life-threatening differential diagnosis for CP. See List 4-3 for broader differential diagnosis.

List 4-2: Must-Not-Miss Differential Diagnosis for Chest Pain

• Acute coronary syndrome	• Cardiac tamponade
• Pneumothorax	• Ruptured esophagus
• Dissecting aortic aneurysm	• Pulmonary emboli

List 4-3: Common Differential Diagnosis for Chest Pain

Cardiac
- ACS – Unstable angina, STEMI, N—STEMI
- Stable angina
- Coronary spasm
- Cardiac tamponade
- Pericarditis
- Myocarditis
- Heart failure

Gastrointestinal
- GERD
- PUD
- Pancreatitis
- Cholecystitis

Pulmonary
- Pulmonary emboli
- Pneumothorax
- Pneumonia

- Pleurisy
- Pulmonary hypertension

Musculoskeletal
- Trauma
- Chest wall pain
- Costrochondritis

Other
- Panic attack
- Psychogenic event

Diagnostic Studies:
For patients who present with intermittent new-onset chest pain the workup should include the following:
- 12-lead ECG
  - Often normal in patients with angina
  - There may be signs of previous myocardial infarction, nonspecific ST and T-wave changes, and or findings consistent with LVH.
  - If ischemia is present, then the characteristic ECG changes include downward sloping.
  - ST segment depression that resolves when the anginal symptoms resolve. T-wave flattening or inversion may also be present.
  - If acute myocardial injury is present, then ST segment elevation in the appropriate contiguous leads will be present.
- Outpatient stress testing
  - Exercise stress testing in the most commonly used noninvasive assessment to evaluate for inducible angina in this patient population.
  - Typically performed on a treadmill but can also be a bicycle in a supine position
  - If patients are not able to perform leg exercises, they are usually evaluated using pharmacologic stress testing.
  - Two basic types of pharmacologic stress testing are (1) simulates exercise with synthetic catecholamines such as dobutamine and (2) uses vasodilator drugs.
  - Exercise stress testing can be combined with other imaging studies such as nuclear, echocardiography, or MRI.
- Fasting lipid panel if not completed in the previous 90 days
- If presentation consistent with heart failure, BNP (brain natriuretic peptide)
- Chest X-ray
  - Only appropriate in the initial workup or if there has been a change in the character or frequency of stable angina
  - Helpful to rule out other diagnosis only
- Echocardiogram
  - It is a noninvasive assessment of cardiac and valvular function.
  - Can detect new wall motion abnormalities
  - Can be used in conjunction with dobutamine as a pharmacologic stress test
- Coronary Angiography
  - Gold standard for evaluating the anatomy of the coronary tree
  - Can be completed as an outpatient with same day discharge
- Cardiac computerized tomography
  - Increasing in use
  - Can detect calcified coronary plaque

Treatment:
- The goal of management of angina is to reestablish a balance between myocardial oxygen demand and supply. Therefore, the practitioner is focused on either decreasing demand or increasing supply.

For Stable Angina:
Lifestyle changes to modify risk factors.
- Smoking cessation
  - Complete cessation of intake of any tobacco products recommended

- Weight management
  - Weight reduction of 10 kg can result in a positive effect on systolic BP up to 20 mm Hg.
- DASH diet
  - Goal less than 2.4 g sodium per day
- Control of HTN
  - According to the Eighth Joint Commission (JNC 8) guidelines treat to maintain BP less than 140/90.
- Control of hyperlipidemia
  - Treatment of hyperlipidemia is longer based on a goal LDL but rather the patient's risk of developing future events and mortality.
  - Hydroxymethyglutaryl coenzyme A (HMG CoA) reductase inhibitors are the drug of choice unless there are contraindications.
  - Intensity of therapy is determined by patient's risk—moderate to high dose recommended unless contraindications are present.
  - Dietary therapy recommended to reduce intake of saturated fats (<7% of total calories), trans-fatty acids (<1% of total calories) and cholesterol (<200 mg/day).
- Control of diabetes
  - A goal A1c of 7% or less for selected patients including those with long life expectancy
  - A goal A1c between 7% and 9% is reasonable for certain patients depending on age, history of hypoglycemia, presence of microvascular complications, or other comorbidities.
- Physical activity
  - Recommended 30 minutes/day of moderate rigorous activity (brisk walking) at least five times per week or vigorous aerobic activity 20 minutes two times weekly.
- Alcohol consumption
  - For males no more than two drinks per day and women one drink per day.

Pharmacological Management
- Nitrates: Can increase myocardial oxygen supply and decrease demand
  - Can be used in an acute attack or prophylactically
  - Available in multiple preparations including spray, buccal, ointment, and short- and long-acting tablets
  - Typical dosing for acute attacks is 0.4 orally q5min for a total of three doses.
  - Prophylactic therapy can be in the form of a patch or ointment. Patch dosing is 0.1 to 0.6 mg/r and ointment is 2%; 0.5 to 2 inches. The development of tolerance can be a significant issue, and it is recommended to allow the patient to have time without nitrates each say.
  - Isosorbide dinitrate (Isordil) can be used prophylactically at 10 to 60 mg t.i.d. with 8 hours needed to be drug free to avoid the development of tolerance
  - Long-acting isorobide mononitrate 20 mg b.i.d. (should be taken at least 7 hours apart)
- β-Blockers (BB): Work to increase myocardial oxygen supply and decrease myocardial oxygen demand. There are multiple choices with differences in efficacy and side effects.
  - Can reduce or eliminate angina attacks and increase exercise tolerance
  - Common dosing using cardioselective BB includes metoprolol 50 to 200 mg daily in two divided doses or atenolol 25 to 200 mg once daily.
  - Major side effects and limited up titration can include bradycardia, hypotension, and worsening of underlying obstructive lung disease
- Calcium channel blockers (CCH): Decrease myocardial oxygen demand by peripheral vasodilation and increase oxygen supply by coronary artery dilatation.
  - The largest group is the dihydropyridine CCHs. Examples include amlodipine, nifedipine, and nicardipine. This group of drugs does not have an effect on heart rate.
  - The second major group of CCHs can lower heart rate. The most commonly prescribed are diltiazem hydrochloride and verapamil.
  - Diltiazem is 120 to 360 mg daily in divided doses.
  - Verapamil 30 to 120 mg daily
- Sodium current inhibitor: Decreases myocardial oxygen demand by partially inhibiting fatty acid oxidation and increased glucose oxidation that results in more adenosine triphosphate for each molecule of oxygen consumed
  - Ranolazine 1,000 to 2,000 mg/day in two divided doses
- Adjunctive medications
  - All patients with coronary disease should take ASA 81 to 325 mg daily unless there are contraindications such as allergy, or gastrointestinal bleeding.

- Selected high-risk patients should take clopidogrel (Plavix)
- See Risk Factor modification for discussion on statins
- Revascularization: Catheter or surgical interventions are indicated when the patient is not able to be controlled medically and to prevent myocardial injury.
- Catheter-based interventions can be performed in a significant number of patients and can include the placement of drug eluting stents, bare metal stents or plain balloon angioplasty.
  - Initial success rates for dilating the coronary arteries is greater than 85%.
  - Principle disadvantage is the risk of restenosis.
- Coronary artery bypass (CABG)
  - Arterial conduits make better graft material than veins.
  - Better outcomes with surgical revascularization of left main obstructions of greater than 50%
  - Recommended in patients with two or three vessel disease and reduced left ventricular function if viable myocardium is present
  - Recommended for coronary disease if there is a concomitant disease that requires surgical intervention such as significant valvular heart disease

Hypertension

Description of the Disease: The JNC 8 was released in 2014 and makes the following recommendations for treatment thresholds for HTN in adult patients:
- BP goal in general population patients aged 60 years and older to be less than 150/90 mm Hg
- BP goal in patients aged 30 through 59 to be less than 140/90 mm Hg
- BP in patients aged less than 30 years to be less than 140/90 mm Hg
- Same thresholds for patients with diabetes or nondiabetes chronic kidney disease (CKD) as for the general population aged less than 60 years (less than 140/90)

Epidemiology:
- Data from the CDC, National Health and Nutrition Survey 2011 to 2012 reports that age-adjusted prevalence among US adults aged 18 years and over was 29.1% in 2011 to 2012, similar to previous data.
- Between men and women the prevalence was similar and increased with age with the highest being in older adults. It was highest in non-Hispanic Black adults at 42%. Of interest, nearly 83% were aware of their diagnosis and nearly 76% were taking their medications with approximately 52% considered controlled.
- HTN is the most common primary care problem and remains an important preventable risk factor for death and disease such as stroke, renal failure, retinopathy, coronary artery disease, and heart failure.

Etiology:
- HTN can be viewed as either primary (unknown etiology, essential HTN, or idiopathic HTN) or secondary—related to other causes. More than 90% of HTN is considered to be primary, without a clear cause. For screening recommendations, see Chapter 1. See List 4-4 for summary of etiologies.

List 4-4: Summary of Etiologies for HTN in Adults

Primary HTN	Secondary HTN
• Onset usually between 25 and 35 years • Exacerbating factors: smoking, excessive ETOH consumption, obesity, use of nonsteroidal anti-inflammatories (sodium retention) • Theories of etiology included increased circulating renin levels, increased sympathetic nervous system activation, increased circulating volume	• CKD • Endocrine abnormalities: hyperaldosteronism, Cushing disease, pheochromocytoma, thyroid or parathyroid disease • Vascular abnormalities: coarctation of the aorta • Pregnancy • Untreated sleep apnea

Risk Factors:
- Exacerbating factors are given in List 4-4

Signs and Symptoms:

Many times there are no obvious clinical symptoms and when there are symptoms they can be a reflection of the secondary causes of HTN. The list below reviews common presentations:
- Elevated BP (depending on age group) on physical examination when measured at rest with arm at heart level with an appropriately sized BP cuff
- Headache may be present, often occurring in the morning and in the suboccipital area
- Chronic untreated HTN may result in left ventricular HTN seen on 12-lead ECG and echocardiogram
- Epistasis with severe uncontrolled HTN
- Visual changes
- S4 present on auscultation reflecting left ventricular hypertrophy
- Displaced PMI associated with left ventricular hypertrophy
- Renal artery bruit may be auscultated when renal artery stenosis is present.

Signs and symptoms associated with secondary causes:
- Renal disease: Hematuria, oliguria, nocturia
- Pheochromocytoma: Flushing, palpitations, tremors, diaphoresis
- Thyroid disease: Tachycardia, flushing, anxiety

Differential Diagnoses:

For the common secondary causes of HTN, differential diagnosis are outlined below:

Renal Disorders
- Renal artery stenosis
- Renal parenchymal disease

Endocrine Disorders
- Pheochromocytoma
- Cushing disease
- Primary aldosteronism
- Hyperthyroidism
- Diabetes

Vascular Disorders
- Coarctation of the aorta
- Carotid stenosis

Other
- Pregnancy
- Sleep apnea

Diagnostic Studies:
- In primary HTN laboratory findings are typically normal; however, baseline BMP and CBC should be ordered in this population.
- Fasting lipid panel and glucose
- Urinalysis—microalbuminuria can be an early sign of target organ damage; hematuria and proteinuria can be present in HTN due to renal vascular disease.
- Chest radiograph—can reveal cardiomegaly (left ventricular hypertrophy) and/or a wide mediastinum which can be consistent with coarctation of the aorta
- 12-lead ECG—can reveal left ventricular hypertrophy changes, rule out dysrhythmias
- Echocardiogram—evaluates left ventricular function, presence of left ventricular hypertrophy
- Angiotensin-converting enzyme inhibitor (ACE-I) stimulation testing to rule out renal vascular HTN
- Renal artery ultrasound to rule out renal artery stenosis
- Aldosterone level if aldosteronism is suspected
- Plasma catecholamine levels if pheochromocytoma is suspected
- Screening thyroid stimulating hormone (TSH) to rule out thyroid abnormalities
- Sleep studies if body habitus and history suggest sleep apnea

Treatment:

Life style Modifications (Continues throughout Management)
- DASH diet—limit sodium intake to less than 2.4 g/day.

- Weight reduction—10 kg weight loss can reduce SBP by up to 20 mm Hg.
- Physical activity—recommend 30 minutes of moderate exercise five times weekly or 20 minute of vigorous exercise two times weekly.
- Alcohol intake—limit to one drink per day for women or two drinks per day for men.

Pharmacological Management (from JNC 8 Recommendations)
- For non-Black general population patients including those with diabetes, start thiazide-type diuretic, ACE-I, angiotensin-receptor blocker (ARB), or CCB, alone or in combination
- For black general population patients including those with diabetes, start thiazide-type diuretic or CCB, alone or in combination
- For patients of all ages with CKD start ACE-I or ARB alone or in combination with another drug class
- ARB and ACE-I should not be used together
- If not at goal BP in 1 month consider increasing the dose of the drug or adding a second agent from a different drug class (thiazide-type diuretic, ACE-I, ARB, CCB)
- Continue to monitor patient and if not at goal on two drugs continue up titration or consider adding a third drug from another class
- If more than three drugs needed or a contraindication exists for one of the recommended drug classes then use another antihypertensive from other classes
- Consider referral to a hypertensive specialist if goal BP is not able to be reached or in complicated patients.
- Ongoing counseling for lifestyle modifications, medication compliance and regular follow-up required

Dyslipidemia

Description of the Disease: Dyslipidemia is an umbrella term used to describe abnormalities in any one or a combination of the measured blood lipids. In particular increased levels of low-density lipoprotein cholesterol (LDL-C), low levels of high-density lipoprotein cholesterol (HDL-C) and or increased levels of triglycerides (TG).

Epidemiology:
- In the USA an estimated 53% of adults have lipid disorders; 27% have high LDL-C, 23% have low HDL-C and 30% have high TG. It is a significant risk factor for the development of coronary heart disease and other vascular disorders.

Etiology:
- Dyslipidemia can be due to a primary gene defect (primary dyslipidemia) or more commonly due to secondary causes such as:
  - Sedentary lifestyle
  - Dietary intake
  - Obesity
  - Liver disease
  - Endocrine disorders—hypothyroidism, hypercortisolism, diabetes
  - CKD
  - Cigarette smoking—increased very-low-density lipoprotein
  - Medications—thiazide-type diuretics, BB, Amiodarone, and estrogen compounds can affect plasma lipids.

Risk Factors:
- The secondary causes listed above place patients at higher risk for developing dyslipidemia.

Signs and Symptoms:
- Frequently this is an asymptomatic disease
- Presentation may be secondary to complications such as coronary artery disease, vascular disease, or pancreatitis from severe hypertriglyceridemia
- If the dyslipidemia is secondary to an endocrine disorder, then the presentation will be driven by the primary endocrine disorder
- In severe dyslipidemia physical examination findings may include xanthomas, corneal arcus, lipdemia retinalis, or prominent earlobe creasing.

Differential Diagnoses:
- Primary dyslipidemia
- Secondary dyslipidemia

Diagnostic Studies:
- Refer to Chapter 1 for the recommended screening for dyslipidemia in adults. The standard initial screening is a fasting lipid panel.
  - LDL-C >190 mg/dL is identified as a patient group at risk that requires treatment.
  - HDL-C <40 mg/dL is considered a cardiac risk factor.
  - HDL-C >60 mg/dL is considered a positive risk factor.
  - Serum triglycerides >150 mg/dL are not linked to cardiac disease but may place the patient at risk for pancreatitis.

Treatment:
- The aim of treatment of dyslipidemia is to decrease the atherosclerotic cardiovascular disease risk including coronary heart disease, stroke, and peripheral arterial disease. Treatment is no longer aimed at reaching a LDL-C or HDL-C goal, but rather risk reduction.
- The 2013 American College of Cardiology (ACC) guidelines identified four statin benefit patient groups and the use of high-intensity or moderate-intensity statin therapy (Stone et al., 2013). See List 4-5.

List 4-5: Summary of Risk Identification and Treatment

Patient Risk Group	Recommended Treatment
• Patients with LDL-C >190 mg/dL	• High-intensity statin (reduce LDL-C by 50%) • Moderate-intensity statin if not candidate for high intensity (reduce LDL-C by 30% to 50%)
• Patients 40 to 75 years old with diabetes and an LDL-C between 70 and 90 mg/dL	• Moderate-intensity statin *If 10-year ASCVD risk > 7.5%, then high-intensity statin.
• Patients with a history of clinical atherosclerotic cardiovascular disease (ASCVD)	• If <75 years high-intensity statin. If not a candidate for high-intensity state then moderate intensity • If >75 years *or* if not a candidate for high-intensity statin then moderate-intensity statin
• Patients between 40 and 75 years of age with a 10-year risk of ASCVD >7.5%	• Moderate- to high-intensity statin

(Stone et al., 2013)

Lifestyle Modifications:
- Critical component of risk reduction
- Dietary intake: Total fat <25% to 30% of total daily intake, saturated fat < 7% of total daily intake, cholesterol <200 mg/day
- Recommended 30 minutes/day of moderate rigorous activity (brisk walking) at least five times per week or vigorous aerobic activity 20 minutes two times weekly

Pharmacologic Management:
Prior to prescribing cholesterol-lowering medication, there should be a discussion of ASCVD risk reduction benefits, adverse effects of therapy, possible drug–drug interactions and patient preferences for treatment.
- High-intensity statin therapy: Atorvastatin 40 to 80 mg daily, rosuvasatin 40 mg daily
- Atorvastatin 80 mg daily starting dose is not recommended by the FDA due to increased risk of myopathy and rhabdomyolysis but was evaluated in the clinical trials.
- Moderate-intensity statin therapy is atorvastatin 10 mg daily, pravastatin 40 mg daily, or simvastatin 20 mg to 40 mg b.i.d.
- No longer support for uptitration on cholesterol-lowering medication to reach a lipid goal
- CK should not be routinely measured in individuals receiving statin therapy.
- Baseline CK measurement is reasonable in the patient population that may be at increased risk for adverse muscle events.
- Reasonable to measure CK if a patient on statin therapy presents with muscle complaints such as pain, tenderness, cramping, weakness, or general fatigue
- Baseline ALT should be performed before starting therapy.
- Repeat measures of ALT should only be ordered if the patient has complaints suggestive of hepatotoxicity.

Congestive Heart Failure

Description of the Disease: Heart failure (HF) is a complex clinical syndrome that results from a structural or functional impairment in either ventricular filling or ejection. The end result is an impaired ability to circulate blood at the rate needed to meet metabolic needs of the body. Cardinal symptoms include dyspnea, fatigue, and fluid retention.

Epidemiology:
- Affects approximately 5 million Americans with an estimated 500,000 new cases diagnosed annually. Although survival has improved, the 5-year mortality is still close to 50%. Heart failure office visits, emergency room visits, and hospital admissions account for a significant portion of the total health care expenditures in the USA.

Etiology:
- Two classifications of HF: Preserved ejection fraction (EF) (formerly diastolic HF); and reduced EF (formerly systolic HF; EF < 40%). Most common causes of HF are as follows:
  - Acute myocardial infarction
  - Valvular heart disease
  - Alcoholic cardiomyopathy
  - Viral cardiomyopathy
  - Pericarditis
  - Systemic bacterial infections
  - Preeclampsia
  - Postpartum cardiomyopathy
  - Autoimmune disorders
  - Toxins
  - Rheumatic or congenital heart disease

Risk Factors:
- See above list

Signs and Symptoms:
- Decompensated heart failure with reduced EF:
  - Dyspnea on exertion and rest
  - Orthopnea
  - Paroxysmal nocturnal dyspnea
  - Elevated jugular venous distention
  - Bibasilar rales or course rales
  - Peripheral edema
  - Ascites
  - Displaced point of maximal impulse
  - Ventricular gallop
  - Systolic murmurs not uncommon
- Heart failure with preserved EF (>50%):
  - Decreased exercise tolerance
  - Dyspnea
  - Fatigue
  - Peripheral edema
  - Jugular venous distention

Differential Diagnoses:
- Acute myocardial infarction
- Pulmonary embolus
- Asthma exacerbation
- COPD exacerbation
- Shock from other causes (for acute HF exacerbations)
- Severe anemia
- Renal disease
- Thyroid disease

Diagnostic Studies:

- Echocardiogram—to evaluate EF, valvular function, wall motion, and diastolic function
- BNP—levels above 80 pg/mL can be consistent with heart failure. Normal ranges can vary based on laboratory.
- CBC—anemia
- BMP—AKI can occur with decreased renal blood flow.
- Cardiac enzymes—if acute ischemic suspected
- 12-lead ECG—ischemia and new-onset dysrhythmias
- CXR—cardiomegaly, pulmonary congestion, Kerley B lines, pleural effusions

Treatment (Lists 4-6 and 4-7):

List 4-6: The Recommended Treatment Based on AHA Staging of HF

Stage of HF		Pharmacologic interventions	Nonpharmacologic interventions
Stage A	• Patients at risk for HF due to disease, cardiotoxins, family history • No evidence of structural disease	• ACE-I as indicated	• Manage underlying disease • Control other risk factors • Weight management • Lifestyle modifications • Regular physical exercise
Stage B	• Patients with structural disease but no symptoms	• ACE-I and BB as appropriate	• All interventions under stage A
Stage C	• Patients with structural disease and symptoms of HF	• Inotropic agents as indicated	• All interventions under stage B • Dietary sodium restriction 2 to 2.5 g/day
Stage D	• Refractory HF		• All measures under Stage C • Ventricular assist devices • Heart Transplant • Hospice

Pharmacologic management for HF with reduced ejection fraction (EF < 40%) is focused on the following targets:

- Symptom management
- Sympathetic nervous system blockade
- Neurohormonal blockade

List 4-7: Summary of Pharmacologic Management of HF with Reduced EF

Symptom Management	Sympathetic nervous system blockade	Neurohormonal Blockade	Vasodilators	Inotropes	Other
Diuretics: • Furosemide (Lasix) 20 to 160 mg p.o. daily • Bumetide (Bumix) 0.5 mg to 10 mg p.o. b.i.d. in divided doses	• Carvedilol 25 mg p.o. b.i.d. as tolerated • Toprol l to 190 mg p.o. daily	• Captopril 6.25 to 50 mg t.i.d. – q.i.d. • Enalapril 2.5 to 40 mg b.i.d. • Lisinopril 2.5 to 10 mg p.o. daily • Eplerenone 12.5 to 50 mg daily • Spironolactone 25 mg daily • Angiotensin-receptor blockers if patient is intolerant to ACE-I	• Hydralazine–nitrate combination (tested in African Americans)	• Digoxin 0.125 mg p.o. daily	• Statins Antiarrythmics Anticoagulation if indicated

Management of the Patient with HF with a Preserved EF:

- Aggressive blood pressure control
- Low-sodium diet (less than 2 to 2.5 g/day)
- Diuretics: Furosemide (Lasix) low dose or thiazide low dose
- Consider ACE-I or ARB
- BB therapy if the patient has had a prior myocardial infarction
- CCHs should be considered.

Peripheral Arterial Disease

Description of the Disease: Peripheral arterial disease (PAD) is a chronic narrowing and in some cases complete obstruction of arterial flow. It is typically caused by atherosclerosis and tends to affect the lower extremities.

Epidemiology:

- According to the most recent statistics published from the American Heart Associate in 2014, PAD affects approximately 8.5 million Americans over the age of 40 years. The highest incidence is in elderly, non-Hispanic Blacks and women. Diabetes, CKD, and smoking were associated with significant increase in the rate of disease.

Etiology:

- Same as that for coronary disease

Risk Factors:

- Similar but not identical to those of coronary heart disease. Diabetes and cigarette smoking are stronger risk factors for PAD.

Signs and Symptoms:

- Claudication: Cramping or tiredness in the calf, thigh, or hip, while walking is a cardinal symptom. Other signs and symptoms are as follows:
  - Diminished femoral and distal pulses
  - Decreased hair and nail growth
  - Audible bruits may be heard over the aorta, iliac, or femoral arteries.
  - Nighttime leg pain in the setting of severe PAD
  - Dependent rubor
  - In severe PAD dry gangrene or poorly healing ulcers

Differential Diagnoses:

- Lumbar disc disorders
- Abdominal aortic aneurysm
- Deep vein thrombosis
- Thrombophlebitis (superficial or septic)
- Trauma or peripheral vascular injuries
- Baker cyst rupture
- Chronic compartment syndrome
- Venous disease
- Muscular strain or injury

Diagnostic Studies:

- Ankle–brachial indexes (ABI) is a screening test that should be used to establish the lower extremity PAD in patients with exertional pain, nonhealing wounds, are >70 years of age or >50 years of age with a history of diabetes and/or smoking. ABI <0.5 suggests severe reduction in flow.
- Routine blood work—CBC, BMP
- Risk factor assessment—fasting lipid profile if not completed in the last 90 days
- Doppler ultrasound primary noninvasive test to determine flow status
- MRA
- CTA

Treatment (both pharmacologic and nonpharmacologic)

Nonpharmacologic

- Smoking cessation

- Consistent exercise
- Surgical intervention—bypass or endovascular

Pharmacologic
- Antiplatelet therapy: Aspirin 75 to 325 mg daily; clopidogrel 75 mg daily as alternative
- Consider cilostazol (Pletal) 100 mg p.o. b.i.d. (contraindicated with HF)
- Consider pentoxifylline (Trental) 400 mg p.o. t.i.d. (increases duration of exercise)

Venous Thromboembolism

Description of the Disease: An alteration in the character of the vein that results in the formation of a thrombus that can be completely or partially occlusive.

Epidemiology:
- Incidence varies in patient groups depending on the risk factors.

Etiology:
- Virchow triad: Venous stasis, vessel injury, hypercoagulability

Risk Factors:
- Recent surgery
- Trauma
- Oral contraceptives particularly in the setting of smoking
- Prolonged immobility
- Malignancy
- Pregnancy
- Postpartum period
- Hypercoaguable states
- Congestive heart failure
- Obesity
- Presence of a long-term venous catheter (upper extremities)

Signs and Symptoms:
- Throbbing or aching pain the affected extremity
- Unilateral extremity swelling
- Low-grade temperature
- Tenderness to palpation
- Warmth to palpation

Differential Diagnoses:
- Baker' cyst
- Muscle strain
- Cellulitis
- Lymphatic obstruction

Diagnostic Studies:
- D-Dimer—in patients without comorbidities that would result in a false positive
- Compression ultrasound of the extremity in question
- Contrast venography if other testing is inconclusive

Treatment:

Nonpharmacologic
- Early ambulation unless pain severity is a limiting factor
- Local heat to the affected extremity

Pharmacologic
- Anticoagulation: Low-molecular-weight heparin with transition to either a factor Xa inhibitor, vitamin K inhibitor (Coumadin), or direct thrombin inhibitor (dabigatran)
- Type of anticoagulation will depend on patient factors and whether or not they are being treated as an outpatient or inpatient.

Inflammatory Cardiac Diseases

Pericarditis

Description of the Disease: Acute pericarditis is an inflammatory disease of the pericardium that can be caused by a variety of conditions including bacterial, fungal, and viral infections.

Epidemiology:
- A viral infection is the most common cause in developed countries with tuberculosis being the most common cause in developing countries and worldwide.

Etiology:
- The pericardium surrounds the surface of the heart and consists of two layers: a serous visceral layer and a fibrous parietal layer. Pericarditis affects 2% to 6% of the general population.

Risk Factors:
- Recent infections particularly viral
- Trauma
- Recent cardiac surgery
- Immunosuppression
- HIV/AIDS
- Immigration from a country where tuberculosis is endemic
- Recent myocardial infarction
- History of chest radiation
- Neoplasia
- Uremia

Signs and Symptoms:
- Chest pain is the primary symptom with varying intensity and nature. It is most often precordial or retrosternal in location.
- Chest pain is characteristically worsened with coughing, deep inspiration, and/or lying flat. Sitting up and leaning forward often lessen the pain.
- Pericardial friction rub on auscultation
- Characteristic ECG changes include PR segment depression and/or widespread ST segment elevation
- Presence of new or worsening pericardial effusion
- High fever
- Dyspnea

Differential Diagnoses:
- Acute coronary syndrome (ACS)
- Bronchitis
- Pneumonia
- Pleurisy
- Pneumothorax

Diagnostic Studies:
- ECG—looking for PR segment depression and/or widespread ST segment elevation
- CBC—leukocytosis with left shift if bacterial
- Erythrocyte sedimentation rate (ESR) and C-reactive protein—elevated
- Echocardiogram—evaluate for cardiac tamponade.
- Cardiac enzymes—may be slightly elevated
- Blood cultures if bacterial infection suspected
- Electrolytes

Treatment:
- Treat the underlying cause if known.
- For idiopathic pericarditis: Nonsteroidal anti-inflammatory drugs (NSAID): Ibuprofen 600 mg p.o. t.i.d. × 10 to 14 days, aspirin 750 to 1,000 mg t.i.d., indomethacin 50 mg t.i.d.
- Corticosteroids may be considered but should be avoided unless necessary to control the severity of symptoms (only after NSAID treatment failure)

- If a bacterial pericarditis is suspected, systemic antibiotics should be started as soon as possible aimed at the possible organisms.
- If tuberculosis is suspected then treatment should be started immediately.
- If cardiac tamponade is present, emergent pericardiocentesis is indicated.

Endocarditis

Description of the Disease: Endocarditis is inflammation or infection of the endothelial layer of the heart that can include the cardiac valves. Hallmarks of infectious endocarditis include fever, positive blood cultures for bacteria or fungi, and the characteristic cardiac lesions on echocardiography.

Epidemiology:
- According to the most recent AHA/ACC Valvular Heart Disease Guidelines (2014) infectious endocarditis still has a very high in-hospital mortality rate of 10% to 20% and a 1-year mortality rate approaching 40% (Nishimura et al., 2014). There is a higher incidence in older patients and in underdeveloped countries is most often associated with rheumatic heart disease.

Etiology:
Most commonly caused by bacteria but can also be fungal in origin.
- Viridans streptococci—accounts for approximately 25% of cases
- taphylococcus aureus—accounts for approximately 33% of cases
- Enterococcal endocarditis—almost all are from *Entercococcus faecalis* and only account for approximately 5% of all cases.
- Gram-negative bacteria—rarely cause endocarditis.
- Fungal endocarditis—can occur in the setting of a compromised immune system and invasive procedures. Candida, *Histoplasma capsulatum*, and Aspergillus account for 80% of all fungal endocarditis cases.

Risk Factors:
- Rheumatic heart disease
- Underlying valvular heart disease
- Prosthetic valve replacement
- Intravenous drug abuse
- Diabetes mellitus
- Immunosuppression
- The presence of an intracardiac device

Signs and Symptoms (Absence of Skin Findings Does Not Rule out Endocarditis):
- Fever lasting several weeks
- Constitutional symptoms: Weight loss, fatigue, general malaise
- Headache
- Dyspnea on exertion
- New or worsening murmur
- Osler's nodes—painful, red nodules in the distal phalanges
- Splinter hemorrhages—linear in appearance, subungual
- Janeway lesions—painless, flat, red macules
- Roth spots—small white retina infarcts
- Pallor
- Generalized petechiae
- Splenomegaly—presence usually indicates endocarditis of at least 10 days

Differential Diagnoses:
- Sepsis from another source
- Congestive heart failure
- Valvular heart disease

Diagnostic Studies:
- Blood cultures—two or three sets of anaerobic or aerobic cultures from a separate venipuncture site
- Transesophageal echocardiogram—more sensitive than transthoracic echocardiography
- CBC with differential—elevated WBC with shift to the left; a normocytic, normochromic anemia may be present

- 12-lead ECG—monitor for prolongation of PR interval that can be an indication of aortic valve abscess formation
- CXR—may be helpful to assess presence or degree of pulmonary edema and to detect septic pulmonary emboli (List 4-8)

List 4-8: Major and Minor Criteria in the Modified Duke Criteria for Diagnosis

Major Criteria for Diagnosis	Minor Criteria for Diagnosis
• At least two positive blood cultures of blood samples drawn 12 hours apart *or* • All of three or majority of greater than four separate blood cultures • Single blood culture positive for *Coxiella bumetti* or antiphase I IgG antibody titer > 1:800	• Predisposing heart condition or IV drug abuse • Fever greater than 100.4° F or 38° C • Vascular complications: ◦ Major arterial emboli ◦ Septic infarcts ◦ Mycotic aneurysms ◦ Janeway lesions ◦ Conjunctival hemorrhages ◦ Intracranial hemorrhage
• Echocardiogram positive for Infectious endocarditis: ◦ Moveable mass on valve or supporting structures ◦ New partial dehiscence of prosthetic valve ◦ New valvular regurgitation	• Immunologic complications: ◦ Glomerulonephritis ◦ Osler nodes ◦ Roth spots ◦ Rheumatoid factor • Microbacterial evidence: ◦ Positive blood cultures that do not meet major criteria ◦ Serologic evidence of infection with an organism consistent with infectious endocarditis

(Nishimura et al., 2014)

Treatment:

- Antibiotic therapy is a mainstay of treatment, and depending the degree of illness, empiric treatment can be initiated once blood cultures are drawn and then narrowed based on sensitivities. A multispecialty team of cardiology, cardiothoracic surgery and infectious disease specialists should determine the need for and timing of surgical intervention. List 4-9 summarizes recommended antibiotic therapy.

List 4-9: Summary of Empiric Antibiotic Recommendations for Infectious Endocarditis

Suspected Staph or Strept:
- Penicillin G 2 million units q8h × 4 weeks with Gentamycin 1 mg/kg IV q8h *or*
- Ceftriaxone (Rocephin) 2 g/day IV × 4 weeks
- For Penn allergic patients: Cefazolin (Ancef) 1 g IV q8h × 4 weeks or vancomycin (Vancocin) 15 mg/kg IV q12h for 4 to 6 weeks

For MRSA:
- Nafcillin (Unipen) 1.5 g q4h for 4 to 6 weeks
- For Pen allergic patients: Vancomycin (Vancocin) 15 mg/kg IV q12h

For Entercocci:
- Gentamycin 1 mg/kg q8h with ampicillin (Omnipen) 2 g OV q4h *or*
- Penicillin G 3 to 5 million units q4h × 4 weeks *or*
- Linezolid (Zyvox) 600 mg IV/p.o. q12h × 2 to 4 weeks
- For Penn allergic patients: Vancomycin (Vancocin) 15 mg/kg IV q12h with gentamicin 1 mg/kg q8h

Review Section

Review Questions with Rationales

1. In a patient with peripheral arterial disease, which of the following lifestyle changes is the most important?

   a. Consistent exercise
   b. Smoking cessation
   c. Weight loss
   d. DASH diet

2. In a patient with heart failure with reduced ejection fraction, which of the following medications blocks the sympathetic nervous output?

   a. Enalapril
   b. Carvediolol
   c. Furosemide
   d. Spironolactone

3. In a patient with coronary heart disease and a history of myocardial infarction and an LDL of 200 mg/dL, total cholesterol of which of the following recommendations in regards to statins?

   a. If there are no contraindications start low-intensity statins.
   b. If there are no contraindications start medium-intensity statins.
   c. If there are no contraindications start high-intensity statins.
   d. Do not start statins order 6 months of lifestyle modifications and then reevaluate.

4. In a patient with complaints of predictable crampy pain with walking that is relieved with rest what is the first screening test?

   a. MRA of the lower extremities
   b. CT angiography of the lower extremities
   c. Ankle–brachial indexes of the lower extremities
   d. Venous ultrasound of the lower extremities

5. A 58-year-old patient presents with dyspnea on exertion, three-pillow orthopnea and PND for the last two nights. He has a history of HF with reduced EF. His weight has increased 2.0 kg over the last week. Which of the following is the most appropriate action?

   a. Increase or start an ACE-I.
   b. Counsel on sodium dietary restrictions.
   c. Increase or start a loop diuretic.
   d. Increase or start spironolactone.

6. A 17-year-old patient with a history and current use of IV drugs presents to the office with fevers for 1 month, 10 lb weight loss, significant fatigue, and malaise. The nurse practitioner should consider which of the following as the most important differential diagnosis to rule out?

   a. Influenza A
   b. Tuberculosis
   c. Pnemonia
   d. Endocarditis

7. When treating a 70-year-old Caucasian male in the office for hypertension, which of the following is the most appropriate threshold to treat?

   a. Start therapy for BP >150/90 mm Hg.
   b. Start therapy for BP >140/90 mm Hg.
   c. Start therapy for BP >160/90 mm Hg.
   d. Do not start therapy in those over the age of 70 years.

8. Which of the following medications is considered high-intensity therapy for dyslipidemia?

   a. Atorvastatin 40 mg p.o. daily
   b. Atorvastatin 10 mg p.o. daily
   c. Simvastatin 20 mg p.o. daily
   d. Pravastatin 40 mg p.o. daily

9. All patients being started on statin therapy should have which baseline laboratories drawn?

   a. CPK
   b. Hgb A1c
   c. Pancreatic enzymes
   d. ALT

10. A patient presents with chest pain; he describes the pain as occurring only when he walks upstairs while carrying groceries; it only lasts 2 to 3 minutes and resolves with rest. Which of the following diagnosis best describes the clinical phenomena?

    a. Stable angina
    b. Unstable angina
    c. Variant angina
    d. Acute coronary syndrome

Answers with Rationales

1. (b) Smoking cessation

   Rationale: Smoking cessation is most important as smoking is a significant risk factor for peripheral arterial disease and continued smoking will further contribute to increase complications.

2. (b) Carvediolol

   Rationale: Carvediolol is a β-blocker that blocks β cells in the sympathetic nervous system.

3. (c) If there are no contraindications start high-intensity statins

   Rationale: The LDL needs to be below 100 mg/dL, so high-intensity statins should be considered as the LDL is 200 in this patient.

4. (c) Ankle–brachial indexes of the lower extremities

   Rationale: This test is done to check for peripheral arterial disease of the legs. This test should be the first test done as it is noninvasive and can be done right in the office setting.

5. (c) Increase or start a loop diuretic

   Rationale: The patient is demonstrating signs and symptoms of increased HF and has a significant weight gain most likely secondary to increased fluid retention. A loop diuretic should be initiated if not started previously and increase if the patient is already on such medication.

6. (d) Endocarditis

   Rationale: IV drug users are at high risk of staph and other infections secondary to nonsterile technique and products utilized to mix drugs. These individuals are at very high risk for the development of endocarditis. The patient's symptoms and IV drug use in this question are suggestive of such a diagnosis.

7. (b) Start therapy for BP >140/90 mm Hg

   Rationale: Patients above 70 are more prone to the development of hypertensive and should be treated early on in order to prevent myocardial problems.

8. (a) Atorvastatin 40 mg p.o. daily

   Rationale: Atorvastatin at the 10 mg dose is mild–intensity therapy for dyslipidemia. Atorvastatin at the 40 mg dose is high-intensity therapy for dyslipidemia.

9. (d) ALT

   Rationale: Statin drugs can cause elevation of liver enzymes. The ALT should be assessed pretreatment and after treatment has been initiated.

10. (a) Stable angina

    Rationale: The patient's symptoms occur on exertion and are relieved in a timely manner with rest, which is suggestive of stable angina.

Suggested Readings

Crawford, M. H. (Ed.). (2014). *Current diagnosis and treatment: Cardiology* (4th ed.). New York, NY: McGraw-Hill Education.

Eckel, R. H., Jakicic, J. M., Ard, J. D., Hubbard, V. S., de Jesus, J. M., Lee, I., . . . Yanovski, S. Z. (2013). 2013 AHA/ACC Guideline on lifestyle management to reduce cardiovascular risk: A report of the American College of Cardiology/American Heart Association task force on practice guidelines. *Circulation, 129,* S76–S99. doi:10.1161/01.cir.0000437740.48606.d1

Fihn, S. D., Gardin, M. J., Abrams, J., Berra, K., Blankenship, J. C., Douglas, P. S., . . . Williams, S. V. (2012). 2012 ACCF/AHA/ACP/AATS/PCNA/SCAI/STS guideline for the diagnosis and management of patients with stable ischemic heart disease. *Journal of the American College of Cardiology, 60*(24), 1–121.

James, P. A., Oparil, S., Carter, B. L., Cushman, W. C., Dennison-Himmelfarb, C., Handler, J., . . . Ortiz, E. (2013). 2014 evidence-based guideline for the management of high blood pressure in adults: Report from the panel members appointed to the Eighth Joint Commission National Committee (JNC 8). *Journal of the American Medical Association, 311*(5), 507–520. doi:10.1001/jama.2013.284427

Mozaffarian, D., Benjamin, E. J., Go, A. S., Arnett, D. K., Blaha, M. J., Cushman, M., . . . Turner, M. B. (2015). Heart disease and stroke statistics—2015 update a report from the American Heart Association. *Circulation, 131,* e1–e294. doi:10.1161/CIR.0000000000000152

Nishimura, R. A., Otto, C. M., Bonow, R. O., Carabello, B. A., Erwin, J. P., Guyton, R. A., . . . Thomas, J. D. (2014). 2014 AHA/ACC guideline for the management of patients with valvular heart disease: A report of the American College of Cardiology/American Heart Association task force on practice guidelines. *Journal of the American College of Cardiology, 63*(22), e57–e185. doi:/10.1016/j.jacc.2014.02.536

Nwankwo, T., Yoon, S. S., Burt, V., Gu, Q. (2013). Hypertension among adults in the United States: National health and nutrition examination survey, 2011–2012. *NCHS Data Brief*, 133, 1–8.

Rooke, T. W., Hirsch, A. T., Misra, S., Sidway, A. N., Beckman, A. J., Findeiss, L. K., . . . Ziegler, R. E. (2011). 2011 ACCF/ AHA focused update of the guidelines for the management of patients with peripheral artery disease (updating the 2005 guideline): A report of the American College of Cardiology foundation/American Heart Association task force on practice guidelines. *Circulation, 124*, 2020–2045. doi:10.1161/ CIR.0b013e31822e80c3

Stone, N. J., Robinson, J., Lichtenstein, A. H., Bairey Mertz, C. N., Blum, C. B., Eckel, R. H., . . . Wilson, P. W. (2013). 2013 ACC/ AHA guideline on the treatment of blood cholesterol to reduce atherosclerotic cardiovascular risk in adults: A report of the American College of Cardiology/American Heart Association Task Force on Practice Guidelines. *Journal of the American College of Cardiology, 63*, 2889–2934. Retrieved from http:// circ.ahajournals.org/

Toth, P. P., Potter, D., & Ming, E. E. (2012). Prevalence of lipid abnormalities in the United States: The national health and nutrition examination survey 2003-2006. *Journal of Clinical Lipidology, 6*(4), 325–330. doi:10.1016/j.jacl.2012.05.002

Yancy, C. W., Jessup, M., Bozkurt, B., Butler, J., Casey, D., Drazner, M. H., . . . Wilkoff, B. (2013). 2013 ACCF/AHA guideline for management of heart failure A report of the American College of Cardiology Foundation/American Heart Association Task Force on practice guidelines. *Circulation, 128*, e240–e327. doi:10.1016/CIR.0b013e31829e8776

Chapter 5

Gastrointestinal Disorders

AtNena Luster-Tucker

Case Presentation

Directions: Carefully review the case study presented below. At the end of the chapter, answer the review questions. Compare your answers to the correct answers listed in the Review Section.

History of Present Illness: A 56-year-old Japanese female presents to the emergency department with complaints of generalized abdominal pain for 12 hours. The patient describes the pain as waxing and waning and difficult to characterize. She also reports nausea with one episode of emesis earlier today. The patient's past medical history includes hypertension, which is uncontrolled. She is uninsured and does not have a primary care provider. Last physical examination was 3 years ago. She reports having similar episodes of pain over the past 4 months of shorter duration and lesser intensity. Previous episodes occurred after eating and resolved spontaneously. She did not seek care for previous episodes of pain due to the lack of health insurance. A 10-lb weight loss and aversion to food has developed in the past 2 months.

Allergies: No known drug allergies

Medications: Over-the-counter "BC Powder" as needed for headaches and back pain

Past Medical History: Uncontrolled hypertension

Past Social History: Tobacco use (50 pack-year history), alcohol use (one to two glasses of wine per night)

Past Surgical History: Cesarean section, hysterectomy

Vital Signs: Blood pressure 105/75, pulse 118, respirations 22, and temperature 98.2°F

Physical Examination:
Physical examination reveals generalized tenderness to the abdomen. No masses are palpable.

Common, Pertinent Clinical Diagnoses + Information

The patient who presents with a gastrointestinal complaint stands to be one of the most complex patients seen in the clinical setting due to the density of the intra-abdominal anatomy as well as the interrelationships of the organs/organ systems. For these reasons, it is imperative that the nurse practitioner complete a thorough history and physical examination. One must also consider gastrointestinal complaints that originate outside of the gastrointestinal tract. Cardiovascular, genitourinary, and gynecologic disorders should also be considered.

Finally, patients with psychosocial and/or mental health issues may present with nonspecific gastrointestinal complaints such as vague abdominal pain, nausea, vomiting, and/or changes in bowel habits. Two primary factors influence the development of a number of gastrointestinal disorders: adequate dietary fiber intake and alcohol consumption in moderation. The recommended amount of dietary fiber intake is based on sex and age.

Sex	Age 50 and Under	Ager 51 and Over
Male	38 g	30 g
Female	25 g	21 g

Alcohol consumption in moderate can be defined as one drink per day for women and up to two drinks per day for men. This aforementioned figure is not intended to be calculated as an average over several days.

Gastroesophageal Reflux Disease

Description of the Disease: Gastroesophageal reflux disease (GERD) is the result of gastric secretions being regurgitated into the esophagus. The acidic nature of the gastric contents results in irritation of the mucosa. Chronic irritation leads damage to the esophageal tissues and places the patient at risk for cancer of the esophagus.

Epidemiology:
- Dietary habits in the United States have contributed to GERD as a common disorder seen in Americans. As many as 40% of Americans have experienced GERD symptoms. Gastroesophageal reflux can occur at any age but is most prevalent in those over the age of 40. Males and females are equally affected.

Etiology:
- Reflux of gastric secretions can be due to a mechanical or functional cause. A functional relaxation of the lower esophageal sphincter can be due to medications, foods, and/or alcohol intake. A defect in the lower esophageal sphincter will result in a mechanical cause.

Risk Factors:
- Obesity
- Nonsteroidal anti-inflammatory drug (NSAID)/aspirin use
- Alcohol intake
- Large meals before bed
- High-fat diet
- Caffeine intake

Signs and Symptoms:
- Abnormal (sour) breath odor
- Burning sensation to the chest
- Burning sensation to the throat
- Indigestion
- Nausea
- Cough
- Tooth decay
- Hoarseness

Differential Diagnoses:
- Barrett esophagus
- Gastritis
- Myocardial infarction
- Angina
- Chronic cough
- *Helicobacter pylori* infection

Diagnostic Studies:
- A clinical diagnosis can be made based on the patient's presentation. The gold standard for diagnosis is esophageal motility studies.

Treatment:
- First-line treatment is lifestyle changes including weight loss and avoidance of aggravating agents. Pharmacologic treatment should be initiated in patients who do not have resolution with lifestyle changes alone. H_2 blockers and proton pump inhibitors can be used with outcomes expected in 4 to 6 weeks.

Extreme cases and those who exhibit worrisome symptoms such as dysphagia and weight loss should be referred to a gastrointestinal specialist for surgical intervention.

Peptic Ulcer Disease

Description of the Disease: Peptic ulcer disease encompasses both gastric and duodenal ulcers.

Epidemiology:
- Approximately 4.5 million Americans suffer from peptic ulcer disease. Duodenal ulcers occur more commonly than gastric ulcers with approximately 10% of the population suffering from a duodenal ulcer at some point. Gastric ulcers have a much higher risk for malignancy.

Etiology:
- The most common cause of peptic ulcer disease is an infection with *H. pylori*. Other causative agents include medications, which disrupt the mucosal layer of the stomach such as NSAIDs and bisphosphonates.

Risk Factors:
- NSAID use
- Bisphosphonate use
- Cigarette smoking
- Alcohol intake
- Gastritis
- GERD

Signs and Symptoms:
- Indigestion
- Bloating
- Chest pain
- Epigastric pain/burning
- Nausea
- Pain related to meals
- Hematemesis
- Melena

Differential Diagnoses:
- GERD
- Gastritis
- Myocardial infarction
- Gastroenteritis

Diagnostic Studies:
- Because the most likely cause of peptic ulcer disease is *H. pylori* infection, *H. pylori* testing is the least invasive method of diagnosing the disorder. The gold standard of diagnosis is endoscopic evaluation to allow for direct visualization.

Treatment:
- Treatment of *H. pylori* using an appropriate medication regiment is necessary for all patients who are *H. pylori* positive. Current regimens include triple therapy for 14 days using a proton pump inhibitor and antibiotic combination. Antibiotic selection should be individualized and can include amoxicillin, clarithromycin, tetracycline, and metronidazole.

Biliary Disease

Description of the Disease: Biliary disease is a general term used to describe disorders that affect the biliary tract of the gastrointestinal tract. The most common diagnosis is cholelithiasis (gallstones) and cholecystitis (inflammation of the gallbladder). For the purpose of this section, we will discuss the aforementioned disorders only.

Epidemiology:
- As many as 20% of Americans have gallstones. Of those with gallstones, one-third will develop acute cholecystitis. Gallstone development is more common in females and during pregnancy. The incidence also increases with age.

Etiology:

- Cholecystitis can be categorized as calculous or acalculous cholecystitis. Calculous cholecystitis is caused by blockage of the cystic duct by a gallstone or biliary sludge. Gallstones are made from small crystals of salt and cholesterol. Acalculous cholecystitis is caused by direct infection or injury to the gallbladder. Choledochal lithiasis is severe complication of cholecystitis and can lead to gangrene of the gallbladder. Choledochal lithiasis is evidenced by dilation of the common bile duct.

Risk Factors:

- Female sex
- Obesity
- Rapid weight loss
- Hormone therapy
- Ethnic race groups
- Pregnancy
- Advanced age
- Diabetes mellitus
- Sickle cell disease
- Cardiovascular disease

Signs and Symptoms:

- Abdominal pain, most commonly to the right upper quadrant
- Radiation of pain to the back and shoulder
- Pain worse after meals
- Nausea
- Vomiting
- Fever
- Diarrhea
- Light-colored stools
- Jaundice (occurs most commonly in the presence of Choledocholithiasis)

Differential Diagnoses:

- Pancreatitis
- Gastritis
- Cholelithiasis
- Choledocholithiasis
- Cholecystitis

Diagnostic Studies:

- Laboratory test
  - Complete blood count (CBC) to evaluate the white blood cell count in the presence of infection
  - Bilirubin level
  - Alkaline phosphatase
  - Aminotransferases (AST and ALT)
- Imaging
  - Ultrasonography is the primary imaging study used for the diagnosis of cholelithiasis and cholecystitis. Computer abdominal tomography (CAT) and radiographic images yield very little help in the diagnosis of biliary disease.

Treatment:

- Treatment of gallstones (cholelithiasis) is primarily controlled by diet. Patients with gallstones should follow a low-fat diet with the avoidance of irritating foods.
- Acute cholecystitis is treated through surgical intervention. Patients will also need intravenous fluid hydration and pain control. Antibiotics are indicated when the patient has a poor clinical appearance.

Diverticular Disease

Description of the Disease: Pouch-like defects that occur in the colon are diagnosed as diverticula. If the diverticula become infected, diverticulitis is present.

Epidemiology:
- The incidence of diverticular disease in the Unites States is relatively high. The risk of diverticula development increases with age. Young adults with diverticular disease are more likely to experience complications related to the disease.

Etiology:
- Diverticula result from a chronic lack of dietary fiber. Once diverticula have developed, the defects cannot be reversed. Infection of the diverticula pouches can result from a number of sources including dietary substances that collect in the pouches as well as intra-abdominal bacteria.
- Diverticulosis is the diagnosis for the presence of diverticula, and the physical examination is without abnormality with a nontender abdomen. Acute diverticulitis is considered an acute abdomen with the presence of rebound tenderness, Rovsing sign, and peritoneal signs on physical examination.

Risk Factors:
- Obesity
- Physical inactivity
- Low dietary fiber intake
- Female gender

Signs and Symptoms:
The patient with diverticula may be asymptomatic. The symptomatic patient may experience the following:
- Bloating
- Abdominal pain
- Constipation
- Diarrhea

Differential Diagnoses:
- Diverticulosis
- Diverticulitis
- Mesenteric ischemia
- Diarrhea
- Gastroenteritis
- Celiac disease

Diagnostic Studies:
- Laboratory tests
  - CBC to evaluate white blood cell count for the presence of infection
  - Reticulocyte count to evaluate the presence of gastrointestinal bleeding
- Imaging
  - CAT with contrast is the primary diagnostic tool. The use of CAT scan can identify diverticula as well as rupture and perforation.

Treatment:
- Diverticulosis is chronic, managed by diet. Patients are instructed to avoid nuts and seeds as well as increase dietary fiber intake. Fiber supplementation may be used.
- Uncomplicated cases of diverticulitis can be managed in the outpatient setting with oral antibiotics and close outpatient follow-up.

Appendicitis

Description of the Disease: Appendicitis can be defined as inflammation of the inner lining of the vermiform appendix.

Epidemiology:
- Appendicitis is one of the most common causes of an acute surgical abdomen in the United States. There are approximately 250,000 cases of acute appendicitis each year. The incidence of appendicitis increases with age. Peak age range is the late teenage years, and a decline is seen in the geriatric population.

Etiology:
- Acute appendicitis occurs when the appendix becomes obstructed with debris and salts. Obstruction can also occur secondary to bacterial infection but is far less common.

Risk Factors:
- Family predisposition
- Extremes of age

Signs and Symptoms:
- Abdominal pain; most commonly in the right lower quadrant and/or umbilical area
- Nausea
- Vomiting
- Anorexia
- Fever
- Rovsing sign (pain elicited in the left lower quadrant when the right lower quadrant is palpated)
- Obturator sign (pain elicited in the right lower quadrant when the right hip is internally and externally rotated)
- Psoas sign (pain elicited in the right lower quadrant when the right hip is extended or flexed against resistance)

Differential Diagnoses:
- Diverticulitis
- Pelvic inflammatory disease
- Ectopic pregnancy
- Urinary tract infection
- Ovarian cyst
- Tubo–ovarian abscess
- Ovarian torsion

Diagnostic Studies:
- Laboratory testing
  - CBC to evaluate white blood cell count which is indicative of infection
  - Urinalysis is used to rule out differential diagnoses such as urinary tract infection and/or renal colic.
  - β-HCG is used to rule out pregnancy and should be performed on all patients of childbearing age.
- Imaging
  - CT scan is the primary diagnostic tool used to identify an acute appendicitis. The current standard is the use of contrast to highlight the intra-abdominal structures. Evidence is emerging to support the use of noncontrast CT scan for the diagnosis of acute appendicitis.
  - When CT scan is not an option or when concern exists over the associated radiation exposure, ultrasonography can be used. Ultrasonography can only be used to identify an enlarged or inflamed appendix as a healthy appendix cannot routinely be seen on ultrasound.

Treatment:
- Removal of the appendix via appendectomy is the only definitive cure for acute appendicitis. All patients with acute appendicitis should be referred for surgical intervention. Antibiotics with aerobic and anaerobic coverage are indicated when the patient exhibits signs of overt infection and/or peritonitis.
- Debate exists over the nonoperative management of acute appendicitis using watchful waiting, hydration, and antibiotics. At the time of this publication, nonoperative management is not considered the standard of care.

Pancreatitis

Description of the Disease: Pancreatitis can be defined as inflammation of the pancreas that is caused by autodigestion of the pancreas by an overproduction of pancreatic enzymes.

Epidemiology:
- The incidence of pancreatitis in the United States is approximately 40 cases per 100,000 adults. The age at the time of occurrence is dependent upon the underlying cause. Pancreatitis due to alcohol and drug abuse is seen more frequently in middle-age adults while pancreatitis secondary to medications and chronic disease is more prominent in the older population.

Etiology:
- There are a number of etiologies that lead to the overproduction of pancreatic enzymes. These causes include alcohol abuse (most common), cholelithiasis, abdominal trauma, abdominal surgery, medications,

toxins, endocrine dysfunction, and viral infections such as mumps and hepatitis. Pancreatitis can be acute or chronic in nature; however, the majority of patients with acute pancreatitis never fully recover.

Risk Factors:
- Alcohol abuse
- Intravenous drug use
- Gallstones
- Male sex

Signs and Symptoms:
- Abdominal pain
- Weight loss
- Fever
- Nausea and vomiting
- Tachycardia
- Diarrhea
- Jaundice
- Steatorrhea
- Indigestion
- Light-colored stools
- Cullen sign (bluish discoloration around the umbilicus that results from inflammation, edema, and/or bleeding into the subcutaneous tissue around the umbilicus)
- Grey Turner sign (reddish-brown discoloration along the flanks that results from retroperitoneal bleeding)

Differential Diagnoses:
- Cholelithiasis
- Cholecystitis
- Hepatitis
- Gastritis
- Mesenteric ischemia
- Peptic ulcer disease
- Pneumonia
- Myocardial infarction
- Pancreatic cancer

Diagnostic Studies:
- Laboratory testing
  - Serum amylase is elevated approximately three times normal in the case of pancreatitis with a return to normal in 48 to 72 hours. A normal amylase does not exclude pancreatitis.
  - Serum lipase is elevated approximately three times normal in the case of pancreatitis with a return to normal in 7 to 14 days. A lipase to amylase ratio >4 is suggestive of alcoholic pancreatitis.
  - Electrolytes include glucose, potassium, calcium, magnesium, and phosphorus.
  - Liver function tests
  - Bilirubin
  - CBC to evaluate WBC in the presence of infection
- Imaging
  - CT scan with contrast is the preferred imaging modality.
  - Abdominal ultrasound can also be used as a noninvasive imaging method.
  - Magnetic resonance imaging can be used when contrast is contraindicated.
  - Endoscopic retrograde cholangiopancreatography (ERCP) and magnetic resonance cholangiopancreatography (MRCP) are more invasive methods of evaluating acute pancreatitis.

Treatment:
- Acute pancreatitis is routinely treated in the inpatient setting with intravenous hydration and nutrition. The patient should also receive parental analgesics. In the case of severe pancreatitis, intensive care services may be warranted due to end-organ damage.
- The mainstay of chronic pancreatitis management is limiting exposure to exacerbating agents such as alcohol, tobacco, and high-fat meals. Pancreatic enzyme replacement may be warranted in the patient with extensive, irreversible pancreas damage.

Gastroenteritis

Description of the Disease: Gastroenteritis is a nonspecific term used to describe inflammation of the gastrointestinal tract.

Epidemiology:
- An exact occurrence is difficult to determine because many patients do not seek medical attention for mild cases. It is estimated that 179 million patients are treated for gastroenteritis each year with no relationship to age, sex, or race.

Etiology:
- The norovirus is the cause of the majority of cases of gastroenteritis. Localized outbreaks of gastroenteritis can occur secondary to the transmission of food-borne, waterborne, environmental, and person-to-person spread of disease. In many cases gastroenteritis is a diagnosis of exclusion, thus should be used cautiously.

Risk Factors:
- Travel to Asia, Africa, and South America
- Day care attendance in children
- Exposure to localized outbreaks
- Immunocompromised state
- Consuming untreated water

Signs and Symptoms:
- Diarrhea
- Nausea
- Vomiting
- Nonspecific abdominal pain
- Bloating
- Anorexia

Differential Diagnoses:
- Acute appendicitis
- Diverticulitis
- Pseudomembranous colitis
- Toxic megacolon
- Intestinal parasites
- Cholecystitis/cholelithiasis

Diagnostic Studies:
Diagnostic testing is focused on ruling out underlying causes and should be tailored to the individual patient presentation. Testing may include the following:
- CBC to evaluate WBC
- Electrolyte panel
- Amylase
- Lipase
- Liver function test
- Urinalysis
- β-HCG
- Radiographic images of the abdomen
- CT scan
- Abdominal ultrasonography

Treatment:
- The goal of treatment is maintaining hydration and electrolyte balance. Meals should be small and frequent until the resolution of symptoms. There is no evidence to withhold food in the case of mild gastroenteritis that is caused by the norovirus.
- Severe cases may require hospitalization for hydration and specialist evaluation.

Inflammatory Bowel Disease

Description of the Disease: Inflammatory bowel disease is a term used to describe a group of diagnoses that results from inflammatory of the lining of the bowel. Crohn disease and ulcerative colitis are the main types.

Epidemiology:
- As many as 2 million American adults have some form of inflammatory bowel disease. Women have a slightly increased incidence over men with the majority of diagnoses occurring in young to middle-aged patients.

Etiology:
- There are three major etiologies associated with the development of inflammatory bowel disease—genetic predisposition, abnormal immune response, and inflammatory response to gut microorganisms. While the later etiologies have been identified, the cause of the response is not understood and thought to be idiopathic in nature.

Risk Factors:
- Cigarette smoking
- Genetic predisposition
- Low-fiber diet

Signs and Symptoms:
Signs and symptoms vary based on the area of the gastrointestinal tract that is involved. Generally speaking, the patient with inflammatory bowel disease may exhibit fever, fatigue, anemia, and body aches. In addition, specific signs and symptoms are more consistent with certain types of inflammatory bowel disease.
- Crohn disease
  - Abdominal cramping
  - Right lower quadrant abdominal pain
  - Diarrhea
  - Malabsorption
  - Weight loss
  - Nausea and vomiting
  - Perianal complications such as fistulas and abscesses
- Ulcerative colitis
  - Constipation
  - Bloody diarrhea
  - Umbilical and/or left lower quadrant abdominal pain
  - Abdominal cramping
  - Irritable bowel syndrome
    - A chronic gastrointestinal disorder that causes cramping, indigestion, abdominal pain, and altered bowel habits is idiopathic in nature.

Differential Diagnoses:
- Celiac disease
- Irritable bowel syndrome
- Lactose intolerance
- Biliary disease
- Gastrointestinal bacterial infections
- Intestinal parasites
- Appendicitis
- Diverticulitis
- Gastroenteritis

Diagnostic Studies:
- Laboratory testing
  - CBC to evaluate the patient for anemia
  - B_{12} evaluation
  - Folate level
  - Iron studies
  - Erythrocyte sedimentation rate (ESR)
  - C-reactive protein (CRP)
  - Stool studies

- Imaging
  - Colonoscopy allows for direct visualization of the bowel mucosa.
  - Flexible sigmoidoscopy can be used to distal ulcerative colitis and proctitis.
  - Abdominal ultrasonography is a valuable, noninvasive tool that can be used for the diagnosis of Crohn disease.
  - CT scan, ultrasonography, and magnetic resonance imaging (MRI) can all be used to identify complications of inflammatory bowel disease such as stenosis and fistulas.

Treatment:
There are four steps associated with the treatment of inflammatory bowel disease, which are as follows:
- Step I: Aminosalicylates
- Step II: Antibiotics
- Step III: Immunomodulators
- Step IV: Clinical trial agents

The typical management of ulcerative colitis includes supportive treatment and stepwise medication implementation until favorable outcomes are produced. The focus of Crohn disease is healing of the mucosal. Hospitalization can provide intravenous hydration and nutrition to allow for NPO status and bowel rest. Surgical intervention is warranted when extensive mucosal damage is present. Corticosteroids can also be used in severe cases.

Gastrointestinal Cancers

Description of the Disease: Gastrointestinal cancers encompass a group of malignancies that develop within the gastrointestinal tract. This includes stomach, colon, pancreatic, anal, rectal, small intestine, appendiceal, and esophageal cancer. For the purpose of this chapter, we will discuss the general principles of gastrointestinal cancers with a focus on colon cancer screening.

Epidemiology:
- The incidence of gastrointestinal cancer increases with age. The rarest of the cancers is anal cancer, with the most common being colon cancer.

Etiology:
- The etiology of cancer development is not clearly understood. While genetics play a role, exposure to carcinogenic agents also contributes.

Risk Factors:
- Tobacco use
- Alcohol intake
- Family history
- Advanced age
- Male sex
- Ethnic race
- Low-fiber, high-fat diet
- Smoked foods and salted meats/fish contain large amounts of nitrates

Signs and Symptoms:
- Abdominal pain
- Weight loss
- Changes in bowel habits
- Nausea and vomiting
- Anorexia
- Fever
- Jaundice

Diagnostic Studies:
- Laboratory testing
  - CBC, reticulocyte count, and iron studies should be used to identify the cause of anemia.
  - Bilirubin
  - Liver function studies

- Imaging
  - Most gastrointestinal cancers can be identified using CT scan, ultrasonography, and MRI.
  - Direct visualization via endoscopy and colonoscopy with biopsy is the method of definitive diagnosis of cancers of the esophagus, stomach, colon, anus, and rectum.

Treatment:

The mainstay of treatment is surgical removal of the malignancy followed by chemotherapy and/or radiation depending on the extent of the cancer. Treatment plans are individualized depending on a number of factors including the cancer stage. Regardless of gastrointestinal cancer type, the key to treatment is early diagnosis and intervention. Colon cancer screening guidelines are in place to facilitate early recognition.

- Colon cancer screening
  - U. S. Preventative Services Task Force (USPSTF) recommends colorectal cancer screening begin at age 50 and continue until age 75 for those at average risk. Colonoscopy is the screening tool of choice due to its ability to detect colon cancer as well as remove colon precancerous colon polyps. Colonoscopies are recommended in 10-year intervals. Annual fecal occult testing is also recommended in conjunction with the screening colonoscopy. Other screening modalities also exist. Benefits and risk vary according to method.
  - Those with risk factors and/or familial history should begin colorectal cancer screening at an earlier age.
  - The decision to continue screening those 76-85 years of age should be an individual decision, based on the patient's history and risk.

Mesenteric Ischemia

Description of the Disease: Mesenteric ischemia is a lack of adequate blood flow to the bowel wall, which leads to peritonitis, gangrene, and necrosis of the bowel if left untreated.

Epidemiology:

- Mesenteric ischemia is largely considered a disease of the elderly due to the association with atherosclerosis. The incidence of mesenteric ischemia is not fully understood because the disorder is grossly misdiagnosed. In the acute care setting, approximately 0.1% of hospitalizations are due to acute mesenteric ischemia.

Etiology:

- Mesenteric ischemia is caused by inadequate blood flow to the mesenteric vessels of the bowel wall. The lack of blood flow can be venous or arterial in nature from embolism or thrombosis. Atherosclerotic vascular disease is the most common. It may also be caused by medications, dehydration, and hypotension.

Risk Factors:

- Smoking
- Hypertension
- Hypercholesterolemia
- Atherosclerotic vascular disease
- Cocaine abuse
- Vasculitis
- Radiation
- Congestive heart failure
- Intra-abdominal malignancy

Signs and Symptoms:

- Chronic intermittent abdominal pain that is consistently associated with meals
- Pain that is disproportional to physical examination
- Food aversion
- Progressive weight loss
- Malnutrition
- Nausea and vomiting
- Bloody diarrhea
- Malaise
- Fever (acute mesenteric ischemia in the later stages)
- Sepsis (acute mesenteric ischemia in the later stages)

Differential Diagnoses:
- Gallbladder disease
- Colitis
- Gastritis
- Acute myocardial infarction

Diagnostic Studies:
- Laboratory testing
  - CBC: May be within range initially with an increase in the white blood cell count seen as the disease progresses
  - Chemistry: Electrolyte abnormalities may occur with metabolic acidosis developed late in the disease.
  - Lactic acid: May be within range. Elevated lactic acid seen in those with tissue death
  - Coagulation studies:
    - Amylase/lipase: Primarily used to rule out differential diagnoses. An elevated amylase may be seen in the patient with mesenteric ischemia.
    - Pregnancy testing: All women of childbearing age with abdominal pain should be tested for pregnancy. Those with a history of tubal ligation should also be tested due to the risk of ectopic pregnancy.
    - Urinalysis: Pyuria can cause abdominal pain as well as generalized symptoms such as malaise, nausea, and fever as in the case of pyelonephritis.
    - ECG: A 12-lead ECG should be performed to rule out cardiac causes.
- Imaging
  - Abdominal X-ray, 2D-view (flat and erect): Used to rule out differential diagnoses such as perforation of the bowel as evidenced by free air in the abdomen, volvulus, ileus, and/or bowel obstruction
  - CT scan of the abdomen and pelvis: CT scan will show evidence of thickened bowel wall, bowel stranding, free fluid in the abdomen can be seen in the patient with mesenteric ischemia. Portal venous air may be seen and is indicative of bowel necrosis.
  - Abdominal CT angiography (CTA): The abdominal CTA is considered to be the diagnostic test of choice due to the noninvasive nature and high specificity. It can also be used as a treatment modality.
  - Ultrasonography: Duplex ultrasonography can be used in the patient with contraindications to CT scan/angiography. Ultrasound lacks the sensitivity seen with CT scan and/or angiography.
  - MRI: MRI is not considered to be a practical diagnostic tool for the patient with suspected mesenteric ischemia due to factors such as cost and time.

Treatment:

Acute Mesenteric Ischemia
- The patient with acute mesenteric ischemia should be referred for emergent surgical evaluation and intervention. The care of the patient with acute mesenteric ischemia includes the following:
  - Resuscitation with intravenous fluids should be aggressive and initiated as soon as the disease is suspected.
  - The patient who is severely hypotensive due to sepsis may require the use of vasopressive medication and is outside of the scope of this presentation.
  - Broad-spectrum antibiotics should be implemented early for the treatment of potential translocation of intestinal bacteria across compromised bowel wall.
  - Parenteral opioid analgesic are indicated to provide adequate pain control.
  - Anticoagulants are indicated for the patient who is identified as having a vasocclussive cause of acute mesenteric ischemia such as portal vein thrombosis.
  - Invasive/operative
    - The mainstays of treatment for the patient with acute mesenteric ischemia are surgical intervention and/or angiography.
    - Angiography is indicated for those with acute mesenteric ischemia without evidence of peritonitis. Angiography is used to identify the cause of the ischemia that may include thromboembolic disease and vasoactive (spasms) and nonocclusive sources. Intra-arterial administration of vasodilating drugs are during the procedure will lead to resolution of the disease.
    - The presence of peritonitis warrants immediate surgical intervention.

Chronic Mesenteric Ischemia
The stable patient who presents with symptoms consistent with chronic mesenteric ischemia should be referred for surgical consultation/evaluation. A vascular surgeon or interventional radiologist will become part of the care treatment to perform the CTA and angiography if necessary.

- Nonpharmacologic
  - Long-term anticoagulants may be warranted based on the etiology of the mesenteric ischemia.
- Invasive/operative
  - Outpatient CTA/angiography is the mainstay of treatment for the stable patient with chronic mesenteric ischemia. The CTA is used to evaluate the patient and localize the source of the ischemia. Subsequent angiography is used to reestablish adequate perfusion via angioplasty or stent placement.

Review Section

Review Questions

1. Colorectal cancer: The nurse practitioner is educating a group of students regarding colorectal cancer. Which of the following statements regarding risk factors for colon cancer is true?

   a. Chronic diarrhea with steatorrhea is a common warning sign for colon cancer.
   b. Having a first-degree relative with colon cancer increases the risk for colon cancer.
   c. The number of colon polyps a patient has an inverse relationship with the risk for colon cancer development.
   d. Performing a thorough abdominal assessment is critical to the diagnosis of colon cancer as most colon masses can be palpated before symptoms are present.

2. Gallbladder: While assessing a 42-year-old Hispanic female with abdominal pain, the nurse practitioner notes pain elicited when he/she deeply palpates the right upper quadrant of the abdomen during inspiration. This finding is most consistent with:

   a. acute cholecystitis.
   b. acute appendicitis.
   c. gastroesophageal reflux disease.
   d. mesenteric ischemia.

3. Appendicitis: The nurse practitioner is assessing a patient who presents with right lower quadrant abdominal pain. Based on the patient's presentation, acute appendicitis is the leading diagnosis. Which of the following would be consistent with the diagnosis of acute appendicitis?

   a. Pain and indigestion after meals
   b. Positive Murphy sign
   c. Weight loss and changes in bowel habits
   d. Positive Psoas sign

4. Diverticulitis: Jackie is a 53-year-old female who presents with left lower quadrant abdominal pain for 5 days. She denies nausea, vomiting, diarrhea, and constipation. Oral intake is adequate. A fever is reported with a temperature maximum of 101.2°F.

The abdominal assessment reveals tenderness to palpation of the left lower quadrant of the abdomen. The remainder of the physical examination is without abnormality. After completion of diagnostic testing, the nurse practitioner diagnoses the patient with acute diverticulitis. Appropriate management of the patient would be:

   a. oral analgesics and NPO status for 24 hours to allow the bowel to rest.
   b. oral antibiotics and outpatient follow-up within 48 hours.
   c. watchful waiting and outpatient follow-up in 1 week.
   d. inpatient hospitalization for intravenous nutrition and surgical intervention.

5. Pancreatitis: Chris is a 42-year-old male who presents to the clinic with abdominal pain, nausea, and vomiting. He has a history of alcoholism and hepatitis B. Based on the patient's history, physical examination, and diagnostic test results, the nurse practitioner diagnoses the patient with pancreatitis. During the physical examination, a bluish discoloration was noted to the periumbilical area of the abdomen. This should be documented in the medical record as:

   a. Grey Turner sign.
   b. obturator sign.
   c. tap sign.
   d. Cullen sign.

6. Celiac Disease: A 20-year-old female presents to the university student health center with complaints of bloating and GI upset. The patient is thin, frail, and underweight according to her BMI. She reports the presence of the aforementioned symptoms beginning in her teenage years. The symptoms worsen after eating desserts and breads. The nurse practitioner is suspicious for:

   a. celiac disease.
   b. acute pancreatitis.
   c. folate deficiency anemia.
   d. Crohn disease.

7. Gastritis: Gastritis is a generic term used to describe irritation of the gastric mucosa. In assessing for possible gastritis, the nurse practitioner understands:

   a. increased dietary fiber is a known risk factor for the development of gastritis.
   b. the uses of nonsteroidal anti-inflammatory medications such as ibuprofen have not been proven to be a contributing factor in the development of gastritis.
   c. dietary modifications is the first line treatment for the patient with gastritis
   d. all patients with gastritis should be referred to a gastrointestinal specialist for monitoring due to the risk of developing gastric cancer secondary to gastritis.

8. GERD: Which of the following would *not* be included in the education given to the patient with gastroesophageal reflux disease (GERD)?

   a. Symptoms such as weight loss, chronic sore throat, and cough are expected side effects of treatment.
   b. Acetaminophen is preferred over ibuprofen as over the counter pain relief.
   c. Caffeine and alcohol should be avoided.
   d. Weight loss can help facilitate the control of symptoms.

9. Abdominal Assessment: The nurse practitioner understands that abdominal pain can be representative of a number of differential diagnoses that originate outside of the gastrointestinal system. Which of the following laboratory tests should be included in the assessment of a geriatric patient with epigastric pain?

   a. Antinuclear antibody test (ANA)
   b. Cardiac enzymes
   c. Reticulocyte count
   d. Rapid plasma reagin (RPR)

10. Fissure/Hemorrhoids: You are assessing a patient who has a history of an umbilical hernia. During the physical examination, a moderate-sized hernia is palpated at the umbilicus. Which of the following physical examination findings would warrant immediate intervention?

    a. Hernia is soft, spongy, and can be manually manipulated back into the abdominal cavity.
    b. Hernia is more prominent when the patient coughs or strains.
    c. Patient complains of mild tenderness when the hernia is manually manipulated back into the abdominal cavity.
    d. Hernia is fixed and unable to be manually pushed back into the abdominal cavity.

Answers with Rationales

1. (a) Having a first-degree relative with colon cancer increases the risk for colon cancer.

   Rationale: Having a first-degree relative with colon cancer places the patient at high risk for colon cancer development. Bowel changes such as alternating diarrhea and constipation are seen with colon cancer with the majority of masses being identified via imaging. Polyposis increases the risk for colon cancer development.

2. (a) Acute cholecystitis

   Rationale: Pain to the right upper quadrant with inspiration during palpation is considered a positive Murphy sign. Murphy sign is consistent with the diagnosis of acute cholecystitis.

3. (d) Positive Psoas sign

   Rationale: Psoas sign is positive when pain is elicited with extension and/or flexion of the thigh. The pain is the result of peritoneal irritation caused by an acute appendicitis.

4. (a) Oral antibiotics and outpatient follow-up within 48 hours.

   Rationale: Mild cases of diverticulitis can be managed on an outpatient basis with oral antibiotics. The key to outpatient management is close follow-up within 48 hours.

5. (c) Tap sign

   Rationale: Cullen sign is a bluish discoloration to the umbilical area of the abdomen that is caused by intraperitoneal hemorrhage, swelling, and/or bruising located in the subcutaneous fatty tissue around the umbilicus.

6. (a) Celiac disease

   Rationale: Celiac disease results in malabsorption due to intolerance to gluten. Symptoms include diarrhea, abdominal pain, and bloating when gluten-containing products are consumed. The patient should avoid wheat, rye, and barley.

7. (c) Dietary modifications is the first-line treatment for the patient with gastritis.

   Rationale: As with GERD, gastritis may be controlled with lifestyle changes such as dietary modifications, making it the first-line treatment. NSAIDs and decreased dietary fiber intake are both known risk factors for gastritis development. Referral to a specialist is warranted when the patient cannot be controlled with traditional measures and/or if diagnostic tests such as an EGD or barium swallow test are needed.

8. (a) Symptoms such as weight loss, chronic sore throat, and cough are expected side effects of treatment.

   Rationale: Weight loss, sore throat, nausea, vomiting, and cough are symptoms of severe GERD and warrant further evaluation. The aforementioned symptoms should be relieved with treatment, not aggravated by it.

9. (b) Cardiac enzymes

   Rationale: Patients with cardiovascular issues can present with abdominal complaints. Geriatric patients, women, and those with chronic health conditions are more likely to have an atypical presentation.

10. (d) Hernia is fixed and unable to be manually pushed back into the abdominal cavity.

    Rationale: The inability to reduce the hernia by manual manipulation is indicative of an incarcerated hernia. Incarcerated hernias warrant immediate surgical intervention.

Chapter 6

Women's Health Review

Kymberlee Montgomery and Owen C. Montgomery

Case Presentation

Directions: Carefully review the case study presented below. At the end of the chapter, answer the review questions. Compare your answers to the correct answers listed in the Review Section.

History of Present Illness: T. M. is a 42-year-old G1 P0010, Caucasian female who presents to the primary care office for a well-woman visit. Upon reviewing her history, T.M. tells the APRN that she has been experiencing irregular vaginal bleeding, right lower quadrant pain, and yellowish, slightly malodorous vaginal discharge for the past week. Her last menstrual period (LMP) was 3 months ago that lasted 7 days with moderate flow. T. M. reports severe menstrual cramping and breast tenderness with her LMP that required Ibuprofen 600 mg every 6 hours for 2 days to alleviate symptoms. Her last women's health examination was 3 years ago for a follow-up visit after a dilatation and evacuation for her incomplete abortion. She also was diagnosed and treated for a chlamydia trachomatis at that time.

Obstetrical History: Single intrauterine pregnancy (IUP) 3 years ago which resulted in a spontaneous abortion at 8 weeks requiring a dilatation and evacuation for prolonged vaginal bleeding.

Gynecologic History: Menarche at age 12; menstrual cycles were at 25- to 30-day intervals lasting 7 days until age 35 accompanied by severe dysmenorrhea and breast tenderness. Menstrual cycle became increasingly irregular at age 35, with periods of amenorrhea lasting 60 to 90 days until her current presentation; used oral contraceptive pills (OCP) off and on beginning at age 16 until age 32 for birth control and severe dysmenorrhea; discontinued OCPs for elevated blood pressure and difficulty adhering to daily regimen; has used male latex condoms irregularly with sexual activity; sexual activity with male partners only; coitarche age 15; 10 lifetime partners; reports two sexual partners in the last year with occasional condom use; denies anal penetration; sexually satisfied but reports dyspareunia with deep penetration; engages in oral sexual activity without protection. History of chlamydia 3 years ago, which was treated; history of genital warts and an abnormal Pap smear at age 24. Patient states that "the warts were burned off" and her repeat Pap smear 3 months after the abnormal Pap was normal. Has not had cervical screening of sexually transmitted infection (STI) screening for 3 years. Never had HIV screening; history of diagnostic laparoscopy at age 28 for right-sided pelvic pain; findings significant for endometriosis treated with cautery. Symptoms improved.

Medical History: Borderline hypertension (HTN) not treated with medication

Surgical History: Impacted wisdom teeth extraction age 16; no complications
Diagnostic laparoscopy age 28; endometriosis; no complications
Dilatation and evacuation age 39; incomplete abortion; no complications

Medications: Herbal Women's Herbal Supplement (unknown) from health food store

Allergies: Penicillin (hives)
Shellfish (anaphylaxis)
Banana (tongue swelling)

Social History: Single; works as a Human Resource Supervisor at a law firm; lives alone in a renovated loft apartment close to work and feels safe at home; denies a history of physical, emotional, and sexual abuse; currently in a sexual relationship with one partner; occasional condom use; feels safe in the relationship

Alcohol: Drinks two to three glasses of wine 3 days a week; reports smoking cigarettes only with alcohol consumption on the weekend; denies recreation drug use; belongs to the neighborhood fitness center but does not go often; has HMO medical insurance through her employer.

Immunizations: Has never received flu or Pneumovax vaccines; does not recall when she received her last tetanus injection

Family History: HTN and osteoporosis: Mother (alive age 79)
                    Colon cancer: Father (deceased age 52)

Review of Systems:
Constitutional: Well-appearing female; denies recent weight loss/gain, fever chills, or fatigue
Integumentary: Denies rashes, lesions, or changes in hair or nails
Head, Eyes, Ears, Nose, Throat (HEENT): Denies head trauma or dizziness; reports occasional headaches with onset of menses; denies eye drainage, redness, or pain; no visual changes, cataracts, glaucoma; wears magnification glasses for reading; last eye examination approximately 5 years ago; denies earaches, vertigo, tinnitus, hearing impairments, ear infections, or discharge; denies nasal congestion, discharge, bleeding, or irritation; reports seasonal allergies to trees
Breast: Denies breast self-examinations; has breast tenderness 2 days before menses; denies lumps or nipple discharge; never had a mammogram
Respiratory: Denies shortness of breath, cough, sputum, or wheezing; denies frequent respiratory illnesses; denies history of asthma, pneumonia, bronchitis
Cardiovascular: Denies chest pain, discomfort, palpitations, orthopnea, or edema
Gastrointestinal: Normal bowel movements once a day; occasional diarrhea when under stress; denies rectal bleeding, black or tarry stools; reports a hemorrhoid during pregnancy that is no longer present; denies liver or gallbladder issues
Genitourinary/Urinary: See HPI; occasional loss of urine when coughing or sneezing if her bladder is full
Musculoskeletal: Denies injury, stiffness, weakness, muscle and joint pain, neck pain, arthritis, or stiffness
Neurologic: Alert and oriented; appropriate affect; denies seizure, numbness, dizziness, vertigo, paralysis, changes in speech, balance, or mental status
Hematologic: Denies history of anemia, blood transfusion, or known blood disorders; denies easy bruising or prolonged bleeding with injury
Endocrine: Denies thyroid issues, excessive sweating, hunger or thirst, cold or heat intolerance
Psychiatric: Denies depression, suicide attempts/ideation; reports mood swings beginning 2 days before menses and lasting most of menses each month

Physical Examination for a Gynecologic Visit:
Vital Signs: Temp = 98.8°F   BP = 148/82   HR = 78 bpm   RR = 20/min
              Height = 5 ft 5 inches   Weight = 198 lbs   BMI = 33   LMP = 3 months ago
General/Neuro/Psych: Pleasant and cooperative female; appropriately groomed and dressed; obese; oriented to person, place, and time
Integumentary: Pink, warm and dry, normal turgor
HEENT: Neck supple; thyroid palpable without nodes or nodules; no adenopathy
Lungs: Clear to auscultation; no wheezing, rales, or rhonchi
Cardiovascular: Regular heart sounds; no murmur. No jugular vein distention or carotid bruits
Breasts: Symmetric without masses, nipple discharge, retraction, or dimpling
Abdomen: Obese, soft, nontender; normal bowel sounds audible in all four quadrants; no masses; no costovertebral angle tenderness (CVAT)
Genitalia: External genitalia without lesions, no evidence of vulvar atrophy; urethra well supported, bladder without prolapse, vagina with scant amount of dark blood in vault and yellow–green eggshell discharge with slight "fishy" odor; cervix is nulliparous. Pap and GC/CT cultures were obtained.

Wet Prep Results:
No evidence of active trichamonids, no hyphae/budding or blastocysts; pH: 5.5
Positive clue cells 3+, multiple RBCs and WBCs; whiff test +

Uterus is anteverted and top normal size, nontender, and mobile.
Adnexa without masses palpated bilaterally but moderate tenderness on the right greater than left with
   tenderness over the right uterosacral ligament
Rectal: Deferred

Introduction

Women comprise more than half of the world's population and make most of the medical choices for their families. Due to increased awareness of the importance of good health, women are living longer and have the ability to enjoy all that life has to offer.

Women's health is paramount to the health of every society. A woman's personal, mental, emotional, and physical health allows for her ability to contribute to the global economy, care for her children, and support her community.

The health of women is therefore an index of the prosperity and well-being of a country. Women often pass on healthy and unhealthy lifestyle choices to their children. Thus, by assisting women to find opportunities to enjoy life and to improve on her health, her entire family will reap the benefits.

Assessment: The Annual Well Woman Examination is a fundamental part of women's health care and is valuable in promoting prevention practices, recognizing risk factors for disease, identifying medical problems, and establishing the clinician–patient relationship.

Common issues presenting in women's health:
- STI
- Vulvovaginitis
- Contraception
- Breast disorders
- Breast cancer screening
- Premenstrual syndrome
- Cervical cancer screening
- Menstrual cycle abnormalities
- Pelvic pain
- Urinary tract infections
- Urinary incontinence
- Perimenopause transition
- Menopause
- Osteoporosis

Well-Woman Visit

In the above case study, T. M. initially presents for a well-woman visit. She reports not having a well-woman visit for over 3 years.

Well-woman assessment recommendations are different depending on the age of the woman (Tables 6-1 to 6-4).

For recommended adult immunization schedule, see Chapter 1, Figure 1-1 from the Center for Disease Control and Prevention (CDC) Immunization Schedule.

Table 6-1: Health Assessment of Women Aged 13 to 18 Years

Screening	Testing	Evaluations/Counseling

Comprehensive History
• Reason for visit
• Health status
  ○ Medical/surgical
  ○ Menstrual
    ▪ Menarche
    ▪ Cycle length
    ▪ Ovulation
• Family medical history
• Dietary/nutrition
• Physical activity
• Medication use (all)
• Tobacco, alcohol, drug use
• Emotional, physical, and sexual abuse
• Sexual practices
  ○ Vaginal, anal, oral sex
  ○ Sexual orientation
  ○ Number of partners
  ○ Contraceptive use
  ○ Sex exchange for drugs or money
  ○ Sexual satisfaction
 	
Physical Examination
• Height
• Weight
• Body mass index (BMI)
• Blood pressure
• Secondary sexual characteristics (Tanner staging)
• Pelvic exam (*a*if indicated by medical history only)
• Abdominal examination
• Additional physical examination as clinically appropriate
	Periodic
	• Chlamydia and gonorrhea testing if sexually active (urine or cervical swab)
	• Human immunodeficiency virus (HIV)
	
	High-Risk Groups
	• Colorectal cancer[a]
	• Diabetes testing
	• Genetic testing/counseling
	• Hemoglobin level assessment
	• Hepatitis B virus testing
	• Hepatitis C virus testing
	• HIV testing (not sexually active)
	• Lipid profile assessment
	• Sexually transmitted infection testing
	• Tuberculosis skin testing
		Sexuality
		• Development
		• High-risk sexual behaviors (number of partners, exchange sex for drugs or money)
		• Preventing unwanted/unintended pregnancy
		• Postponing sexual involvement
		• Contraceptive options, including emergency contraception, and long-acting reversible contraception (LARC)
		• Sexually transmitted infections—barrier protection
		• Internet/phone safety
		
		Fitness and Nutrition
		• Physical activity
		• Dietary/nutrition (including eating disorders and obesity)
		• Multivitamin with folic acid
		• Calcium intake
		
		Psychosocial Evaluation
		• Suicide: Depressive symptoms
		• Interpersonal/family relationships
		• Sexual orientation and gender identity
		• Personal goal development
		• Behavioral/learning disorders
		• Emotional, physical, and sexual abuse by family or partner
		• School experience
		• Peer relationships
		• Acquaintance rape prevention
		• Bullying
		
		Cardiovascular Risk Factors
		• Family history
		• Hypertension
		• Dyslipidemia
		• Obesity (BMI > 30)
		• Diabetes mellitus
		• Personal history of preeclampsia, gestational diabetes, or pregnancy-induced hypertension
		
		Health/Risk Assessment
		• Hygiene (including dental), fluoride supplementation
		• Injury prevention
		• Exercise and sports safety
		• Weapons, including firearms
		• Hearing
		• Occupational hazards
		• Recreational hazards
		• Safe driving practices (seat belt use, no distracted driving, texting, or driving while under the influence of substances)
		• Helmet use
		• Skin exposure to ultraviolet rays
		• Tobacco, alcohol, other drug use
		• Piercing and tattooing

[a] Only for those with a family history of familial adenomatous polyposis or 8 years after the start of pancolitis.

Adapted from The American Congress of Obstetricians and Gynecologists (ACOG). *Well–woman recommendations*. Retrieved from http://www.acog.org/About-ACOG/ACOG-Departments/Annual-Womens-Health-Care/Well-Woman-Recommendations

Table 6-2: Health Assessment of Women Aged 19 to 39 Years

Screening	Testing	Evaluations/Counseling

History
• Reason for visit
• Health status: Medical/surgical, menstrual, reproductive health
• Family medical history
• Dietary/nutrition assessment
• Physical activity
• Use of complementary and alternative medicine
• Tobacco, alcohol, other drug use
• Abuse/neglect
• Sexual practices
  ○ Vaginal, anal, oral sex
  ○ Sexual orientation
  ○ Number of partners
  ○ Contraceptive use
  ○ Sex exchange for drugs or money
  ○ Sexual satisfaction
• Urinary and fecal incontinence
 	
Physical Examination
• Height
• Weight
• Body mass index (BMI)
• Blood pressure
• Neck: Adenopathy, thyroid
• Breasts (clinical breast examination every 1–3 yr beginning at age 20)
• Abdomen
• Pelvic examination: Ages 19–20 yr when indicated by the medical history; age 21 or older, periodic pelvic examination
• Additional physical examinations as clinically appropriate
	Periodic
	• Cervical cytology:
	  ○ **Age 21–29 yr**: Screen every 3 yr with cytology alone
	  ○ **Age 30 yr or older**: Preferred—cotest with cytology and HPV testing every 5 yr; option—screen with cytology alone every 3 yr
	• Chlamydia and gonorrhea testing (if aged 25 yr or younger and sexually active)
	• Human immunodeficiency virus (HIV) testing—providers should be aware of and follow their states' HIV screening requirements.
	
	High-Risk Groups
	• Bone mineral density screening
	• Colorectal cancer screening
	• Diabetes testing
	• Genetic testing/counseling
	• Hemoglobin level assessment
	• Hepatitis C virus testing
	• Lipid profile assessment
	• Mammography
	• Sexually transmitted infection testing
	• Thyroid-stimulating hormone (TSH) testing
	• Tuberculosis skin testing
		Sexuality and Reproductive Planning
		• Contraceptive options for prevention of unwanted pregnancy, including emergency contraception
		• Discussion of a reproductive health plan
		• High-risk behaviors
		• Preconception and genetic counseling
		• Sexual function
		• Sexually transmitted infections—barrier protection
		
		Fitness and Nutrition
		• Physical activity
		• Dietary/nutrition assessment (including eating disorders and obesity)
		• Folic acid supplementation
		• Calcium intake
		
		Psychosocial Evaluation
		• Interpersonal/family relationships
		• Intimate partner violence
		• Acquaintance rape prevention
		• Work satisfaction
		• Lifestyle/stress
		• Sleep disorders
		
		Cardiovascular Risk Factors
		• Family history
		• Hypertension
		• Dyslipidemia
		• Obesity
		• Diabetes mellitus
		• Personal history of preeclampsia, gestational diabetes, or pregnancy-induced hypertension
		• Lifestyle
		
		Health/Risk Assessment
		• Breast self-awareness (may include breast self-examination)
		• Chemoprophylaxis for breast cancer (for high-risk women aged 35 yr or older)
		• Hygiene (including dental)
		• Injury prevention
		  ○ Exercise and sports involvement
		  ○ Firearms
		  ○ Hearing
		  ○ Occupational hazards
		  ○ Recreational hazards
		  ○ Safe driving practices (seat belt use, no distracted driving, texting, or driving while under the influence of substances)
		• Skin exposure to ultraviolet rays
		• Suicide: Depressive symptoms
		• Tobacco, alcohol, other drug use

Adapted from The American Congress of Obstetricians and Gynecologists (ACOG). *Well–woman recommendations.* Retrieved from http://www.acog.org/About-ACOG/ACOG-Departments/Annual-Womens-Health-Care/Well-Woman-Recommendations

Table 6-3: Health Assessment of Women Aged 40 to 64 Years

Screening	Testing	Evaluations/Counseling

History
 • Reason for visit
 • Health status: Medical/ surgical, menstrual, reproductive health
 • Family medical history
 • Dietary/nutrition assessment
 • Physical activity
 • Use of complementary and alternative medicine
 • Tobacco, alcohol, other drug use
 • Pelvic prolapse
 • Menopausal symptoms
 • Abuse/neglect
 • Sexual practices
   ○ Vaginal, anal, oral sex
   ○ Sexual orientation
   ○ Number of partners
   ○ Contraceptive use
   ○ Sex exchange for drugs or money
   ○ Sexual satisfaction
 • Urinary and fecal incontinence
 	
 Physical Examination
 • Height
 • Weight
 • Body mass index (BMI)
 • Blood pressure
 • Neck: Adenopathy, thyroid
 • Breasts and axillae (yearly clinical breast examination)
 • Abdomen
 • Pelvic examination
 • Additional physical examinations as clinically appropriate
	Periodic
	 • Cervical cytology:
	   ○ Preferred—cotest with cytology and HPV testing every 5 yr; option—screen with cytology alone every 3 yr
	 • Colorectal cancer screening: Preferred—beginning at age 50 yr: colonoscopy every 10 yr[a]
	 • Diabetes testing—every 3 yr after age 45 yr
	 • Hepatitis C virus testing— one-time testing for persons born from 1945 through 1965 and unaware of their infection status
	 • Human immunodeficiency virus (HIV) testing— providers should be aware of and follow their states' HIV screening requirements.
	 • Lipid profile assessment— every 5 yr beginning at age 45 yr
	 • Mammography—annually
	 • Thyroid-stimulating hormone (TSH) testing—every 5 yr beginning at age 50 yr
	
	 High-Risk Groups
	 • Bone mineral density screening
	 • Colorectal cancer screening
	 • Diabetes testing
	 • Hemoglobin level assessment
	 • Lipid profile assessment
	 • Sexually transmitted infection testing
	 • TSH testing
	 • Tuberculosis skin testing
		Sexuality: Preconception and genetic counseling is appropriate for certain women in this age group.
		 • High-risk behaviors
		 • Contraceptive options for prevention of unwanted pregnancy, including emergency contraception
		 • Sexual function
		 • Sexually transmitted infections—barrier protection
		
		 Fitness and Nutrition
		 • Physical activity
		 • Dietary/nutrition assessment (including eating disorders and obesity)
		 • Folic acid supplementation
		 • Calcium intake
		
		 Psychosocial Evaluation
		 • Family relationships
		 • Intimate partner violence
		 • Work satisfaction
		 • Lifestyle/stress
		 • Sleep disorders
		 • Advance directives
		
		 Cardiovascular Risk Factors
		 • Family history
		 • Hypertension
		 • Dyslipidemia
		 • Obesity
		 • Diabetes mellitus
		 • Personal history of preeclampsia, gestational diabetes, or pregnancy-induced hypertension
		 • Lifestyle
		
		 Health/Risk Assessment
		 • Aspirin prophylaxis to reduce the risk of stroke (ages 55–79 yr)[b]
		 • Breast self-awareness (may include breast self-examination)
		 • Chemoprophylaxis for breast cancer (for high-risk women)
		 • Hormone therapy
		 • Hygiene (including dental)
		 • Injury prevention
		   ○ Exercise and sports involvement
		   ○ Firearms
		   ○ Hearing
		   ○ Occupational hazards
		   ○ Recreational hazards
		   ○ Safe driving practices (seat belt use, no distracted driving, texting, or driving while under the influence of substances)
		 • Sun exposure
		 • Suicide: Depressive symptoms
		 • Tobacco, alcohol, other drug use

[a] Colorectal cancer screening for African American women should begin at age 45 years.

[b] The recommendation for aspirin prophylaxis must weigh the benefits of stroke prevention against the harm of gastrointestinal bleeding. Visit the U.S. Preventive Services Task Force at http://www.uspreventiveservicestaskforce.org/Page/Document/UpdateSummaryFinal/aspirin-for-the-prevention-of-cardiovascular-disease-preventive-medication for more information

Adapted from The American Congress of Obstetricians and Gynecologists (ACOG). *Well–woman recommendations*. Retrieved from http://www.acog.org/About-ACOG/ACOG-Departments/Annual-Womens-Health-Care/Well-Woman-Recommendations

Table 6-4: Health Assessment of Women Aged 65 Years and Older

Screening	Testing	Evaluations/Counseling

History
• Reason for visit
• Health status: Medical/surgical, menstrual, reproductive health
• Family medical history
• Dietary/nutrition assessment
• Physical activity
• Pelvic prolapse
• Menopausal symptoms
• Use of complementary and alternative medicine
• Tobacco, alcohol, other drug use, and concurrent medication use
• Abuse/neglect
• Sexual practices
  ○ Vaginal, anal, oral sex
  ○ Sexual orientation
  ○ Number of partners
  ○ Barrier protection
  ○ Sex exchange for drugs or money
  ○ Sexual satisfaction
• Urinary and fecal incontinence
 	
Physical Examination
• Height
• Weight
• Body mass index (BMI)
• Blood pressure
• Neck: Adenopathy, thyroid
• Breasts and axillae (yearly clinical breast examination)
• Abdomen
• Pelvic examination[a]
• Additional physical examinations as clinically appropriate
	Periodic
	• Bone mineral density screening.[b] (In the absence of new risk factors, screen no more frequently than every 2 yr.)
	• Cervical cytology: Discontinue in women with evidence of adequate negative prior screening results (three consecutive negative cytology results or two consecutive negative cotest results within the previous 10 yr, with the most recent test performed within the past 5 yr) and no history of CIN 2 or higher.
	• Colorectal cancer screening[c]:
	  ○ Colonoscopy every 10 yr
	    Or
	  ○ Fecal occult blood testing or fecal immunochemical test, annual patient-collected
	    Or
	  ○ Flexible sigmoidoscopy every 5 yr
	    Or
	  ○ Double-contrast barium enema every 5 yrs
	    Or
	  ○ Computed tomography colonography every 5 yr
	    Or
	  ○ Stool DNA
	• Diabetes testing (every 3 years)
	• Hepatitis C virus testing (one-time testing for persons born from 1945 through 1965 and unaware of their infection status)
	• Lipid profile assessment (every 5 yr)
	• Mammography annually
	• Thyroid-stimulating hormone (TSH) testing (every 5 yr)
	• Urinalysis
	
	High-Risk Groups
	• Hemoglobin level assessment
	• Human immunodeficiency virus (HIV) testing
	• Sexually transmitted infection testing
	• TSH testing
	• Tuberculosis skin testing
		Sexuality
		• Sexual function
		• Sexual behaviors
		• Sexually transmitted infections—barrier protection
		
		Fitness and Nutrition
		• Physical activity
		• Dietary/nutrition assessment (including eating disorders and obesity)
		• Calcium intake
		
		Psychosocial Evaluation
		• Neglect/abuse
		• Intimate partner violence
		• Lifestyle/stress
		• Depression/sleep disorders
		• Family relationships
		• Advance directives
		
		Cardiovascular Risk Factors
		• Hypertension
		• Dyslipidemia
		• Obesity
		• Diabetes mellitus
		• Personal history of preeclampsia, gestational diabetes, or pregnancy-induced hypertension
		• Sedentary lifestyle
		
		Health/Risk Assessment
		• Aspirin prophylaxis (for women aged 79 yr or younger)[d]
		• Breast self-awareness (may include breast self-examination)
		• Chemoprophylaxis for breast cancer (for high-risk women)
		• Hearing
		• Hormone therapy
		• Hygiene (including dental)
		• Injury prevention
		  ○ Exercise and sports involvement
		  ○ Firearms
		  ○ Occupational hazards
		  ○ Prevention of falls
		  ○ Recreational hazards
		  ○ Safe driving practices (seat belt use, no distracted driving, texting, or driving while under the influence of substances)
		• Skin exposure to ultraviolet rays
		• Suicide: Depressive symptoms
		• Tobacco, alcohol, other drug use
		• Visual acuity/glaucoma

[a] When a woman's age or other health issues are such that she would not choose to intervene on conditions detected during the routine examination, it is reasonable to discontinue pelvic examinations.

[b] In the absence of new risk factors, screen no more frequently than every 2 years.

[c] ACOG supports stopping routine screening at age 75 years.

[d] The recommendation for aspirin prophylaxis must weigh the benefits of stroke prevention against the harm of gastrointestinal bleeding. Visit the U.S. Preventive Services Task Force at http://www.uspreventiveservicestaskforce.org/Page/Document/UpdateSummaryFinal/aspirin-for-the-prevention-of-cardiovascular-disease-preventive-medication for more information.

Adapted from The American Congress of Obstetricians and Gynecologists (ACOG). *Well–woman recommendations.* Retrieved from http://www.acog.org/About-ACOG/ACOG-Departments/Annual-Womens-Health-Care/Well-Woman-Recommendations

Sexually Transmitted Infections

Introduction: An STI includes over 30 different bacteria, viruses, and parasites that are transmitted through sexual contact, including vaginal, oral, and anal sex. The consequences of an STI can be devastating physically (infertility, ectopic pregnancy, chronic pelvic pain, cancer, and death) and psychologically (distress, depression, anxiety, etc.). Over 1 million individuals will acquire a STI in 1 day. The most common sexually transmitted diseases will be covered in this section. Trichomoniasis will be covered in the section on Vaginitis.

Prevention: All health care professionals that provide health services to women and their support systems need to educate on preventative measures to protect against STIs.

- Abstinence
- Delaying the onset of sexual activity
- Limiting number of sexual partners
- Limiting high risk sexual practices
- Immunization
- Emphasizing the use of condoms
- Partner notification and treatment
- Reporting of STIs according to the laws in each state

Bacterial Sexually Transmitted Infections

GENITAL CHLAMYDIA INFECTION

Description: A chlamydial infection is the most frequently reported sexually transmitted bacterial infection in the United States; sequelae may result in conjunctivitis, urethritis, cervicitis, pelvic inflammatory disease (PID), infertility, ectopic pregnancy, and chronic pelvic pain.

Epidemiology and Etiology:

- Caused by obligate intracellular, gram-negative bacterium *Chlamydia trachomatis*
- Estimated 2.8 million new infections occur each year/most are unreported
- Highest prevalence in young women ages 15 to 25 years (highest in Hispanic and African American women)
- Frequently found in conjunction with Neisseria gonorrhoeae infection

Risk Factors:

- Unprotected sexual contact/inconsistent latex condom use
- Sharing sex toys
- New sexual partner
- Multiple partners
- Drug and alcohol use
- History of previously acquired STIs
- Sex for money or drug exchange

Signs and Symptoms:

- **Subjective Complaints:**
  - Can be vague or asymptomatic
  - Abnormal vaginal discharge
  - Irregular, intermenstrual vaginal bleeding
  - Postcoital bleeding
  - Dysuria
  - Dyspareunia
  - Pelvic cramping/pelvic pain
  - Dysmenorrhea
  - Infertility
- **Physical Examination Findings:**
  - May be normal
  - Cervicitis/friable cervix
  - Mucopurulent vaginal discharge (green or yellow)
  - Edematous and hyperemic endocervical tissue
  - Cervical motion tenderness (PID)
  - Blood in vaginal vault

Differential Diagnosis:
- PID (and/or salpingitis/endometritis)
- Urinary tract infection
- Urethritis
- Vaginitis
- Gonococcal cervicitis
- Reiter syndrome

Diagnostic Studies:
- Annual screening of all sexually active women aged ≤25 years is recommended; screen women >25 with the above risk factors
- Diagnosed by testing urine or by collecting swab specimens from the endocervix or vagina
- Culture, direct immunofluorescence, EIA, nucleic acid hybridization tests for endocervical swabs
- Nucleic acid amplification tests (NAATs) are the most sensitive tests and are FDA-cleared for use with urine, endocervical swab, or vaginal swab; self- or provider-collected vaginal swab is highest recommended specimen; urine testing may miss up to 10% of infection when compared to swab.
- Certain NAATs have also been FDA-cleared for use on liquid-based cytology specimens; individuals who undergo testing and are diagnosed with chlamydia should be tested for other STIs (Table 6-5).

Treatment:
- Pharmacologic: Patients infected with *C. trachomatis* frequently are coinfected with N. gonorrhoeae; this finding has led to the recommendation that patients treated for chlamydia also be treated routinely with a regimen that is effective against uncomplicated genital N. gonorrhoeae infection (Table 6-5).

Follow-Up (FU) and Referral:
- Individuals treated for chlamydia should be instructed to abstain from sexual intercourse for 7 days after single-dose therapy or until completion of a 7-day regimen.
- To minimize the risk for reinfection, patients also should be instructed to abstain from sexual intercourse until all of their sex partners have been treated.
- With the exception of pregnant women, test of cure is not advised for patients treated with the recommended or alternative regimens, unless therapeutic compliance is in question, symptoms persist, or reinfection is suspected.
- *Chlamydia*-infected women and men should be retested approximately 3 months after treatment, regardless of whether they believe that their sex partners were treated.
- If retesting at 3 months is not possible, providers should retest whenever persons next present for medical care in the 12 months following initial treatment.
- Instruct patients to refer their sex partners for evaluation, testing, and treatment if they had sexual contact with the patient during the 60 days preceding onset of the patient's symptoms or chlamydia diagnosis.

Special Considerations:
- All patients should be counseled on prevention, transmission, treatment, follow-up, and safe sex practices; using latex condoms
- Screen patient for all STI/HIV coinfections.
- Some women who have uncomplicated cervical infection already have subclinical upper reproductive tract infection upon diagnosis.

Table 6-5: CDC Treatments for Uncomplicated Chlamydial Infections

Recommended Regimens	Alternative Regimens
• **Azithromycin** 1 g orally in a single dose Or • **Doxycycline** 100 mg orally twice a day for 7 d	• **Erythromycin** base 500 mg orally four times a day for 7 d Or • **Erythromycin ethylsuccinate** 800 mg orally four times a day for 7 d Or • **Levofloxacin** 500 mg orally once daily for 7 d Or • **Ofloxacin** 300 mg orally twice a day for 7 d

Adapted from Centers for Disease Control and Prevention. *2015 STD treatment guidelines.* Retrieved from http://www.cdc.gov/std/tg2015/chlamydia.htm

GONORRHEA GONOCOCCAL INFECTION

Description: A gonorrhea gonococcal infection is the second most commonly reported sexually transmitted bacterial infection in the United States; sequelae may result in urethritis, cervicitis, PID, infertility, ectopic pregnancy, and chronic pelvic pain; if left untreated, gonorrhea can become systemic and/or disseminated.

Epidemiology and Etiology:
- Caused by gram-negative diplococcus bacterium *N. gonorrhoeae*
- Estimated 700,000 new infections occur each year in the United States
- Highest prevalence in young women ages 15 to 24 years; varies widely among communities and populations
- Frequently found in conjunction with *C. trachomatis* infection

Risk Factors:
- Unprotected sexual contact/inconsistent latex condom use
- Sharing sex toys
- New sexual partner
- Multiple partners
- Drug and alcohol use
- History of previously acquired STIs
- Sex for money or drug exchange
- Maternal–child transmission at birth

Signs and Symptoms:
- **Subjective Complaints:**
  - Frequently vague or asymptomatic
  - Abnormal vaginal discharge
  - Abnormal urethral discharge
  - Irregular, intermenstrual vaginal bleeding
  - Postcoital bleeding
  - Dyspareunia
  - Dysuria
  - Pelvic cramping/pelvic pain
  - Dysmenorrhea
  - Rectal discharge
  - Sore throat with discharge
  - Rash
  - Painful joints
  - Infertility
- **Physical Examination Findings:**
  - May be normal
  - Cervicitis/friable cervix
  - Mucopurulent vaginal discharge (green or yellow)
  - Mucopurulent urethral discharge (green or yellow)
  - Edematous and hyperemic endocervical tissue
  - Cervical motion tenderness (PID)
  - Blood in vaginal vault
  - Bartholin's and/or Skene gland abscess/discharge

Differential Diagnosis:
- PID (and/or salpingitis/endometritis)
- Urinary tract infection
- Nongonococcal cervicitis, vaginitis, urethritis
- Nongonococcal pharyngitis or arthritis
- Septic arthritis
- Reiter syndrome
- Fitz–Hugh–Curtis syndrome (perihepatitis)

Diagnostic Studies:
- Annual screening of all sexually active women aged ≤25 years is recommended; screen women >25 with the above risk factors

- Pharyngeal and anorectal infections should be considered based on information regarding sexual practices elicited from the sexual history.
- Diagnosed by testing urine or by collecting swab specimens from the endocervix or vagina
- Culture, direct immunofluorescence, EIA, and NAATS for endocervical swabs
- NAATs are the most sensitive tests and are FDA-cleared for use with urine, endocervical swab, or vaginal swab; self- or provider-collected vaginal swab is highest recommended specimen; urine testing may miss up to 10% of infection when compared to swab.
- Certain NAATs have also been FDA-cleared for use on liquid-based cytology specimens; individuals who undergo testing and are diagnosed with gonorrhea should be tested for other STIs.
- NAAT tests are not FDA-cleared for use in the rectum, conjunctiva, and pharynx.

Treatment:
- Pharmacologic: Patients infected with *N. gonorrhoeae* frequently are coinfected with *C. trachomatis*; this finding has led to the recommendation that patients treated for gonococcal infection also be treated routinely with a regimen that is effective against uncomplicated genital *C. trachomatis* infection (Table 6-6).

Pregnancy: Pregnant women infected with *N. gonorrhoeae* should be treated with a recommended or alternate cephalosporin. Azithromycin 2 g orally can be considered for women who cannot tolerate a cephalosporin. Either azithromycin or amoxicillin is recommended for treatment of presumptive or diagnosed *C. trachomatis* infection during pregnancy (Table 6-7).

Follow-Up (FU) and Referral:
- Individuals treated for gonorrhea should be instructed to abstain from sexual intercourse for 7 days after single-dose therapy or until completion of a 7-day regimen.

Table 6-6: CDC Treatments for Uncomplicated Gonococcal Infections of the Cervix, Urethra, and Rectum

Recommended Regimens	Alternative Regimens
• **Ceftriaxone** 250 mg in a single intramuscular dose *Plus* • **Azithromycin** 1 g orally in a single dose *Or* • **Doxycycline** 100 mg **orally** twice a day for 7 d	• **Cefixime** 400 mg in a single oral dose *Plus* • **Azithromycin** 1 g orally in a single dose *Or* • **Doxycycline** 100 mg orally twice daily for 7 d *Plus* • Test of cure in 1 wk If the patient has severe cephalosporin allergy: • **Azithromycin** 2 g in a single oral dose *Plus* • Test of cure in 1 wk

Adapted from Centers for Disease Control and Prevention. *2015 STD treatment guidelines.* Retrieved from http://www.cdc.gov/std/tg2015/gonorrhea.htm

Table 6-7: CDC Treatments for Uncomplicated Gonococcal Infections of the Pharynx

Recommended Regimens
• **Ceftriaxone** 250 mg in a single intramuscular dose *Plus* • **Azithromycin** 1 g orally in a single dose *Or* • **Doxycycline** 100 mg orally twice daily for 7 d

Adapted from Centers for Disease Control and Prevention. *2015 STD treatment guidelines.* Retrieved from http://www.cdc.gov/std/tg2015/gonorrhea.htm

- To minimize the risk for reinfection, patients also should be instructed to abstain from sexual intercourse until all of their sex partners have been treated.
- With exception of pregnant women, test of cure is not advised for patients treated with the recommended regimen, unless therapeutic compliance is in question, symptoms persist, or reinfection is suspected.
- Gonorrhea-infected women and men should be retested approximately 3 months after treatment, regardless of whether they believe that their sex partners were treated.
- If retesting at 3 months is not possible, providers should retest whenever persons next present for medical care in the 12 months following initial treatment.
- Instruct patients to refer their sex partners for evaluation, testing, and treatment if they had sexual contact with the patient during the 60 days preceding onset of the patient's symptoms or gonorrhea diagnosis.
- Cephalosporin resistant *N. gonorrhoeae* has been recognized nationally; Cephlosporin treatment options are not recommended for the treatment of gonococcal infections.

Special Considerations:

- All patients should be counseled on prevention, transmission, treatment, follow-up, and safe-sex practices/using latex condoms.
- Screen patient for all STI/HIV coinfections.
- Severe complications can include a disseminated infection causing endocarditis, perihepatitis, and acute arthritis.
- Some women who have uncomplicated cervical infection already have subclinical upper reproductive tract infection upon diagnosis.

PELVIC INFLAMMATORY DISEASE

Description: PID is an infection where bacteria move upward from the cervix into areas of the upper female genital tract, which can include the uterus, the fallopian tubes, and the ovaries. The surrounding tissues such as pelvic ligaments and peritoneum may also be affected.

Epidemiology and Etiology:

- Caused by the two main sexually transmitted bacteria listed above, namely, *C. trachomatis and N. Gonorrhoeae*; studies show *T. vaginalis* also found in acutely symptomatic women.
- Other bacterial organisms isolated in the upper reproductive tract of women diagnosed with PID include such as *bacterial vaginosis, group B Streptococcus, Staphylococcus, Bacteroides, Clostridium, Mycoplasma hominis, Ureaplasma urealyticum, Escerichia coli, and Actinomyces*; PID is usually polymicrobial (Table 6-8).

Table 6-8: CDC Treatments for Mild to Moderately Severe Acute PID: Oral Options

Recommended Regimens

- **Ceftriaxone** 250 mg IM in a single dose
  Plus
- **Doxycycline** 100 mg orally twice a day for 14 d
  With or *Without*
- **Metronidazole** 500 mg orally twice a day for 14 d
  Or
- **Cefoxitin** 2 g IM in a single dose and **Probenecid** 1 g orally administered concurrently in a single dose
  Plus
- **Doxycycline** 100 mg orally twice a day for 14 d
  With or *Without*
- **Metronidazole** 500 mg orally twice a day for 14 d
  Or
- **Other parenteral third-generation cephalosporin** (e.g., ceftizoxime or cefotaxime)
  Plus
- **Doxycycline** 100 mg orally twice a day for 14 d
  With or *Without*
- **Metronidazole** 500 mg orally twice a day for 14 d

Adapted from Centers for Disease Control and Prevention. *2015 STD treatment guidelines*. Retrieved from http://www.cdc.gov/std/tg2015/pid.htm

- Symptoms can appear days to week following.
- Estimated over 1 million infections occur each year in the United States.
- Highest prevalence in young women under the age of 25 years
- Timing of cervical infection in relation to the menstrual cycle is crucial: progesterone dominance in the cycle produces increased endocervical resistance to upward spread of infection.
  - Oral contraceptives, and progesterone-only contraceptives depot medroxyprogesterone acetate, *Norplant*, and *Implanon* may mimic effect and can have protective benefit.
  - Presence of sperm or intrauterine device (IUD) strings lessens protective benefit.
  - After diagnosis of initial infection, susceptibility increases to reinfection, infertility, and ectopic pregnancy.

Risk Factors:
- History of previous PID
- Untreated chlamydia and/or gonorrhea (10% to 40% will progress to acute PID)
- Adolescence
- Unprotected sexual contact/inconsistent or no latex condom use
- Sharing sex toys
- New sexual partner
- Multiple partners
- Drug and alcohol use
- History of previously acquired sexually transmitted infections
- Sex for money or drug exchange

Signs and Symptoms:
- **Subjective Complaints:**
  - Can be vague or asymptomatic
  - Abnormal vaginal discharge
  - Irregular, intermenstrual vaginal bleeding
  - Postcoital bleeding
  - Dysuria
  - Dyspareunia
  - Pelvic cramping/pelvic pain
  - Abdominal pain
  - Dysmenorrhea
  - Fever
  - Tachycardia
  - Nausea/vomiting
  - Infertility
- **Physical Examination Findings:** Providers should maintain low threshold for diagnosis (due to potential of damage to reproductive health).
  - Muscular guarding
  - Cervical motion tenderness (CMT)
  - Uterine tenderness
  - Adnexal tenderness
  - Rebound abdominal/pelvic tenderness
  - Cervicitis/friable cervix
  - Mucopurulent vaginal discharge (green or yellow)
  - Edematous and hyperemic endocervical tissue
  - Blood in vaginal vault
  - Fitz–Hugh–Curtis syndrome (perihepatitis)
  - Tubo–ovarian abscess
  - Leukocytes in vaginal secretions on microscopy

Differential Diagnosis:
- Ectopic pregnancy
- Septic incomplete abortion
- Acute appendicitis
- Diverticular disease

- Adnexal torsion
- Appendicitis
- Fibroidal degeneration

Treatment:

- Minimum Criteria: Empiric treatment for PID should be initiated in sexually active young women and other women at risk for STIs if they are experiencing pelvic or lower abdominal pain, if no cause for the illness other than PID can be identified, and if *one or more* of the following minimum criteria are present on pelvic examination:
  - Cervical motion tenderness
  - Uterine tenderness
  - Adnexal tenderness

Note: The presence of signs of lower genital tract inflammation in addition to one of the above findings increases the specificity of the PID diagnosis:
  - Oral temperature >101°F (>38.3°C)
  - Abnormal cervical or vaginal mucopurulent discharge
  - Presence of abundant numbers of WBC on saline microscopy of vaginal fluid
  - Elevated erythrocyte sedimentation rate
  - Elevated C-reactive protein
  - Laboratory documentation of cervical infection with *N. gonorrhoeae* or *C. trachomatis*
- Definitive Criteria:
  - Endometrial biopsy with histopathologic evidence of endometritis
  - Transvaginal sonography or magnetic resonance imaging (MRI) techniques showing thickened, fluid-filled tubes with/without free pelvic fluid or tubo–ovarian complex
  - Laparoscopic abnormalities consistent with PID
- Pharmacologic: Women with mild or moderate clinical severity of PID, outpatient therapy yields clinical outcomes similar to inpatient therapy.
- The decision to hospitalize a patient should be based on the judgment of the provider and whether the patient meets any of the following suggested criteria:
  - Unable to exclude surgical emergencies (i.e., appendicitis)
  - Patient is pregnant
  - Patient fails to respond clinically to oral antimicrobial therapy.
  - Patient is unable to follow or tolerate an outpatient oral regimen.
  - Patient has severe illness, nausea and vomiting, or high fever.
  - Patient has a tubo–ovarian abscess.

All treatment regimens should be effective against *both N. gonorrhoeae* and *C. trachomatis.*

Follow-Up (FU) and Referral:

- Provider–patient communication within 72 hours after initiation of treatment; patients should demonstrate substantial clinical improvement within 3 days after initiation of therapy; those who do not improve within this period will require hospitalization, additional diagnostic tests, and surgical intervention.
- Repeat testing of all women who have been diagnosed with chlamydia or gonorrhea is recommended 3 to 6 months after treatment, regardless of whether their sex partners were treated.
- Male sex partners of women with PID should be examined and treated if they had sexual contact with the patient during the 60 days preceding the patient's onset of symptoms.
- Abstain from sexual intercourse until therapy is completed and until they and their sex partners no longer have symptoms.

Special Considerations:

- All patients should be counseled on prevention, transmission, treatment, follow-up, and safe sex practices/use of latex condoms.
- Screen for concurrent STIs/HIV.
- Discuss treatment plans, strict adherence, and follow-up.
- Discuss increased risk for ectopic pregnancy, infertility, and reinfection.
- Women using an IUD for contraception have increased risk for PID during first 3 weeks after insertion; the IUD does not need to be removed but the patient needs to be closely followed.

SYPHILIS

Description: Syphilis is a serious, systemic sexually acquired infection that can cause significant damage all over the body; difficult to diagnose at times as the signs and symptoms can be found in many other disease processes.

Epidemiology and Etiology:
- Caused by the spirochete *Treponema pallidum*
- Incidence in the US is higher than HIV; 56,000 reported new cases in 2013
- Transmission is from individual to individual by direct contact through a syphilitic sore, known as a chance (seen mainly on the external genitals, nipples, vagina, anus, rectum, lips, and mouth); also can be transmitted through vertical transmission, or transplacentally (infected pregnant woman to fetus)
- *T. pallidum* enters the circulatory system through skin and mucous membranes, and can access the lymphatic and central nervous systems.
- Four stages of sequelae: Primary, secondary, latent, and neurosyphilis

Risk Factors:
- Anogenital-to-anogential, oral-to-anogenital, or anogential-to-oral contact with an individual with known or unknown syphilis
- Unprotected sexual contact/inconsistent/no latex condom use
- New sexual partner
- Multiple partners
- Drug and alcohol use
- History of previously acquired STIs
- Sex for money or drug exchange

Signs and Symptoms:
- **Subjective Complaints:**
  - Primary syphilis (10 to 60 days after infection)
    - Painless sore
    - Adenopathy
  - Secondary syphilis (4 to 8 weeks after chancre appears)
    - Skin rash on the palms and soles of the feet
    - Malaise
    - Wart-like papules in warm areas/folds of the body (condylomata lata)
    - Alopecia
    - Mucous patches in the mouth, pharynx, larynx, and genitalia
    - Flu-like symptoms
    - Fever
  - Latent syphilis
    - Usually asymptomatic
    - Can have paralysis numbness, gradual blindness, dementia, difficulty coordinating muscle movements
  - Neurosyphilis
    - Can be asymptomatic
    - Ophthalmic complaints
    - Headache
    - Altered behavior
    - Auditory complaints
    - Stroke-like syndromes with seizures
  - Teritary syphilis
    - Rubbery lesions on the abdomen, breast, eyes, and mucous areas
- **Physical Examination Findings:**
  - Primary syphilis
    - Indurated, painless papule or ulcer at site of inoculation
    - Regional lymphadenopathy (rubbery, painless, and bilateral)
  - Secondary syphilis
    - Rash palms and soles (macular, popular, squamous, pustualar, or combination)
    - Lymphadenopathy
    - Mucous patches

- ○ Condylomata lata
- ○ Alopecia (patchy, occipital or bitemporal, lateral eyebrows)
- ○ Fever
- ○ Splenomegaly
- ○ Hepatitis
- ○ Meningitis
- ○ Glomerulonephritis
- Latent syphilis
  - ○ Early (<1-year duration)
    - ○ Usually no clinical signs
  - ○ Late (≥1-year duration)
    - ○ May be asymptomatic with no appreciable clinical signs of infection
    - ○ Can have an array of abnormal findings related to damage to any body systems
  - ○ Neurosyphilis (few months to a few years after infection; can occur at any stage)
    - ○ Acute meningitis
    - ○ Basilar meningitis
    - ○ Endarteritis
    - ○ Paresis
    - ○ Tabes dorsalis
    - ○ Ocular issues
  - ○ Tertiary syphilis
    - ○ Gummas; destructive rubbery lesions in skeletal, spinal, and mucosal areas, eyes, and viscera
    - ○ Aortic aneurysm
    - ○ Aortic insufficiency
    - ○ Coronary ostial stenosis

Differential Diagnosis:
- Primary syphilis
  - Herpes
  - Neoplastic lesions
  - LGV
  - Chancroid
  - Granuloma inguinale
- Secondary syphilis
  - Dermatologic symptomology that includes a rash
  - Hepatitis
- Latent syphilis
  - Vague as any organ system can be involved
- Tertiary syphilis
  - Vague as any organ system can be involved; significant disease

Diagnostic Studies:
- Definitive diagnostic testing:
  - Dark-field microscopy (no longer common)
  - Direct fluorescent antibody test (DFA-TP) of lesions or exudate
- Screening tests/presumptive diagnosis:
  - Nontreponemal serologic testing: A fourfold change in titer, equivalent to a change of two dilutions (e.g., from 1:16 to 1:4 or from 1:8 to 1:32) is considered necessary to demonstrate a clinically significant difference.
  - Venereal Disease Research Laboratory (VDRL)
  - Rapid plasma reagin card (RPR) test
  - Automated Reagin Test
  - Treponemal serologic testing: most often positive for life
    - ○ Fluorescent treponemal antibody absorption (FTA-ABS)
    - ○ *Treponema pallidum* particle agglutination (TP-PA)
    - ○ Microhemagglutination assay for antibodies to *Treponema pallidum* (MHA-TP)
  - CSF evaluation for those with neurologic or ophthalmic symptoms, evidence of tertiary syphilis, or treatment failure

Treatment (Table 6-9):

- Be aware of the Jarisch–Herxheimer reactions: a self-limited reaction to antitreponemal therapy that is characterized by fever, malaise, nausea, and vomiting. It may be associated with chills and exacerbation of secondary rash and occurs within 24 hours after therapy and usually resolves within 24 hours.

Follow-Up (FU) and Referral:

- Patients treated for primary or secondary syphilis should be reexamined clinically and serologically 6 months and 12 months following treatment.
- Patients with latent syphilis should be followed up clinically and serologically at 6, 12, and 24 months.
- HIV-infected patients should be evaluated more frequently (i.e., at 3, 6, 9, 12, and 24 months for HIV-infected patients with primary or secondary syphilis; at 6, 12, 18, and 24 months for HIV-infected persons with latent syphilis).
- Follow-up titers should be compared to the maximum or baseline nontreponemal titer obtained on day of treatment.

Special Considerations:

- Patients with primary, secondary or early latent syphilis, or syphilis of unknown duration with a high nontreponemal serologic test titer (i.e., >1:32), should be referred to the local health department STI program for interview, partner elicitation, and partner follow-up.
- Follow-up of patients with early syphilis is a public health priority. Laws and regulations in all states require that persons diagnosed with syphilis be reported to public health authorities.
- Reporting can be provider-based or laboratory-based.
- Screen for STI/HIV coinfection.
- All patients should be counseled on prevention, transmission, treatment, follow-up, and safe sex practices/ use of latex condoms.
- Discuss treatment plans, strict adherence, and follow-up.
- Correct and consistent use of latex condoms use may decrease the spread of syphilis infections but does not eradicate it.

Table 6-9: CDC Treatments for Syphilis

Stage	Treatment
Primary, secondary, and early latent syphilis without neurologic involvement	**Benzathine penicillin G**, intramuscularly, 2.4 million units in a single dose **If penicillin allergic (one of the following):** • **Doxycycline** 100 mg orally twice daily for 2 wk • **Tetracycline** 500 mg orally four times daily for 2 wk
Late latent or latent syphilis of unknown duration without neurologic involvement	**Benzathine penicillin G** 7.2 million units total, administered as three doses of 2.4 million units intramuscularly each at 1-wk intervals **If penicillin allergic (one of the following):** • **Doxycycline** 100 mg orally twice daily for 28 d • **Tetracycline** 500 mg orally four times daily for 28 d
Tertiary (late) syphilis without neurologic involvement	**Benzathine penicillin G** 7.2 million units total, administered as three doses of 2.4 million units intramuscularly each at 1-wk intervals **If penicillin allergic:** • Treat according to treatment for late latent syphilis.
Neurosyphilis	**Aqueous crystalline penicillin G** 18–24 million units/d, administered as 3–4 million units intravenously every 4 hr or continuous infusion for 10–14 d intravenously **Alternative regimen (if compliance can be ensured):** • **Procaine penicillin** 2.4 million units intramuscularly once daily *Plus* • **Probenecid** 500 mg orally four times a day, both for 10–14 d

Adapted from Centers for Disease Control and Prevention. *2015 STD treatment guidelines.* Retrieved from http://www.cdc.gov/std/tg2015/syphilis.htm

Viral Sexually Transmitted Infections

Viral STIs have no cure available; the goals are to reduce symptomology and reduce spread.

GENITAL HERPES

Description: Genital herpes is a lifelong, chronic, highly transmitted viral infection characterized by multivesicular or ulcerative, painful lesions.

Epidemiology and Etiology:
- Caused by herpes simplex virus (HSV), a double-stranded DNA virus surrounded by an envelope of lipid glycoprotein; the types are distinguished by the proteins on their surfaces
  - HSV Type 1 (HSV-1): Primarily oral lesions; increasing culprit of genital lesions (50% of all new genital cases)
  - HSV Type 2 (HSV-2): Primarily genital lesions; can be responsible for oral lesions
- Estimated that over 50 million individuals in the United States are infected with HSV-2; anogenital herpes infections attributed to HSV-1 are increasing
- Approximately 776,000 new cases of HSV-2 in the United States annually
- Many individuals infected with HSV-2 do not experience symptoms and transmit the virus through asymptomatic shedding.
- HSV is transmitted through body fluids or from exposure to the fluid from a herpetic lesion.
- The median recurrence rate is highly variable; approximately 4.5 outbreaks per year in the first year of HSV-2 infection.

Risk Factors:
- Anogenital to anogenital, oral to anogenital, or anogenital to oral contact with an individual with known or unknown HSV
- Unprotected sexual contact/inconsistent/no latex condom use
- Sharing sex toys
- New sexual partner
- Multiple partners
- Drug and alcohol use
- History of previously acquired sexually transmitted infections
- Sex for money or drug exchange

Transmission: HSV penetrates susceptible mucosal surfaces, open wounds, or cracks in the skin surface; once transmission occurs, the virus is transported along peripheral nerve axons to the nerve cells located in sacral ganglia and paraspinous ganglia; the virus remains in latency in these areas indefinitely; neonatal transmission via exposure during childbirth possible.

Signs and Symptoms:
- **Physical Examination Findings:** See Table 6-10
  - Many patients will present with the above symptoms, some may present in the predrome with no visible lesions; others may exhibit lesions anywhere in the lesion cycle described above; approximately 70% to 90% of primary HSV-2 infections will also present with HSV cervicitis demonstrating ulcerative lesions, redness, and/or friability of the cervix; in some patients, a clear, copious, watery discharge may also be noted.

Differential Diagnosis:
- Syphilis
- Chancroid
- Herpes zoster
- Candidiasis
- Carcinoma
- Lymphagranuloma venereum (LGV)
- Granuloma inguinale/donovanosis
- Chlamydia
- Gonorrhea
- Vaginitis
- Asymptomatic meningitis

Table 6-10: Signs and Symptoms of Genital Herpes Infection

First Clinical Episode (Primary Infection)	Recurrent Symptomatic Infection
• Occurrence of numerous bilateral painful genital lesions that last an average of 12 d • Lesions, usually bilateral, begin as painful papules; papules progress into vesicles; vesicles progress into pustules; pustules progress into ulcers; the ulcers dry out and crust over and turn into healed tissue • Lesion bases are smooth and red • Pain and itching at site • Dysuria • Vaginal or urethral discharge • Tender, inguinal adenopathy • Neck adenopathy • Fever • Chills • Malaise • Dyspareunia • Headaches	• Prodromal symptoms of localized tingling, burning, and/or irritation 12–24 hr before lesions occur; can have prodrome without lesions • Lesions tend to be unilateral, last 4–6 d, and be less extensive than primary infection unless the individual is immunocompromised • Lesion bases are smooth and red

Diagnostic Testing:
- Virologic Testing
  - Viral culture: The gold standard (viral recovery for early vesicles is approximately 90%; ulcers approximately 70%, and crusted lesions approximatley 30%)
  - Antigen detection: Moderately sensitive (>85%) in symptomatic shedders; better for detecting HSV in healing lesions
  - Cytology (Tzanck or Pap): Identifies typical HSV-infected cells (multinucleated giant cells and eosinophilic inclusion bodies) in exfoliated cells or biopsies (not reliable)
  - Polymerase chain reaction (PCR) assays for HSV DNA: Highly sensitive and are increasingly used in many settings; FDA-cleared for testing of anogenital specimens
  - Always test for concomitant STIs in women and their partners.
- Type Specific Serologic Test (not indicated for the general population)
  - HSV-1 (gG1) and HSV-2 (gG2) are antigen specific and are the only serologic testing commercially available to distinguish HSV-1 from HSV-2
    - Useful in the following situations:
      - Recurrent or atypical genital HSV-like symptoms with negative cultures
      - A clinical diagnosis of genital herpes without laboratory confirmation
      - An intimate partner with a genital herpes
      - As part of a comprehensive evaluation for STI for a woman with multiple sex partners, HIV infection, or a history of high risk behaviors

Treatment (Table 6-11):
- IV therapy is also available for serious disease and complications; may require hospitalization.
- Topical analgesics may be used for relief of painful lesions and dysuria.

Special Considerations:
- HSV can be transmitted when lesions are not present, and most cases are transmitted during asymptomatic periods.
- Partners of infected individuals should be evaluated and counseled; suppressive therapy should also be considered.
- Periods of stress to the body can induce an outbreak (i.e., illness, menses, life situations).
- Correct and consistent use of latex condoms may decrease the spread of HSV infections but does not eradicate it.
- All women should be counseled on the natural history of the disease, prevention, transmission, strict adherence to treatment plans, follow-up, and safe sex practices.

Table 6-11: CDC Treatments for Herpes Simplex Virus

First Clinical Episode (Primary Infection)	Episodic Therapy for Recurrent Symptomatic Infection	Suppressive Therapy for Recurrent Genital Herpes
• **Acyclovir** 400 mg orally three times day for 7–10 d *Or* • **Acyclovir** 200 mg orally five times a day for 7–10 d *Or* • **Famciclovir** 250 mg orally three times a day for 7–10 d *Or* • **Valacyclovir** 1 g orally twice a day for 7–10 d	• **Acyclovir** 400 mg orally three times a day for 5 d *Or* • **Acyclovir** 800 mg orally twice a day for 5 d *Or* • **Acyclovir** 800 mg orally three times a day for 2 d *Or* • **Famciclovir** 125 mg orally twice daily for 5 d *Or* • **Famciclovir** 1,000 mg orally twice daily for 1 day *Or* • **Famciclovir** 500 mg once, followed by 250 mg twice daily for 2 d *Or* • **Valacyclovir** 500 mg orally twice a day for 3 d *Or* • **Valacyclovir** 1 g orally once a day for 5 d	• **Acyclovir** 400 mg orally twice a day *Or* • **Famciclovir** 250 mg orally twice a day *Or* • **Valacyclovir** 500 mg orally once a day *Or* • **Valacyclovir** 1 g orally once a day

Adapted from Centers for Disease Control and Prevention. *2015 STD treatment guidelines.* Retrieved from http://www.cdc.gov/std/tg2015/herpes.htm

- Discuss increased risk for ectopic pregnancy, infertility, and reinfection.
- Hand washing with soap and water inactivates HSV; encourage women to keep good hygiene to help prevent transmission.
- Educate on recognition of prodromal symptoms and to avoid sexual activity when prodromal symptoms or lesions are present.
- Stomatitis, pharyngitis, radicular pain, sacral paresthesias, transverse myelitis, autonomic dysfunction, disseminated infection, fulminant hepatitis, ocular involvement (more common with HSV-1), and herpetic whitlow (more common with HSV-1) are rare complications that have been reported with herpes infections.
- Partners of infected individuals should be evaluated and counseled; suppressive therapy should also be considered.

CONDYLOMATA ACUMINATA (GENITAL WARTS)

Description: Condylomata acuminata are wart-like growths on the skin of the anogenital area

Epidemiology and Etiology:
- Caused by the human papillomavirus (HPV)
- More than 150 known strains of HPV; over 40 strains are sexually transmitted through direct skin to skin contact during vaginal, anal, and oral sexual activity; virus has affinity for skin (keratinized squamous epithelium) and the mucous membranes (nonkeratinized squamous epithelium).
- Most common and contagious STI in the US; approximately 6.2 million new cases annually; over 20 million currently infected with one or more strains.
- More than 50% of sexually active individuals are infected with one or more HPV types in their lifetime; ages 15 to 30 have the highest incidence.
- Estimated 360,000 new cases of genital warts each year (highly underreported)
- Approximately 43% of women have genital HPV infections and less than 7% have oral HPV infections.

- Sexually transmitted HPV categories:
  - Low risk HPV: Nononcogenic types that cause anogenital warts; HPV types 6 and 11 are responsible for over 90% of all anogenital warts and have been also associated with conjunctival, nasal, oral, and laryngeal warts.
  - High risk HPV: Oncogenic types that are responsible for the majority of genital/cervical cancers; HPV types 16 and 18 are predominately detected in cervical cancer (99.7%) in the United States and cause 70% of cancers worldwide; HPV types 31, 33, and 35 are increasing in prevalence but are found occasionally in genital warts.

Risk Factors:
- Anogenital to anogenital, oral to anogenital, or anogenital to oral contact with an individual with known or unknown HPV
- Unprotected sexual contact/inconsistent or no latex condom use
- Sharing sex toys
- New sexual partner
- Multiple partners
- Drug and alcohol use
- History of previously acquired sexually transmitted infections
- Sex for money or drug exchange

Signs and Symptoms:
- **Subjective Complaints:**
  - Can be vague or asymptomatic
  - Wart-like growths in the anogenital region
  - May experience pain, pruritus, or burning
  - Depending on location: Dyspareunia and bleeding
- **Physical Examination Findings:**
  - Flat, popular, or pedunculated growths on the anogenital skin or mucosa; usually keratinized; may also be visualized inside the vagina and on the cervix (with and without colposcopy)
  - Often described to resemble the heads of broccoli or cauliflower

Differential Diagnosis
- Neoplastic lesions (i.e., verrucous carcinoma, squamous cell carcinoma)
- Skin conditions (i.e., actinic keratosis, moles, psoriasis, skin tags)
- Condyloma latum
- Vestibular papillomatosis
- Granuloma inguinale
- Molluscum contagiosum
- Hymenal remnants
- Hemorrhoids

Diagnostic Testing
- Visual inspection
- Tissue biopsy
- Pap smear of cervix (screening discussed in Chapter 1)
- Screen for concomitant infections

Treatment:
- Goal is to alleviate symptoms, relieve cosmetic concern, and removal of warts; factors that determine treatment include wart size, wart number, anatomical place of wart, patient preference, cost, convenience, side effects, and provider experience (Tables 6-12 and 6-13).
- Lesions >2 cm should be treated by surgical modalities (cryotherapy, cautery, or laser treatment).

Special Considerations:
- Prevention through vaccination
  - Gardasil: Immunization indicated for females aged 9 to 26
    - Prevents against HPV types 6, 11, 16, and 18
    - May be given to sexually active female even if they have been diagnosed with HPV; if the individual is already positive for one or more types, the vaccine will not eradicate the disease, it will however prevent against the above types in which individual has not been previously exposed.
    - Immunization schedule includes a series of 3 IM injections at baseline, 2 months, and 6 months.
    - Do not give to those severely allergic to yeast.

Table 6-12: CDC Recommended Regimens for the Treatment of External Genital Warts: Patient Applied

Treatment	Directions	Considerations
Podofilox 0.5% solution or gel	Cotton swab twice a day for 3 d, followed by no treatment for 4 d; cycle can be repeated up to 4 cycles.	• The total wart area treated should not exceed 2 cm. • Total volume of podofilox should be limited to 0.5 mL/d. • The health-care provider should apply the initial treatment to demonstrate the proper application technique and identify which warts should be treated. • Mild to moderate pain or local irritation might develop after treatment. • Safety use in pregnancy not established.
Imiquimod 5% cream	Once a day at bedtime, three times a week for up to 16 wk; wash with soap and water 6–10 hr after application	• Local inflammatory reactions, including redness, irritation, induration, ulceration/erosions, hypopigmentation, and vesicles are common. • Imiquimod might weaken latex condoms and vaginal diaphragms. • Safety use in pregnancy not established.
Sinecatechins 15% ointment	Three times daily (0.5-cm strand of ointment to each wart) using a finger to ensure coverage with a thin layer of ointment until complete clearance of warts; should not be continued for longer than 16 wk	• Do not wash off medication after use. • Avoid sexual contact while the ointment is on the skin. • Common side effects: Erythema, pruritus/burning, pain, ulceration, edema, induration, and vesicular rash. • May weaken latex condoms and diaphragms. • Safety use in pregnancy, with immunocompromised persons, or with clinical herpes is not established.

Adapted from Centers for Disease Control and Prevention. *2015 STD treatment guidelines.* Retrieved from http://www.cdc.gov/std/tg2015/warts.htm

Table 6-13: CDC Recommended Regimens for the Treatment of External Genital Warts: Provider Applied

• **Cryotherapy** with liquid nitrogen or cryoprobe. Repeat applications every 1–2 wk.
  Or
• **Trichloroacetic** acid (TCA) or **Bichloroacetic** acid (BCA) 80%–90%
  Or
• **Surgical removal** either by tangential scissor excision, tangential shave excision, curettage, or electrosurgery

Adapted from Centers for Disease Control and Prevention. *2015 STD treatment guidelines.* Retrieved from http://www.cdc.gov/std/tg2015/candidiasis.htm

• Cervarix: Immunization indicated for female aged 9 to 25
  ○ Prevents against HPV types 16 and 18.
  ○ May be given to sexually active female even if they have been diagnosed with HPV; if the individual is already positive for one or more types, the vaccine will not eradicate the disease, it will however prevent against the above types in which individual has not been previously exposed
  ○ Immunization schedule includes a series of 3 IM injections at baseline, 2 months, and 6 months.
  ○ Do not give to those anaphylactic to latex; prepackaging contains latex.
• All patients should be counseled on prevention, transmission, treatment, follow-up, and safe sex practices/use of latex condoms.
• Discuss treatment plans, strict adherence, and follow-up.
• Correct and consistent use of latex condoms may decreases the spread of HSV infections but does not eradicate it.
• Educate on importance of Pap smears and abnormal sequelae.

- HPV has a high asymptomatic viral shedding and is extremely contagious.
- See Chapter 1 for prevention of cervical cancer; smoking increases the risk of cervical cancer; counsel smokers regarding smoking cessation modalities.
- See http://www.asccp.org/Guidelines-2/Management-Guidelines-2 for management of abnormal Pap smear guidelines.

Vaginitis

Introduction: A normal vagina contains bacterial colonies that keep vaginal environment healthy and at a pH level of 3.8 to 4.2. Normal vaginal discharge is clear to white in color and odorless and contains lactobacilli organisms to aid in fighting off other bacteria and viruses. Vaginal symptomology is one of the most frequent reasons that women visit a health care provider. This portion will explore three common causes of vaginitis: bacterial vaginosis, vulvovaginal candidiasis, and trichomoniasis, and atrophy.

Definition: Vaginitis is a variety of conditions that cause vulvovaginial symptoms such as pruritus, irritation, burning, discomfort, and discharge.

Trichomoniasis

Description: Trichomoniasis is one of the most common curable STI.

Epidemiology/Etiology:
- Caused by *Trichomoniasis vaginalis (T. vaginalis)*, the only known protozoan parasite that infects the genital tract; single-celled flagellated anaerobic organism
- Over 3.7 million individuals with trichomoniasis in the US; 7.4 million new cases annually
- Highest prevalence in non-Hispanic Black women
- Associated with adverse pregnancy outcomes, including premature rupture of membranes and preterm labor, pelvic inflammatory disease, and increased risk for HIV infection

Risk Factors:
- Unprotected sexual contact/inconsistent or no latex condom use
- Sharing sex toys
- New sexual partner
- Multiple partners
- Drug and alcohol use
- History of previously acquired sexually transmitted infections
- Sex for money or drug exchange

Signs and Symptoms:
- **Subjective Complaints**
  - Often asymptomatic
  - Vaginal discharge
  - Vaginal pruritus
  - Vaginal odor
  - Postcoital bleeding
  - Vaginal burning
  - Dysuria
  - Dyspareunia
- **Physical Examination Findings:** (speculum examination)
  - Frothy gray or yellow–green discharge
  - Cervical petechiae ("strawberry cervix")
  - Edematous and hyperemic endocervical/vaginal tissue
  - Cervical friability

Differential Diagnosis:
- Bacterial vaginosis
- Chlamydia

- Gonorrhea
- Herpes genitalis
- Atrophic vaginitis
- Retention of foreign body (tampon)
- Desquamative inflammatory vaginitis
- Vulvodynia
- Vulvar dermatologic conditions
- Allergic reaction (spermicides, deodorants, soaps, etc.)

Diagnostic Studies: Be sure to take sample from lateral walls of the vagina
- **Mobile** trichamonads visualized on saline microscopy (poor sensitivity)
- Vaginal pH > 4.5
- Culture
- DNA probe
- NAAT (highest sensitivity and specificity; detects five times more *T. vagnalis* than microscopy)
- OSOM Trichomonas rapid test

Treatment (Table 6-14):
- Patients should be advised to avoid alcohol consumption while taking the above medications and for 24 hours after the completion of Metronidiazole or 72 hours after completion of Tinidazole.

Special Considerations:
- Consider rescreening 3 months after initial infection.
- Male partners are usually asymptomatic: sex partners of patients with *T. vaginalis* should be treated.
- Abstain from sex until both patient and partners are treated and asymptomatic.
- All patients should be counseled on prevention, transmission, treatment, follow-up, and safe sex practices and the use of latex condoms.
- Douching may worsen vaginal discharge.
- Discuss treatment plans, strict adherence, and follow-up.
- Screen for concomitant STIs.
- Educate patients that trichomoniasis has been associated with adverse outcomes during pregnancy (preterm delivery, low birth weight, and premature rupture of membranes).
- The treatment regimens are safe for use anytime during a pregnancy.
- If repeated treatment fails, refer to specialist or through free consultation with the CDC.

Table 6-14: CDC Recommended Regimens for the Treatment of Trichomoniasis

Recommended Regimens

- **Metronidazole** 2 g orally in a single dose
  Or
- **Tinidazole** 2 g **oral** in a single dose
  Or
- **Metronidazole** 500 mg twice a day for 7 d (alternative regimen)

Treatment Failure:
If the recommended treatment fails, the following treatment failure regimen is recommended:
- **Metronidazole** 500 **mg** orally twice a day for 7 d (if initial treatment was 2 g orally in a single dose)
  Or
- **Tinidazole** 2 g **orally** single dose.
With failure of either regimen, consider treatment with:
- **Metronidazole** or **Tinidazole** 2 g orally once a day for 5 day

Adapted from Centers for Disease Control and Prevention. *2015 STD treatment guidelines.* Retrieved from http://www.cdc.gov/std/tg2015/warts.htm

Bacterial Vaginosis

Description: Most common polymicrobial infection in the vagina

Epidemiology/Etiology:
- Caused by a lack of normal hydrogen peroxide producing lactobacilli and an overgrowth of facultative anaerobic organisms in the vagina
  - *G. vaginalis, Mycoplasma homonis, Bacteriods species, Peptostreptococcus species, Fusobacterium species, Prevotella species, Atopobium vaginae,* and others (these are found in the normal vaginal flora as well)
- Not reportable; estimated prevalence is 29% with an average recurrence rate of 20% to 40% at one month; 30% in 3 months
- May be related to sexually activity but is not considered an STI

Signs and Symptoms:
- **Subjective Complaints**
  - Often asymptomatic
  - Vaginal discharge
  - Vaginal pruritus
  - Vaginal odor (usually fishy) may be worse after intercourse and after menses
  - Postcoital bleeding
  - Vaginal burning
  - Dysuria
  - Dyspareunia
- **Physical Examination Findings:** (speculum examination)
  - Watery, homogenous gray–white to yellow discharge usually adherent to the vaginal walls
  - Edematous/irritated vaginal tissue

Differential Diagnosis:
- Trichomoniasis
- Chlamydia
- Gonorrhea
- Herpes genitalis
- Atrophic vaginitis
- Retention of foreign body (tampon)
- Desquamative inflammatory vaginitis
- Vulvodynia
- Vulvar dermatologic conditions
- Allergic reaction (spermicides, deodorants, soaps, etc.)

Diagnostic Studies: Be sure to take sample from lateral walls of the vagina
- The clinical diagnosis of BV requires three out of the four Amsel criteria:
  - Abnormal gray discharge
  - Vaginal pH > 4.5
  - Positive amine test: Adding a few drops of KOH to the discharge produces an amine or fishy odor (whiff test)
  - More than 20% of cells visualized with saline microscopy are clue cells (bacteria clumping on the borders of epithelial cells and "ground glass" appearance to the cytoplasm)
- Gram stain (gold standard)
- DNA probe

Treatment (Table 6-15):
- Patients should be advised to avoid alcohol consumption while taking the above medications and for 24 hours after the completion of Metronidiazole or 72 hours after completion of Tinidazole.

Special Considerations:
- Follow-up is unnecessary; return if symptoms reoccur.
- Using a different treatment regimen might be an option in patients who have a recurrence; however, re-treatment with the same topical regimen is another acceptable approach for treating recurrent BV during the early stages of infection.
- Routine treatment of a sexual partner is not recommended.

Table 6-15: CDC Recommended Regimens for the Treatment of Bacterial Vaginosis

Recommended Regimens	Alternative Regimens

• **Metronidazole** 500 mg orally twice a day for 7 d
  Or
• **Metronidazole gel** 0.75%, one full applicator (5 g) intravaginally, once a day for 5 d
  Or
• **Clindamycin cream** 2%, **one** full applicator (5 g) intravaginally at bedtime for 7 d
	• **Tinidazole** 2 g orally once daily for 2 d
	  Or
	• **Tinidazole** 1 g orally once daily for 5 d
	  Or
	• **Clindamycin** 300 mg orally twice daily for 7 d
	  Or
	• **Clindamycin ovules** 100 mg intravaginally once at bedtime for 3 d

Adapted from Centers for Disease Control and Prevention. *2015 STD treatment guidelines.* Retrieved from http://www.cdc.gov/std/tg2015/trichomoniasis.htm

- Douching may worsen symptoms.
- BV may be associated with PID and postoperative infections; educate patient on signs and symptoms of PID.
- Educate patients that BV has been associated with adverse outcomes during pregnancy (preterm delivery, and premature rupture of membranes).

Candidiasis

Definition: Vulvocandidiasis (VVC) is the second most common vaginal infection caused by fungi; commonly known as a yeast infection.

Epidemiology/Etiology:
- Most cases are caused by *Candida albicans* (85% to 90%); *C. glabrata*, and *C. parapsilosis*
- Estimated that 75% of women will have at least one VVC episode and 40% to 45% will have two or more episodes of VVC in their lifetime.
- Yeast grows as oval budding cells (budding) and chains of cells (pseudohyphae).
- Can be associated with diabetes, corticosteroid use, antibiotic use, hormonal changes (menses, pregnancy, hormone containing pharmaceuticals, etc.); vaginal environmental changes (moisture, temperature, douching, etc); not considered sexually transmitted
- Divided into two categories:
  - Uncomplicated VVC
    - Sporadic episodes
    - Mild to moderate symptom
    - Usually related to a *Candida albicans* infection
    - Nonimmunocompromised/nonpregnant women
  - Complicated VVC
    - Recurrent episodes (four or more per year)
    - Severe symptoms
    - Usually related to nonalbicans candida infections
    - Women with diabetes, severe medical illness, debilitation, immunosuppression, and other vulvovaginal conditions are at higher risk
    - Pregnancy

Signs and Symptoms:
- **Subjective Complaints**
  - May be asymptomatic
  - Vaginal discharge
  - Vaginal pruritus
  - Vaginal soreness
  - Dyspareunia
  - Dysuria
  - Vaginal burning
  - Postcoital bleeding

- **Physical Examination Findings:** (speculum examination)
  - Thick, white, and clumpy vaginal discharge ("cottage-cheese-like")
  - Usually adherent to the vaginal walls
  - Edematous/irritated vaginal tissue
  - Vulvar excoriation
  - Fissures

Differential Diagnosis:
- Trichomoniasis
- Bacterial vaginosis
- Chlamydia
- Gonorrhea
- Herpes genitalis
- Atrophic vaginitis
- Retention of foreign body (tampon)
- Desquamative inflammatory vaginitis
- Vulvodynia
- Vulvar dermatologic conditions
- Allergic reaction (spermicides, deodorants, soaps, etc.)

Diagnostic Studies:
- Visualization of pseudohyphae and/or budding on saline microscopy when mixed with 10% KOH (unless *C. glabrata*)
- Gram stain
- Cultures
- Vaginal pH 4.0 to 4.5

Treatment (Tables 6-16 and 6-17):
- Maintenance: Oral fluconazole (i.e., 100-, 150-, or 200-mg dose) weekly for 6 months is the first line of treatment.
- Compromised host: 7 to 14 days of topical therapy

Table 6-16: CDC Recommended Regimens for the Treatment of Uncomplicated Vulvovaginal Candidiasis

Over-the-Counter Intravaginal Agents	Prescription Intravaginal Agents	Oral Agents
• **Butoconazole** 2% cream 5 g intravaginally for 3 d Or • **Clotrimazole** 1% cream 5 g intravaginally for 7–14 d Or • **Clotrimazole** 2% cream 5 g intravaginally for 3 d Or • **Miconazole** 2% cream 5 g intravaginally for 7 d Or • **Miconazole** 4% cream 5 g intravaginally for 3 d Or • **Miconazole** 100 mg vaginal suppository, one suppository for 7 d Or • **Miconazole 200** mg vaginal suppository, one suppository for 3 d Or • **Miconazole** 1,200 mg vaginal suppository, one suppository for 1 day Or • **Tioconazole** 6.5% ointment 5 g **intravaginally** in a single application	• **Butoconazole** 2% cream (single-dose bioadhesive product), 5 g intravaginally for 1 day Or • **Nystatin** 100,000-unit vaginal tablet, one tablet for 14 d Or • **Terconazole** 0.4% cream 5 g intravaginally for 7 d Or • **Terconazole** 0.8% cream 5 g intravaginally for 3 d Or • **Terconazole** 80 mg vaginal suppository, one suppository for 3 d	• **Fluconazole** 150 mg oral tablet, one tablet in single dose

Adapted from Centers for Disease Control and Prevention. *2015 STD treatment guidelines.* Retrieved from http://www.cdc.gov/std/tg2015/bv.htm

Table 6-17: CDC Recommended Regimens for the Treatment of Complicated Vulvovaginal Candidiasis

Recurrent Vulvovaginal Candidiasis (RVVC)	Severe Vulvovaginal Candidiasis (VVC)	Nonalbicans VVC
• Seven to 14 d of topical therapy or a 100-, 150-, or 200-mg oral dose of fluconazole every third day for a total of three doses [day 1, 4, and 7]) • Consider Maintenance Regimen	• Seven to 14 d of topical "azole" • Fluconazole 150 mg repeated in 72 hr	• Optimal treatment unknown • 7 to 14 d of nonfluconazole azole drug • Boric acid 600 mg in a gelatin capsule administered vaginally once daily for 2 wk

Adapted from Centers for Disease Control and Prevention. *2015 STD treatment guidelines.* Retrieved from http://www.cdc.gov/std/tg2015/candidiasis.htm

Special Considerations:
- Patients should be instructed to return for follow-up visits only if symptoms persist or recur within 2 months of onset of the initial symptoms.
- Topical agents usually cause no systemic side effects; local burning or irritation can occur, mimicking original symptoms.
  - Therapy with the oral "azoles" has been associated rarely with abnormal elevations of liver enzymes.
  - Be sure complete medication history is accurate: significant interactions can occur when oral agents are administered with other drugs, including astemizole, calcium channel antagonists, cisapride, cyclosporin A, oral hypoglycemic agents, phenytoin, protease inhibitors, tacrolimus, terfenadine, theophylline, trimetrexate, rifampin, and warfarin.
  - Consider referring to a vulvovaginitis specialist for complicated VVC if treatment is not effective.
  - Creams and suppositories in this regimen are oil-based and may weaken latex condoms and diaphragms.
  - Douching may worsen symptoms.
  - Abstain from sex until both patient and partners are treated and asymptomatic.
  - All patients should be counseled on prevention, transmission, treatment, follow-up, and safe sex practices (use of latex condoms).
  - Discuss treatment plans, strict adherence, and follow-up.
  - Screen for concomitant STIs.

Atrophic Vaginitis

Definition: Atrophic vaginitis, or vaginal atrophy, is inflammation and thinning of the vaginal epithelium; can also affect the urinary tract.

Epidemiology/Etiology:
- Cause is from decrease in estrogen levels (estrogen deficiency); common and underreported.
- Decrease or absence of estrogen causes a loss of cellular glycogen and lactic acid; the epithelium becomes thinned and less elastic; the vagina becomes short and narrow; the pH increases; mechanical weakness occurs and causes predisposition to infection.
- Usually observed in perimenopausal, menopausal, and postmenopausal women; also seen in conditions and medical therapy that decrease ovarian estrogen (i.e., radiation therapy, chemotherapy, oophorectomy, lactation, and antiestrogen medications).

Signs and Symptoms:
- **Subjective Complaints**
  - May be asymptomatic
  - Vulvovaginal pruritus
  - Decrease in vaginal lubrication
  - Dyspareunia
  - Vaginal dryness
  - Vaginal irritation/burning
  - Vague pressure sensation
  - Hematuria
  - Urinary urgency, frequency

- Stress incontinence
- Yellow vaginal discharge with odor
- Postcoital bleeding
- **Physical Examination Findings**
  - Pale, smooth, and shiny vaginal epithelium
  - May see areas of inflammation
  - Friability
  - Watery, yellow discharge
  - Dryness of labia/recession of labia minora
  - Decrease of vaginal rugae
  - Urethral caruncle
  - Stenotic vaginal introitus
  - Minor lacerations
  - Organ prolapse (cystocele, rectocele, etc.)

Differential Diagnosis:
- Trichomoniasis
- Bacterial vaginosis
- Chlamydia
- Gonorrhea
- Herpes genitalis
- Candidiasis
- Retention of foreign body (tampon)
- Desquamative inflammatory vaginitis
- Vulvodynia
- Vulvar dermatologic conditions
- Allergic reaction (spermicides, deodorants, soaps, etc.)
- Urinary tract infection
- Organ prolapse
- Neoplasm

Diagnostic Studies:
- Most by physical examination
- Vaginal pH > 4.7

Treatment:
- Over-the-counter, water-based preparations
- Topical or oral estrogen therapy

Special Considerations:
- Many women do not spontaneously discuss vaginal dryness issues.
- Some women self-treat for a vaginal yeast infection due to similarity of symptoms prior to consulting a provider.
- Dyspareunia related to vaginal atrophy may be very emotionally distressing and difficult for some women.
- Active diagnosis and intervention may help prevent, manage, or eliminate symptoms.
- Encourage safe and healthy sexual relationships.
- All patients should be counseled on prevention, transmission, treatment, follow-up, and safe sex practices (use of latex condoms).
- Discuss treatment plans, adherence, and follow-up if needed.
- Screen for concomitant STIs.

Contraception

Introduction: Approximately 50% of all pregnancies in the United States are unintended; most of the unplanned pregnancies occur in adolescence or in women aged 40 and older, one third of unplanned pregnancies in the middle reproductive years; 50% of intended pregnancies result from not using a birth control method while the other 50% result from contraceptive failure.

In order to assist women and their partner to choose the best personal methods, the providers must:
- Discuss an ongoing reproductive health plan at each visit.
- Elicit a comprehensive contraceptive and sexual history.
- Screen for reproductive and sexual coercion.
- Screen for intimate partner violence.
- Provide full counseling on options/methods.
  - Risks/benefits
  - Ascertain latex allergy.
  - Efficacy and failure rates
  - Ease of use
  - Noncontraceptive benefits
  - Explain and emphasize use of barrier methods for prevention of STIs.
  - Explain emergency contraception options.
  - Consider benefits and risks to women with coexisting medical conditions.
- Understand and consult the United States Medical Eligibility Criteria (US MEC) for contraceptive use for guidance on the safety of contraceptive method use for women with specific medical conditions (Table 6-18).

Female Sterilization

Description: Invasive fallopian tube occlusion via methods of cauterization, blocking, or ligation to prevent fertilization.
- Surgical methods (usually done by laparoscopy; can be done via laparotomy)
  - Tubal ligation
  - Electrocauterization
  - Occlusion by rings or clips

Effectiveness:
- Failure rate: 0.5%

Risks:
- Any potential risks associated with surgery (bleeding, infection, etc.) and anesthesia

Precautions:
- MEC Operative Female Sterilization
  - No categorical contraindications
  - Eligibility restrictions include known or suspected allergy/hypersensitivity to materials used for surgery; women who have conditions that would classify them as a high surgical risk; uncertainty to end fertility.
- Pregnancy (Table 6-19)

Special Considerations:
- Counsel patients that sterilization is for desired lifetime infertility; although reversal may be possible, there is a low success rate and high cost.
- Latex condom use is necessary for prevention of STIs.
- Any woman who becomes pregnant after surgical sterilization requires a full workup for an ectopic pregnancy.

Table 6-18: US Medical Eligibility Criteria: Categories

1	No restriction for the use of the contraceptive method
2	Advantages of using the method generally outweigh the theoretical or proven risks
3	Theoretical or proven risks of the method usually outweigh the advantages; not usually recommended unless more appropriate methods are not available or acceptable
4	Unacceptable health risk if the contraceptive method is used; method not to be used

Adapted from Centers for Disease Control and Prevention. *Summary of the U.S. medical eligibility criteria for contraceptive use.* Retrieved from http://www.cdc.gov/mmwr/preview/mmwrhtml/rr5904a1.htm

Table 6-19: Advantages, Disadvantages, Side Effects, and Noncontraceptive Benefits of Surgical Female Sterilization

Advantages	Disadvantages	Side Effects	Noncontraceptive Benefits
• Highly effective • Immediately effective • No need for backup method • No hormonal changes • No maintenance costs	• Requires surgery and risks involved • No protection against STIs	• Increases risk for ectopic pregnancy • Pain at incision site • Possible regret	• Reduces risk of ovarian cancer • May protect against PID

- Nonsurgical Methods
  - Tubal micro inserts (Essure)
    - Two small metal coils enwrapped in a mesh (polyethylene terephthalate (PET) are placed in the fallopian tube under local anesthesia or sedation).
    - Coils expand to prevent movement of the device.
    - PET fibers cause an inflammatory reaction causing tissue growth in the fallopian tube walls.
    - Tubal occlusion occurs within 3 to 6 months after placement.

Effectiveness:
Failure rate of 0.2%

Risks:
- Improper placement
- Possible uterine or tubal perforation during procedure
- Allergy to contrast medium used during a follow-up hysterosalpingogram

Precautions/Contraindications:
- MEC for Operative Female Sterilization
  - No categorical contraindications
  - Eligibility restrictions include known or suspected allergy/hypersensitivity to nickel; uncertainty to end fertility.
- Current PID
- Previous delivery, miscarriage or abortion within 6 weeks
- Taking immunosuppressive medications
- Known inaccessibility to uterus and fallopian tubes
- Previous tubal ligation (Table 6-20)

Special Considerations:
- Counsel patients that sterilization is for desired lifetime infertility; Essure is not designed for removal.
- Backup contraception is necessary for 3 to 6 months or until tubal occlusion is verified.
- Latex condom use is necessary for prevention of STIs.
- Patients with Essure should notify providers that they have microinserts before any intrauterine procedure.
- Any woman who becomes pregnant after microinsert sterilization requires a full workup for an ectopic pregnancy.

Barrier Methods

Description: Methods that provide an obstruction between the sperm and the egg; oldest and most widely used contractive methods; can be carried in purse or pocket
- Condoms
- Diaphragms
- Cervical cap
- Sponge
- Spermicides

Condoms: Sheaths worn over the penis or inside the vagina to prevent sperm from reaching the cervix and upper genital tract

Table 6-20: Advantages, Disadvantages, Side Effects, and Noncontraceptive Benefits of Nonsurgical Female Sterilization

Advantages	Disadvantages	Side Effects	Noncontraceptive Benefits
• Highly effective • Immediately effective • No need for backup method • No hormonal changes • No maintenance costs • No surgery required	• No protection against STIs • Requires follow up hysterosalpingogram to document tubal occlusion • Requires 3–6 mo of backup method until tubal occlusion can be verified	• Possible regret • Cramping during and post procedure	• Reduces risk of ovarian cancer • May protect against PID

MALE CONDOM

Description: Available in latex, natural animal membranes, polyurethane, silicone, and other synthetic materials
- *Only latex condoms prevent against HIV.*

Effectiveness:
- Failure rate: Highly dependent on correct and consistent use
  - Perfect use: 2%
  - Typical use: 18%

Risks: Unintended pregnancy
- Inconsistent or nonuse: Possible STI acquisition as transmission can occur with a single sex act with an infected partner
- Incorrect use: Protective effect of condoms is decreased leading to condom breakage, slippage, or leakage; more commonly entails a failure to use condoms *throughout the entire* sex act, from the beginning (of sexual contact) to the end (after ejaculation).

Precautions/Contraindications
- No contraindications
- Eligibility restrictions include known or suspected allergy/hypersensitivity to materials used in condom (i.e., latex) or in the spermicide (nonoxynol-9) (Table 6-21).

Special Considerations:
- Correct use of condoms is essential to their effectiveness; education of patients by providers is essential.
- Male condoms and female should not be used simultaneously as they can adhere to each other causing slippage or breakage of one or both devices.
- Recommending reservoir tip condoms may decrease condom breakage or leave ½ inch of empty space at tip of condom.
- Oil-based lubricants should be avoided as they can damage the condom and increase breakage (polyurethane is not affected); use water based lubrication if necessary.
- Counsel patients to check expiration dates on condom packaging; latex can degrade over time.
- Emergency contraception should be readily available.

FEMALE CONDOM

Description: Available in polyurethane or nitrile; coated internally and externally with silicone based lubricant; can be inserted into the vagina up to 8 hours before intercourse and removed directly after intercourse.

Effectiveness:
- Failure rate
  - Perfect use: 5%
  - Typical use: 21%

Risks:
- Unintended pregnancy
- Inconsistent or nonuse: Possible STI acquisition as transmission can occur with a single sex act with an infected partner
- Incorrect use: Leads to condom breakage, slippage, or leakage; more commonly entails a failure to use condoms *throughout the entire* sex act, from the beginning (of sexual contact) to the end (after ejaculation).

Table 6-21: Advantages, Disadvantages, Side Effects, and Noncontraceptive Benefits of the Male Condom

Advantages	Disadvantages	Side Effects	Noncontraceptive Benefits
• Over the counter • Easy to use • Easily reversible	• New condom required with every act of intercourse • Breakage/slippage • Requires male cooperation • Can cause vaginal irritation • Interruption of foreplay	• Possibly allergy to latex/spermicide that can cause anaphylaxis • Decreased sensation for males	• Reduces risk of STIs, including HIV (latex) • Delays premature ejaculation • Prevents allergy to semen

Table 6-22: Advantages, Disadvantages, Side Effects, and Noncontraceptive Benefits of the Female Condom

Advantages	Disadvantages	Side Effects	Noncontraceptive Benefits
• Over the counter • Can be used during menses • Woman controlled • Easily reversible • Can be placed before initiation of intercourse	• New condom required with every act of intercourse • Breakage/slippage • Can be noisy • Can cause vaginal irritation and discomfort • Can cause penile irritation • Expensive	• Possible hypersensitivity to materials and lubricant	• Reduces risk of STIs, including HIV

Precautions/Contraindications:
- No contraindications
- Eligibility restrictions include known or suspected allergy/hypersensitivity to materials used in condom or lubricant (Table 6-22).

Special Considerations:
- Correct use of condoms is essential to their effectiveness; education of patients by providers is essential.
- Educate to check the expiration date on the condom packaging; condoms are more likely to break if used after the expiration date.
- Male condoms and female should not be used simultaneously as they can adhere to each other causing slippage or breakage of one or both devices.
- Emergency contraception should be readily available.

DIAPHRAGM

Description: Small, latex or silicone covered, dome shaped device; one teaspoon of spermicide fills dome and additional spermicide coats the rim of the device to create a spermicidal barrier prior to placement; placed into the vagina, over the cervix, and behind the pubis symphysis; provider fitting necessary with sizes ranging from 50 to 95 mm.
- Types
  - Flat metal spring (for women with firm vaginal muscle tone)
  - Coil metal spring (for women with average vaginal muscle tone)
  - Arcing spring (for women with decreased vaginal muscle tone)
  - Wide seal (for women with average or decreased vaginal muscle tone)

Effectiveness:
- Failure rate
  - Perfect use: 6%
  - Typical use: 12%

Risks:
- Unintended pregnancy
- Higher incidence of urinary tract infection (UTI), bacterial vaginosis, vaginal candidiasis

- Birth control methods that need spermicides to be effective should only be used if the woman is at low risk of HIV infection; frequent use of spermicides may increase the risk of getting HIV from an infected partner
- Increased risk of toxic shock syndrome if the diaphragm is left in for more than 24 hours

Precautions/Contraindications:
- MEC Category 4:
  - High risk for HIV infection
- MEC Category 3:
  - High risk for HIV infection or AIDS
  - History of toxic shock syndrome
  - Antiretroviral therapy
  - Allergy to latex
  - Allergy to spermicides
- History of recurrent UTIs
- Not recommended for patients with significant anatomical conditions (i.e., cystocele, rectocele, uterine prolapse) (Table 6-23)

Special Considerations:
- Correct use and placement of diaphragm is essential to effectiveness; education of patients by providers is essential
  - Teach application of spermicide, placement, and removal; practice in office with provider available to check.
  - Insert the diaphragm up to 6 hours before intercourse; leave it in place for at least 6 hours but no more than 24 hours after the last act of intercourse.
  - Additional acts of intercourse before 6 hours have elapsed require insertion of fresh spermicide onto the rim of the diaphragm with her finger without removing the device.
  - Must be left in place for 6 to 8 hours
  - Once removed, wash with warm soap and water, dry thoroughly, inspect for holes and tears, store in cool, clean, and dark environment.
- Oil-based lubricants should be avoided as they can damage the condom and increase breakage.
- Emergency contraception should be readily available.
- Diaphragm needs to be refit after:
  - Childbirth
  - Pelvic surgery
  - Weight changes of 10 to 15 lbs

CERVICAL CAP

Description: Smaller version of the diaphragm; device fits snugly over the cervix; spermicide is placed inside the bowl and groove around the outside of the device and inserted into the vagina; cap is pressed up against cervix to form a tight seal; only available cap in the United States is made of silicone (latex free).

Table 6-23: Advantages, Disadvantages, Side Effects, and Noncontraceptive Benefits of the Diaphragm

Advantages	Disadvantages	Side Effects	Noncontraceptive Benefits
• Can be inserted 6 hr before intercourse and must be left in place for 6–8 hr afterward • Cost effective (used for up to 2 yr) • No hormonal effects • Can be used while breast-feeding beginning 6 wk after childbirth	• Requires a visit to a trained provider for sizing and instruction • Required with every act of intercourse • Insertion and removal may be difficult for some women • Requires additional spermicide insertion into vagina another act of intercourse occurs within 6 hr	• Possible hypersensitivity to materials and spermicide • UTI • Bacterial vaginosis • Vaginal candidiasis • Increases risk of toxic shock • Pelvic discomfort or vaginal irritation	• May reduce risk of STIs • May lower risk of cervical neoplasia

- Sizes:
  - 22 mm (nulliparous women)
  - 26 mm (women with history of pregnancy, regardless of outcome)
  - 30 mm (multiparous women with history of full term vaginal delivery)

Effectiveness:
- Failure rate
  - Approximately 14% among nulliparous women
  - Approximately 29% among women with a history of vaginal delivery

Risks:
- Unintended pregnancy
- Higher incidence of bacterial vaginosis and vaginal candidiasis
- Birth control methods that need spermicides to be effective should only be used if the woman is at low risk of HIV infection; frequent use of spermicides may increase the risk of getting HIV from an infected partner
- Increased risk of toxic shock syndrome if the cap is left in for more than 24 hours
- Not recommended for patients with significant anatomical conditions (i.e., cystocele, rectocele, uterine prolapse) (Table 6-24)

Special Considerations:
- Correct use and placement of the cervical cap is essential to effectiveness; education of patients by providers is essential.
  - Teach application of spermicide, placement, and removal; practice in office with provider available to check.
  - Must fit snugly over the cervix; leave it in place for at least 6 hours but no more than 48 hours after the last act of intercourse.
  - Must be left in place for 6 to 8 hours.
  - Once removed, wash with warm soap and water, dry thoroughly, inspect for holes and tears, store in cool, clean, and dark environment.
- Do not prescribe until 6 weeks postpartum or post abortion.
- Does not protect against STIs; latex condoms should be used.
- Emergency contraception should be readily available.

SPONGE

Description: Small, doughnut-shaped device containing 1 g of nonoxynol-9 spermicide that fits over the cervix; made of polyurethane and has a loop for easy removal

Table 6-24: Advantages, Disadvantages, Side Effects, and Noncontraceptive Benefits of the Cervical Cap

Advantages	Disadvantages	Side Effects	Noncontraceptive Benefits
• Cost effective. No hormonal effects • No need to insert more spermicide with additional acts of intercourse • Woman controlled	• High degree of cap displacement with intercourse • Requires a visit to a trained provider for sizing and instruction • Required with every act of intercourse • Must be left in place for 6–8 hr afterward • Insertion and removal may be difficult for some women • Should not be worn for more than 48 hr	• Possible hypersensitivity to materials, sulfites, and spermicide • Bacterial vaginosis • Vaginal candidiasis • Increases risk of toxic shock • Pelvic discomfort or vaginal irritation	• None

Effectiveness:
- Failure rate
  - Perfect use 9% and typical use 12% among nulliparous women
  - Perfect use 20% and typical use 24% among parous women

Risks:
- Unintended pregnancy
- Higher incidence of bacterial vaginosis and vaginal candidiasis
- Increased risk of toxic shock syndrome if the sponge is left in for more than 24 hours
- Birth control methods that need spermicides to be effective should only be used if the woman is at low risk of HIV infection; frequent use of spermicides may increase the risk of getting HIV from an infected partner
- Not recommended for patients with significant anatomical conditions (i.e., cystocele, rectocele, uterine prolapse) (Table 6-25)

Special Considerations:
- Correct use and placement of the sponge is essential to effectiveness; education of patients by providers is essential.
  - Must fit snugly over the cervix; leave it in place for at least 6 hours after last act of intercourse
  - Must be left in place for 6 to 8 hours
  - Must be removed after 48 hours
  - Discard after removal.
- Does not protect against STIs; latex condoms should be used
- Emergency contraception should be readily available.

SPERMICIDE

Description: Foam, jelly, cream, film, or suppository inserted into the vagina used to destroy sperm; used often with other forms of contraception

Effectiveness:
- Failure rate
  - Perfect use: 18%
  - Typical use: 28%

Risks:
- Unintended pregnancy
- Higher incidence of bacterial vaginosis and vaginal candidiasis
- Birth control methods that need spermicides to be effective should only be used if the woman is at low risk of HIV infection; frequent use of spermicides may increase the risk of getting HIV from an infected partner (Table 6-26)

Special Considerations:
- Needs to be placed high in the vagina (close to cervix)
- Does not protect against STIs/HIV; latex condoms should be used.
- Emergency contraception should be readily available.
- Spermicide should be left in vagina for 6 hours past intercourse; no washing or douching.

Table 6-25: Advantages, Disadvantages, Side Effects, and Noncontraceptive Benefits of the Sponge

Advantages	Disadvantages	Side Effects	Noncontraceptive Benefits
• Over the counter • Can be inserted before intercourse • No hormonal effects • No need to insert more spermicide with additional acts of intercourse • Woman controlled • Effective for 24 hr	• Can be only used once • Required with every act of intercourse • Must be left in place for 6–8 hr afterward • Insertion and removal may be difficult for some women • Should not be worn for more than 24 hr	• Possible hypersensitivity to materials and spermicide • Bacterial vaginosis • Vaginal candidiasis • Increases risk of toxic shock • Pelvic discomfort or vaginal irritation • Vaginal dryness	• None

Table 6-26: Advantages, Disadvantages, Side Effects, and Noncontraceptive Benefits of Spermicide

Advantages	Disadvantages	Side Effects	Noncontraceptive Benefits
• Cost effective • Over the counter • No hormonal effects • Woman controlled	• Required with every act of intercourse • Each form of spermicide has own set of directions; must read and follow directions carefully • Does not protect against STIs/HIV	• Possible hypersensitivity/allergy to spermicide • Bacterial vaginosis • Vaginal candidiasis • Pelvic discomfort or vaginal irritation	• None

COITUS INTERRUPTUS (WITHDRAWAL)

Description: During intercourse, penis is withdrawn from the vagina prior to ejaculation; known as "pulling out"

Effectiveness:
- Failure rate
  - Typical use: 27%
  - Perfect use: 4%

Risks:
- Unintended pregnancy
- STIs/HIV (Table 6-27)

Special Considerations:
- Emergency contraception should be readily available
- Counsel for STI/HIV testing

HORMONAL CONTRACEPTIVES

Description: The use of hormones (estrogen and progestin) to prevent pregnancy; delivery systems include: oral birth control pills; contraceptive patch, injections, implants, vaginal rings, and IUDs; approximately one third of all sexually active women in the United States, including 50% of women aged 20 to 24 years, use OCP.

Combination Oral Contraceptives (COC): Pill taken orally every day for contraception and/or for noncontraceptive benefits; contains various combinations of estrogen and progestin.
- Monophasic preparations: Delivers same amount of hormones throughout cycle
- Multiphasic preparations: Delivers a varying amount of hormones throughout the cycle

Hormonal mechanism of action: Important for providers to understand the mechanisms of action and the effects of the common hormones in order to select most appropriate and acceptable formulation.

Estrogen—Enhances Cycle Control:
- Suppression of the hypothalamic gonadotropin-releasing factors
- Suppression of the pituitary production of follicle stimulating hormone (FSH)
  - Inhibits ovulation
- Alters secretions within the uterus to produce edema and dense cellularity
  - Decreases chance of implantation
- Prevents follicle maturation
- Stabilizes the endometrium
- Potentiates progestin effect
  - Ethinyl estradiol

Progestin—Provides Major Contraceptive Effect
- Suppression of the hypothalamic gonadotropin-releasing factors
- Suppresses secretion of luteinizing hormone (LH)
  - Inhibits ovulation

Table 6-27: Advantages, Disadvantages, Side Effects, and Noncontraceptive Benefits of Coitus Interruptus

Advantages	Disadvantages	Side Effects	Noncontraceptive Benefits
• No costs • No hormonal effects • No devices • No chemicals	• Male controlled; must be able to accurately predict ejaculation • Does not protect against STIs/HIV • May diminish sexual pleasure	• None	• None

- Thickens cervical mucous
- Inhibits sperm migration
- Creates atrophic endometrium for implantation

Common Progestins
- First generation: Good potency; well tolerated; choice when low levels of progestins are desirable; may cause increased break through bleeding (BTB)
  - Norethindrone, norethindrone acetate, ethynodiol diacetate
- Second generation: Higher potency; longer half-life; higher androgenic activity; may increase libido but may also potentiate acne, hirsutism, and dyslipidemia
  - Norgesterel and levonorgesterel
- Third generation: Maintain increased progestational activity; reduce androgen activity; potentiate estrogenic activity with low androgens and increase sex hormone–binding globulin (SHBG);
  - Decrease cystic acne;
  - Possible increase in risk of thrombotic events (due to estrogen activity)
  - Desogestrel, norgestimate, gestodene
- Fourth generation: Come from spironolactone, a potassium sparing diuretic; have antimineralocorticoid and antiandrogenic properties
  - Drospirenone

Effectiveness:
- Failure rate
  - Perfect use: 0.3%
  - Typical use: 8%

Risks (Tables 6-28 to 6-30):

Special Considerations:
Educate Patients:
- Pill should be taken same time each day.
- Take pills with meals or at bedtime to reduce nausea.
- Latex condoms should be used for prevention of STIs.

Initiation: Please see MEC for contraindications and precautions.
- Comprehensive health history
- BP
- Weight and BMI

Timing: COCs can be initiated at any time as long as the woman is not pregnant (Quick Start); two common initiation times.
- Start on the first day of menstrual.
- Start on the first Sunday after menstrual bleeding begins.

Backup Contraception:
- If COCs are started within first 5 days of onset of menstrual bleeding, no additional contraceptive protection is needed.
- If COCs are started >5 days of onset of menstrual bleeding, abstinence or additional contraceptive protection is needed for the next 7 days.

Switching from another contraceptive method:
- COCs can be started immediately as long as the woman is not pregnant.

Table 6-28: Combined Oral Contraceptives: Summary of the US Medical Eligibility Criteria for Contraceptive Use

Category 1	Category 2	Category 3	Category 4
• Age <40 yr • Anemia: Thalassemia and iron deficiency • Benign ovarian tumors • Benign breast disease • Family history of cancer • Cervical ectropion • Mild cirrhosis • Minor surgery without immobilization • Depressive disorders • History of gestational diabetes mellitus • Endometrial cancer • Endometrial hyperplasia • Endometriosis • Epilepsy (watch drug interactions) • Gestational trophoblastic disease • Headaches: Nonmigrainous • History of bariatric surgery: Restrictive procedures • History of pelvic surgery • HIV • Malaria • Ovarian cancer • Parity • Past ectopic pregnancy • PID • Postabortion • Postpartum >42 d • Severe dysmenorrhea • STIs • Vaginitis • Varicose veins • Thyroid disorders • TB • Uterine fibroids • Vaginal bleeding: Irregular pattern • Viral hepatitis carrier • Antiretroviral therapies • Antimicrobial therapies (broad spectrum antibiotics, antifungals, antiparasitics)	• Diabetes without vascular disease • Gall bladder disease: Asymptomatic or treated by cholecystectomy • Migraines without aura and age <35 yr • Pregnancy-related hypertension • Pregnancy-related cholestasis • Hyperlipidemias (can be category 3 depending on severity) • IBD • Liver tumor: Focal nodular hyperplasia • Obesity • ≥30 kg/m² BMI • Menarche to <18 yr and ≥30 kg/m² BMI • Postpartum without other factors for VTE • Rheumatoid arthritis • Smoking age <35 • Solid organ transplant (uncomplicated) • Systemic lupus: Severe thrombocytopenia; immune-suppressive therapy; none of the previous two • Unexplained vaginal bleeding • Uncomplicated valvular heart disease • Major surgery without immobilization • Superficial thrombophlebitis • Family history of DVT/PE (first degree) • Cervical cancer • Breast-feeding for 1 mo or more • Undiagnosed breast mass • Sickle cell disease	• Age ≥40 yr • Breast-feeding (<1 mo postpartum) • Breast-feeding postpartum • 21 to <30 d with or without other risk factors for VTE • *30–42 d, with other risk factors for VTE • Postpartum, not breast-feeding, with other risks for VTE (21–42 d postpartum) • Smoking if age ≥35 yr and <15 cigarettes a day • Gastric bypass or known malabsorptive disease/procedures (COC only) • Hypertension • Known hyperlipidemias • Previous breast cancer (no disease for 5 yr) • Gall bladder disease • Migraine without aura • Rifampin or rifabutin therapy • IBD if moderate to severe • History of cholestasis (if COC related) • Certain antiretroviral and anticonvulsant medications (i.e., phenytoin, carbamazepine, barbiturates, primidone, topiramate, oxcarbazepine)	• Postpartum (<21 d) • Smoking if age ≥35 yr and ≥15 cigarettes a day • Venous thrombosis (DVT/PE) • Known thrombogenic mutations protein S, C, or antithrombin deficiency, Factor V Leiden, prothrombin mutations • Current breast cancer • Hypertension (systolic ≥160 mm Hg or diastolic ≥ 100 mm Hg) • Pregnancy • Ischemic heart disease • Acute viral hepatitis • Malignant liver tumor • Hepatocellular adenoma • Solid organ transplant (complicated) • Migraine with aura • Severe cirrhosis • Diabetes with nephropathy, retinopathy, neuropathy, other vascular disease of >30 yr duration (can be category 3 depending on severity of disease) • Structural heart disease • Major surgery with prolonged immunization • Multiple risk factors for CVD • Breast-feeding <21 d • Stroke • Systemic lupus with positive or unknown antiphospholipid antibodies

Adapted from the CDC MMWR Recommendations and Reports. *U.S. Selected Practice Recommendations for Contraceptive Use, 2013.* Retrieved from http://www.cdc.gov/mmwr/pdf/rr/rr6205.pdf

Table 6-29: Advantages, Disadvantages, and Noncontraceptive Benefits for Combined Oral Contraceptives

Advantages	Disadvantages	Noncontraceptive Benefits
• Menses is shorter, less painful, and predictable • Highly effective when taken properly • Rapid reversibility (within 2 wk) • Reduction in PMS • Eliminates discomfort related to ovulation (mittelschmertz)	• May be costly • Daily administration with strict adherence • No protection against STIs/HIV	• Lowers incidence of endometrial and ovarian cancer • Lowers incidence of breast and ovarian disease, and pelvic infection • Lowers incidence of anemia • Decreased functional ovarian cysts • Reduces risk of ectopic pregnancy • Decreases symptoms of menopause • May reduce menstrual migraines related to estrogen withdrawal • Improve acne and hirsutism • Reduce symptoms of endometriosis, osteoporosis

Table 6-30: Side Effects of Estrogen, Progesterone, and Androgen

Estrogen	Progesterone	Androgen
• Weight gain • Early or midcycle BTB • Hypomenorrhea • Nausea • Headaches • Enlarged breasts • Breast tenderness • Melasma • Telangiectasia • Increase in gall bladder cholesterol • Hypertension • Thromboembolic events • CVA	• Weight gain (cyclic) • Late cycle BTB • Headaches • Fatigue • Mood alterations • Hypertension • Increase insulin resistance	• Acne • Hirsutism • Weight gain (slow) • Increased appetitie • Libido changes • Enlarged breasts • Breast tenderness • Increased LDL • Decreased HDL

- If it has been >5 days of onset of menstrual bleeding, abstinence or additional contraceptive protection is needed for the next 7 days.
- If the woman is switching from an IUD.
- If the woman has had sexual intercourse since the start of her current menstrual cycle and it has been >5 days since menstrual bleeding started (residual sperm may cause fertilization), consider:
  - Advise the women to retain the IUD for at least 7 days after combined hormonal contraceptives are initiated and return for IUD removal.
  - Advise the woman to abstain from sexual intercourse or use barrier contraception for 7 days before removing the IUD and switching to the new method.

Follow-Up:
Recommendations for follow-up are user and situation specific; *NO* follow-up visit is required for health women; frequent follow-up plans may be necessary for adolescents and for those with medical conditions.
- Women should return at any time to discuss side effects, issues, or changes.
- At all routine visits, all providers participating in the care of women using COCs should:
  - Assess the woman's satisfaction with her contraceptive method and whether she has any concerns about method use.
  - Assess any changes in health status, including medications, that would change the appropriateness of combined hormonal contraceptives for safe and effective continued use based on US
  - Assess blood pressure.
  - Consider assessing weight changes and discuss weight changes related to COCs

- In case vomiting or diarrhea occurs due to illness, efficacy may be compromised.
  - Vomiting or diarrhea (for any reason, for any duration) that occurs within 24 hours after taking a hormonal pill
  - Vomiting or diarrhea, for any reason, continuing for 24 to 48 hours after taking hormonal pill
  - Continue taking pills daily at the usual time (if possible); no additional contraceptive protection is needed
    - Emergency contraception is not usually needed but can be considered as appropriate.
    - No need to redose to make up for the pill lost
    - Vomiting or diarrhea, for any reason, continuing for $\geq$48 hours after taking any hormonal pill
  - Continue taking pills daily at the usual time.
  - Use backup contraception or abstinence until hormonal pills have been taken for 7 consecutive days after vomiting or diarrhea has resolved.
  - If vomiting or diarrhea occurs in the last week of hormonal pills, omit the hormonal free interval by finishing the hormonal pills in the current pack and starting a new pack the following day or if woman is unable to start a new pack immediately, use backup or abstinence until hormonal pills from a new pack have been taken for 7 consecutive days.
- Emergency contraception should be considered if vomiting or diarrhea occurred within the first week of a new pill pack and unprotected sexual intercourse occurred within the previous 5 days.
- Late or missed COCs: A dose is considered late if it has been <24 since the dose was due; a dose is considered missed if $\geq$24hours have elapsed since the dose was due.
  - One pill is late or if one pill is missed:
    - Take the late or missed pill as soon as possible.
    - Continue taking the remaining pills as prescribed, at the usual time (even if it means taking two pills on the same day).
    - No additional contraceptive protection is needed.
    - Emergency contraception is not usually needed but can be considered if hormonal pills were missed earlier in the cycle or in the last week of the previous cycle.
  - If two or more consecutive hormonal pills are missed:
    - Take the most recent missed pill as soon as possible (only one).
    - Continue taking remaining pills at the usual time.
    - Use backup contraception or abstain from sexual intercourse until hormonal pills have been taken for 7 consecutive days.
    - If pills were missed in the last week of hormonal pills, omit the hormonal free interval by finishing the hormonal pills in the current pack and starting a new pack the following day or if woman is unable to start a new pack immediately, use back up or abstinence until hormonal pills from a new pack have been taken for 7 consecutive days.
      - Emergency contraception should be considered if vomiting or diarrhea occurred within the first week of a new pill pack and unprotected sexual intercourse occurred within the previous 5 days.

Break Though Bleeding with COCs:
- Educate and reassure patients that unscheduled spotting or bleeding is common within the first 3 to 6 months on COCs.
- Consider an underlying gynecologic problems (i.e., incorrect/inconsistent use, interactions with medications, STIs, pregnancy, cigarette smoking, or any new or undiagnosed pathologic uterine conditions.
- No underlying gyn problem found:
  - Discontinue combined hormonal contraceptive use for 3 to 4 consecutive days and restart a new pack.
  - Offer alternative contraceptive options.

Counsel on Severe COC Warnings: (ACHES)
- A—Abdominal pain (severe)
- C—Chest pain (severe), cough, shortness of breath, or sharp pain upon inhalation
- H—Headache (severe), dizziness, weakness, or numbness (especially if one sided)
- E—Eye problems (vision loss or blurring), speech problems
- S—Severe leg pain (calf or thigh)

Progestin Only Oral Contraceptives (POP)

Description: OCP that contains a progestin only; no estrogen content; thickens cervical mucus to make it impermeable to sperm; see Progestin

Effectiveness:
- Failure rate
  - Perfect use: 0.3%
  - Typical use: 8%

Risks: Important to know contraindications and precautions
- Possible increase of thromboembolic conditions in users of POPs that contain desogestrel (Tables 6-31 and 6-32)

Table 6-31: Progesterone Only Oral Contraceptives: Summary of the US Medical Eligibility Criteria for Contraceptive Use

Category 1	Category 2	Category 3	Category 4
• Menarche to >45 • Mild cirrhosis • DVT/PE: Family history (first-degree relative) • Major surgery without prolonged immobilization • Minor surgery without immobilization • Depressive disorders • Anemia • Benign ovarian tumors • Benign breast disease • Family history of breast cancer • Breast-feeding (1 mo or more) postpartum • Cervical cancer • Cervical ectropion • Cervical intraepithelial neoplasia • Mild cirrhosis • DVT/PE: Family history (first-degree relative) • Major surgery without prolonged immobilization • History of gestational diabetes • Endometrial cancer • Endometrial hyperplasia • Epilepsy • Gestational trophoblastic disorder • Headaches (nonmigrainous) • Headaches without aura • History of bariatric surgery: Restrictive procedures • History of pregnancy-related cholestasis • History of pregnancy-induced hypertension • History of pelvic surgery • HIV/AIDS • Malaria • Rheumatoid arthritis • Severe dysmenorrhea • STIs • Smoking • Obesity • Ovarian cancer • Parity • PID • Peripartum cardiomyopathy • Postabortion • Postpartum • Antiretroviral therapy • Antimicrobial therapy	• Breast disease: Undiagnosed mass • Breast-feeding (<1 mo postpartum) • DVT/PE • Major surgery with pro-longed immobilization • Diabetes mellitus • Gall bladder disease • Headaches without aura age <35 • Headaches with aura, any age • History of cholestasis with past COC use • Hyperlipidemias • Hypertension systolic ≥160 mm Hg or diastolic ≥100 mm Hg • Vascular disease • IBS • Ischemic heart disease • Liver tumors: Focal nodular hyperplasia • Solid organ transplant • Stroke • Multiple risk factors for arte-rial CVD • Past ectopic pregnancy • Peripartum cardiomyopathy • Antiretroviral therapy • Systemic lupus: Severe thrombocytopenia/immune-suppressive treatment • Thrombogenic mutations • Unexplained vaginal bleeding • Heavy or prolonged bleeding	• Past and no evidence for current disease for 5 yr • Severe cirrhosis • History of bariatric surgery: Malabsorptive procedure • Ischemic heart disease (severe) • Hepatocellular adenoma • Malignant liver tumors • Headaches with aura, any age • Stroke • Systemic lupus: (positive or unknown) anitphospholipid antibodies • Antiretroviral therapy • Anticonvulsant therapy medications (i.e., phenytoin, carbamazepine, barbiturates, primidone, topiramate, oxcarbazepine) • Rifampin or rifabutin therapy	• Current breast cancer

Adapted from the CDC MMWR Recommendations and Reports. *U.S. selected practice recommendations for contraceptive use, 2013.* Retrieved from http://www.cdc.gov/mmwr/pdf/rr/rr6205.pdf

Table 6-32: Advantages, Disadvantages, and Noncontraceptive Benefits of Progesterone Only Oral Contraceptive Pills

Advantages	Disadvantages	Noncontraceptive Benefits
• Highly effective when taken properly • Simple fixed regimen (same pill every day, no hormone-free week) • May be used for contraception for women who have contraindications to estrogen • Can be used in lactating women between 6 wk and 6 mo postpartum • Immediate reversibility • Reduction in PMS • Can cause amenorrhea	• See progesterone side effects in Table 6-31. • Daily administration with strict adherence • May cause abnormal menstrual patterns • Increase incidence of ovarian cysts • No protection against STIs/HIV • Can cause amenorrhea • Ovulation still occurs in about 40% of POP users	• May lower painful crisis related to sickle cell disease • May lower incidence of anemia • May be used to treat estrogen-related dermatitis

Special Considerations:

  Educate Patients:
- Pill should be taken same time each day.
- Take pills with meals or at bedtime to reduce nausea.
- Latex condoms should be used for prevention of STIs.

Initiation: Please see MEC for contraindications and precautions.
- Weight and BMI (useful but not necessary)

Timing: POPs can be initiated at any time as long as the woman is not pregnant (Quick Start).

Backup Contraception:
- If POPs are started within first 5 days of onset of menstrual bleeding, no additional contraceptive protection is needed.
- If POPs are started >5 days of onset of menstrual bleeding, abstinence or additional contraceptive protection is needed for the next 2 days.

Switching from Another Contraceptive Method:
- POPs can be started immediately as long as the woman is not pregnant.
- If it has been >5 days of onset of menstrual bleeding, abstinence or additional contraceptive protection is needed for the next 2 days.
- If the woman is switching from an IUD.
- If the woman has had sexual intercourse since the start of her current menstrual cycle and it has been >5 days since menstrual bleeding started (residual sperm may cause fertilization), consider:
  - Advise to retain the IUD for at least 2 days after combined hormonal contraceptives are initiated and return for IUD removal.
  - Advise to abstain from sexual intercourse or use barrier contraception for 2 days before removing the IUD and switching to the new method.
  - Advise to use ECPs at the time of IUD removal.

Follow-Up:
Recommendations for follow-up are user and situation specific; *NO* follow-up visit is required for healthy women; frequent follow-up plans may be necessary for adolescents and for those with medical conditions.
- Women should return at any time to discuss side effects, issues, or changes.
- At all routine visits, all providers participating in the care of women using POPs should:
  - Assess the woman's satisfaction with her contraceptive method and whether she has any concerns about method use.
  - Assess any changes in health status, including medications, that would change the appropriateness of POPs for safe and effective continued use based on US.
  - Assess blood pressure.
  - Consider assessing weight changes and discuss weight changes related to POPs.

Vomiting or severe diarrhea (occurring within 3 hours after taking regularly scheduled POP)
- Take another pill as soon as possible.
- Continue taking pills daily, one each day, at the same time each day.
- Use backup contraception or avoid sexual intercourse until 2 days after vomiting or diarrhea has resolved.
- Emergency contraception should be considered if the woman has had unprotected sexual intercourse.

Missed POPs: A dose is considered missed if it has been <3 hours since the dose was due:
- Take one pill as soon as possible/as soon as remembered.
- Continue taking the remaining pills as prescribed, at the usual time (even if it means taking two pills on the same day).
- Use backup contraception or abstinence until pills have been taken correctly, on time, for 2 consecutive days.
- Emergency contraception should be considered if the woman has had unprotected sexual intercourse.

CONTRACEPTIVE PATCH

Description: Square transdermal patch (1.75 sq inch) applied to a woman's abdomen, buttock, upper outer arm, or upper torso; not for placement on the breasts; contains three layers: a beige outer polyester layer (protection; a middle medicated adhesive layer; and a clear liner) mimics the 28 days dosing schedule of COC's with 21 days of active hormones; three consecutive patches are applied week followed by 1 week patch-free interval; mechanism of action is same as COC above.

Hormones Released Daily:
- Ethinyl estradiol (estrogen) 20 mcg
- Norelgestromin: (progestin) (active metabolite of norgestimate) 150 mcg

Effectiveness:
- Failure rate
  - Perfect use: 0.3%
  - Typical use: 9%

Note: Efficacy may be decreased in women weighing >198 lbs (90 kg).

Risks:
   MEC for Contraceptive Use:
- Contraceptive patch criteria are the same as for COCs. See Table 6-28.
  - Important to know contraindications and precautions (Table 6-33)

Table 6-33: Advantages, Disadvantages, Side Effects, and Noncontraceptive Benefits of the Contraceptive Patch

Advantages	Disadvantages	Side Effects	Noncontraceptive Benefits
• Convenient • Menses is shorter, less painful, and predictable • Highly effective when used properly • Forgiving: Each patch can inhibit ovulation for 9 d, allowing time if a patch change was missed for up to 2 d • No significant weight gain • Tolerated well by women who cannot tolerate oral administration or who have abnormal/limited abdominal drug absorption • Rapid reversibility • Reduction in PMS • Eliminates discomfort related to ovulation (mittelschmertz)	• Visible • Skin irritation • May be costly • Daily administration with strict adherence • No protection against STIs/HIV • Possible slight increase in risk of VTE (increased serum estrogen levels)	• Skin reactions • Breast symptoms: Tenderness, pain, enlargement • Headaches • Nausea	Same as COCs: • Lowers incidence of endometrial and ovarian cancer • Lowers incidence of breast and ovarian disease, and pelvic infection • Lowers incidence of anemia • Decreased functional ovarian cysts • Reduces risk of ectopic pregnancy • Decreases symptoms of menopause • May reduce menstrual migraines related to estrogen withdrawal • Improve acne and hirsutism • Reduce symptoms of endometriosis, osteoporosis

Special Considerations:

Educate Patients:
- Patch should be replaced every week for 3 consecutive weeks.
- Apply to dry, clean skin; do not use lotions or oils.
- If the patch falls off or becomes partially detached, a new patch should be applied immediately; if patch was off or partially detached for more than 24 hours, a new patch cycle should be started immediately and additional backup contraception is required.
- To discard the patch, fold it in half (closed on itself) on the adhesive side; discard in the trash; do not flush down toilet.
- Rotate patch sites to decrease inflammation.
- Patch can be used continuously by skipping the hormonal free week and applying an active patch.
- Latex condoms should be used for prevention of STIs.

Initiation:
- Please see MEC for contraindications and precautions (Table 6-28).
- Weight and BMI; caution with patients weighing over 198 lbs

Timing:
- The patch can be initiated at any time as long as the woman is not pregnant (Quick Start); two common initiation times
- Start on the first day of menstrual cycle.
- Start on the first Sunday after menstrual bleeding begins.

Missed or Forgotten Patches:
- First week: Forgotten or placed late
  - Place patch immediately.
  - Additional contraception method or abstinence until the patch is in place for 7 consecutive days.
  - Provide emergency contraception if woman has engaged in unprotected sexual intercourse.
  - Remind patient to change patch each week on the same day of the week that she replaced the patch.
- Second to third week:
  - 1 to 2 days late
    - Remove patch and replace it with new patch.
    - No additional contraception necessary
  - >2 days late
    - Remove old patch and replace it with new patch.
    - Provide emergency contraception if woman has engaged in unprotected sexual intercourse.
    - Use backup method of contraception or abstain from intercourse until the patch has been correctly applied for 7 consecutive days.
    - Remind patient to change patch each week on the same day of the week that she replaced the patch.
- Fourth week:
  - Remove patch.
  - Replace patch on the usual day.
  - No backup method of contraception needed.

Follow-Up:
Recommendations for follow-up are user and situation specific; *NO* follow-up visit is required for healthy women; frequent follow-up plans may be necessary for adolescents and for those with medical conditions.
- Women should return at any time to discuss side effects, issues, or changes.
- At all routine visits, all providers participating in the care of women using the patch should:
  - Assess the woman's satisfaction with her contraceptive method and whether she has any concerns about method use.
  - Assess any changes in health status, including medications, that would change the appropriateness of hormonal contraceptives for safe and effective continued use.

CONTRACEPTIVE RING

Description: A soft, transparent, and flexible ring that is inserted into the vagina; made of ethylene vinyl acetate copolymer; outer diameter of 54 mm; placed vaginally every 28 days; stays in place for 21 days and is removed for 7 days to induce a withdrawal bleed; inhibits ovulation (see COC)

Hormones Released Daily:
- Ethinyl estradiol 15 mcg
- Etonogestrel 120 mcg (metabolite of desogestrel)

Effectiveness:
- Failure rate
  - Perfect use: 0.3%
  - Typical use: 9%

Risks:

MEC for Contraceptive Use:
- Same as COCs; see Table 6-22.
- Important to know contraindications and precautions (Table 6-34)
- Pregnancy
- STIs/HIV

Special Considerations:

Educate Patients:
- Woman must be comfortable touching her vagina.
- Providers can teach insertion and removal techniques in the office setting.
- Ring should be removed every 21 days; a new ring should be inserted 1 week later.
- For continuous contraception, the ring can be removed on day 21 and a new ring can be inserted for another 21 days.
- Latex condoms should be used for prevention of STIs.

Table 6-34: Advantages, Disadvantages, Side Effects, and Noncontraceptive Benefits of the Contraceptive Ring

Advantages	Disadvantages	Side Effects	Noncontraceptive Benefits
• Convenient • Vaginal delivery hormonal system increases bioavailability and lowers side effects • Does not require provider fitting • Menses is shorter, less painful, and predictable • Excellent cycle control with less BTB • Highly effective when used properly • Forgiving: Each patch can inhibit ovulation for 35 d, allowing time if a ring change was missed for up to 2 wk • Can remove from vagina for up to 3 hr without a decrease in effectiveness • Tolerated well by women who cannot tolerate oral administration, the adhesive of the patch or who have abnormal/limited abdominal drug absorption • Rapid reversibility (17–19 d) • Rapid effectiveness (3 d) • Reduction in PMS • Eliminates discomfort related to ovulation (mittelschmertz) • No weight gain • Can use with tampons • Safe in women with latex allergies	Same as COCs and: • No protection against STIs/HIV • Possible slight increase in risk of VTE (increased serum estrogen levels) • Expulsion during intercourse, constipation, removal of a tampon • Possible increased risk of VTE	Same as COCs and: • Vaginitis • Leukorrhea • Vaginal discomfort	Same as COCs: • Lowers incidence of endometrial and ovarian cancer • Lowers incidence of breast and ovarian disease, and pelvic infection • Lowers incidence of anemia • Decreased functional ovarian cysts • Reduces risk of ectopic pregnancy • Decreases symptoms of menopause • May reduce menstrual migraines related to estrogen withdrawal • Improves acne and hirsutism • Reduces symptoms of endometriosis and osteoporosis

Initiation:
- Please see MEC for contraindications and precautions (Table 6-28).

Timing:
- The vaginal ring can be initiated at any time as long as the woman is not pregnant (Quick Start); two common initiation times.
  - Start on the first day of menstrual.
  - Start on the first Sunday after menstrual bleeding begins.

Delayed Insertion or Reinsertion:
- <48 hours since a ring should have been inserted.
  - Insert ring as soon as possible.
  - Keep the ring in until the scheduled ring removal day.
  - No additional contraceptive protection is needed.
  - Emergency contraception is not usually needed but can be considered if delayed insertion or reinsertion occurred earlier in the cycle or in the last week of the previous cycle.
- ≥48 hours since a ring should have been inserted.
  - Insert ring as soon as possible.
  - Keep the ring in until the scheduled ring removal day.
  - Use backup contraception or abstinence until a ring has been worn for 7 consecutive days.
- If the ring removal occurred in the third week of ring use:
  - Omit the hormone-free week by finishing the third week of ring use and starting a new ring immediately.
  - If unable to start a new ring immediately, use backup contraception until a ring has been worn for 7 consecutive days.
- Emergency contraception should be considered if the delayed insertion or reinsertion occurred within the first week of ring use and unprotected sexual intercourse occurred in the previous 5 days.
- If removal takes place but the woman is unsure of how long the ring has been removed, consider the ring to have been removed for ≥48 hours since a ring should have been inserted or reinserted.

Follow-Up:
Recommendations for follow-up are user and situation specific; *NO* follow-up visit is required for healthy women; frequent follow-up plans may be necessary for adolescents and for those with medical conditions.
- Women should return at any time to discuss side effects, issues, or changes.
- At all routine visits, all providers participating in the care of women using the ring should:
  - Assess the woman's satisfaction with her contraceptive method and whether she has any concerns about method use.
  - Assess any changes in health status, including medications, that would change the appropriateness of hormonal contraceptives for safe and effective continued use.

INJECTABLE HORMONAL CONTRACEPTIVES

Description: A progesterone only, 3 month interval injectable contraceptive that contains depot medroxyprogesterone (DMPA); inhibits ovulation (see Hormonal Contraception: Progestin)

Two Formulations:
- DMPA 150 mg for intramuscular injection
- DMPA 104 mg for subcutaneous injection

Effectiveness
- Failure rate
  - Perfect use: 0.2%
  - Typical use: 6%

Risks (Tables 6-35 and 6-36):
Special Considerations:
- Counsel patients on the high incidence of uterine bleeding for the first 3 months while using DMPA.
- Counsel patients on the high incidence of amenorrhea after the subsequent injections.
- DMPA may not be an appropriate choice for women planning a pregnancy within 1 year.

Initiation:
- Please see MEC for contraindications and precautions (Table 6-29).
- Baseline weight and BMI (useful but not necessary)

Table 6-35: Injectable Hormonal Contraceptives: Summary of the US Medical Eligibility Criteria for Contraceptive Use

Category 1	Category 2	Category 3	Category 4
• Age 18–45 • Anemia • Benign ovarian tumors • Benign breast disease • Family history of breast cancer • Breast-feeding (1 mo or more postpartum) • Cervical ectropion • Cirrhosis (mild) • DVT/PE: Family history of first-degree relative • Major surgery without prolonged immobilization • Minor surgery without immobilization • Ovarian cancer • Postabortion • Postpartum • Thyroid disorder • Viral hepatitis • Uterine fibroids • Tuberculosis • Superficial venous thrombosis • Parity • Past ectopic pregnancy • Severe dysmenorrhea • STIs • Smoking • PID • Peripartum cardiomyopathy • Depressive disorders • Obesity • History of gestational diabetes • Malaria • History of pregnancy-induced hypertension • History of pelvic surgery • HIV/AIDS • History of bariatric surgery • Endometrial hyperplasia • Endometrial cancer • Epilepsy • Gestational trophoblastic disease • Headaches (nonmigrainous) • History of pregnancy-related cholestasis • Antiretroviral therapy • Anticoagulant therapy • Antimicrobial therapy • Rifamicin or rifabutin therapy	• Menarche to <18 • Age >45 yr • Breast disease: Undiagnosed mass • Breast-feeding (<1 mo postpartum) • Cervical cancer • Cervical intraepithelial neoplasia • DVT/PE • Major surgery with prolonged immunization • Diabetes: Insulin and noninsulin dependent • Liver tumor focal nodular hyperplasia • Gallbladder disease • Migraine headaches with or without aura age ≥35; with aura any age may be a category 3 depending on severity and age • Solid organ transplant • Thrombogenic mutations • Rheumatoid arthritis (may be category 3 if severe) • Peripartum cardiomyopathy (moderate to severe) • History of COC-related cholestasis • Obesity: Menarche to ≤18 yr and 30 kg/m² BMI • Hyperlipidemia • IBS • Hypertension: Systolic 140–159 mm Hg or diastolic 90–99 mm Hg	• History of breast cancer with no recurrent disease for 5 yr) • Cirrhosis (severe) • Diabetes mellitus with nephropathy, retinopathy/neuropathy; other vascular disease or diabetes >20 yr duration • Hypertension: Systolic ≥160 mm Hg or diastolic ≥100 mm Hg • Vascular disease • Ischemic heart disease • Hepatocellular adenoma • Malignant liver tumor • Multiple risk factors for CAD • Stroke • Systemic lupus (may be category 2 if not severe) • Unexplained vaginal bleeding • Heavy, irregular vaginal bleeding patterns	• Current breast cancer

Adapted from the CDC MMWR Recommendations and Reports. *U.S. selected practice recommendations for contraceptive use, 2013.* Retrieved from http://www.cdc.gov/mmwr/pdf/rr/rr6205.pdf

Table 6-36: Advantages, Disadvantages, Side Effects, and Noncontraceptive Benefits of Injectable Hormonal Contraceptives

Advantages	Disadvantages	Side Effects	Noncontraceptive Benefits
• Convenient: Does not require daily compliance • Highly effective • Woman controlled • Can be used by women who have contraindications to estrogen • Infrequent dosing • Reduces risk of ectopic pregnancy • Absence of menstruation • Decrease in ovulation pain, cramps, mood changes, menstrual headaches, breast tenderness, and nausea • Minimal drug interactions • Reversible • May use while breast-feeding	• High incidence of prolonged uterine bleeding or spotting • Requires visit to a provider for injection • Weight gain: Approx. 3.5 lb in the first year • Possible increase in depression • Delayed fertility • Long-term users may develop decreased, reversible bone density • No protection against STIs/HIV	• Severe allergic reactions may occur • Irritation/infection at injection site • May have initial prolonged uterine bleeding • Headaches • Nervousness • Decreased libido • Breast discomfort • May decrease HDL cholesterol	• Decreases incidence of grand mal seizures • May decrease anemia • Reduces pain associated with endometriosis • Decreases fibroid (myoma)-associated bleeding • Decreases risk of PID • Decreases risk of endometrial cancer

Timing:

DMPA can be given at any time as long as the woman is not pregnant.

- If DMPA is started within the first 7 days since menstrual bleeding started, no additional contraceptive protection is needed.
- If DMPA is started >7 days since menstrual bleeding started, abstinence or use additional contraceptive method for the next 7 days.

Follow-Up:

Recommendations for follow-up are user and situation specific; *NO* follow-up visit is required for healthy women; frequent follow-up plans may be necessary for adolescents and for those with medical conditions.

- Women should return at any time to discuss side effects, issues, or changes.
- At all routine visits, all providers participating in the care of women using DMPA should:
  - Assess the woman's satisfaction with her contraceptive method and whether she has any concerns about method use.
  - Assess any changes in health status, including medications, that would change the appropriateness of DMPA for safe and effective continued use
  - Women must return every 13 weeks for injection.

Early Injection:

- Can be given early when necessary

Late Injection:

- May be given up to 2 weeks late without requiring additional contraceptive protection (15 weeks from last injection)
- If the woman is >2 weeks late (>15 weeks from the last injection) for a repeat DMPA injection, she can have the injection if she is not pregnant; abstinence from sexual intercourse or use additional contraceptive method for the next 7 days.
- Consider the use of emergency contraception if appropriate.

Educate on DMPA Warning Signs:

- Repeated, intense headaches
- Heavy bleeding
- Depression
- Severe lower abdominal pain
- Signs and symptoms of injection site infection: Prolonged pain, redness, itching, or bleeding, pus like exudate

IMPLANTABLE HORMONAL CONTRACEPTIVES

Description: Single rod or tube containing a progesterone hormone; inserted in the subdermal tissue of the arm; etonogestrel 68 mg (same progestin that is contained in the vaginal ring) is slowly released over 3 years to suppress ovulation (see Progestins); contains barium to allow location/position via X-ray

Effectiveness:
- Failure rate
  - Perfect use: 0.05%
  - Typical use: 0.05%

Risks (Tables 6-37 and 6-38):

Special Considerations:
- Counsel patients on the high incidence of uterine bleeding or amenorrhea with implants.
- May be a good option for women with conditions with alterations in carbohydrate metabolism (i.e., diabetics)
- Make sure women know the date of replacement.

Table 6-37: Implantable Hormonal Contraceptives: Summary of the US Medical Eligibility Criteria for Contraceptive Use

Category 1	Category 2	Category 3	Category 4
• Age 18–45 • Anemia • Benign ovarian tumors • Benign breast disease • Family history of breast cancer • Breast-feeding (1 mo or more postpartum) • Cervical ectropion • Multiple risk factors for CAD • Cirrhosis (mild) • DVT/PE: Family history of first-degree relative • Major surgery without prolonged immobilization • Minor surgery without immobilization • Ovarian cancer • Postabortion • Postpartum • Thyroid disorder • Viral hepatitis • Uterine fibroids • Tuberculosis • Rheumatoid Superficial venous thrombosis • Parity • Past ectopic pregnancy • IBS • Severe dysmenorrhea • STIs • Smoking • Hypertension: Controlled • Hypertension: Systolic 140–159 mm Hg or diastolic 90–99 mm Hg • PID • Peripartum cardiomyopathy • Depressive disorders • Obesity	• Menarche to <18 • Age >45 yr • Breast disease: Undiagnosed mass • Breast-feeding (<1 mo postpartum) • Cervical cancer • Cervical intraepithelial neoplasia • DVT/PE • Major surgery with prolonged immunization • Diabetes: Insulin and non-insulin dependent • Vascular disease • Liver tumor: Focal nodular hyperplasia • Gallbladder disease • Migraine headaches with or without aura age ≥35; with aura any age may be a category 3 depending on severity and age • Solid organ transplant • Thrombogenic mutations • Peripartum cardiomyopathy (moderate to severe) • History of COC-related cholestasis • Hyperlipidemia • Antiretroviral therapy • Anticonvulsant therapy • Antimicrobial therapy • Rifamicin or rifabutin therapy	• History of breast cancer with no recurrent disease for 5 yr • Cirrhosis (severe) • Diabetes mellitus with nephropathy, retinopathy/neuropathy; other vascular disease or diabetes >20 yr duration • Hypertension: Systolic ≥160 mm Hg or diastolic ≥100 mm Hg • Ischemic heart disease • Hepatocellular adenoma • Malignant liver tumor • Stroke • Systemic lupus (may be category 2 if not severe) • Unexplained vaginal bleeding • Heavy, irregular vaginal bleeding patterns	• Current breast cancer

(*continued*)

Table 6-37: Implantable Hormonal Contraceptives: Summary of the US Medical Eligibility Criteria for Contraceptive Use (*continued*)

- History of gestational diabetes
- Malaria
- History of pregnancy-induced hypertension
- History of pelvic surgery
- HIV/AIDS
- History of bariatric surgery
- Endometrial hyperplasia
- Endometrial cancer
- Epilepsy
- Gestational trophoblastic disease
- Headaches (nonmigrainous)
- History of pregnancy-related cholestasis
- Antiretroviral therapy

Adapted from the CDC MMWR Recommendations and Reports. *U.S. selected practice recommendations for contraceptive use, 2013.* Retrieved from http://www.cdc.gov/mmwr/pdf/rr/rr6205.pdf

Table 6-38: Advantages, Disadvantages, Side Effects, and Noncontraceptive Benefits of Implantable Hormonal Contraceptives

Advantages	Disadvantages	Side Effects	Noncontraceptive Benefits
• Convenient • Highly effective • Rapid insertion: 1 min for insertion; 3 min for removal • Easy use after insertion • Reversible: Immediate fertility return after removal • High incidence of amenorrhea • Used in women where estrogen is contraindicated • Woman controlled • Reduction in PMS • Eliminates discomfort related to ovulation (mittelschmertz) • Cost effective • High continuation rate • Can be used while breast-feeding • Provides contraception for 3 yr	• High incidence of prolonged uterine bleeding or spotting • High incidence of amenorrhea • Requires visit to a provider for placement • Insertion or removal complications • Does not protect against STIs/HIV • Possible weight gain • Possible increased risk of VTE	• Acne • Breast symptoms: Tenderness, pain, enlargement • Headaches • Depression	• Provides relief of pelvic pain due to endometriosis • No impact on carbohydrate metabolism

Initiation:
- Please see MEC for contraindications and precautions.
- Baseline weight and BMI (useful but not necessary)

Timing:
- Contraceptive implants can be placed at any time as long as the woman is not pregnant.
  - If the implant is inserted within the first 5 days since menstrual bleeding started, no additional contraceptive method is needed.
  - If the implant is inserted >5 days since menstrual bleeding started, abstinence or use additional contraceptive method for the next 7 days.

Follow-Up:

Recommendations for follow-up are user and situation specific; *No* follow-up visit is required for healthy women; frequent follow-up plans may be necessary for adolescents and for those with medical conditions.

- Women should return at any time to discuss side effects, issues, or changes.
- At all routine visits, all providers participating in the care of women using the implant should:
  - Assess the woman's satisfaction with her contraceptive method and whether she has any concerns about method use.
  - Assess any changes in health status, including medications, that would change the appropriateness of hormonal contraceptives for safe and effective continued use.

INTRAUTERINE DEVICES

Description: Small "T" shaped device that is placed in the uterine cavity to provide long acting contraception; most commonly used reversible contraception worldwide.

Hormonal IUD Delivery System: Progestin Influence

LNG 52 IUS: Levonorgesterol 52 mg; released into the uterine cavity at 20 mcg daily

- Approved for 5 years of use
- Thickens cervical mucous
- Impairs sperm function
- Suppresses the endometrium causing atrophy
- Ovulation may be impaired due to the absorption of levonorgestrel in the system (see Progestins).

LNG 13.5 IUS: Levonorgesterol 13.5 mg; relaeased into the uterine cavity at 14 mcg daily

- Approved for 3 years of use
- Thickens cervical mucous
- Impairs sperm function
- Suppresses the endometrium causing atrophy
- Ovulation may be impaired due to the absorption of levonorgestrel in the system (see Progestins)

Nonhormonal IUD Delivery System:

Copper T 380A IUD: Contains polyethylene and copper along the horizontal arms and the vertical stem

- Approved for 10 years of use
- Causes an increase in copper ions, enzymes, prostaglandins and white blood cells (immune response) in tubal fluids; inhibits sperm motility and the acrosomal reaction necessary for fertilization
- Rarely inhibits implantation; does not interrupt an implanted pregnancy

Effectiveness:

- Failure rate
  - LNG IUD
    - Perfect use: 0.6%
    - Typical use: 0.8%
  - Copper T
    - Perfect use: 0.2%
    - Typical use: 0.2%

Risks:

Please see Tables 6-39 to 6-41 for MEC for contraceptive use: Important to know contraindications and precautions

- Differences between the hormonal and nonhormonal systems
- Chance of uterine perforation on insertion
- Possibility of expulsion (2% to 10% in first year/3.2% in 3 years causing unintended pregnancy if expulsion is unknown); more likely at time of menses
- Women with purulent cervicitis, current chlamydia or gonorrhea infections, and those at a very high individual likelihood of STI exposure should not have IUD placement delayed until undergoing appropriate testing and treatment.
- Latex condoms should be used to prevent STIs/HIV (Tables 6-39 to 6-41).

Special Considerations:

- Counsel women on the high incidence of uterine bleeding or amenorrhea.
- Make sure women know the date of replacement.
- Teach women how to check for string placement.

Table 6-39: LNG-IUD: Summary of the US Medical Eligibility Criteria for Contraceptive Use

Category 1	Category 2	Category 3	Category 4
• Age: Menarche to ≥20 • Anemia • Benign ovarian tumors • Benign breast disease • Family history of breast cancer • Cervical ectropion • Multiple risk factors for CAD • Cirrhosis (mild) • DVT/PE: Family history of first-degree relative • Major surgery without prolonged immobilization • Minor surgery without immobilization • Ovarian cancer • Postabortion • Thyroid disorder • Viral hepatitis • Tuberculosis • Postpartum ≥4 wk • Rheumatoid Superficial venous thrombosis • Parity • Past ectopic pregnancy • IBS • Severe dysmenorrhea • STIs • Smoking • Hypertension: Controlled • Hypertension: Systolic 140–159 mm Hg or diastolic 90–99 mm Hg • PID • Depressive disorders • Obesity • History of gestational diabetes • Malaria • History of pregnancy-induced hypertension • History of pelvic surgery • History of bariatric surgery • Endometrial hyperplasia • Endometrial cancer • Epilepsy • Heavy, irregular vaginal bleeding patterns • Headaches (nonmigrainous) • History of pregnancy-related cholestasis • Anticonvulsant therapy • Rifamicin or rifabutin therapy	• Age: Menarche to <20 • Breast disease: Undiagnosed mass • HIV • Cervical cancer • Cervical intraepithelial neoplasia • DVT/PE • Major surgery with prolonged immunization • Diabetes: Insulin and non-insulin dependent • Vascular disease • Liver tumor: Focal nodular hyperplasia • Gallbladder disease • Migraine headaches with or without aura age ≥35; with aura any age may be a category 3 depending on severity and age • Solid organ transplant • Stroke • Postpartum • Thrombogenic mutations • Peripartum cardiomyopathy (moderate to severe) • History of COC-related cholestasis • Hyperlipidemia • Antimicrobial therapy • Nulliparous • PID without subsequent pregnancy • Uterine fibroids • Peripartum cardiomyopathy • Postabortion: Second trimester	• History of breast cancer with no recurrent disease for 5 yr • AIDS • Gestational trophoblastic disease: Decreasing or undetectable BhCG • Cirrhosis (severe) • Diabetes mellitus with nephropathy, retinopathy/neuropathy; other vascular disease or diabetes >20 yr duration • Hypertension: Systolic ≥160 mm Hg or diastolic ≥100 mm Hg • Ischemic heart disease • Hepatocellular adenoma • Malignant liver tumor • Systemic lupus (may be category 2 if not severe) • Unexplained vaginal bleeding • Increased risks of STI (may also be category 2 depending on severity)	• Current breast cancer • Cervical cancer: Awaiting treatment • Distorted uterine cavity • Endometrial cancer • Gestational trophoblastic disease with persistently elevated B-hCG levels • Current PID • Immediately post septic abortion • Pregnancy • STI with current purulent cervicitis • Gonorrhea or Chlamydial infection • Tuberculosis (pelvic) • Unexplained vaginal bleeding • Puerperal sepsis

Adapted from the CDC MMWR Recommendations and Reports. *U.S. selected practice recommendations for contraceptive use, 2013.* Retrieved from http://www.cdc.gov/mmwr/pdf/rr/rr6205.pdf

Table 6-40: Copper-IUD: Summary of the US Medical Eligibility Criteria for Contraceptive Use

Category 1	Category 2	Category 3	Category 4
• Age: Menarche to ≥20 • Benign ovarian tumors • Current breast cancer • Breast disease: Undiagnosed mass • Benign breast disease • Gallbladder disease • Thrombogenic mutations • Stroke • Systemic lupus (may be category 2) • Liver tumor: Focal nodular hyperplasia • Migraine headaches with or without aura age ≥35; with aura any age • Diabetes: Insulin and noninsulin dependent • Hepatocellular adenoma • Malignant liver tumor • Ischemic heart disease • Hyperlipidemia • Vascular disease • DVT/PE • History of COC-related cholestasis • Cervical intraepithelial neoplasia • Family history of breast cancer • Cervical ectropion • Multiple risk factors for CAD • Cirrhosis • DVT/PE: Family history of first-degree relative • Endometriosis • Major surgery without prolonged immobilization • Minor surgery without immobilization • Ovarian cancer • Postabortion • Thyroid disorder • Viral hepatitis • Tuberculosis • Postpartum ≥4 wk • Rheumatoid Superficial venous thrombosis • Parity • Past ectopic pregnancy • IBS • Severe dysmenorrhea • STIs • Smoking • Hypertension: Controlled	• Age: Menarche to <20 • Anemia • HIV • Cervical cancer • Major surgery with prolonged immunization • Acute DVT/PE • Solid organ transplant • Postpartum • Peripartum cardiomyopathy (moderate to severe) • Antimicrobial therapy • Nulliparous • PID without subsequent pregnancy • Uterine fibroids • Peripartum cardiomyopathy • Postabortion: Second trimester • Endometriosis	• History of breast cancer with no recurrent disease for 5 yr • AIDS • Gestational trophoblastic disease: Decreasing or undetectable BhCG • Diabetes mellitus with nephropathy, retinopathy/neuropathy; other vascular disease or diabetes >20 yr duration • Hypertension: Systolic ≥160 mm Hg or diastolic ≥100 mm Hg • Unexplained vaginal bleeding • Increased risks of STI (may also be category 2 depending on severity)	• Cervical cancer: Awaiting treatment • Distorted uterine cavity • Endometrial cancer • Gestational trophoblastic disease with persistently elevated B-hCG levels • Current PID • Immediately post septic abortion • Pregnancy • STI with current purulent cervicitis • Gonorrhea or Chlamydial infection • Tuberculosis (pelvic) • Unexplained vaginal bleeding • Puerperal sepsis

(continued)

Table 6-40: Copper-IUD: Summary of the US Medical Eligibility Criteria for Contraceptive Use (*continued*)

- Hypertension: Systolic 140–159 mm Hg or diastolic 90–99 mm Hg
- PID
- Depressive disorders
- Obesity
- History of gestational diabetes
- Malaria
- History of pregnancy-induced hypertension
- History of pelvic surgery
- History of bariatric surgery
- Endometrial hyperplasia
- Endometrial cancer
- Epilepsy
- Heavy, irregular vaginal bleeding patterns
- Headaches (nonmigrainous)
- History of pregnancy-related cholestasis
- Anticonvulsant therapy
- Rifamicin or rifabutin therapy

Adapted from the CDC MMWR Recommendations and Reports. U.S. selected practice recommendations for contraceptive use, 2013. Retrieved from http://www.cdc.gov/mmwr/pdf/rr/rr6205.pdf

Table 6-41: Advantages, Disadvantages, Side Effects, and Noncontraceptive Benefits of IUD Contraceptives

Advantages	Disadvantages	Side Effects	Noncontraceptive Benefits
• Highly effective • Can be used for women of all ages and parity • Long-term method • Rapid return to fertility after removal • Excellent safety record • Woman controlled • Convenient • Visible on X-ray, MRI, and ultrasound • Used in women where estrogen is contraindicated • Can use while breast-feeding • Tampon use is fine	• Menstrual disturbances • Requires a visit to a provider for insertion • Cramping and discomfort • Possibility of expulsion • Infection • Uterine perforation/device migration • Pregnancy complications • No protection against STIs/HIV	• Cramping and abnormal bleeding on insertion • Copper T: Increases dysmenorrhea and heavy bleeding with menses • LNG: Amenorrhea • Actinomycosis may be seen on Pap smear	• Reduction in endometrial cancer • LNG: Reduces menstrual blood loss up to 50% (anemia) • LNG: Possible prevention of PID (see Progestins) • Lowers incidence of ectopic pregnancy

PID Considerations: Slight increase in risk of PID within the first 20 days after insertion; PID occurring after 3 months is considered and STI; Women at high risk for STIs should be screened prior to insertion; positive cultures in an asymptotic woman should be treated per guidelines (see STI) promptly; the IUD does not need to be removed during treatment unless there is evidence of spread or treatment failure.

Initiation:
Please see MEC for contraindications and precautions.
- Comprehensive history
- Bimanual examination and cervical inspection

- STI screening according to guidelines
- Baseline weight and BMI (useful but not necessary)
- Women with known medical problems or other special conditions might need additional examinations or tests before being determined to be appropriate candidates for a particular method of contraception.
- No antibiotic treatment is needed at the time of insertion unless infection is suspected.

Timing:

LNG IUD and the Copper T can be inserted at any time as long as the woman is not pregnant and:

- Anytime or immediately postpartum
- Within the first 7 days immediately post abortion (excluding septic abortion)
- Anytime for patients with amenorrhea
- Anytime while breast-feeding

LNG IUD:

- Insertion within the first 7 days since menstrual bleeding started, no additional contraceptive method is needed.
- Insertion >7 days since menstrual bleeding started, abstinence or use additional contraceptive method for the next 7 days.

Copper T:

- Can also be inserted within 5 days of the first act of unprotected sexual intercourse as an emergency contraception; can be inserted >5 days after sexual intercourse as long as insertion does not occur >5 days after ovulation; no additional contraceptive method is needed after Copper T insertion

Follow-Up:

Recommendations for follow-up are user and situation specific; *NO* follow-up visit is required for healthy women; frequent follow-up plans may be necessary for adolescents and for those with medical conditions

- Women should return at any time to discuss side effects, issues, or changes.
- At all routine visits, all providers participating in the care of women using the IUD should:
  - Assess the woman's satisfaction with her contraceptive method and whether she has any concerns about the IUD.
  - Assess any changes in health status, including medications, that would change the appropriateness of the IUD for safe and effective continued use.
  - Consider performing an examination to check for the presence of the IUD strings.
  - Consider assessing weight changes and counseling women who are concerned about weight changes perceived to be associated with their contraceptive method.
  - IUS can safely be removed when the srings are visible outside of cervical os by gently pulling on the strings; advise prompt medical attention for heavy bleeding, cramping, pain, vaginal discharge, or fever.

Management of IUD Issues and Complaints:

- Menstrual abnormalities
- Unscheduled spotting is common during the first 3 to 6 months.
  - Persistent irregularities more common with Copper T; uncommon with LNG
  - Consider underlying gynecologic issue (IUD displacement, STIs, pregnancy, polyps, etc.).
  - If no underlying issues found
    - NSAID for 5 to 7 days
    - Counsel on alternative methods if unacceptable.
- Amenorrhea
- Reassurance; common with LNG
  - If bleeding pattern changes quickly to amenorrhea, consider pregnancy testing.
  - Counsel on alternative methods if unacceptable.
- PID in IUD users:
  - Appropriately treat the PID.
  - Provide comprehensive management for STIs; educate on latex condom use.
  - IUD does not need to be removed.
  - Reassess in 48 to 72 hours; if no improvement, continue antibiotics and consider IUD removal.
  - For IUD removal, wait until antibiotics have been initiated to prevent increased risk for bacterial spread from the removal procedure.
  - Consider ECPs; discuss alternate contraceptive methods.

Pregnancy Occurring with IUD in Place:
- Evaluate for ectopic pregnancy.
- Counsel on the increased risk for SAB and preterm delivery if IUD is left in place; removal provides some reduction of risk.
- If desire is to not continue with pregnancy, provide options counseling.
- If desire is to continue pregnancy, advise prompt medical attention for heavy bleeding, cramping, pain, vaginal discharge, or fever.

IUD Strings Not Visible
- Ultrasound to confirm location of IUD
  - No confirmation; consider expulsion or perforation through uterine wall.
  - Ultrasound confirms correct IUD placement; advise prompt medical attention for heavy bleeding, cramping, pain, vaginal discharge, or fever.
- IUD warning signs: (PAINS)
  - P—Period is late
  - A—Abdominal cramps
  - I—Increase body temperature (fever)
  - N—Noticeable vaginal discharge
  - S—Spotting

EMERGENCY CONTRACEPTION

Description: Methods used by women after sexual intercourse to prevent pregnancy
- Copper T 380 IUD (see Copper T 380 A IUD)
- Oral preparations: Taken orally as soon as possible within 5 days of unprotected sexual intercourse
  - Levonorgestrel 1.5 mg: Can take as a single dose or can split the dose by taking 0.75 mg followed by a repeat dose 12 hours later)
  - Ulipristal acetate (UPA) 30 mg in a single dose
  - Combined estrogen and progestin in two doses
- Yuzpe regimen: One dose of ethinyl estradiol 100 μg plus levonorgestrel 0.50 mg followed by a second dose of ethinyl estradiol 100 μg plus levonorgestrel 0.50 mg 12 hours later

Effectiveness Failure Rate
- Copper T 380 A: <0.1%
- ECP: difficult to measure

Risks:
Same as for Copper IUD; See COCs for absolute contraindications for ECP (Table 6-42)
- Pregnancy
- STIs/HIV

Special Considerations:
- Counsel all women on the availability and types of emergency contraception
- Use of latex condoms is necessary to reduce the risk of STIs/HIV
- If vomiting occurs within 3 hours of ECP dose; another dose should be taken as soon as possible; antiemetic should be considered; UPA and levonorgestrel cause less nausea and vomiting

Table 6-42: Advantages, Disadvantages, Side Effects, and Noncontraceptive Benefits Emergency Contraception

Advantages	Disadvantages	Side Effects	Noncontraceptive Benefits
• May be highly effective • Woman controlled • Some available over the counter with no age restriction	• No protection against STIs/HIV • May need a visit to provider for IUD • Prescription • See IUD disadvantages	• Nausea • Vomiting • Abdominal pain/cramping • Fatigue • Headaches • See IUD side effects	• See IUD

FERTILITY AWARENESS METHODS

Description: Methods of contraception to prevent pregnancy by abstinence of sexual intercourse around ovulation or using knowledge of the time of ovulation to augment with other methods (Table 6-43)

Risks:

Please see Tables 6-18 to 6-42 for MEC for contraceptive use: Important to know contraindications and precautions
- Unintended pregnancy
- STIs/HIV (Table 6-44)

Special Considerations:

May not be a reliable method for women who have:
- Irregular menses
- Anovulatory cycles (i.e., PCO)
- Recently discontinued hormonal contraceptive methods
- Recurrent vaginal infections accompanied by spotting
- Entered perimenopause
- Recently delivered (postpartum)
- Difficulty reading a thermometer, accessing cervical mucous, abstaining from intercourse, or using barrier methods for fertility periods

Table 6-43: Fertility Awareness Methods

Type	Instructions	Effectiveness
Standard days method	• Count first day of menses as day 1 of cycle • Avoid intercourse or use barrier methods during days 8–19 of cycle	Perfect use: 5% Typical use: 12%
Calendar method	• Chart menses for 6 mo to calculate fertile time • Subtract 18 d from total length of the shortest menstrual cycle (first day of fertile period) • Subtract 11 d from the total length of the longest cycle • Avoid intercourse or use barrier method during these days	Perfect use: 5% Typical use: 25%
Basal body temperature method (BBT)	• Check temperature daily upon awakening by same route each day (before getting out of bed) • Record on a graph or a BBT chart • Rise in baseline temperature of 0.4°F lasting for 3 d indicates ovulation • Avoid intercourse or use barrier methods during the 3-day temperature rise	Perfect use: 3% Typical use: 22%

Cervical mucous method/ billing method	• Assess cervical mucous daily and noting changes surrounding ovulation
	  ○ Thick, sticky vaginal mucous appears after menstruation
	  ○ Thin, stretchy (elastic), clear vaginal mucous (spinnbarkeit) occurs prior to ovulation; last day of wetness or "peak day"; usually coincides with ovulation
	  ○ Thick, sticky vaginal mucous reappears after ovulation
	• Avoid intercourse or use barrier during the days of spinnbarkeit until 4 d past the peak day
		Perfect use: 3%
		Typical use: 25%

Symptothermal Method	• Combines cervical mucous method with BBT method • Uses other possible ovulation indicators such as abdominal cramping (mittleschmerz), spotting, breast tenderness, changes in position or firmness of the cervix to predict fertile period • Avoid intercourse at the first sign of ovulation until 3 d after a temperature rise or 4 d after peak cervical mucous	Perfect use: 0.4% Typical use: 13%–20%

Table 6-44: Fertility Awareness Methods: Advantages and Disadvantages

Advantages	Disadvantages
• Low or no cost • No hormonal effects • No allergic reactions to latex/spermicide/materials • Can be used to pinpoint ovulation for conception	• Requires periods of abstinence from intercourse or the use of barrier methods • No protection against STIs/HIV • Requires comprehensive understanding of the menstrual cycle, the method, and instructions (thermometer usage, cervical mucous evaluation, etc.) • Requires couple agreement and participation

Breast Disorders

Benign breast disease: Changes in the breast that are not cancer
- Mastalgia
- Nipple Discharge
- Breast Masses

Epidemiology and Etiology:
Mastalgia:
- Breast pain; can be cyclic (related to the menstrual cycle), noncyclic (not related to the menstrual cycle), and extramammary (not related to breast tissue)

Nipple Discharge:
- Fluid leaking from the breast that is not related to breast-feeding; usually benign but may be indicative of neoplastic process; color, consistency, and whether discharge is bilateral or unilateral is important to diagnosis and cause; nonspontaneous, nonbloody, bilateral discharge is usually related to fibrocystic changes

Note: nipple discharge that is unilateral and bloody may indicate invasive ductal carcinoma, intraductal papilloma, or an invasive ductal carcinoma and needs to be referred to specialist for evaluation

- Ductal ectasia: A breast condition that is characterized by dilation of the mammary ducts, periductal fibrosis, and inflammation; green, yellow, or brown nipple discharge
- Endocrinologic abnormalities: Milky nipple discharge that is not related to lactation; can signal hypoprolactinemia or hypothyroidism; can be related to hormonal contraceptive use and tricyclic antidepressants
- Mastitis or Abscess: Purulent nipple discharge

Breast Masses:
Lesions within the breast that are found during a clinical or breast self-examination
- Nonproliferative breast lesions:
  - Fibrocystic changes of the breast: Variances found in the normal breast tissue
  - Breast cysts: Fluid filled sacs with the breast tissue; may be tender
  - Fibrosis: Scar tissue and inflammation in the breast tissue; related to cyst rupture or resolution
  - Adenosis: Enlarged breast lobules due to an increasing number of breast glands
  - Lacatational adenomas: Painless, firm, and rubbery lesions found usually in late pregnancy or postpartum; mobile; increases in size due to increasing estrogen levels; regress after pregnancy and lactation
  - Fibroadenomas: Common round, solid, and rubbery tumors found in women in their late teens or early twenties; mobile; can enlarge under hormonal influence and cause discomfort
- Proliferative breast lesions without atypia: Usually do not cause palpable mass; visualized on mammography; refer to breast or oncology specialist
  - Epithelial hyperplasia: Overgrowth of the myoepithelial and luminal cells of the breast
  - Sclerosing adenosis: Increased fibrosis and extra tissue in the breast lobules; compresses and distorts epithleium
  - Radial scar: Complex sclerosing lesions that have a fibroelastic core; radial extension to the peripheral ducts and tissue
  - Papillomas: Small wart-like, intraductal growths; common in women aged 35 to 55 years

- Proliferative breast lesions with atypia: Neoplastic cells replace normal tissue within the breast without affecting the basement membrane; found on mammography; refer to breast or oncology specialist
  - Lobular carcinoma in situ (LCIS): Malignant cells replace the normal epithelium of the lobules
  - Ductal carcinoma in situ (DCIS): Malignant cells replace the normal epithelium of the ducts

Signs and Symptoms:
- **Subjective Complaints:**
  - Breast tenderness
    - Cyclic: Usually begins with the luteal phase of the menstrual cycle and ends with menses; usually bilateral
    - Noncyclic: Not associated with the menstrual cycle; can be related to tumors, mastitis, breast cysts, previous breast surgery, medications (antidepressants and antihypertensives) and hormonal therapies; may have unknown etiology
    - Extramammary: Pain with various causes unrelated to the breast tissue (chest wall trauma, fractures, fibromyalgia, angina, shingles, etc); women frequently complain of pain deeper than breast tissue, around and under the bra line, and around the rib cage
  - Fluid or discharge found on clothing; may or may not be elicited with nipple stimulation
  - Lump or a change in breast consistency
- **Physical Examination Findings:**
  - Breast examination can be normal.
  - May find areas of fibrocystic changes with or without masses in the tissue
  - Small, round, rubbery, firm, mobile tissue; usually less than 2 cm
  - Nipple discharge (see above)

Differential Diagnosis:
- Neoplastic process
- Endocrine disorders
- Fat necrosis
- Breast injury

Diagnostic Studies:
- None may be indicated
- Breast ultrasound: Can distinguish between a cyst and a solid mass
- Mammography (see Table 6-45 and Chapter 1): X-ray technique; able to detect changes in the breast approximately 2 years before they become palpable; can be screening or diagnostic
- Magnetic Resonance Imaging (MRI): Adjunct for early detection of breast cancer for women at extremely high risk; may not detect microcalcifications; helpful in post cancer evaluations
- Fine needle aspiration (FNA): Determines if a palpable lump is a simple cyst; drained fluid is evaluated by pathology
- Core needle biopsy: Large gauge needle is used to obtain tissue sample from large, solid breast masses
- Excisional biopsy: Definitive test; removal of lesion (Table 6-45)

Treatment:
- Pharmacologic (for mastalgia):
  - Treatment may be unnecessary
  - Danazol
  - Bromocriptine
  - Gonadotropin-releasing hormone antagonists
  - Tamoxifen
  - Oral and injectable hormonal contraceptives (for cyclic mastalgia)
- Nonpharmacologic:
  - Properly fitting bra/sports bra
  - Low salt diet
  - Vitamin E (controversial)
  - Vitamin B (controversial)
  - Evening primrose oil (controversial)
  - Avoidance of caffeine
  - Exercise

Table 6-45: Mammogram BI-RADS Classification

BI-RADS Classification	Recommendation	Explanation
0	Additional imaging evaluation and/or comparison to prior mammograms is needed	Possible abnormality may not be clearly seen or defined; additional imaging by spot compression, magnified views, or ultrasound is needed
1	Negative; no significant abnormality	Breasts appeal normal
2	Benign findings	No significant abnormality; the radiologist chooses to describe a benign finding such as lymph nodes in the breast, benign calcifications, or fibroadenomas; assist with comparing breast changes to future studies
3	Probably benign finding—Follow-up in a short time frame is suggested	Finding suggests a lesion with a high chance (>98%) to be benign; follow-up suggested to ensure stability
4	Suspicious abnormality—Biopsy should be considered • 4A: Low suspicion of cancer • 4B: Intermediate suspicion of cancer • 4C: Moderate concern of cancer	Abnormality that raises suspicion and needs to be further evaluated by biopsy
5	Highly suggestive of malignancy—Appropriate action should be taken	Finding shows a high probability of cancer (at least 95%); biopsy is strongly recommended; refer to breast specialist
6	Known biopsy-proven malignancy—Appropriate action should be taken	Finding on a mammogram has already been proven cancer by biopsy; used to evaluate treatment response

Adapted from the American Cancer Society. Retrieved from http://www.cancer.org/treatment/understandingyourdiagnosis/examsandtestdescriptions/mammogramsandotherbreastimagingprocedures/mammograms-and-other-breast-imaging-procedures-mammo-report

Special Considerations:
- Any suspicious findings or testing should be sent for evaluation and referred to a breast specialist.
- For benign conditions, provide education and reassurance.
- Instruction on breast self-examination and breast self-awareness
- Women should have a clinical breast examination yearly.
- See Chapter 1 for preventive services and mammography screening.
- Nipple smear for cytologic evaluation of discharge

Breast Cancer

Description: A malignant neoplasm on the breast tissue

Epidemiology/Etiology
- The most common cancer in women regardless of race or ethnicity
- Most common cause of death in Hispanic women
- Second most common cause of death from cancer in White, Black, Asian/Pacific Islander, and American Indian/Alaska Native women

Risk Factors:
- Increasing age (single largest risk factor); majority over the age of 50
- Personal history of breast cancer
- Family history of first-degree relative with breast cancer
- Long-term use of hormone replacement therapy
- Alcohol intake
- Diet high in fat
- Early menarche

- Never breastfed
- Menopause after the age of 55
- Nulliparity
- Delayed childbearing
- Exposure to radiation therapy
- Dense breasts; findings of atypical hyperplasia or lobular carcinoma in situ
- Obesity
- Positive *BRCA1* and *BRCA2* gene mutations

Signs and Symptoms
- **Subjective Complaints:**
  - May be asymptomatic
  - New lump in breast of axilla; usually painless
  - Redness or flaky skin in the nipple area
  - Pulling in or pain in the nipple
  - Changes in size or shape of breast
  - Irritation on the skin of the breast
  - Nipple discharge
- **Physical Examination Findings:**
  - May not have any physical findings
  - Firm, painless, nonmobile lump in the breast or axilla
  - Dimpling
  - Retraction
  - Skin irritations, eczema, or ulcerations
  - Pain with palpation
  - Nipple discharge
  - Diffuse nodularity
  - Lymphadenopathy
  - Fungating mass (rare)

Differential Diagnosis:
- Breast cyst
- Fibroademona
- Fat necrosis
- Intraductal papilloma
- Mastitis
- Dermatitis
- Cellulitis
- Fibrocystic breast disease/changes
- Breast abscess

Diagnostic Studies:
- Mammogram
- Ultrasound
- FNA
- Core needle biopsy
- Excisional biopsy
- Hormone-receptor studies
- Full bodywork up to check for metastasis

Treatment:
- Refer to breast specialist/oncologist (specialty team).
- Treatment may include surgical and/or medical therapies (chemotherapy, radiation, aromatase inhibitors, etc.).

Special Consideration:
- Provide support, education, assistance, and guidance to women and their supports systems.
- Encourage women and support systems to ask questions and express concerns.
- Educate about support groups and counseling.
- Emphasize follow care and further prevention strategies.

Premenstrual Syndrome (PMS)

Description: Wide variety of physical, behavioral, and emotional symptoms that usually occur during the luteal phase of the menstrual cycle; cyclic and regular; may interfere with the lives of women and their support systems

Epidemiology/Etiology:
- Many theories; cause unknown
- 90% of women experience menstrual related discomfort; 20% to 30% affect daily activities; 3% to 8% of women qualify for a psychiatric disorder
- Estimated 43 to 55 million women experience some type of PMS symptoms.
- Proposed factors include low progesterone levels, fluctuations in serotonin, vitamin deficiencies, fluid retention, hypoglycemia, and nutritional deficiencies.
- Worsens over reproductive years

Risk Factors:
- Family history of PMS
- Age; more common for women in their thirties
- Personal history of anxiety, depression, or mental illness
- Lack of exercise
- High caffeine intake
- High stress levels
- Low vitamin and mineral levels
- High salt diet/high sugar diet

Signs and Symptoms:
- More than 200 symptoms associated with PMS (Table 6-46)

Table 6-46: Common Signs and Symptoms of PMS

Physiologic	Emotional
• Breast pain	• Marked irritability
• Breast swelling	• Mood swings
• Back pain	• Anger
• Abdominal pain	• Anxiety
• Headaches	• Feelings of hopelessness/despair
• Weight gain	• Sad
• Muscle aches	• Tension
• Bloating	• Restlessness
• Extremity edema	• Loneliness
• Skin changes	• Confusion
• Gastrointestinal issues	• Depression
	• Insomnia/hypersomnia
	• Fatigue
	• Lack of energy
	• Aggression
	• Food cravings
	• Dizziness
	• Decrease interest in normal activities
	• Difficulty concentrating
	• Tearful
	• Social withdrawal

Differential Diagnosis:
- Depression
- Anxiety
- Perimenopause
- Chronic fatigue syndrome
- Irritable bowel syndrome
- Thyroid disease

Diagnostic Studies:
- Thyroid profile
- Complete metabolic panel
- Hormonal panel
- Fasting blood sugar

The American Congress of Obstetricians and Gynecologists (ACOG) has developed the following diagnostic criteria for PMS:
- Women report at least one of each of the following affective and somatic symptoms during the 5 days before menses in three consecutive menstrual cycles, end within 4 days after menses begins, and interfere with normal activities:

Affective
- Depression, angry outburst, irritability, anxiety, confusion, and social withdrawal

Somatic
- Breast tenderness or swelling, abdominal bloating, headache, joint or muscle pain, weight gain, and swelling of extremities

Treatment:
- Pharmacologic:
  - Serotonin reuptake inhibitors (Fluoxetine, Sertraline, Paroxetine, Citalopram)
  - Anxiolytic agents
  - Spironolactone
  - Prostglandin inhibitors
  - Hormonal suppression with oral contraception or gonadotropin-releasing hormone agonists
- Nonpharmacologic:
  - Complex carbohydrate diet
  - Aerobic exercise
  - Nutrition supplements (calcium)
  - PMS support groups

Special Considerations:
- PMS can exacerbate already diagnosed disorders (i.e., seizures)
- Comprehensive history is crucial to determining patterns

Abnormal Cervical Screening

Description: Results of the Papanicolaou (Pap) smear show abnormalities (dysplasia) ranging from insignificant changes to cervical neoplasia; dysplasia can be mild, moderate, or severe

Epidemiology/Etiology:
HPV is the major cause of abnormal Pap smears and is the etiologic agent found in 99.7% of cervical cancers (see Genital Warts); cofactors present in persistence: cigarette smoking, an immune-compromised system, and HIV infection
- Incidence of cervical cancer has decreased over 50% in the last 30 years due to cervical screening tests
- Approximately 12,000 new cases of cervical cancer/year and 4,000 deaths/year
- Joint screening recommendations from the American Cancer Society (ACS), the American Society for Colposcopy and Cervical Cancer (ASCCP), and the American Society for Clinical Pathology (ASCP) as well as updated guidelines from the US Preventative Services Task Force (USPSTF) reduce cervical cancer incidences markedly.
- Most HPV infections are transient; persistent infections beyond 1 to 2 years increase the risk of cervical cancer.

- HPV 16 and 18 has highest cervical carcinogenic potential.
- Most common in teenagers and women in their early 20s but decreases as women age; the normal immune system of women <21 years of age usually clears/reduces viral load of HPV infection in an average of 8 to 24 months; usually acquired shortly after initiation of vaginal intercourse.
- Most types of HPV related cancers take approximately 3 to 7 years to progress to cervical cancer.

Risk Factors:
- Smoking/history of smoking
- HIV
- History of cervical cancer or high grade squamous intraepithelial lesions
- Infrequent or absent Pap smear tests
- More than one sexual partner
- Male sexual partner who has had sex with >1 person
- First intercourse at an early age
- STIs
- Male sexual partner that has had a sexual partner with cervical cancer

Signs and Symptoms:
- **Subjective Complaints:**
  - Usually asymptomatic
  - Postcoital bleeding
  - Abnormal discharge
- **Physical Examination Findings:**
  - Visualization of the cervix is usually normal
  - Condyloma on the cervix
  - Friable cervix

Differential Diagnosis
- Cervicitis
- Vaginal carcinoma
- Endometrial carcinoma
- Vaginitis
- HSV
- PID

Diagnostic Studies:
Pap smear and HPV testing (joint organization screening recommendations):
- Cervical cancer screening should begin at age 21 years; women younger than age 21 years should not be screened regardless of the age of sexual initiation or the presence of other behavior-related risk factors.
- Women aged 21 to 29 years should be tested with cervical cytology alone every 3 years; cotesting for HPV should not be performed in women younger than 30 years.
- For women aged 30 to 65 years, cotesting with cytology and HPV testing every 5 years is preferred.
- In women aged 30 to 65 years, screening with cytology alone every 3 years is acceptable; annual screening should not be performed.
- Women who have a history of cervical cancer, have HIV infection, or are immune-compromised should not follow routine screening guidelines.
- Both liquid-based and conventional methods of cervical cytology collection are acceptable for screening
- In women who have had a hysterectomy with removal of the cervix (total hysterectomy) and have never had moderate dysplasia or higher, routine cytology screening and HPV testing should be discontinued and not restarted for any reason.
- Screening by any modality should be discontinued after age 65 years in women with evidence of adequate negative prior screening results and no history of CIN 2 or higher; adequate negative prior screening results are defined as three consecutive negative cytology results or two consecutive negative cotest results within the previous 10 years, with the most recent test performed within the past 5 years.
- To find full cervical cancer screening recommendation please see USPSTF website: http://www .uspreventiveservicestaskforce.org/uspstf/uspscerv.htm; to view the ACS recommendation statement, please see http://www.cancer.org/Cancer/news/News/new-screening-guidelines-for-cervical-cancer
- Pap smear results: See Table 6-47.

Table 6-47: Bethesda System for Reporting Cervical Cytology

Item	Clarification
Specimen type	• Conventional test (Pap test), liquid-based preparation, or other
Specimen adequacy	• Satisfactory for evaluation (describe presence/absence of endocervical/transformation zone component and any other quality indicators, i.e., partially obscuring blood, inflammation, etc.) • Unsatisfactory for evaluation (specify reason) • Specimen rejected/not processed (specify reason) • Specimen processed and examined, but unsatisfactory for evaluation of epithelial abnormality because of (specify reason)
General categorization (optional)	• Negative for intraepithelial lesion or malignancy • Other: See interpretation/result (e.g., endometrial cells in a woman aged 40 yr or older) • Epithelial cell abnormality: See interpretation/result (specify "squamous" or "glandular" as appropriate)

Interpretation/result	• Negative for intraepithelial lesion or malignancy (when there is no cellular evidence of neoplasia, state this in the General Categorization above, in the interpretation/result section of the report, or both–whether or not there are
	• Organisms (or other nonneoplastic findings)
	  ○ Organisms
	    ▪ Trichomonas vaginalis
	    ▪ Fungal organisms morphologically consistent with Candida species
	    ▪ Shift in flora suggestive of bacterial vaginosis
	    ▪ Bacteria morphologically consistent with Actinomyces species
	    ▪ Cellular changes consistent with HSV
	  ○ Other nonneoplastic findings (optional to report; list not inclusive)
	    ▪ Reactive cellular changes associated with inflammation (includes typical repair), radiation, IUDs
	    ▪ Glandular cells status posthysterectomy
	    ▪ Atrophy
	• Other (list not comprehensive)
	  ○ Endometrial cells (in a woman aged 40 yr or older) (specify if negative for squamous intraepithelial lesion)
	• Epithelial cell abnormalities
	  ○ Squamous cell
	    ▪ Atypical squamous cells (ASC)
	    ▪ of undetermined significance (ASC-US)
	    ▪ Cannot exclude HSIL (ASC-H)
	    ▪ Low-grade squamous intraepithelial lesion (LSIL) (encompassing: HPV/mild dysplasia/cervical
	    ▪ Intraepithelial neoplasia (CIN) 1
	    ▪ High-grade squamous intraepithelial lesion (HSIL) (encompassing: moderate and severe dysplasia, carcinoma in situ; CIN 2 and CIN 3)
	    ▪ With features suspicious for invasion (if invasion is suspected)
	    ▪ Squamous cell carcinoma
	  ○ Glandular cell
	    ▪ Atypical endocervical cells (not otherwise specified or specify in comments)
	      ▪ Endometrial cells (not otherwise specified or specify in comments)
	      ▪ Glandular cells (not otherwise specified or specify in comments)
	    ▪ Atypical
	      ▪ Endocervical cells, favor neoplastic
	      ▪ Glandular cells, favor neoplastic
	    ▪ Endocervical adenocarcinoma in situ (AIS)
	    ▪ Adenocarcinoma
	      ▪ Endocervical
	      ▪ Endometrial
	      ▪ Extrauterine
	      ▪ Not otherwise specified
	      ▪ Other malignant neoplasms (specify)

(continued)

Table 6-47: Bethesda System for Reporting Cervical Cytology (*continued*)	
Ancillary testing	• Provide a brief description of the test method(s) and report the result so that the clinician easily understands it. • Automated Review If case examined by automated device, specify device and result.
Educational notes and suggestions (optional)	• Suggestions should be concise and consistent with clinical follow-up guidelines published by professional organizations (references to relevant publications may be included).

Adapted from the American College of Obstetricians and Gynecologists. Practice Bulletin Number 131, Clinical Management Guidelines for Obstetrician-Gynecologists.

Treatment:
- Cytology alone
  - Negative or ASCUS cytology and HPV negative: Screen again in 3 years or maintain age appropriate screening practices
  - All others: Refer to ASCCP guidelines at http://www.asccp.org/guidelines-2/management-guidelines-2
  - Infection: Treat infection
- HPV Cotesting
  - Cytology negative, HPV negative or ASCUS cytology and HPV negative: Screen again in 5 years or maintain age appropriate screening practices
  - Cytology negative and HPV positive
    - 12-month follow-up with cotesting
    - Test for HPV-16 or HPV-16/18 genotypes:
      - If positive results from test for HPV-16 or HPV-16/18, referral for colposcopy
      - If negative results from test for HPV-16 or HPV-16/18, 12-month follow-up with cotesting
  - All others: Refer to the ASCCP guidelines

Treatments may include follow-up, colposcopy, loop electrical excision procedure (LEEP), and cold knife cone biopsy; carcinoma in situ should be referred to a gyn specialist or oncologist.

Special Considerations:
- Even if woman has had HPV vaccination, she should receive an appropriate Pap smear screening.

Amenorrhea

Description: Abnormal cessation or the absence of menstruation; normal menstrual state of a woman prior to menarche and after menopause and during pregnancy

Primary Amenorrhea: The absence of the onset of menstrual periods in a young woman aged 14 years who lacks other evidence of pubertal development or a woman aged 16 years even in the presence of pubertal signs

Secondary Amenorrhea: The condition where a woman who had previously menstruated but has been without a menstrual period for 3 cycles or 6 months

Epidemiology/Etiology:
- Affects 2% to 5% of all childbearing age women
- Approximately 3% to 4% of the population will be diagnosed with pathologic amenorrhea
- Causes arise from pregnancy, hypothalamic–pituitary dysfunction, ovarian dysfunction, and alterations of the genital outflow tract (Table 6-48)

Signs and Symptoms:
- **Subjective Complaints**: Depends on cause
  - Absence of menarche (primary)
  - Abnormalities in puberty/growth/development (primary)
  - Missed menses at regularly schedule time (secondary)

Table 6-48: Common Causes of Amenorrhea	
Primary	**Secondary**
Mullerian agenesis	Pregnancy (most common)
Hypergonadotropic hypogonadism	Menopause
Androgen insensitivity	Breast-feeding
Vaginal septum	Gonadal failure: High follicle stimulating hormone (FSH)
Pituitary tumors	Weight loss
Imperforate hymen	Poor nutrition
Puberty delay	Excessive exercise
Labial agglutination	Contraceptive methods
Cervical stenosis	Anorexia/bulimia
Abnormal karyotype	Obesity
Prolactinomas	Chronic anovulation
Kallman syndrome	Hypo-/hyperthyroidism
Turner syndrome	Cushing syndrome
Stress	Asherman syndrome
Weight changes (loss)	Addison disease
Anorexia/bulimia	PCOS
PCOS	Ovarian tumor
Head trauma	Pituitary tumor
Congenital hyperplasia	Sheehan syndrome
	Abnormal karyotype
	Cervical stenosis

- **Physical Examination Findings:** Depends on cause
  - May be normal
  - Need to take a comprehensive medical history with focus on family history, history of medications, psychosocial history, sexual history, and menstrual history
  - Breast and pelvic examination: Finds may or may not corroborate complaints

Differential Diagnosis
- Pregnancy (always rule out pregnancy as possible cause first)
- See Table 6-48.

Diagnostic Studies
- Primary laboratory studies
  - β-HCG to rule out pregnancy
  - FSH to differentiate hypogonadotropic versus hypergonadotropic hypogonadism
  - LH
  - Estradiol to differentiate hypogonadotropic versus hypergonadotropic hypogonadism
  - Prolactin to diagnose hyperprolactinemia, adenomas
  - Thyroid stimulating hormone (TSH) to diagnose thyroid disease (hypothyroidism)

- Secondary laboratory tests include:
  - Testosterone to help diagnose PCOS and to exclude an ovarian tumor
  - DHEAS to exclude an adrenal tumor
  - 17-OH-P to diagnose late-onset CAH
  - 2-hour glucose tolerance test, fasting lipid panel to diagnose PCOS
  - Karyotype and autoimmune testing to diagnose Premature ovarian failure

Radiologic Evaluation:
- Pelvic ultrasound: Diagnosis of PCOS or to determine the presence of a uterus
- HSG or saline infusion sonography: To rule out Mullerian anomalies or intrauterine synechiae
- MRI: To diagnose Mullerian anomaly or hypothalamic–pituitary disease

Treatment:
Usually refer primary amenorrhea to specialist
- Pharmacologic:
  - Progesterone challenge test to induce menstrual withdrawal:
    - Progesterone in oil 100 mg intramuscularly
    - Medroxyprogesterone acetate 10 mg p.o. every 12 hours for 5 days
    - Micronized progesterone 400 mg p.o. daily for 14 days
    - If no withdrawal bleeding occurs then estrogen is given along with additional progesterone to establish the patency of the outflow tract.
  - Estrogen therapy is required for estrogen deficiency in premature ovarian failure.
  - Oral contraceptive or hormone therapy (HT) until the age of 50 years
- Nonpharmacologic:
  - Surgical correction may be warranted.

Geriatric Considerations:
- Amenorrhea is the normal menstrual state in a postmenopausal woman.
- Menstruation after 12 months of amenorrhea (menopause) requires evaluation for uterine and pelvic neoplasm.

Abnormal Uterine Bleeding

Description: Abnormal uterine bleeding (AUB)—any menstrual flow that is not of normal volume, duration, regularity, or frequency; not related to pregnancy; uterine bleeding pattern and etiology of bleeding
- Normal menses: About 5 to 7 days in duration with cycle length of 21 to 35 days
- Heavy menstrual bleeding: ([AUB/HMB] previously called *menorrhagia*) menstrual blood loss greater than 80 ccs; also can be defined by the women's perception
  - Passing clots greater than an inch or changing sanitary protection more than every 3 hours
- Intermenstrual bleeding: ([AUB/IMB] previously called *metrorrhagia*) bleeding between menses
- Combination of both HMB IMB previously called *menometrorrhagia*
- Polymenorrhea: Bleeding that occurs more than every 21 days
- Oligomenorrhea: Bleeding that occurs less frequently than every 35 days (Table 6-49)

Table 6-49: PALM-COEIN is the Internationally Accepted Definition System of AUB with Descriptive Terms*

AUB-**P**—Polyps	AUB-**C**—Coagulopathy
AUB-**A**—Adenomyosis	AUB-**O**—Ovulatory dysfunction
AUB-**L**—Leiomyoma "Lsm" submucosal or "Lo" for other myoma	AUB-**E**—Endometrial
	AUB-**I**—Iatrogenic
AUB-**M**—Malignancy and hyperplasia	AUB-**N**—Not yet classified

*Dysfunctional uterine bleeding, the term previously used to describe AUB without a definable cause, is no longer a recommended term and not part of the PALM-COEIN system.

Epidemiology/Etiology:

One of the most common reasons for gynecologic visits; representing one third of outpatient visits and two thirds of consultations in the perimenopausal and postmenopausal years; may affect 10% to 30% percent of reproductive aged women and 50% of perimenopausal women; less likely in prepubertal and menopausal women.

- Common causes:
  - Uterine pathologies such as polyps (AUB-P), adenomyosis (AUB-A), leiomyoma (AUB-L), and hyperplasia or carcinoma (AUB-M)
- Less common causes:
  - Coagulopathies such as Von Willebrand disease (AUB-C) and ovulatory dysfunction (AUB-O)
  - Anatomic causes and normal ovulation (AUB-P, AUB-L, AUB-M than AUB-O) after a woman's normal during adolescent years.
- AUB-O includes a spectrum of disorders ranging from amenorrhea to heavy and irregular menses (AUB/HMB).
  - Polycystic ovarian syndrome (PCOS) is the most common endocrinopathy causing AUB-O from unopposed estrogen stimulation to the endometrium (80%).
- In AUB with normal ovulation and no other pathology, 20% of AUB-O (old DUB diagnosis) the hypothalamic pituitary ovarian pathway is intact and bleeding is likely from local endometrial factors including fibrinolytic activity, tissue plasminogen activator activity, and abnormal prostaglandin synthesis.

Signs and Symptoms:

- AUB of any type requires a thorough history and physical examination and appropriate laboratory and imaging tests depending on her age.
- History includes the woman's age of menarche and LMP, cycle length, menstrual bleeding pattern(s), duration, frequency, volume of blood loss, abnormal bleeding other than menses, any associated pain and any previous or current medical or surgical therapy.
- Important to elicit a medication history that may include anti coagulants: warfarin, heparin, aspirin, NSAIDs, hormonal preparations, contraceptive agents, and herbal preparations.
- A family history to rule out inherited coagulopathy.
- **Subjective Complaints:**
  - Uterine bleeding as described above
  - Fatigue
  - Shortness of breath
  - Heart palpitations
- **Physical Examination Findings:**
  - May be normal
  - Obesity or excess weight
  - PCOS signs including hirsutism, acne, thyroid nodule or insulin resistance, acanthosis nigrans on neck
  - Bruising or swollen joints
  - Abnormal uterine size or shape
  - Blood in vaginal vault
  - Visible pathology including cervical or endometrial polyps
  - Severe atrophic changes with erosion
  - Ulcerative lesion of vagina

Differential Diagnosis:

Most likely diagnosis varies by age group but excluding pregnancy and neoplasia and identification of any underlying pathology is the mandate.

- **Ages 13 to 18**: Usually associated with normal anatomy but due to either persistent anovulation from immaturity of the hypothalamic–pituitary–ovarian axis or from coagulation defects; consider pregnancy, sexually transmitted infections, and sexual abuse; may be due to nonideal use of oral contraceptives, or reaction to long acting reversible contraceptives (LARC)
- **Ages 19 to 39**: Pregnancy and STIs are more common than in 13 to 18 age group; anatomic abnormalities such as polyps and leiomyoma are more common; anovulatory cycles, PCOS, hormone contraception, endometrial pathology, and hyperplasia; endometrial cancer is rare in this age group unless additional risk factors such as obesity or chronic unopposed estrogen; postcoital bleeding, cervicitis, chlamydial infection, and cervical intraepithelial neoplasia must be considered.

- **Ages 40 to 65**: Increasingly in this perimenopausal transition age group, anovulatory bleeding from declining ovarian reserves and hypothalamic–pituitary–ovarian dysfunction is more common than pregnancy and STIs; rule out intrauterine pathology such as endometrial hyperplasia/adenocarcinoma, endometrial polyps, and myomas.
- **Ages 65 and older:** Menopause—average age is 51.5 years; amenorrhea for 12 months after a woman's final menstrual period (FMP); bleeding 12 months after a woman's FMP (postmenopausal bleeding) must be investigated to rule out premalignant or malignant endometrial pathology.
- Atrophic changes of the endometrium
- Atrophic changes of the vagina
- Vaginal malignancy with ulceration of the vagina and vulva, and serosanginous fallopian
- Ovarian malignancy

Diagnostic Studies:
- Laboratory studies:
  - Pregnancy test: Urine usually accurate and sufficient but blood test when quantitative is needed
  - Complete blood count including platelets
  - Additional screening for bleeding disorders based on family or personal history
  - TSH
  - Pap smear
  - Chlamydia trachomatis testing as age appropriate
  - Wet prep as needed (trichamoniasis)
  - STI cultures of cervix
  - Office endometrial sampling or biopsy (age >35 years or with additional risks factor such as obesity, unopposed estrogen)
  - Hysteroscopic directed endometrial biopsy when appropriate
- Imaging studies:
  - Ultrasound/transvaginal ultrasound: Anatomic growths,
  - Saline Infusion sonohysterography: Polyps and intrauterine pathology
  - MRI: For differentiating adenomyosis and myomas
  - Hysteroscopy: Office, saline, CO_2, or hospital based

Treatment:
- Pharmacologic:
  - NSAIDs
  - Combination oral contraceptives: Twice to four times a day for an acute bleed, then taper for 21 days
  - Oral progestins: Norethindrone acetate 5 mg p.o. every 4 hours until bleeding stops, then taper over 21 days very effective
  - Progestin containing IUD
  - IV Premarin: 25 mg IV every 4 hours for 3 doses as emergency
  - Androgens
  - Antifibrinolytic agents: Tranexamic acid 500 mg p.o. twice a day for 5 days (50% effective)
  - GnRH agonists
  - Iron therapy, oral and IV to treat the anemia
- Nonpharmacologic therapy:
  - Uterine artery embolization (UAE) is an interventional radiologic procedure to reduce bleeding from myomas, AUB-L (after pregnancy and malignancy have been ruled out).
  - If pharmacologic therapy has failed UAE may also be used to treat AUB-C and AUB-O.
  - Surgical therapy: Includes dilatation and curettage (D and C), endometrial ablation or resection, myomectomy and hysterectomy
  - Dilatation and curettage with hysteroscopy
  - Endometrial ablation/resection
  - Hysterectomy is the definitive therapy.
    - Patient satisfaction rate is 85%.
    - 600,000 done per year in the United States.
    - Risk benefit includes operative complications, costs, and recovery time.

Geriatric Considerations:
- Postmenopausal bleeding defined as bleeding 12 months after the FMP (described above)
- Must have tissue sampling (biopsy) for risk of uterine malignancy

- Bleeding with HT is common in the first 6 months and does not have the same risk of malignancy; decreases risk of endometrial malignancy with HT

Pelvic Pain and Dysmenorrhea

Description: Female pelvic pain can be divided into two general types: acute and chronic

Acute Pelvic Pain:
- Usually of sudden onset
- Less than 7 days duration
- Intense
- Associated with other signs and symptoms including possible unstable vital signs and significant abnormalities on history and physical examinations
- Morbidity and even mortality can result for the incorrect diagnosis which includes:
  - Appendicitis
  - Ectopic pregnancy
  - Ovarian torsion.

Chronic Pelvic Pain:
- Caused by multiple organ systems including pelvic organs and neurologic system
- Usually of long-standing, 6 months or more
- Affects quality of life and function requiring medical care

Cyclic Pelvic pain
- Associated with the menstrual cycle

Dysmenorrhea:
- Pain associated with menstruation
- Most common cyclic pain affecting 60% of menstruating women

Primary Dysmenorrhea:
- Pain with menstrual cycles from early after menarche, usually 1 to 2 years
- Young women predominate
- Unrelated to pelvic pathology

Secondary Dysmenorrhea:
- Pain associated with menses that begins sometime after menses has been established.
- Underlying pathology with a differential diagnosis similar to chronic pelvic pain

Dyspareunia:
- Persistent or recurrent genital pain associated with sexual intercourse causing marked distress or interpersonal difficulty
- Deep dyspareunia is frequently associated with endometriosis.
- Treated by treating the underlying pathology
- Insertional dyspareunia is associated with vulvar vestibulitis: treated medically with topical agents or occasionally surgical removal of vestibular glands.

Epidemiology/Etiology:

Acute Pelvic Pain
- Can be an emergency if severe.
- Correct diagnosis is critical to avoid morbidity and mortality.
- Pregnancy-related complications including ectopic pregnancy and incomplete abortion must be ruled out.
- Ovarian pathology including ruptured ovarian cysts and torsion may be the presenting problem with acute onset of pelvic pain.
- Appendicitis lifetime incidence is 7%, the most common cause of GI source of pelvic pain and of the need for surgery.

Chronic Pelvic Pain
- Affects 12% to 20% of women in the United States
- Endometriosis is the most common finding in women with chronic pelvic pain.
- Diagnosed in 15% to 40% of laparoscopies performed for pelvic pain.
- 18% to 35% of women with chronic pelvic pain have history of PID.
- Irritable bowel syndrome (IBS) is found in 5% to 80% of women with chronic pelvic pain.

Signs and Symptoms:

Acute Pelvic Pain Associated with:

- Infection, ischemia and inflammation
- Invokes the autonomic nervous system response including symptoms of
  - Fever
  - Chills
  - Diaphoresis
  - Abnormal vaginal bleeding
  - Dizziness
  - Syncope
  - Emesis
  - Significant diarrhea
  - Obstipation
  - Dysuria
  - Hematuria
  - Hematochezia

Signs Indicative of an Acute Process:

- Elevated temperature
- Tachycardia
- Orthostasis
- Abdominal distention
- Abnormal bowel sounds
- Ascites
- Peritonitis
- Abnormal pregnancy

Primary Dysmenorrhea Presents with:

- Spasmodic colicky pain 1 to 3 days before the menstrual cycle
- Nausea, fatigue, nervousness, dizziness, diarrhea and headache in 50% to 90% of women

Chronic Pelvic Pain:

- Not associated with the autonomic nervous system and usually does not present with fever, nausea or diaphoresis.
- Pain may be out of proportion to the amount of tissue damage and reflects chronic neurogenic inflammation with multiple somatic and psychological symptoms.

Physical Examination Findings:

Acute Pelvic Pain:

- Tachycardia
- Fever
- Orthostasis
- Acute abdomen with rebound and or guarding
- Cervical motion tenderness
- Tender pelvic mass
- Vaginal bleeding
- Purulent vaginal discharge

Chronic Pelvic Pain:

- Pain on pelvic examination even with gentle touch
- Pain with palpation of the pelvic floor muscle
- Cervical motion tenderness
- Pain with deep palpation of the vaginal fornix
- Pelvic masses uterine or ovarian
- Uterine enlargement consistent with myomas
- Pelvic fixation or scarring consistent with pelvic malignancy or previous surgery

Differential Diagnosis

Acute Pelvic Pain:

- Gynecologic origin:
  - Dysmenorrhea
  - Ectopic pregnancy or

- Incomplete abortion/miscarriage
- Pelvic inflammatory disease or tubo–ovarian abscess
- Ovarian torsion of cyst or mass
- Mittelschmerz
- Gastrointestinal origin:
  - Appendicitis
  - Irritable bowel syndrome
  - Colitis and inflammatory bowel disease
  - Small bowel obstruction
  - Diverticulitis
  - Mesenteric adenitis
  - GI malignancy
- Urologic origin:
  - Acute cystitis
  - Pyelonephritis
  - Kidney or ureteral stone
- Musculoskeletal origin:
  - Peritonitis
  - Complicated hernia
  - Pelvic or abdominal trauma
- Infectious and other origin:
  - Herpes zoster
  - Sickle cell crisis
  - Vasculitis

Chronic Pelvic Pain:
- Gynecologic origin:
  - Endometriosis
  - Adenomyosis
  - Myomas
  - Malignancy
  - Ovarian mass or ovarian remnant
  - Chronic PID
  - Endometritis
- Psychological origin:
  - History of physical or sexual abuse
- Urologic origins:
  - Interstitial cystitis
  - Detrusor dyssynergia (irritable bladder)
  - Chronic UTI
  - Malignancy
  - Radiation cystitis
  - Urinary tract stone
- Gastrointestinal origin:
  - Irritable bowel syndrome
  - Diverticular disease
  - Colitis and inflammatory bowel disease
  - Celiac disease
  - Malignancy
- Musculoskeletal origin:
  - Hernias
  - Spinal-related disease: Disc rupture, compression
  - Degenerative joint disease
  - Fibromyositis
- Neurologic origins:
  - Neuralgia of pelvic nerves: Ilioinguinal or genitofemoral
  - Spinal tumor

Diagnostic Studies
- Initial laboratory tests:
  - CBC with differential
  - ESR sedimentation rate
  - Urinalysis
  - Urine pregnancy test
  - Serum pregnancy test if indicated
  - Gonorrhea and chlamydia tests
- Radiologic tests:
  - Pelvic ultrasound
  - CT scan with and without contrast
  - Abdominal X-rays

Treatment
- Pharmacologic:
  - Nonsteroidal anti-inflammatory drugs (NSAIDS) for primary dysmenorrhea
    - Ibuprofen 600 mg every 4 to 6 hours maximum dose 3,200 mg in 24 hours
    - Naproxen sodium 550 mg every 12 hours
  - Oral contraceptives to reduce dysmenorrhea: Standard 28 days cycle or continuous extended fashion with cycles every 90 days
  - Ovulation suppression with gonadotropin-releasing hormone (GnRH) agonists to treat chronic pelvic pain associated with endometriosis
  - *Lupron Depo* 3.75 mg IM monthly for 6 months
  - Treatment of PID with antibiotics per guidelines (See PID)
  - Inpatient or outpatient
- Nonpharmacologic:
  - Chronic pelvic pain: A multidisciplinary team approach to address anxiety and depression associated with the chronic pain and disruption of their lives.
    - Heat
    - Acupuncture
    - Transcutaneous electrical nerve stimulation TENS for dysmenorrhea
  - Diagnostic laparoscopy:
    - Most chronic pelvic pain patients with normal ultrasound are managed medically/conservatively.
    - If the presentation includes an acute abdomen, adnexal mass or ectopic pregnancy then a diagnostic laparoscopy is both diagnostic and therapeutic.
    - 60% to 80% of women with chronic pelvic pain have no intraperitoneal pathology.
  - Laparotomy may be needed if:
    - Large pelvic mass
    - Ileus
    - Bowel obstruction
  - Hysterectomy, oophorectomy, and salpingectomy (TAH BSO):
    - Disabling pelvic pain after a woman no longer desires fertility
    - Hysterectomy and BSO reduce the recurrence of pelvic pain six fold.

Geriatric Considerations:
- Rarely found in postmenopausal women:
  - Acute and chronic pain associated with menstrual cycles
  - Pregnancy
  - Endometriosis
- Gastrointestinal causes and urologic causes are more likely in geriatric population.
  - Diverticulitis
  - Bowel obstruction
  - Kidney stones
  - Pelvic malignancy
- Musculoskeletal causes of chronic pelvic pain especially hip related pain referred to the pelvis.
- Signs and symptoms may be more subtle.
- Elderly patients may present later than young women.

- Radiologic imaging including CT scan and ultrasound are critical diagnostic tools to evaluate the older women with pelvic pain.
- In one study of elderly women:
  - 60% of elderly patients seen in the Emergency Room were admitted to the hospital.
  - 20% required surgery; and there was a
  - 5% mortality.
- Pelvic masses must be evaluated and, if needed, removed to rule out ovarian and other malignancies

Urinary Tract Issues

Urinary Tract Infections (UTIS)

Description: UTIs are among the most common bacterial infections found in adults; may involve the lower and/or upper urinary tract

Asymptomatic bacteriuria: Presence of significant bacteria in the urine without symptoms.

Acute cystitis: The presence of bacteria in the bladder and the presence of symptoms which may include dysuria, frequency, urgency, suprapubic tenderness and occasionally hematuria

Acute pyelonephritis: An infection in the upper urinary tract associated with significant bacteria with fever and flank pain

Recurrent UTI: Reinfection with the same bacteria after adequate therapy or with a new bacteria after proven negative culture

Epidemiology/Etiology:
- Estimated 11% of women will report at least one provider diagnosed UTI every year; probability of 60% of all women will be diagnosed once in their lifetime with up to 5% multiple times.
- 80% of UTIs are found in women.
- *Escherichia coli* is common cause (80% to 90%) of UTIs in women; ascends into the bladder from the vagina and urethra as a result of sexual intercourse or instrumentation; less common causes: *Staphylociccus saprophyticus, proteus, Pseudomonas, Klebsiella, Enterobacter, and Group B Strep*
- May result from hematogenous or lymphatic spread (rare)

Risk Factors for UTIs:
- Premenopausal women:
  - Previous history of UTIs
  - Recent or frequent sexual activity
  - Diabetes
  - Obesity
  - Anatomic congenital abnormalities
  - Sickle cell trait
  - Increasing parity
  - Urinary tract calculi
  - Diaphragm and spermicide use
  - Poor hygiene
  - Neurologic conditions that require catheterization
- Postmenopausal women:
  - Recent UTI
  - Diabetes
  - Atrophic urogenital tract
  - Pelvic floor relaxation
  - Poor hygiene
  - Incomplete emptying that occurs from the prolapse of the bladder and pelvic floor

Signs and Symptoms:
- **Subjective Complaints:**
  - May be asymptomatic
  - Dysuria
  - Nocturia

- Urinary urgency
- Urinary frequency
- Hematuria
- Suprapubic pain
- Dyspareunia
- Fever/chills(upper UTIs)
- Flank pain (upper UTIs)
- Fatigue (upper UTIs)
- Nausea/vomiting/diarrhea (upper UTIs)
- **Physical Examination Findings:**
  - Negative pelvic examination
  - Palpated suprapubic tenderness
  - May find CVA tenderness, fever, and tachycardia with upper tract infections only

Differential Diagnosis

- Acute cystitis versus acute pyelonephritis
- Vaginitis
- STIs (gonorrhea, chlamydia, trichamoniasis)
- PID
- HSV
- Renal calculi
- Overactive bladder (OAB)
- Appendicitis
- Pregnancy/ectopic pregnancy

Diagnostic Studies:

- UTI: A clean catch urine specimen sent for urinalysis and culture and sensitivity sensitive to 100,000 colonies per milliliter
  - Bacteriuria is diagnosed with between 1,000 and 10,000 bacteria per milliliter.
- Urine dip stick testing: Positive nitrites, blood, and leukocytes on dipstick test (false-negative tests are common)
- Microscopy: Pyuria ($\geq$10 leukocytes/HPF) and bacteriuria

Treatment

- Uncomplicated UTIs: (if culture and sensitivity test positive, treat appropriate bacteria); first-generation cephalosporins and amoxicillin are less effective in the treatment of acute uncomplicated cystitis.
  - Single-dose regimen: Fosfomycin tromethamine 3 g p.o. once
  - Three-day regimens: 90% successful treatment regimens
    - Trimethoprim: 160 mg one tablet p.o. twice a day for 3 days
    - Sulfamethoxazole: 800 mg one tablet p.o. twice a day for 3 days
    - Ciprofloxin: 250 mg one tablet p.o. twice a day for 3 days
    - Levofloxin: 250 mg one tablet p.o. once a day for 3 days
  - Seven-day regimens: 90% successful treatment regimens
    - Nitrofurantoin monohydrate 100 mg p.o. twice a day for 7 days
  - Consider adding phenazopyridine hydrochloride 200 mg p.o. three times a day (p.r.n.) for 2 days to decrease discomfort related to UTI (may change urine color to bright orange, red, or blue depending on preparation).
- Acute pyelonephritis: Important to know resistance organisms in the community; most women can be treated as an outpatient; fluorquinolones for a full 7 day treatment, or first generation cephalosporins, or amoxicillin/clavulanate for a full 14 day treatment is appropriate.

Recurrent UTI Prevention:

- Techniques may include improved hygiene around sexual intercourse, post coital voiding, and increased hydration (no supportive published data); Cranberry juice and cranberry tablets have been shown to be effective in reducing recurrent UTIs; return to office if symptom not resolved after complete therapy.

Postcoital Prevention:

- UTIs related to sexual activity
- Single dose antibiotic therapy especially post coital has been shown to reduce recurrence 95%.

Geriatric Considerations:
- Urinary tract infections are more common in older women; incidence of asymptomatic bacteriuria is as high as 20% in women over 65 years of age.
- Recurrence rates are higher.
- Should have culture proven UTI
- Cause is the hypoestrogenic state of the vaginal epithelium which along with prolapse and impaired voiding increase the risk of UTIs.
- Older women with asymptomatic bacteriuria may present with symptoms of urinary incontinence or already ill from septic shock or urosepsis.

Urinary Incontinence (UI)

Description: Loss of bladder control

Epidemiology/Etiology:
- Urinary incontinence affects 10% to 70% of women living in a community setting and up to 50% of nursing home residents.
- Prevalence increases gradually during young adult life, has a broad peak around middle age (also as a result pregnancy), and then steadily increases in the elderly.
- Can have transient causes (UTIS, medication side effects, atrophic urethritis and atrophic vaginitis, pregnancy, psychological issues, delirium, functional issues including immobility and stool impaction)
- Can also be the result of anatomical abnormalities, such as a congenital ectopic ureter or fistulas, and physical changes such as pelvic relaxation and prolapse.
- Abnormal growths such as polyps, bladder stones, or less commonly, bladder cancer can cause urinary incontinence.
- Abnormal growths often cause urge incontinence and may be associated with blood in the urine.
- Pelvic support problems are a frequent cause of UI as pelvic organs are held in place by supportive tissues and muscles; these supporting tissues may become torn or stretched, or they may weaken due to aging; if the tissues that support the urethra, bladder, uterus, or rectum become weak, these organs may drop down or prolapse, causing urine leakage or making it hard to pass urine.
- Fistulas can allow urine to leak out through the vagina.
- Neuromuscular disorders can interfere with the transmission of signals from the brain and spinal cord to the bladder and urethra.

Stress Urinary Incontinence (SUI):
- Loss of urine when a woman coughs, laughs, or sneezes; Leaks with activity that increases intra-abdominal pressure to the bladder(i.e., walking, running, or exercising); it is caused by a weakening of the tissues that support the bladder or the muscles of the urethra; most common diagnosis in noninstitutionalized women (29% to 75%)

Urge Incontinence (UI):
- Leakage of urine caused by overactive detrusor muscles that cause uninhibited detrusor contractions and changes within pressures in the bladder; usually involves neurologic component; represents 7% to 33% of the cases of UI

Mixed Incontinence:
- A combination of both stresses and urge incontinence symptoms represents the remaining causes common in the older population.

Overflow Incontinence:
- It is a steady loss of small amounts of urine when the bladder does not empty all the way during voiding; causes include obstruction of the urethra, or neurologic defects that prevent the woman from feeling the urge to void.

Signs and Symptoms:
- **Subjective Complaints:**
  - Leaking urine
  - Urgency
  - Frequency
  - Nocturia
  - Dysuria
  - Enuresis

- **Physical Examination Findings:**
  - May be normal
  - Pelvic floor relaxation
  - Irritated vaginal tissue due to urine leakage

Differential Diagnosis:
- Urinary obstruction
- Multiple Sclerosis
- UTI
- Pelvic support defects (cystocele, rectocele, etc.)
- Vaginitis
- Neurologic conditions

Diagnostic Studies:
- History, physical, and direct observation of urine loss
- Postvoid residual volume (PVR)
- Urodynamic testing: Measures pressure and volume of bladder as it fills and the flow rate as it empties
- Cystourethroscopy: Bladder scope

Treatment:
- Nonpharmacologic:
  - Lifestyle changes
  - Behavior therapy: Bladder training and pelvic training
  - Physical therapy
  - Devices
  - Weight loss if overweight
  - Kegel exercises
    - Instruct women to squeeze pelvic floor muscles (the muscles to stop the flow of urine); hold for up to 10 seconds, then release; repeat 10 to 20 times in a row at least 3 times a day; do not perform Kegels while exercising.
- Pharmacologic:
  - Oxybutynin chloride orally
  - Tolterodine orally
  - Trospium chloride orally
  - Derifenacin orally
  - Solifenacin orally
  - Oxybutin patch to skin of abdomen
- Anti-incontinence procedures:
  - Botox injections
  - Sacral nerve stimulator
  - Periurethral bulking agents injection
- Surgical (SUI only):
  - Burch colposuspension
  - Sling procedures
  - Anterior colporrhaphy (poor long-term results)
  - Needle urethropexy
  - Paravaginal defect repair

Geriatric Considerations:
- Over 50% of women over age 50 have complaints of UI.
- Most women do not seek help for mild UI.
- 11% of women aged 65 years and older have a surgical procedure for UI symptoms of OAB very common.
- Mild incontinence in early perimenopause tends to decline in the first 5 years after menopause.
- HT does not improve stress urinary incontinence but does improve urgency incontinence when the urgency is from estrogen deficient urethral tissue.
- UI is a significant problem for custodial care and is one of the main reasons for admission into nursing homes.
- Up to 50% of nursing home residents suffer from UI.

Perimenopause and Menopause Transition

Description:
- Menopause:
  - Absence of menstrual periods for 12 consecutive months after a woman's FMP
  - Permanent end of menstruation and fertility
  - Normal, natural event associated with reduced functioning of the ovaries; resulting in lower levels of ovarian hormones (primarily estrogen)
  - Symptoms vary from woman to woman in severity of presentation.
- Perimenopause:
  - Typically lasting 6 years or more; span of time that begins with the onset of menstrual cycle changes and other menopause-related symptoms and extends through menopause (FMP) to 1 year after menopause
  - Experienced only with spontaneous (natural) menopause, not with induced menopause
  - Frequently called the menopause transition
  - Associated with decline in fertility
  - Progressive decline in mood
- Postmenopause:
  - Span of time after menopause, remainder of life after the FMP
- Premature menopause:
  - Occurrence of menopause at or before the age of 40; resulting from genetics, autoimmune disorders, or medical procedures or treatments
- Induced menopause:
  - Cessation of menstruation that occurs as the result of surgical removal of both ovaries
  - Iatrogenic ablation of ovarian function through chemotherapy or radiation therapy

Epidemiology/Etiology:
- Average age of menopause in the United States is 51.5 years with a range of normal menopause from 40 to 58 years of age.
- Estimated 50 million women will be postmenopausal in the United States in 2020 with almost 500 million worldwide.
- Life expectancy of 72 years worldwide and 82 years in developed countries by 2025
- Natural aging process of the ovary resulting in the decrease of hormones estradiol and estrone; FSH and LH are released in compensation in higher levels from pituitary.

Signs and Symptoms:
- Sleep pattern changes due to declining estrogen
- Vasomotor instability: Hot flashes
- Skin changes with dryness and hair loss on scalp and body
- Genitourinary changes: Dyspareunia from decreased lubrication, lower libido
- Vaginal pH change makes more prone to vaginal and urinary infections, urinary leakage
- Depressed state, cognitive declines
- Heart palpitations, pounding in the chest and arrhythmias
- Joint pains and aches
- Headaches, hormonal in nature

Differential Diagnosis: (causes of amenorrhea around the time of the perimenopause)
- Secondary amenorrhea
- Premature menopause
- Premature ovarian failure
- Pregnancy

Diagnostic Studies:
- Must rule out pregnancy: Urine pregnancy test fast and inexpensive, serum blood test for accuracy and quantification
- Serum tests for hormonal markers: Low estradiol and elevated FSH and LH
- Age-appropriate cancer screening (see Chapter 1)
- Screening for osteoporosis consistent with the recommendations of the National Osteoporosis Foundation (Box 6-1)

Box 6-1: Normal Levels of Postmenopausal Hormones		
Estradiol:	Premenopausal level	30–400 pg/mL
	Postmenopausal level	0–30 pg/mL
Follicle stimulating hormone (FSH):	Premenopausal level	4.7–21.5 mIU/mL
	Postmenopausal level	25.8–134.8 mIU/mL
Luteinizing hormone (LH):	Premenopausal level	5–25 IU/L
	Postmenopausal level	14.2–52.3 IU/L

Treatment:
- Pharmocologic: (dose is dependent on brand name)
  - Hormone therapy:
    - Oral estrogen: Premarin, Estrace
    - Oral progesterone: Provera, Aygestin, Prometrium
    - Oral combo progesterone/estrogen: Premphase, Prempro, Femhrt, Activella
    - Estrogen patch: Climara, Alora, Vivelle, Minivelle
    - Estrogen/progesterone patch: Combipatch, Climara Pro
    - Estrogen ring: E string, Fem ring
    - Estrogen cream: Premarin cream
    - Transdermal estrogen: Divigel, Estrogel, Elestrin
  - Nonhormone therapy:
    - Antidepressants: To ease hot flashes and help with sleep issues
      - Venlafaxine (Effexor)
      - Fluoxetine (Prozac)
      - Paroxetine (Paxil)
      - Escitalopram (Lexapro)
      - Clonidine (Catapress)
  - Menopausal osteoporosis prevention: (see Osteoporosis)
    - Alendronate (Fosamax)
    - Risedronate (Actonel)
    - Ibandronate (Boniva)
    - Raloxifene: If risk of using estrogen products
  - Nonpharmacologic:
    - Watch triggers of smoking, stress, tight clothes, and heat; avoid these.
    - Diet changes: Avoid caffeine, spicy foods, and alcohol.
    - Increase isoflavones such as soy products, chick peas, lentils to diet.
    - Life changes: Increase exercise, add yoga for stress and sleep issues, dress in layers, keep room cooler.
    - Many women try either Mexican or Chinese wild yam cream or gel rubbed into the skin to relieve hot flashes.
    - Acupuncture and yoga have been successful in relieving the symptoms of menopause in some women.
    - Over-the-counter medications to reduce symptoms: (all with phytoestrogen properties)
    - Vitamin E in high doses
    - Black cohosh
    - Evening primrose oil
    - Red clover
    - Ginseng
    - St John wort (for emotional symptom management)
    - Vaginal lubricants are very useful to ease dyspareunia (Boxes 6-2 and 6-3)

Approved Prescription Products for Menopausal Symptoms in the United States
- Oral estrogen products
  - 17β-estradiol (Estrace and generics) 0.5, 1.0, 2.0 mg/day
  - Conjugated estrogens (Premarin) 0.3, 0.45, 0.625, 0.9, 1.25 mg/day

Box 6-2: International Menopause Society: Global Consensus Position Statement on the Use of Menopausal Hormone Therapy

- Menopausal hormone therapy (MHT) is the most effective treatment for vasomotor symptoms associated with menopause at any age, but benefits are more likely to outweigh risks for symptomatic women before the age of 60 years or within 10 years after menopause.
- MHT is effective and appropriate for the prevention of osteoporosis-related fractures in at-risk women before age 60 years or within 10 years after menopause.
- Randomized clinical trials and observational data as well as meta-analyses provide evidence that standard-dose estrogen-alone MHT may decrease coronary heart disease and all-cause mortality in women younger than 60 years of age and within 10 years of menopause.
- Data on estrogen plus progestin MHT in this population show a similar trend for mortality, but in most randomized clinical trials no significant increase or decrease in coronary heart disease has been found.
- Local low-dose estrogen therapy is preferred for women whose symptoms are limited to vaginal dryness or associated discomfort with intercourse.
- Estrogen as a single systemic agent is appropriate in women after hysterectomy, but additional progestin is required in the presence of a uterus.
- The option of MHT is an individual decision in terms of quality of life and health priorities as well as personal risk factors such as age, time since menopause and the risk of venous thromboembolism, stroke, ischemic heart disease, and breast cancer.
- The risk of venous thromboembolism and ischemic stroke increases with oral MHT, but the absolute risk is rare below age 60 years. Observational studies point to a lower risk with transdermal therapy.
- The risk of breast cancer in women over 50 years associated with MHT is a complex issue. The increased risk of breast cancer is primarily associated with the addition of a progestin to estrogen therapy and related to the duration of use.
  ○ The risk of breast cancer attributable to MHT is small, and the risk decreases after treatment is stopped.
  ○ The dose and duration of MHT should be consistent with treatment goals and safety issues and should be individualized.
  ○ In women with premature ovarian insufficiency, systemic MHT is recommended at least until the average age of the natural menopause.
  ○ The use of custom-compounded bioidentical hormone therapy is not recommended.
  ○ Current safety data do not support the use of MHT in breast cancer survivors.

Adapted from De Villers, T. J., Gass, M., Haines, C. J., Hall, J., Pierroz, D., & Rees, M. (2013). Global consensus statement on menopausal hormone therapy. *Climacteric*, 16, 203–204.

- Synthetic conjugated estrogens (Enjuvia) 0.3, 0.45, 0.625, 0.9, 1.25 mg/day
- Esterified estrogens (Menest) 0.3, 0.625, 1.25, 2.5 mg/day
- Estropipate (Ogen and generics) 0.625, 1.25, 2.5 mg/day
- Transdermal estrogen 17β-estradiol patch
  - Climara 0.025 to 0.1 mg/day dose once a week
  - Menostar 0.014 mg/day dose once a week
  - Estraderm 0.05 to 0.1 mg/day dose twice a week
  - Minivelle and Vivelle-Dot 0.0375 to 0.1 mg/day dose twice a week
- Transdermal products (gel or spray)
  - 17β-estradiol (Divigel 0.25, 0.5, 1.0 mg/day) (Elestrin 0.52, 1.04 use lowest effective dose)
  - 17β-estradiol (Evamist spray 1.53 mg/spray use 1 to 3/day adjust dosage by response)
- Vaginal estrogen products
  - Topical or vaginal creams
    ○ 17β-estradiol (*Estrace Vaginal Cream*) indication is Vulvovaginal atrophy
    ○ Initial: 2 to 4 g/day for 1 to 2 weeks
    ○ Maintenance: 1 g two to three times per week (0.1 mg active ingredient/g)
    ○ Conjugated estrogens (*Premarin Vaginal Cream*) indication is atrophic vaginitis and moderate to severe dyspareunia 0.5 to 2 g/day (0.625 mg active ingredient/g) or topically twice a week.
  - Vaginal Rings
    ○ 17β-estradiol (Estring) indication is moderate to severe symptoms of vulvar and vaginal atrophy due to menopause.
    ○ 2 mg (releases 7.5 μg/day) for 90 days
    ○ Estradiol acetate (Femring) indication is moderate to severe vasomotor symptoms due to menopause and moderate to severe vulvar and vaginal atrophy due to menopause.
    ○ 50 or 100 μg/day estradiol for 90 days (systemic levels and require a progestogen if intact uterus)

Box 6-3: NIH STRAW + 10 Classifications of the Stages of Reproductive Aging

Stage	Menarche −5	−4	−3b	−3a	−2	−1	FMP (0) +1a	+1b	+1c	+2
Terminology	Reproductive				Menopausal Transition		Postmenopause			
	Early	Peak	Late		Early	Late	Early			Late
					Perimenopause					
Duration	*Variable*				*Variable*	1–3 years	2 years (1 + 1)		3–6 years	*Remaining life span*
Principal Criteria										
Menstrual Cycle	Variable to regular	Regular	Regular	Subtle changes in Flow/Length	Variable Length Persistent ≥7-day difference in length of consecutive cycles	Interval of amenorrhea of ≥60 days				
Supportive Criteria										
Endocrine										
FSH			Low	Variable*	↑Variable*	↑ >25 IU/L**	↑Variable		Stabilizes	
AMH			Low	Low	Low	Low	Low		Very Low	
Inhibin B				Low	Low	Low	Low		Very Low	
Antral Follicle Count			Low	Low	Low	Low	Very Low		Very Low	
Descriptive Characteristics										
Symptoms						Vasomotor symptoms *Likely*	Vasomotor symptoms *Most Likely*			*Increasing symptoms of urogenital atrophy*

*Blood draw on cycle days 2–5 ↑ = elevated.

**Approximate expected level based on assays using current international pituitary standard.

From Harlow, S. D., Gass, M., Hall, J. E., Lobo, R., Maki, P., Rebar, R. W., . . . de Villiers, T. J. (2012). Executive summary of the Stages of Reproductive Aging Workshop + 10: Addressing the unfinished agenda of staging reproductive aging. *Fertility and Sterility, 97*(4), 843–851, with permission.

- Vaginal Tablets
  - Estradiol (*Vagifem*)
  - 10 µg tablet vaginally, one tablet/day for 2 weeks
  - Maintenance: One tablet twice/week
- Combination estrogen–progestin products
  - Conjugated estrogens (E) + medroxyprogesterone acetate (P) (*Premphase*)

    0.625 mg E + 5.0 mg P (two tablets: E and E + P) (E alone days 1 to 14, E + P days 15 to 28)

  - Conjugated estrogens (E) + medroxyprogesterone acetate (P) (*Prempro*)

    0.3 or 0.45 mg E + 1.5 mg P, 0.625 mg E + 2.5 or 5.0 mg P

  - Ethinyl estradiol (E) + norethindrone acetate (P) (*Femhrt or FemHRT Lo*)

    2.5 µg E + 0.5 mg P or 5 µg E + 1 mg P

  - 17β-estradiol (E) + norethindrone acetate (P) (*Activella*)

    0.5 mg E + 0.1 mg P, or 1 mg E + 0.5 mg P

  - 17β-estradiol (E) + drospirenone (P) (*Angeliq*)

    1 mg E + 0.5 mg P*, 0.5 mg E + 0.25 mg P* p.o. daily

- Transdermal continuous combined
  - 17β-estradiol (E) + norethindrone acetate (P) (*CombiPatch*)

    0.05 mg E + 0.14 mg P twice/week or 0.05 mg E + 0.25 mg P twice/week

  - 17β-estradiol (E) + levonorgestrel (P) (*Climara Pro*)

    0.045 mg E + 0.015 mg P once/week

- Progestins
  - Medroxyprogesterone acetate (Provera) 2.5, 5, 10 mg/day
  - Micronized progesterone (Promethium) 100, 200 mg/day
- Nonestrogen progesterone oral products
  - Conjugated estrogens + bazedoxifene (Duavee) 0.45 (E) + 20 (bazedoxifene) mg/day
- Indication: Moderate to severe vasomotor symptoms
  - Ospemifene (Osphena) 60 mg/day
- Indication: Moderate to severe dyspareunia, a symptom of vulvar and vaginal atrophy, due to menopause
  - Paroxetine (Brisdelle) 7.5 mg/day
- Indication: Moderate to severe vasomotor symptoms

Geriatric Considerations:
- Menopausal transition starts at the FMP and continues for the remainder of life; significant health issues continue to be
  - Cardiovascular health
  - Detection and prevention of malignancy
  - Prevention and detection of osteoporosis
- Recommendations for
  - Healthy diet, regular exercise, and supplements as needed for heart and bone health.
- Pregnancy is not a concern.
- Sexually transmitted infections remain an important issue for evaluation and treatment.
- Cancer screening is addressed in Chapter 1 and cardiovascular health in Chapter 4.

Osteopenia and Osteoporosis

Description: Osteopenia and osteoporosis are skeletal bone disorders; predisposes women to increased bone fracture risks
- Osteopenia: Low mineral bone density; decrease in the amount of calcium and phosphorous
- Osteoporosis: Compromised bone strength

- Bone strength:
  - Bone density: Grams of mineral per area or volume; determined by peak bone mass and amount of bone loss in any given individual
  - Bone quality: Architecture. Turnover, damage accumulation, and mineralization
- World Health Organization (WHO) definitions based on bone mineral density test results:
  - Normal: T score greater than or equal to -1.0
  - Low bone mass (osteopenia): T score between -1.0 and -2.5
  - Osteoporosis: T score less than or equal to -2.5 (and lower)

Epidemiology and Etiology:
- Osteoporosis is a serious health threat for aging postmenopausal women due to lower estrogen levels postmenopause; decreased estrogen accounts for about two-third of bone loss during the 5 to 7 years around menopause.
- Decreased estrogen production in groups of young women: eating disorders, elite athletes, etc.
- 13% to 18% of White American women $\geq$age 50 have osteoporosis of the hip.
- Women account for 80% (8 million) of the population diagnosed with osteoporosis (total of 10 million).
- Approximately one in two women over age 50 will break a bone because of osteoporosis.
- A woman's risk of breaking a hip is equal to her combined risk of breast, uterine, and ovarian cancer.

Risk Factors:
- Used in FRAX 10-year calculator (Box 6-4)

Signs and Symptoms:
- **Subjective Complaints:**
  - Usually asymptomatic
  - Pain related to fracture
  - Unexplained bone or joint pain
- **Physical Examination Findings:**
  - May be asymptomatic
  - Stooped posture
  - Kyphosis
  - Fracture
  - Loss of height

Differential Diagnosis:
- Atraumatic compression fracture
- Osteomalacia
- Osteonecrosis
- Metastatic bone disease

Diagnostic Testing:
The National Osteoporosis Foundation recommends a Bone Mineral Density (BMD) test for women using a DXA (dual energy X-ray absorptiometry)scan:
- Over 65 years of age
- Postmenopausal women under age 65 with risk factors

Box 6-4: Risk Factors for Osteoporosis

Advanced age (ages 50–90)
Parental history of fragility fracture
Female sex
Rheumatoid arthritis
Low femoral neck BMD
Coexisting medical conditions associated with bone loss
Alcohol intake >3 units daily
Current tobacco smoking
Low body weight; small and thin body type
Long-term use of glucocorticoids
Losing height
Prior fracture (not traumatic)

- Women going through menopause with risk factors
- Women who break a bone after age 50
- Women with specific medical conditions or taking certain medications such as glucocorticoids, antiseizure medications, gonadotropins, excess thyroid medication
- Postmenopausal women who have stopped taking HT

Treatment:
- Lifestyle changes
- Medications to prevent future fractures and increase bone mineral density
- Calcium- and vitamin D-rich diet (Tables 6-50 and 6-51)
- Daily exercise
- Indications for medical therapy and lifestyle changes:
  - Postmenopausal women who have had vertebral or hip fracture
  - Postmenopausal women with T scores ≤−2.5 at the lumbar spine, femoral neck, or total hip
  - Postmenopausal women with T scores from −1.0 to −2.5 and 10-year FRAX risk of major osteoporotic fracture of at least 20% or of hip fracture of at least 3%
- Approved medications for the prevention or treatment
  - Bisphosphonates are approved for both prevention and treatment of postmenopausal osteopenia and osteoporosis; can treat bone loss and can build bone mass; inhibits osteoclast reabsorption
- Alendronate 5 to 10 mg/day or 35 to 70 mg/week
- Risedronate 5 mg/day, 35 mg/week, 150 mg/month
- Ibandronate 150 mg once a month, or 3 mg IV every 90 days
- Zoledronic acid 5 mg IV over 15 minutes yearly
  - SERMs are selective estrogen receptor modulators; estrogen agonists/antagonists; inhibits bone reabsorption and turnover; indicated for prevention and treatment
- Raloxifene 60 mg/day
  - Calcitonin is a naturally occurring hormone that can help slow the rate of bone loss; inhibits osteoclast bone reabsorption
- Natural occurring 200 IU daily intranasal spray
  - Monoclonal antibody: Inhibits RANKL (protein that causes bone loss); inhibits the maturation of osteoclasts
- Denosumab single ampoule IM injection every 6 months by health care provider
  - Parathyroid hormone
- Teraparatide parathyroid hormone (PTH) daily self-injection for 2 years
  - Menopausal hormone therapy (MHT): Estrogen decreases the rate of bone reabsorption; promotes activity of osteoblasts
- The Food and Drug Administration (FDA) recommends taking the lowest possible dose of MHT for the shortest time to meet treatment goals; discuss using alternative osteoporosis medications instead.

Geriatric Considerations:
- High-risk group for fall-related fractures
- Hip fracture has up to a 20% mortality.
- Major reason for admission to residential nursing homes
- Avoid excess alcohol.
- Avoid smoking.
- Appropriate diet, nutrition, and exercise

Table 6-50: Daily Calcium Requirements	
Age	**Milligrams (mg)/day**
9–18	1,300
19–50	1,000
51 and older	1,200

Table 6-51: Daily Vitamin D Requirements	
Age	**International Units (IU)/day**
1–70	600
71+	800

Review Section

Review Questions

1. A 63-year-old female, G3 P3 comes to your office for a well-woman examination. She states she has not had a gynecologic examination or screenings for over 10 years due to loss of insurance. Her last menstrual period was at the age of 52 and she has had no vaginal bleeding ever since. She reports that she has not been sexually active for over 5 years. She takes no medications and has no significant medical history. What well-woman screenings are appropriate for this woman?

   a. Pap smear, mammogram, Dexa scan, and a urine culture
   b. Pap smear with HPV, mammogram, lipid profile, colonoscopy
   c. Pap smear with HPV, mammogram, HSV-1 and -2 serology, and urinalysis
   d. Pap smear, breast MRI, Dexa scan, and colonoscopy

2. A woman presents with a yellow vaginal discharge with a fishy odor accompanied by vaginal burning for 1 week. She tells you that it started after she used a new soap she bought at the store. Her examination shows an irritated vagina with the presence of watery, yellow discharge. The vaginal pH is 5.0, and the wet prep shows clue cells and has a positive whiff test. She has no known drug allergies. Which medication is the best choice to treat this patient?

   a. Terconazole 0.4% cream 5 g intravaginally for 7 days
   b. Azithromycin 1 g orally once
   c. Doxycycline 100 mg orally twice a day for 7 days
   d. Metronidazole 500 mg orally twice a day 7 days

3. A 37-year-old female, G5 P3023 comes into your office to discuss birth control options. She tells you that she does not think she wants any more children in the future but would like to keep her options open. Her husband refuses to use condoms, and she is currently using the withdrawal method, which makes her nervous. She smokes half pack of cigarettes a day, and her medical history is significant for exercise-induced asthma. Based on the CDC Medical Eligibility Criteria (MEC) for Contraception, which option would be the best choice for this woman?

   a. Tubal ligation
   b. Vaginal contraceptive ring
   c. IUD
   d. Combined Oral Contraceptive (COC) pill

4. A Dexa scan result shows a T score of −2.4 in both the hip and the spine of a 66-year-old female. This result is indicative of:

   a. osteoporosis.
   b. normal bone density.
   c. osteogenisis.
   d. osteopenia.

5. The Pap smear result for M. K., a 55-year-old female, shows atypical squamous cells of undetermined significance (ASC-US) with a negative high-risk HPV cotesting result. She has no significant medical history other than controlled high blood pressure. The appropriate management for this woman would be:

   a. repeat Pap and HPV screening in 3 years.
   b. repeat Pap and HPV screening in 6 months.
   c. repeat Pap and HPV screening in 1 year.
   d. refer for colposcopy.

6. A 40-year-old woman comes into your office for an annual examination. Her last menstrual period started 3 days ago, and it is just beginning to taper off. She tells you that occasionally, when her bladder is full, she loses some urine when she coughs or sneezes. The urine dip stick in the office shows positive for RBCs and leukocytes. Your next step for treatment includes:

   a. referral to urologist for a stress incontinence workup.
   b. treat her UTI with ciprofloxacin 250 mg orally twice a day for 3 days.
   c. obtain a urine specimen by catheterization and send it to the laboratory for culture and sensitivity.
   d. recommend regular Kegel exercises and frequent voiding.

7. A 42-year-old female patient comes to your office with a history of 3 months of amenorrhea. She now presents with irregular vaginal bleeding and mild pelvic cramping for 1 week. Her pregnancy test in the office is negative. Your initial evaluation should include:

   a. order a FSH, LH, and estradiol to confirm menopause.
   b. obtain a sample of her endometrium to rule out hyperplasia.
   c. refer to a gynecologist to schedule a laparoscopy for pelvic pain.
   d. immediate referral to the emergency room to rule out any ectopic pregnancy.

8. J. P., a 28-year-old female comes to your office because her partner informed her that he went to a health-care provider for a yellow discharge coming from his penis. He was given antibiotics and told to tell his partner to "get checked." J. P. admits to only occasional condom use with this partner. Inspection and speculum examination shows a small amount of mucopurulent vaginal discharge, a slightly friable cervix, and no lesions. The rest of her physical examination is unremarkable. Vaginal pH is 5.0, and wet prep shows motile *Trichomonas vaginalis,* RBCs, and WBCs. The appropriate management for this patient would be:

   a. serology for HIV and HPV, Ceftriaxone 250 mg IM once, and acyclovir 400 mg orally three times a day for 7 days.
   b. metronidiazole 500 mg orally twice a day for 7 days.
   c. cultures for gonorrhea and chlamydia, offer STI serology, metronidazole 2 g orally in a single dose, ceftriaxone 250 IM once, and azithromycin 1 g orally once.
   d. cultures for gonorrhea and chlamydia, offer STI serology, metronidazole 2 g orally in a single dose, and azithromycin 1 g orally once.

9. In regard to the use of menopausal hormone therapy (MHT), the nurse practitioner understands that research indicates:

   a. MHT is the most effective treatment for vasomotor symptoms associated with menopause at any age, but benefits are more likely to outweigh risks for symptomatic women before the age of 60 years or within 10 years after menopause.
   b. MHT causes breast cancer in women over 40 and should be avoided unless the woman has been diagnosed with osteoporosis.
   c. compound bioidentical hormones are much safer in symptomatic women and should be initiated as primary treatment.
   d. standard-dose estrogen-alone MHT may increase coronary heart disease and all-cause mortality in women younger than 60 years of age and within 10 years of menopause.

10. L.V., a 21-year-old female, comes to your office for a well-woman examination. She had a Copper T IUD placed 1 year ago for birth control and has no complaints. Her menses is monthly, and lasts for 7 days with moderate cramping. She takes ibuprofen 400 mg orally p.r.n., and she feels it works well. She is sexually active with one partner and she faithfully uses latex condoms. She has had all three *Gardasil* injections. Regarding a Pap smear at this visit:

   a. she does not need a Pap smear at this visit since she had all of the three injections of the HPV vaccination.
   b. she does not need a Pap smear at this time; perform HPV testing only.
   c. she will need a Pap smear with and HPV contesting at this visit.
   d. she will need a Pap smear only at this visit.

Answers with Rationales

1. (b) Pap smear with HPV, mammogram, lipid profile, colonoscopy

   Rationale: A pap smear with HPV cotesting, a mammogram, a lipid profile, and a colonoscopy are all normal screenings for women aged 40 to 60 years. A Dexa scan is indicated for women who are at high risk for osteoporosis prior to the age of 65. A bone mineral density screening begins at age 65 years in the absence of risk factors and should be done no more frequently than every 2 years. Breast MRIs, urine cultures, and HSV serology are not appropriate well-woman screening for this woman.

2. (d) Metronidazole 500 mg orally twice a day for 7 days

   Rationale: This woman presents with the symptoms, physical findings, and diagnostic testing (pH, clue cells, whiff test) for bacterial vaginosis. The CDC recommends metronidiazole 500 mg orally twice a day for 7 days as appropriate treatment. Terconazole is the treatment for yeast, azithromycin 1 g orally once is the appropriate treatment for chlamydia, and doxycycline 100 mg orally twice a day for 7 days can be used to treat uncomplicated gonoccocal infections.

3. (c) IUD

   Rationale: This woman is over the age of 35 and is a smoker. Estrogen-containing contraception is a contraindication for smokers over the age of 35. The vaginal ring and COCs both contain estrogen. She wishes to keep her fertility options open; thus, a tubal ligation would not be an appropriate choice. Either the Copper T or the progestin-containing IUD is appropriate for this woman.

4. (d) osteopenia.

   Rationale: A T score between -1.0 and -2.5 is indicative of osteopenia; a T score less than or equal to -2.5 (and lower) is indicative of osteoporosis.

5. (a) repeat Pap and HPV screening in 3 years.

   Rationale: An ASC-US Pap with negative cotesting should be repeated in the normal screening sequence (3 years). The ACS, USPTFS, ASCCP, ASCP, and ACOG all agree that any additional screening or further testing before this time is unnecessary.

6. (d) recommend regular Kegel exercises and frequent voiding.

   Rationale: This woman comes to the office with her menses. Any urine specimen would be contaminated with blood and leukocytes, rendering the dip stick inaccurate. She is not complaining of any UTI symptoms; thus, treating an infection is inappropriate. She is experiencing stress incontinence when her bladder is full. Kegel exercises and more frequent bladder emptying would improve her leakage situation.

7. (b) obtain a sample of her endometrium to rule out hyperplasia.

   Rationale: The provider should perform a pregnancy test first to rule out a pregnancy (ectopic, missed abortion, or normal pregnancy). If negative, an endometrial biopsy for a sampling of the uterus should be performed in patients with irregular vaginal bleeding aged 35 years and older. This woman has not met the definition of menopause nor the criteria for an ectopic pregnancy.

8. (c) cultures for gonorrhea and chlamydia, offer STI serology, metronidazole 2 g orally in a single dose, ceftriaxone 250 IM once, and azithromycin 1 g orally once.

   Rationale: The provider has diagnosed trichomoniasis on the wet prep; in addition, the woman does not know the condition for which her partner has been treated. Penile discharge can be present in men with gonorrhea; thus, this patient should be treated for trichomoniasis, chlamydia, and gonorrhea to prevent PID. Cultures should be done in the office, and the woman should be offered serology testing for STIs (HIV, hepatitis, etc.).

9. (a) MHT is the most effective treatment for vasomotor symptoms associated with menopause at any age, but benefits are more likely to outweigh risks for symptomatic women before the age of 60 years or within 10 years after menopause.

   Rationale: The International Menopause Society issued a global consensus on the safety of MHT rooted in sound empirical research and analysis. Option A is the only true option based on the research findings. Option B is false as although some studies indicate that MHT may be associated with breast cancer in women over 50, it is usually associated with the addition of a progestin to estrogen therapy and related to duration of use (a viable option for some women). Custom-compound bioidentical hormones are not recommended as there are limited studies based on their safety. Lastly, MHT may decrease coronary heart disease in women younger than 60 years of age.

10. (d) she will need a Pap smear only at this visit.

    Rationale: During a well-woman visit for a woman aged 21, a Pap smear (cervical cytology) alone is indicated. HPV cotesting does not begin until the age of 30 years.

Suggested Readings

American Cancer Society. (2015a). *Cervical cancer screening guidelines.* Retrieved from http://www.cancer.org/healthy/informationforhealthcareprofessionals/acsguidelines/cervicalcancerscreeningguidelines/index

American Cancer Society. (2015b). *Guidelines for the early detection of cancer.* Retrieved from http://www.cancer.org/healthy/findcancerearly/cancerscreeningguidelines/american-cancer-society-guidelines-for-the-early-detection-of-cancer

American Cancer Society. (2015c). *Understanding your mammogram report – BI-RADS categories.* Retrieved from http://www.cancer.org/treatment/understandingyourdiagnosis/examsandtestdescriptions/mammogramsandotherbreastimagingprocedures/mammograms-and-other-breast-imaging-procedures-mammo-report

American College of Obstetricians and Gynecologists (ACOG). (2012a). Clinical management guidelines for obstetrician-gynecologists: Breast cancer screening. *Practice Bulletin, 122.* Washington, DC: ACOG.

American College of Obstetricians and Gynecologists (ACOG). (2012b). Clinical management guidelines for obstetrician-gynecologists: Osteoporosis. *Practice Bulletin, 129.* Washington, DC: ACOG.

American College of Obstetricians and Gynecologists (ACOG). (2012c). Clinical management guidelines for obstetrician-gynecologists: Screening for cervical cancer, *Practice Bulletin, 131.* Washington, DC: ACOG.

American College of Obstetricians and Gynecologists (ACOG). (2012d). Well woman visit. *Practice Bulletin, 534.* Washington, DC: ACOG. Retrieved from http://www.acog.org/About-ACOG/ACOG-Departments/Annual-Womens-Health-Care/Well-Woman-Recommendations

American College of Obstetricians and Gynecologists (ACOG). (2013). Clinical management guidelines for obstetrician-gynecologists: Management of abnormal uterine bleeding associated with ovulatory dysfunction. *Practice Bulletin, 136*. Washington, DC: ACOG.

American College of Obstetricians and Gynecologists (ACOG). (2014a). Clinical management guidelines for obstetrician-gynecologists: Management of menopausal symptoms. *Practice Bulletin, 141*. Washington, DC: ACOG.

American College of Obstetricians and Gynecologists (ACOG). (2014b). *Guidelines for women's health care: A resource manual* (4th ed.). Washington, DC: ACOG.

American Society for Colposcopy and Cervical Cancer. (n.d.). *Management guidelines*. Retrieved from http://www.asccp.org/Guidelines-2/Management-Guidelines-2

Association of Reproductive Health Professionals. (2014). *Quick reference guide for clinicians: Choosing a birth control method*. Retrieved from https://www.arhp.org/publications-and-resources/quick-reference-guide-for-clinicians/choosing

Beckmann, C., Ling, F., Herbert, W., Laube, D., Smith, R., Casonova, R., ... Weiss, P. M. (2014). *Obstetrics and gynecology* (7th ed.). Philadelphia, PA: Wolters Kluwer & Lippincott Williams & Wilkins.

Berek, J. (2012). *Berek and Novak's gynecology*. Philadelphia, PA: Lippincott, Williams, & Wilkins.

Centers for Disease Control and Prevention. (2010). *U.S. Medical Eligibility Criteria for contraceptive use, 2010*. Retrieved from http://www.cdc.gov/reproductivehealth/UnintendedPregnancy/USMEC.htm

Centers for Disease Control and Prevention. (2012). U.S. Medical Eligibility Criteria for contraceptive use, 2010: Revised recommendations for the use of hormonal contraception among women at high risk for HIV and infected with HIV. *Morbidity and Mortality Weekly Report, 61*(24), 449–452. Retrieved from http://www.cdc.gov/mmwr/preview/mmwrhtml/mm6124a4.htm?s_cid=mm6124a4_e%0d%0a

Centers for Disease Control and Prevention. (2014). *Recommended adult immunization schedule-US 2014*. Retrieved from http://www.cdc.gov/vaccines/schedules/downloads/adult/adult-schedule.pdf

Centers for Disease Control and Prevention. (2015). *Sexually transmitted diseases*. Retrieved from http://www.cdc.gov/std/

De Villers, T. J., Gass, M., Haines, C. J., Hall, J., Pierroz, D., & Rees, M. (2013). Global consensus statement on menopausal hormone therapy. *Climacteric, 16*, 203–204.

Harlow, S. D., Gass, M., Hall, J. E., Lobo, R., Maki, P., Rebar, R. W., ... de Villiers, T. J. (2012). Executive summary of the Stages of Reproductive Aging Workshop + 10: Addressing the unfinished agenda of staging reproductive aging. *Fertility and Sterility, 97*(4), 843–851.

Hatcher, R., Trussell, J., Nelson, A., Cates, W., Kowal, D., & Policar, M. (2011). *Contraceptive technology* (20th Rev. ed.). New York, NY: Ardent Media.

Hoffman, B., Schorge, J., Schaffer, J., Halvorson, L., Bradshaw, K. Cunningham, F.G. (2012). *Williams gynecology*. New York, NY: McGraw-Hill.

Munro, M., Critchley, H., Broder, M., & Fraser, I. (2011). FIGO classification system (PALM-COEIN) for causes of abnormal uterine bleeding in nongravid women of reproductive age. *International Journal of Gynecology and Obstetrics, 113*, 3–13.

National Osteoporosis Foundation. (2014). *Clinician's guide to prevention and treatment of osteoporosis*. Washington, DC: National Osteoporosis Foundation.

North American Menopause Society. (NAMS). (2010). *Menopause practice: A clinician's guide* (4th ed.). Mayfield Heights, OH: NAMS.

North American Menopause Society. (NAMS). (2012). The 2012 hormone therapy position statement of The North American Menopause Society. *Menopause, 19*(3), 257–271.

United States Preventative Services Task Force (USPSTF). (2002 to 2016). *Recommendations for primary care practice*. Retrieved from http://www.uspreventiveservicestaskforce.org.

Chapter 7

Men's Health

Al Rundio

Case Presentation

Directions: Carefully review the case study presented below. At the end of the chapter, answer the review questions. Compare your answers to the correct answers listed in the Review Section.

History of Present Illness: Mr. R is a 61-year-old male, who presents to the urologist office with a complaint of urinary urgency and frequency, pain on urination and voiding in decreased amounts. He states that he has had these symptoms for around 3 months now. He has a history of frequent occurrences of acute prostatitis. He has taken a course of Cipro 500 mg b.i.d. for 1 month, and then he took Cipro 500 mg once daily for 1 month. Within 2 to 3 d after stopping the Cipro the symptoms reoccur.

Past Medical History:
Recurrent prostatitis every 2 to 3 years for the past 15 years
GERD (gastroesophageal reflux disease) for the past 25 years

Past Surgical History:
Tonsillectomy and adenoidectomy at age 7
Appendectomy at age 9

Family History:
Mother: NIDDM, HTN, abdominal aortic aneurysm (resected), colon resection for adenocarcinoma in situ of the colon and diverticula
Father: Right inguinal herniorrhaphy with postoperative staphylococcal infection, penile carcinoma resected, prostate cancer successfully treated with Lupron Rx and radiation therapy, coronary artery disease, Parkinson disease, Alzheimer disease
Sister: Healthy
Paternal Grandfather: COPD, atherosclerosis—deceased at age 84
Paternal Grandmother: Depression—deceased at age 62
Maternal Grandmother: Pancreatic cancer with whipple surgical procedure—deceased at age 52
Maternal Grandfather: Lung cancer—deceased at age 62

Social History:
Married to same spouse for 43 years
Two children alive and healthy
One grandson alive and healthy
Nonsmoker. Social drinker—two to four glasses of wine weekly; one to two beers weekly
Employed full time as an Associate Dean in a major university

Sexual History:
Monogamous heterosexual relationship for over 44 years
Reports decreased sexual activity
No history of sexually transmitted infections

Physical Examination:

Vital Signs: BP = 122/80   Pulse 64   RR = 15   Temperature = 97.6°F oral

General: Alert, healthy-appearing male in no acute distress. Affect is appropriate. No obvious signs of distress

Focused Exam: Abdomen is soft, not distended, bowel sounds, no pain or tenderness, no masses

Genital Examination: Penis normal, no masses. Testes are descended, no masses. Tanner stage V.

Rectal Examination: No blood. Stool Hematest negative. No masses. Prostate firm, not boggy, no masses, moderate enlargement, no tenderness

Urine dipstick: No blood. Negative on other parameters

Differential Diagnoses: Urinary tract infection, enlarged prostate—benign prostatic hypertrophy.

Plan: PSA, clean catch midstream urinalysis, urine culture and sensitivity, urine flow study, bladder ultrasound, Levaquin 500 mg p.o. once daily at 30 d after urine c and s specimen is collected.

Benign Prostatic Hyperplasia/Hypertrophy:

Benign prostatic hyperplasia/hypertrophy (BPH) is an enlarged prostate gland.

The prostate gland surrounds the urethra. As the prostate becomes larger, it may partially block the urethra. This often causes problems with urinating.

BPH occurs in a significant number of men as they age. About half of all men older than 75 have some symptoms. BPH is probably a normal part of the aging process in men, caused by changes in hormone balance and cell growth. BPH causes urinary problems as follows:

- Trouble getting a urine stream started and completely stopped (dribbling)
- Often feeling like one needs to urinate. Voiding at night time
- A weak urine stream
- A sense that the bladder is not completely empty after urination

In a small number of cases, BPH may cause the bladder to be blocked, making it impossible or extremely hard to urinate. This problem may cause urinary retention with a retrograde backflow of urine that can lead to bladder infections, stones, or kidney damage.

For mild symptoms, home treatment strategies may work, such as given below:

- Practice "double voiding." Urinate as much as one can, relax for a few moments, and then urinate again.
- Avoid caffeine and alcohol.
- Avoid medications that can make urination difficult, such as over-the-counter antihistamines, decongestants (including nasal sprays), and allergy pills. If home treatment does not help, BPH can be treated with medication (see information under BPH in this chapter). Medication can reduce the symptoms.

Case Progression:

Mr. R's urine c and s was negative. The urine flow study demonstrated a decreased urinary flow. The bladder ultrasound demonstrated no masses or lesions. Residual urine postvoiding was estimated at 50%. PSA value was measured at 0.9.

Follow-up appointment was made with the patient to discuss the testing results. It was determined that Mr. R's BPH was causing partial obstruction of urinary flow. The treatment plan was revised to include adding Flomax 0.4 mg once daily at bedtime (refer to information on Flomax in this chapter).

Follow-Up:

Flomax worked well for this patient. Repeat ultrasounds and flow studies demonstrated marked improvement. The patient's symptoms resolved, and he has had no repeat episodes of a urinary tract infection. The patient continues to be monitored every 6 months.

Men's Health Part I

Describe common disorders of the male genitourinary tract.

Discuss the pharmacologic agents and other treatments utilized for treating common disorders of the male genitourinary tract in men. Male anatomy as shown in Figure 7-1.

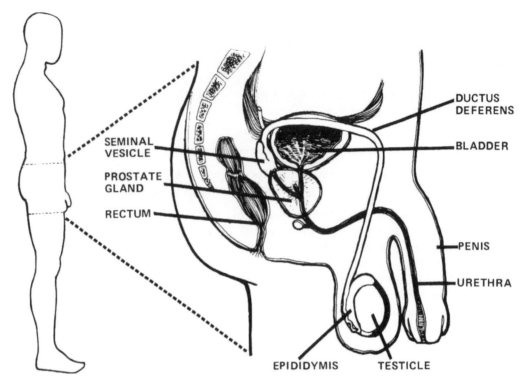

Figure 7-1: Male reproductive system.
Source: Centers for Disease Control Prevention Atlanta, GA.

Average Life Expectancy:
- Women = 81 years of age
- Men = 76 years of age

Why?
- Women pay more attention to their health.
- Women are more apt to see a provider early on when they have a symptom.

Trust can be better achieved if questions are gender neutral.
- Tell me about your living situation.
- Are you sexually active?
- Are your partners men, women, or both?
- Are you married?
- Do you have a girlfriend/boyfriend?
- Have you ever been treated for a sexually transmitted disease?
- Have you ever experimented with illegal drugs and/or alcohol?

Sexual History:
- Sexual behavior or other feelings
- Concerns with sexual identity
- Sexual behavior that increases the risk of disease or of experiences that involve harassment of or by others
- Worry about masturbating or even touching the body

Topics of Discussion—Sexually Transmitted Diseases

SYPHILIS

- Primary
- Secondary
- Latent

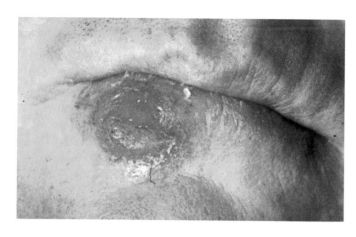

Figure 7-2: Oral chancre, lower lip.
Source: Public Health Agency of Canada, Centers for Disease Control Prevention Atlanta, GA.

Syphilis Stages and Organism Identity:
Chancre of Syphilis
- Clean
- Painless
- Hard base
- Highly contagious
- Heals spontaneously
- Appears at site of inoculation

Note: The chancre of syphilis is represented in Figure 7-2. Rashes also are common on the plantar and palmar surfaces as represented in Figure 7-3.

Serologic Markers:
- Venereal Disease Research Laboratory (VDRL) test
- Rapid plasma reagin (RPR) test
- Fluorescent treponemal antibody absorption (FTA-ABS) test (fluorescent *Treponema* antibody)

Treatment:
Center for Disease Control and Prevention Treatments for Syphilis

Stage	Treatment
Primary, secondary, and early latent syphilis without neurologic involvement	**Benzathine penicillin G**, intramuscularly, 2.4 million units in a single dose **If penicillin allergic (one of the following):** • **Doxycycline** 100 mg orally twice daily for 2 wk • **Tetracycline** 500 mg orally four times daily for 2 wk
Late latent or latent syphilis of unknown duration without neurologic involvement	**Benzathine penicillin G** 7.2 million units total, administered as three doses of 2.4 million units intramuscularly each at 1-wk intervals **If penicillin allergic (one of the following):** • **Doxycycline** 100 mg orally twice daily for 28 d • **Tetracycline** 500 mg orally four times daily for 28 d
Tertiary (late) syphilis without neurologic involvement	**Benzathine penicillin G** 7.2 million units total, administered as three doses of 2.4 million units intramuscularly each at 1-wk intervals **If penicillin allergic:** Treat according to treatment for late latent syphilis.
Neurosyphilis	**Aqueous crystalline penicillin G** 18–24 million units/day, administered as 3–4 million units intravenously every 4 hours or continuous infusion for 10–14 d intravenously **Alternative regimen (if compliance can be ensured):** • **Procaine penicillin** 2.4 million units intramuscularly once daily *Plus* • **Probenecid** 500 mg orally four times a day, both for 10–14 d

Adapted from Centers for Disease Control and Prevention. *2015 STD treatment guidelines.* Retrieved from http://www.cdc.gov/std/tg2015/syphilis.htm

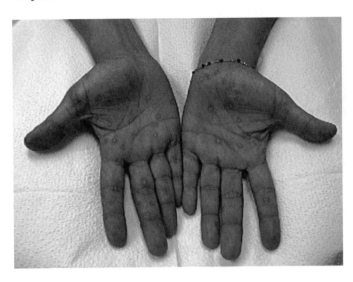

Figure 7-3: Palmar rash.
Source: Dr. John Toney, Southeast STD/HIV Prevention Training Center Centers for Disease Control Prevention Atlanta, GA.

CHANCROID

- Causative organism is a gram-negative bacillus, *Haemophilus ducreyi*.
- Incubation period is 3 to 5 d.
- Vesicopustule breaks down to form a painful, soft ulcer with a necrotic base, surrounding erythema, and undermined edges.
- Multiple lesions and inguinal adenitis is common.
- Health education and safe-sex practices should be encouraged.
- Serologic testing for syphilis, HIV, and all other STIs should be performed; retesting 3 months later if test results are negative
- HIV-positive patients may fail single-dose therapy.

Treatment:
- For treatment with antibiotics, the Centers for Disease Control and Prevention (CDC) recommends the following:
  - Azithromycin 1 g p.o. single dose
  - Ceftriaxone 250 mg IM single dose
  - Erythromycin 500 mg p.o. q.i.d. for 7 d
  - Ciprofloxacin 500 mg p.o. b.i.d. for 3 d
  - Streptomycin and ceftriaxone have been shown to be synergistic in the treatment of chancroid.

Treatment:
- Single-dose ciprofloxacin (92% cure rate) and azithromycin are effective.
- Treatment of partners is similar to that of the source patient.
- Patients should not engage in sexual activity until the ulcers are healed.

GONORRHEA

- Incubation 2 to 10 d
- Causative organism is the *Neisseria gonorrhoeae*.

Symptoms include the following:
- Extremely white, yellow, or green purulent discharge (see Figure 7-4), burning during urination, painful intercourse, vaginal bleeding/discharge
- Can cause ophthalmic gonorrhea
- Can be disseminated

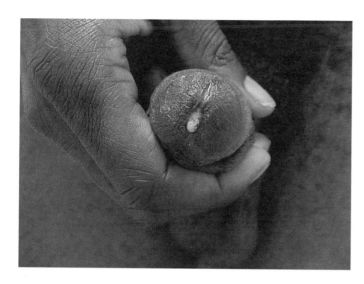

Figure 7-4: Penile discharge, gonorrhea. Source: Cincinnati STD/HIV Prevention Training Center Centers for Disease Control Prevention Atlanta, GA.

Center for Disease Control and Prevention Treatments for Uncomplicated Gonococcal Infections of the Cervix, Urethra, and Rectum

Recommended Regimens	Alternative Regimens
• **Ceftriaxone** 250 mg in a single intramuscular dose *Plus* • **Azithromycin** 1 g orally in a single dose *Or* • **Doxycycline** 100 mg orally twice a day for 7 d	• **Cefixime** 400 mg in a single oral dose *Plus* • **Azithromycin** 1 g orally in a single dose *Or* • **Doxycycline** 100 mg orally twice daily for 7 d *Plus* • Test of cure in 1 wk If the patient has severe cephalosporin allergy: • **Azithromycin** 2 g in a single oral dose *Plus* • Test of cure in 1 wk

Adapted from Centers for Disease Control and Prevention. *2015 STD treatment guidelines.* Retrieved from http://www.cdc.gov/std/tg2015/gonorrhea.htm

GONOCOCCAL INFECTIONS OF THE PHARYNX

See Box 7-1.

Treatment:
- Since chlamydial infection is more common than GC, if GC is present it is assumed that chlamydia is present.
- Should give either doxycyline 100 mg p.o. b.i.d. $\times$ 7 d or azithromycin 1 g p.o. concurrently
- For ophthalmic infection, ceftriaxone 1 g IM.

Box 7-1: Center for Disease Control and Prevention Treatments for Uncomplicated Gonococcal Infections of the Pharynx

Recommended Regimens

- **Ceftriaxone** 250 mg in a single intramuscular dose
  Plus
- **Azithromycin** 1 g orally in a single dose
  Or
- **Doxycycline** 100 mg orally twice daily for 7 d

Adapted from Center for Disease Control and Prevention. *2010 STD treatment guidelines.* Retrieved from http://www.cdc.gov/std/treatment/2010/gonococcal-infections.htm

HERPES ZOSTER

Treatment:
- Caused by herpes simplex virus (HSV)-1 or -2
- Painful blisters or open sores
- Lesions may be preceded by tingling or burning sensation in the legs, buttocks, or genital region.
- Lesions may disappear spontaneously within a few weeks.
- Virus remains in body and may reoccur from time to time.

GENITAL HERPES

- Caused by HSV-1 or -2
- Painful blisters or open sores
- Lesions may be preceded by tingling or burning sensation in the legs, buttocks, or genital region.
- Lesions may disappear spontaneously within a few weeks.
- Virus remains in body and may reoccur from time to time.

Treatment:
Center for Disease Control and Prevention Treatments for Herpes Simplex Virus

First Clinical Episode (Primary Infection)	Episodic Therapy for Recurrent Symptomatic Infection	Suppressive Therapy for Recurrent Genital Herpes
• **Acyclovir** 400 mg orally three times a day for 7–10 d *Or* • **Acyclovir** 200 mg orally five times a day for 7–10 d *Or* • **Famciclovir** 250 mg orally three times a day for 7–10 d *Or* • **Valacyclovir** 1 g orally twice a day for 7–10 d.	• **Acyclovir** 400 mg orally three times a day for 5 d *Or* • **Acyclovir** 800 mg orally twice a day for 5 d *Or* • **Acyclovir** 800 mg orally three times a day for 2 d *Or* • **Famciclovir** 125 mg orally twice daily for 5 d *Or* • **Famciclovir** 1,000 mg orally twice daily for 1 day *Or* • **Famciclovir** 500 mg once, followed by 250 mg twice daily for 2 d *Or* • **Valacyclovir** 500 mg orally twice a day for 3 d *Or* • **Valacyclovir** 1 g orally once a day for 5 d	• **Acyclovir** 400 mg orally twice a day *Or* • **Famciclovir** 250 mg orally twice a day *Or* • **Valacyclovir** 500 mg orally once a day *Or* • **Valacyclovir** 1 g orally once a day

Adapted from Centers for Disease Control and Prevention. *2015 STD treatment guidelines.* Retrieved from http://www.cdc.gov/std/tg2015/herpes.htm

- Intravenous (IV) therapy is also available for serious disease and complications; may require hospitalization
- Topical analgesics may be used for relief of painful lesions and dysuria.

ACYCLOVIR

- Genital herpes simplex (treatment and prophylaxis)
- Herpes simplex labialis (cold sores)
- Herpes zoster (shingles)
- Acute chickenpox both in nonimmunocompromised patients and immunocompromised patients
- Herpes simplex encephalitis
- Acute mucocutaneous HSV infections in immunocompromised patients (i.e., AIDS)

Indications:

- Herpes simplex keratitis (ocular herpes)
- Herpes simplex blepharitis (not to be mistaken with ocular herpes)
- Prophylaxis against herpes viruses in immunocompromised patients (such as patients undergoing cancer chemotherapy; HIV patients)
- The most common adverse drug reactions ($\geq$1% of patients) associated with systemic acyclovir therapy (oral or IV) and include:
  - Nausea
  - Vomiting
  - Diarrhea
  - Headache
  - In high doses, hallucinations have been reported.

Adverse Reactions:

Availability

- Acyclovir has been associated with renal failure; this can be fatal.
- Patients receiving acyclovir should be adequately hydrated to prevent renal toxicity secondary to crystal urea. IV acyclovir should not exceed a concentration of 7 mg/mL. Infusion should be over 1 hour to minimize crystallization of drug in the renal tubules.

Precautions

- Chlamydia: Parasitic sexually transmitted disease; intracellular obligate which closely resembles a gram-negative bacteria
  - Produces serious reproductive tract complications in either sex.

CHLAMYDIA

- Males
- Often asymptomatic
- Thick, cloudy, penile discharge
- Dysuria
- Testicular pain

Signs and Symptoms—Males:

- Laboratory/diagnostics
  - Culture is most definitive but takes 3 to 9 d.
  - EIA for screening; results in 30 to 120 minutes.

Etiology/Incidence:

- *Chlamydia trachomatis*
- One of the most common bacterial STDs in the United States
- Over 4 million infections annually
- Abnormal genital discharge and burning with urination.
- Many individuals have few to no symptoms.

Center for Disease Control and Prevention Treatments for Uncomplicated Chlamydial Infections

Recommended Regimens	Alternative Regimens
• **Azithromycin** 1 g orally in a single dose *Or* • **Doxycycline** 100 mg orally twice a day for 7 d	• **Erythromycin** base 500 mg orally four times a day for 7 d *Or* • **Erythromycin ethylsuccinate** 800 mg orally four times a day for 7 d *Or* • **Levofloxacin** 500 mg orally once daily for 7 d *Or* • **Ofloxacin** 300 mg orally twice a day for 7 d

Adapted from Centers for Disease Control and Prevention. *2015 STD treatment guidelines.* Retrieved from http://www.cdc.gov/std/tg2015/chlamydia.htm

HUMAN PAPILLOMA VIRUS

- Human papilloma virus (HPV)
- Genital warts
- Approximately 20 million Americans are currently infected with HPV. Another 6 million people become newly infected each year.
- HPV is so common that at least 50% of sexually active men and women get it at some point in their lives.
- Genital HPV is the most common sexually transmitted infection (STI) in the world.
- There are more than 40 HPV types that can infect the genital areas of males and females. These HPV types can also infect the mouth and throat. Most people who become infected with HPV do not even know they have it.
- Transmission is by sexual contact.
- Most people with HPV do not develop symptoms or health problems from it. In 90% of cases, the body's immune system clears HPV naturally within 2 years.
- Certain types of HPV can cause genital warts in males and females. Rarely, these types can also cause warts in the throat called recurrent respiratory papillomatosis (RRP).
- Other HPV types can cause cervical cancer. These types can also cause other, less common but serious cancers, including cancers of the vulva, vagina, penis, anus, and head and neck (tongue, tonsils, and throat).
- The types of HPV that can cause genital warts are not the same as the types that can cause cancer (Box 7-2).
- There is no way to know which people who get HPV will go on to develop cancer or other health problems.

HPV Screening

- Pap smears for women
- Gardasil vaccination
- Anal paps for men
- Consultation/referral for positive results

Treatment:

CDC Recommended Regimens for the Treatment of External Genital Warts: Patient Applied

Treatment	Directions	Considerations
Podofilox 0.5% solution or gel	Cotton swab twice a day for 3 d, followed by no treatment for 4 d; cycle can be repeated up to four cycles.	• The total wart area treated should not exceed 2 cm. • Total volume of podofilox should be limited to 0.5 mL/day. • The health-care provider should apply the initial treatment to demonstrate the proper application technique and identify which warts should be treated. • Mild to moderate pain or local irritation might develop after treatment. • Safety use in pregnancy not established
Imiquimod 5% cream	Once a day at bedtime, three times a week for up to 16 weeks; wash with soap and water 6–10 hours after application.	• Local inflammatory reactions, including redness, irritation, induration, ulceration/erosions, hypopigmentation, and vesicles are common. • Imiquimod might weaken latex condoms and vaginal diaphragms. • Safety use in pregnancy not established
Sinecatechins 15% ointment	Three times daily (0.5-cm strand of ointment to each wart) using a finger to ensure coverage with a thin layer of ointment until complete clearance of warts; should not be continued for longer than 16 weeks	• Do not wash off medication after use. • Avoid sexual contact while the ointment is on the skin. • Common side effects: Erythema, pruritus/burning, pain, ulceration, edema, induration, and vesicular rash • May weaken latex condoms and diaphragms • Safety use in pregnancy, with immunocompromised persons, or with clinical herpes, is not established.

Adapted from Centers for Disease Control and Prevention. *2015 STD treatment guidelines.* Retrieved from http://www.cdc.gov/std/tg2015/warts.htm

> **Box 7-2: CDC Recommended Regimens for the Treatment of External Genital Warts: Provider Applied**
>
> - **Cryotherapy** with liquid nitrogen or cryoprobe. Repeat applications every 1–2 weeks.
>   *Or*
> - **Podophyllin** resin 10%–25% in a compound tincture benzoin
>   *Or*
> - **Trichloroacetic** acid (TCA) or **Bichloroacetic** acid (BCA) 80%–90%
>   *Or*
> - **Surgical removal** either by tangential scissor excision, tangential shave excision, curettage, or electrosurgery

Adapted from Center for Disease Control and Prevention. *2010 STD treatment guidelines.* Retrieved from http://www.cdc.gov/std/treatment/2010/pid.htm

Men's Health Part II

Male anatomy as shown in Figure 7-4.

Erectile Dysfunction

- Erectile dysfunction (ED) is a condition that affects men. More than 50% of men over the age of 40 have ED.
- ED presents with the following:
  - Difficulty getting an erection
  - Maintaining an erection long enough for sex
  - Also known as ED or impotence
  - The etiology is not enough blood flow to the penis, thus preventing an erection.

Treatment:
- A PDE5 inhibitor medication that is used to treat ED
- Other PDE5 inhibitors on the market are sildenafil (Viagra), tadalafil (Cialis), and vardenafil (Levitra). Prior to any of these medications, men should have a complete urologic workup to rule out other disease states that may cause erective dysfunction, for example, decreased testosterone levels.
- Other medications:
  - Caverject (alprostadil—a penile injection) and Yocon (yohimbine—a herbal)

Source: Edmunds and Mayhew (2013, p. 368).

Benign Prostatic Hyperplasia

- Benign prostatic hyperplasia (BPH):
  - More cells; increases by 10% each decade starting at age 50
  - Compresses urethra
- Presents with:
  - Hesitancy, urgency, decreased force of stream, and increased risk of infection
  - Backflow to kidneys can lead to destruction of kidney cells

BPH Management:
- TURP, transurethral laser prostatectomy
- TUR microwave thermotherapy
- Increase fluids, home catheter use, void when you have the urge (do not wait).
- Medications: Flomax, Proscar, Cardura, Hytrin, Minipress, Avodart, UroXatral;
- Herbs: Saw Palmetto, B-Sitosterol plant extract, Pygeum Africanum, rye grass pollen, vitamins and nutrients (pumpkin seed oil, zinc)

Source: Edmunds & Mayhew (2013, pp. 368 & 369).

Prostatitis

- An inflammation or infection of the prostate gland
- Most commonly diagnosed urologic disease in men
- About 50% of men will be treated for prostatitis in the United States.

Etiology:
- Infections by bacteria or other organisms cause 50% to 70% of cases.
- Bacteria may result from a bladder infection or sexual contact with a partner who is infected with an STI.
- Another cause is a chemical reaction secondary to BPH; some of the urine may remain in the urethra after urination and back up into the prostate gland.
- Urate irritates the tissues of the prostate gland.
- In addition to urinary reflux, there are several pathways through which the infective organism or irritating chemical may reach the prostate gland.
- It may descend from the kidney or bladder, or ascend from the seminal vesicles.

Risk Factors:
- Iatrogenic: Recently had a medical instrument inserted into the urinary tract
- Engaged in anal intercourse
- Abnormalities in the urinary tract
- Had a recent or recurrent bladder infection
- BPH

Types:
- Three major types of prostatitis exist
  - Bacterial prostatitis (acute and chronic)
  - Nonbacterial prostatitis
  - Prostatodynia

Diagnosis:
- Digital rectal examination (DRE): one of the most important diagnostic tools
- Prostate massage: Clinician massages the prostate gland to expel fluid; fluid is then analyzed for microorganisms.
- Sequential urine test: Includes three samples
  - Measured amount of urine
  - Second sample of any discharge after prostate massage
  - Final sample of urine after massage
- Needle biopsy
- Prostate-specific antigen (PSA): Blood test that measures the levels of PSA (a substance produced by the prostate) in the blood
  - USPSTF: Value of this test is not determined. PSA elevates after DRE.
- Imaging tests: Includes ultrasound, IVP, MRI, and CT scans

Treatment:
- Acute and chronic bacterial prostatitis
  - Antibiotics such as fluoroquinolones (i.e., Cipro 500 mg p.o. b.i.d., Levaquin 500 mg p.o. o.d., Floxacin), Bactrim DS b.i.d., doxycycline 100 mg b.i.d.
- Nonbacterial prostatitis
  - NSAIDS, drugs to shrink the prostate gland such as Proscar, Hytrin, Cardura, hyperthermotherapy
- Prostatodynia
- Drugs may be prescribed to prevent muscle spasms in the bladder and urethra such as Baclofen, Detrol XR, NSAIDS, hyperthermotherapy.

Alternative Treatments:
- Heat: Warm sitz baths, hot compresses (not recommended for patients with acute bacterial prostatitis), whirlpool baths
- Alternate hot and cold therapy
- Herbal therapies such as zinc, saw palmetto, pumpkin seed oils, essential fatty acids
- Anxiety treatment such as meditation, biofeedback, yoga, and moderate exercise

Epididymitis

- Inflammation of the epididymis
- *C. trachomatis* is the major cause in sexually active heterosexual men under age 35, which accounts for about 70% of cases.
- *N. gonorrhea* causes the majority of the remaining cases.
- Some men have a combination of both infections.
- *Pseudomonas aeruginosa* is the most common cause in men over age 35.

Symptoms:
- Unilateral scrotal pain
- Fever
- Epididymal tenderness and/or swelling
- *Plus* Cremasteric sign
- Must rule out testicular torsion promptly by radionuclide scan, Doppler flow study, or surgical exploration in a teenager or young adult who presents with acute unilateral testicular pain without urethritis

Treatment:
- Treatment is rest, scrotal support, Jockey short underwear, and antimicrobial therapy such as Cipro, Floxacin.
- The possibility of testicular tumor or chronic infection (such as tuberculosis) must be excluded when a patient with unilateral intrascrotal pain and swelling does not respond to appropriate antimicrobial therapy.

Testicular Cancer

- Testicular: #1 killer of 15- to 35-year-olds

Treatment:
- Orchiectomy, chemotherapy, and radiation
- Sperm banking
- Should begin self-examinations (warm shower q monthly)

Source: McPhee and Papadakis (2010, p. 1484).

Prostate Cancer

- Most common noncutaneous malignancy in men in the United States and the second most common cause of cancer death in men above the age of 55 (lung and colon cancer precede prostate deaths)
- In the United States, there are approximately 218,000 newly diagnosed cases and about 27,000 deaths annually.
- Disease is rare before age 50; incidence increases with age
- Frequency of disease varies in different parts of the world.
  - High in North America and European countries
  - Intermediate in South America
  - Low in the Far East (suggesting environmental or dietary etiology to the disease)

Source: McPhee and Papadakis (2010, p. 1484).

Symptoms:
- Asymptomatic in 80% of patients
- Symptoms may include dysuria, difficulty voiding, increased urinary frequency, complete urinary retention, back and/or hip pain, and hematuria.
- Advanced disease may include spinal cord compression from intradural metastases, deep vein thrombosis, pulmonary emboli, and myelophthisis.

Histologic Grading:
- Over 95% of prostatic carcinomas are adenocarcinomas that arise in the prostatic acini.
- Adenocarcinomas may begin anywhere in the prostate gland but have an affinity for the periphery of the gland.
- The area of tumor that is most poorly differentiated with highest histologic grade appears to determine its biologic behavior.

Source: McPhee and Papadakis (2010, p. 1484).

Diagnosis:
- DRE: Posterior surfaces of the lateral lobes, where carcinoma begins most frequently in men, are easily palpable on DRE.
- Carcinoma is characteristically hard, nodular, and irregular.
- Local extraprostatic extension of tumor into the seminal vesicles can often be detected by the DRE.
- Scrotal and/or lower extremity lymphedema indicates extensive disease.

Source: McPhee and Papadakis (2010, p. 1484).

Biochemical Markers:
Prostate-Specific Antigen
- The serum PSA is an imperfect tumor marker for the early detection of prostatic cancer.
- Approximately 18% to 30% of men with intermediate degrees of elevation (4.1 to 10 ng/mL) will be found to have prostate cancer.
- PSA levels are generally higher in African Americans and men with BPH.
- Normal value is <4 ng/mL.
- Increasing values on different tests or a level >10 is indicative of recommending a prostatic biopsy.
- Imaging
- Transrectal prostatic biopsy with a rapid-fire spring-loaded needle under sonography provides the most accurate sampling.

Treatment:
- Surgery: Total prostatoseminovesiculectomy is the oldest treatment for carcinoma of the prostate.
  - Radical perineal prostatectomy and radical retropubic prostatectomy are other types of surgical procedures. Great risk of impotence with these procedures.
- Robotic surgery (DaVinci prostatectomy): Procedure is nerve-sparing.
- Radiation: Colitis and cystitis can result from radiation treatment. A Gleason score of 7 has less risk of metastasis.
- Cryosurgery
- Implantation of radium seeds
- Chemotherapy
- Proton therapy
- Watchful waiting (wait and see; low-grade tumors not necessarily being treated today)
- Androgen deprivation (Lupron (leuprolide))
- Lupron injection (5 mg/mL for daily subcutaneous injection)
- Lupron Depot (7.5 mg/vial for monthly intramuscular depot injection)
- Lupron Depot 22.5 mg for 3-month, 30 mg for 4-month, and 45 mg for 6-month administrations are prescribed for the palliative treatment of advanced prostate cancer.
- Viadur 72 mg yearly subcutaneous implant
- PROVENGE (sipuleucel-T) is approved by the FDA as an autologous cellular immunotherapy for the treatment of asymptomatic or minimally symptomatic metastatic hormone refractory prostate cancer.
- PROVENGE is the first medication in a new class of therapy termed autologous cellular immunotherapy.
- The active component of PROVENGE consists of its own antigen-presenting cells (APCs) that have been cultured with a recombinant antigen (PAP–GM–CSF, comprised of PAP, an antigen expressed in most prostate cancers, and GM–CSF, an immune cell activator) to stimulate the body's immune system against prostate cancer.

Mechanism of Action of Provenge:
- Activate T cells, which then proliferate to target prostate cancer cells.
- Stimulate an immune response against prostate cancer (measured out to 26 weeks in clinical trials).
- This is an extremely expensive medication costing around $91,000 for three required doses.
- Check with patient's insurance carrier to assure reimbursement.
- Prolongs life approximately by 6 months; however, the drug has only been available since 2010 so more data on life expectancy is needed.

Bladder Cancer

- Second-most common urologic cancer
- More common in men than women
- Mean age of patients at diagnosis is 65.

- Cigarette smoking and exposure to industrial dyes or solvents are risk factors.
- 98% of bladder cancers are epithelial malignancies.

Source: McPhee and Papadakis (2010, p. 1489).

Essentials of Diagnosis:
- Gross or microscopic hematuria
- Urinary frequency and urgency
- Positive urinary cytology
- Filling defect within bladder observed on imaging studies

Diagnosis:
- Imaging (ultrasound, CT, or MRI)
- Cystourethroscopy and biopsy
- Pathology and staging

Treatment:
- Transurethral resection
- Partial cystectomy
- Radical cystectomy
- Intravesical chemotherapy (common agents are thiotepa, mitomycin, doxorubicin, and BCG)
  - BCG (Bacillus Calmette–Guerin) has demonstrated to be the most efficacious. This medication was used to vaccinate individuals to prevent tuberculosis. It has been found to be an effective treatment for bladder cancer.
- Radiotherapy

Source: McPhee and Papadakis (2010, p. 1489).

Review Section

Review Questions

1. Mr. J presents with blood in his semen. Rectal examination reveals an extremely tender, boggy prostate with no masses or lesions palpated. The most likely diagnosis is:

   a. bladder cancer.
   b. acute bacterial prostatitis.
   c. torsion of the left testicle.
   d. UTI.

2. Treatment for Mr. J would be:

   a. prostate massage.
   b. Cipro 500 mg p.o. b.i.d. for 30 d.
   c. Cipro 500 mg p.o. for 7 d.
   d. EES 500 mg p.o. for 14 d.

3. A frequently presenting symptom of a patient with BPH is:

   a. frequent nocturia.
   b. good urine stream.
   c. rectal pain.
   d. constipation.

4. John J., a 13-year-old, presents with an acute onset of right testicular pain. On examination, the patient is in excruciating pain and there is a noted difference in testicular decent. What is the most likely diagnosis?

   a. Epididymitis
   b. Torsion of the right testicle
   c. Right inguinal hernia
   d. UTI

5. In Question 4, the *best* intervention is:

   a. referral to a urologist ASAP.
   b. routine urine analysis.
   c. rectal examination.
   d. administer a pain medication.

6. In Question 4, the *best* test to perform is:

   a. PSA.
   b. routine urine analysis.
   c. stat testicular ultrasound.
   d. rectal examination.

7. A nurse practitioner diagnoses a patient with gonorrhea. This patient should also be treated for which of the following?

    a. Syphilis
    b. Chancroid
    c. Herpes
    d. Chlamydia

8. What would be the best treatment regimen for the patient in Question 7?

    a. Cipro 500 mg p.o. b.i.d. for 10 d
    b. Doxycycline 100 mg p.o. b.i.d. for 7 d
    c. Flagyl 500 mg p.o. b.i.d. for 7 d
    d. EES 500 mg p.o. b.i.d. for 7 d

9. A patient's PSA level has been increasing for the past 3 years by 0.7 ng/mL. The readings are the following: 2013—PSA = 0.9; 2014—PSA = 1.6; 2015—PSA = 2.3. The best treatment plan for this patient is:

    a. Cipro 500 mg p.o. b.i.d. for 10 d.
    b. repeat serum PSA level in 1 week.
    c. doxycycline 100 mg p.o. b.i.d. for 10 d.
    d. referral to urologist for further evaluation.

10. In Question 9, the urologist will most likely order:

    a. a repeat PSA.
    b. a complete metabolic panel.
    c. a prostate needle biopsy.
    d. reevaluate patient in 6 months.

Answers with Rationales

1. (b) Acute bacterial prostatitis

    Rationale: A tender, boggy prostate is the classic assessment finding for acute bacterial prostatitis.

2. (b) Cipro 500 mg p.o. b.i.d. for 30 d

    Rationale: The fluoroquinolone class of antibiotics is the preferred medication to order. The prostate gland is difficult to penetrate with antibiotic therapy, so generally an initial course of antibiotics is prescribed for 21 to 30 d.

3. (a) Frequent nocturia

    Rationale: One of the classic signs of BPH is having to void frequently at night time.

4. (b) Torsion of the right testicle

    Rationale: Torsion of the testes most frequently occurs in adolescents. The typical presenting symptom is an acute sudden onset of pain in the affected testicle.

5. (a) Referral to a urologist ASAP

    Rationale: Surgical intervention must be done quickly in order to release the torsion; otherwise, the lack of blood flow to the testicle can cause testicular death.

6. (c) Stat testicular ultrasound

    Rationale: A testicular ultrasound can determine if blood flow to the testicle is present or compromised.

7. (d) Chlamydia

    Rationale: Chlamydia is the most common STI, and oftentimes, individuals who present with gonorrhea also have a coexisting infection with *Chlamydia*.

8. (b) Doxycycline 100 mg p.o. b.i.d. for 7 d

    Rationale: Doxycycline is one of the preferred treatment regimens for chlamydia.

9. (d) Referral to urologist for further evaluation

    Rationale: A PSA that increases consistently by 0.7 ng/mL/year could be a sign of prostate cancer.

10. (c) A prostate needle biopsy

    Rationale: In order to determine if the patient has prostate cancer, a prostate needle biopsy is the preferred procedure/test.

Suggested Readings

Edmunds, M. W., & Mayhew, M. S. (2013). *Pharmacology for the primary care provider* (4th ed.). St. Louis, MO: Elsevier/Mosby.

McPhee, S. J., & Papadakis, M. A. (Eds). (2016). *Current medical diagnosis & treatment* (49th ed.). New York, NY: McGraw-Hill.

Chapter 8

Musculoskeletal System

Jennifer L. Mondillo

Case Presentation

Directions: Carefully review the case study presented below. At the end of the chapter, answer the review questions. Compare your answers to the correct answers listed in the Review Section.

History of Present Illness:

Mrs. Masterman, a 62-year-old woman with a history of hypertension, has had intermittent left knee pain and general achiness for several months. The pain is alleviated with rest and acetaminophen, but it interferes with her daily activities. Her family history is significant for osteoarthritis. Her hypertension is well-controlled on 10 mg of lisinopril daily. On examination, there is mild decreased and limited range of motion of the left knee with mild effusion and palpable crepitus, but not erythema or warmth. At this visit, the provider gives her the diagnosis of osteoarthritis and acetaminophen was recommended for pain.

Mrs. Masterman returns her follow-up visit 3 months later and explains to her provider that her pain is no longer well-controlled and acetaminophen is not working. The provider discusses various types of pharmacologic and nonpharmacologic management for pain. She discusses with her provider that because she is "favoring" her left knee, her right knee has been painful as well.

Physical Examination:

Vital Signs: Temperature = 98.6   Pulse = 70   Respirations = 18   Blood pressure = 128/72

Knee Examination:

Observe: Mrs. Masterman has difficulty with walking and is unable to climb onto the table and requests to sit on the chair. Denies crepitus with right knee, but significant crepitus with left knee increasing over last 6 months.

Inspect for any edema, erythema, bruising, muscle atrophy of bilateral quadraceps.

Palpate: *Always* begin with nonaffected limb first:

  Right knee: No warmth, redness, effusion, or point tenderness

  Left knee: No warmth, redness, mild effusion, medium point tenderness generalized area of knee

Assess:

  Right knee: Full range of motion with flexion and extension. No crepitus; no effusions; no edema or erythema. Negative Lachman test; negative anterior and posterior drawer signs; negative valgus and varus stress tests; negative McMurray test

  Left knee: Limited range of motion with extension, full range of motion with flexion; positive crepitus; no effusions or erythema; positive for mild edema generalized knee joint; negative Lachman test; negative anterior and posterior drawer signs; negative valgus and varus stress tests; negative McMurray test

  Hip examination: Full range-of-motion bilateral hips and negative point tenderness

Differential Diagnosis:
Osteoarthritis
Knee strain
Rheumatoid arthritis
Gout/pseudogout
Systemic lupus erythematosus

Treatment:
Osteoarthritis: It is a chronic condition, and treatment is aimed at working toward minimizing and limiting pain and optimizing functional abilities.
Pharmacologic Treatment:
- *Acetaminophen:* First line of treatment for mild to moderate pain associated with osteoarthritis
  - Dosing up to 4 g daily (may be split throughout 24 hours)
  - Minimal risk of nephrotoxicity and hepatotoxicity if taken as directed
- **NSAIDS (nonsteroidal anti-inflammatory drugs)**
- **Patient education** is important to facilitate an understanding of their condition and their abilities to minimize their pain as they will not be pain-free daily.
- **Exercise programs** such as walking, resistance training, and water therapy can help reduce pain and prolong disability.
- **Physical therapy** and use of ice/heat have possible benefits.
  - Knee braces/sleeves provide possible pain relief.
  - Transcutaneous electrical nerve stimulation (TENS) units have posed possible pain relief, but research is conflicting.
- **Intra-articular steroid injections:** To be considered if knee joint is edematous and painful
  - Cannot have more than three injections per year and no more than one injection per month
  - Dosing: 1 mL of steroid with 3 to 4 mL of local anesthetic
  - 24 hours of immobilization will maximize effects of medication, but mobility and ambulation encouraged after initial 24 hours.
- **Referral to orthopedic surgeon:** To to be considered if all treatment methods have been exhausted and pain is increasing. X-rays and MRIs prior to consult should be performed.

Osteoarthritis

Description of Disease: Noninflammatory degenerative disorder of movable joints, especially the hands, knees, hips, and spine. It occurs when the protective cartilage on the distal ends of your bones degenerates over time causing joint destruction. Formation of osteophytes, cysts, and hypertrophy can occur.

Epidemiology:
- Osteoarthritis (OA) is the most common joint disorder in the United States. Symptomatic knee OA occurs in 10% of men and 13% of women aged 60 years or older. The number of people affected with symptomatic OA is likely to increase due to the aging of the population and the obesity epidemic.

Etiology:
- Idiopathic: Occurs without obvious cause
- Higher incidence in women over 50
- Affects over 27 million adults
- Possibly results from secondary causes such as
  - Metabolic/endocrine
  - Congenital
  - Trauma

Risk Factors:
- Older age: Risk increases with age.
- Sex: Women are more likely to develop OA.

- Obesity: Added stress is put on weight-bearing joints, such as hips and knees. In addition, fat tissue produces proteins that may cause harmful inflammation in and around joints.
- Joint injuries and bone composition: Injuries may increase the risk of OA.
- Certain occupations: A job that includes tasks with repetitive stress on a particular joint, that joint may eventually develop OA.
- Genetics
- Comorbidities: Diabetes or other rheumatic diseases such as gout and rheumatoid arthritis (RA) can increase your risk of OA.

Signs and Symptoms:
- Pain: Joint pain aggravated during or after movement.
- Tenderness: Joint is tender when applying light pressure to it.
- Stiffness: Joint stiffness in the arm most noticeable upon waking up or after a period of inactivity
- Loss of flexibility: Decrease in range of motion as disease progresses
- Grating sensation: Felt or heard when using the joint
- Bone spurs: These extra bits of bone, which feel like hard lumps, may form around the affected joint.
- Hands
  - Heberden nodes: Enlargement of DIP joints
  - Bouchard nodes: Enlargement of PIP joints

Differential Diagnoses:
- Crystalline arthropathies (i.e., gout and pseudogout)
- Inflammatory arthritis (e.g., RA)
- Seronegative spondyloarthropathies (e.g., psoriatic arthritis and reactive arthritis)
- Rheumatic disease
- Fibromyalgia
- Tendonitis

Diagnostic Studies:
- X-rays: Reveals cartilage loss by a narrowing of the space between the bones in the joint. Bone spurs around a joint can be visualized.
- Laboratory tests: Analyzing your blood or joint fluid can help pinpoint the diagnosis.
  - Blood tests may help rule out other causes of joint pain, such as RA.
- Joint fluid analysis: Examining and testing the fluid can determine if there's inflammation and if pain is caused by gout or an infection.

Treatment:
- Preserving function and minimizing pain are primary goals of treatment—encourage range of motion exercises.
- Exercise: Educate on body mechanics, muscle strengthening.
- Weight management
- Rest and joint care
- Nonpharmacologic management: Ice to improve range of motion and heat to decrease muscle spasm
- Complementary and alternative therapies: Physical therapy
- Medications
  - Acetaminophen: 500 mg to 1 g t.i.d. or q.i.d.
    - May cause GI upset and liver toxicity
  - NSAIDS
    - Ibuprofen 400 to 800 mg t.i.d.
    - Indomethacin 50 to 200 mg/day up to 1 g/day q.i.d.
    - Cox-2 inhibitors (Celebrex) 100 to 200 mg/day
    - Educate on side effects especially with GI symptoms.
- Intra-articular injections of hyaluronic acid
  - Hyalgan
  - Synvisc
- Surgery: Refer to orthopedics for procedures such as fusion or joint replacements.

Osteoporosis

Description of Disease: A demineralization of the bone, resulting in decrease in bone mass with otherwise-normal structural components. It is a medical condition in which the bones become brittle and fragile from loss of tissue, typically as a result of hormonal changes, or deficiency of calcium or vitamin D.

Epidemiology:

- Due to its prevalence worldwide, osteoporosis is considered a serious public health concern. Currently it is estimated that over 200 million people worldwide suffer from this disease. Aging of populations worldwide will be responsible for a major increase in the incidence of osteoporo   menopausal women.

Etiology:

- Most common metabolic bone disease in the United States. Affects o 5 million men in the United States (currently diagnosed). Currently af years and after—age 40 to death.

Risk Factors:

Uncontrollable Risk Factors

- Being over age 50
- Being female
- Menopause
- Family history of osteoporosis
- Low body weight/being small and thin
- Broken bones or height loss
- Lack of estrogen

Controllable Risk Factors

- Not getting enough calcium and vitamin D
- Not eating enough fruits and vegetables
- Getting too much protein, sodium, and caffeine
- Having an inactive lifestyle
- Smoking
- Excessive alcohol intake
- Losing weight

Signs and Symptoms:

- Backache of joint pains
- Spontaneous fracture of vertebral collapse
- Loss of height
- Kyphosis (Dowager hump)
- Reoccurrence of fractures that occur easily

Differential Diagnoses:

- Hyperthyroidism
- Mastocytosis
- Multiple myeloma
- Osteomalacia and renal osteodystrophy
- Paget disease
- Scurvy
- Sickle cell anemia

Diagnostic Studies:

- Bone density tests: Is the only test that can diagnose osteoporosis before a broken bone occurs. This test helps to estimate the density of your bones and your chance of breaking a bone. NOF recommends a bone density test of the hip and spine by a central DXA machine to diagnose osteoporosis. DXA stands for dual-energy X-ray absorptiometry.
- Blood and urine tests can be used to identify possible causes of bone loss. Some of these tests include the following:
  - Blood calcium levels
  - 24-hour urine calcium measurement

- Thyroid function tests
- Parathyroid hormone levels
- Testosterone levels in men
- 25-hydroxyvitamin D test to determine whether the body has enough vitamin D. Biochemical marker tests, such as NTX and CTX
- Biochemical marker tests of the blood and/or urine may help to estimate how fast you are losing or making bone.
- X-rays and vertebral fracture assessments (VFAs) can show breaks in the spine.
- Nuclear bone scans, CT scans, or MRIs can show changes that may be caused by cancer, bone lesions, inflammation, new broken bones, or other conditions. They are often used to help find the cause of back pain or to follow up on abnormalities seen on an X-ray.

Treatment:
- Prevention is key. Severity of disease, age, and comorbidities must be taken into consideration.
- Balanced diet—protein not to exceed greater than 20% of total calories. Diet education to include diets high in calcium and low in fat
- Exercise
  - Weight-bearing exercises of at least 30 minutes three to four times a week
  - Strength training such as lifting weights, swimming
  - Mild to moderate walking exercises with those currently diagnosed
  - Active and/or passive range of motion for bedridden patients
- Osteoporosis medications: Osteoporosis treatments come in several forms. Many should be started during childhood; others include prescription drugs to treat osteoporosis.
  - Actonel, Binosto, Boniva, and Fosamax (also available as generic) work by inhibiting cells that break down bone and slowing bone loss. Actonel, Binosto, and Fosamax are usually taken once a week, while Boniva is taken once a month. There are strict ways to take these medications, since if taken incorrectly, they can lead to ulcers in the esophagus. Another osteoporosis medication of the same class is Reclast, which is given as a once-yearly 15-minute infusion in a vein. Reclast is said to increase bone strength and reduce fractures in the hip, spine and wrist, arm, leg, or rib.
  - Evista is an osteoporosis drug that has some actions similar to estrogen, such as the ability to maintain bone mass. However, studies have shown that it does not increase the risk of breast or uterine cancers like estrogen. Evista can cause blood clots and often increases hot flashes.
  - Forteo is a medication used for the treatment of osteoporosis in postmenopausal women and men who are at high risk for a fracture. A synthetic form of the naturally occurring parathyroid hormone, Forteo is the first drug shown to stimulate new bone formation and increase bone mineral density. It is self-administered as a daily injection for up to 24 months. Side effects include nausea, leg cramps, and dizziness.
  - Prolia is a monoclonal antibody—a fully human, laboratory-produced antibody that inactivates the body's bone-breakdown mechanism. It is the first "biologic therapy" to be approved for osteoporosis treatment. Prolia is approved for postmenopausal women with osteoporosis and high risk of fracture, and when other osteoporosis medicines have not worked.
  - Menopausal hormone replacement therapy—either estrogen alone or a combination of estrogen and progestin—is known to help preserve bone and prevent fractures. The drug Duavee (estrogen and bazedoxifene) is a type of HRT approved to treat menopause-related hot flashes. Duavee may also prevent osteoporosis in high-risk women who have already tried nonestrogen treatment.
  - HRT is no longer prescribed for osteoporosis alone because of other health risks long-term hormone therapy poses. In women who have been on hormone replacement therapy in the past and then stopped it, the bone begins to thin again—at the same pace as during menopause.
- Alcohol and smoking should be avoided.
- Elderly patients should be protected from falls—education to family and caretakers should occur.

Rheumatoid Arthritis

Description of Disease: It is a chronic inflammatory autoimmune disease in which the body's immune system mistakenly attacks your joints. The abnormal immune response causes inflammation, damaging joints and organs, such as the heart. Early diagnosis and prompt treatment is the key to preventing joint destruction and organ damage.

Epidemiology:

- About 1.5 million people in the United States have RA. Nearly three times as many women have the disease as men. In women, RA most commonly begins between ages 30 and 60. In men, it often occurs later in life.

Etiology:

- Cause remains unknown and diseases of joints such as OA and gout may predispose to RA. About half of patients have progressive disease.

Risk Factors:

- Smoking: Smokers are at increased risk.
- Sex: Females are at increased risk.
- Family history: Genetic predisposition has higher risk.
- Age: Middle-age persons (aged 30 to 60) are at increased risk.

Signs and Symptoms:

- Tenderness and pain on passive motion
- Fatigue
- Warm, swollen, reddish joints
- Long periods of joint stiffness in the morning are common.
- Inflammation in the small joints of the wrist and hand is common.
- Most often affects joints bilaterally
- Permanent deformity in chronic disease
- Synovial cysts can be visualized and palpated—baker cysts are common findings in chronic disease

Differential Diagnoses:

- Gout
- OA
- Systemic lupus erythematosus
- Rheumatic fever
- Ankylosing spondylitis
- Lyme disease
- Reiter syndrome

Diagnostic Studies:

- Elevated erythrocyte sedimentation rate (ESR or sed rate) indicates the presence of an inflammatory process in the body.
- Other common blood tests: look for rheumatoid factor and anticyclic citrullinated peptide (anti-CCP) antibodies.
  - Higher predictive value than rheumatoid factor
  - Not all patients are anti-CCP positive.
- Rheumatoid factor: Isolated in 70% to 80% of cases at some point in disease
  - Not specific to RA
  - First 6 months have less than 50% positive factor.
  - Once positive, no need to check again.
- Complete Blood Count (CBC): Mild to moderate normocytic anemia
- Radiographs: Track the progression of RA in your joints over time.
  - Able to assess degree of joint destruction and progression

Treatment:

- Primary treatment goals are to delay disease progression with DMARDs (disease-modifying antirheumatic drugs).
- Suspected RA medications include methotrexate preferred, supplemented with folate 1 mg daily or 7 mg weekly.
- Education on methotrexate: Abstain from alcohol and not to be taken during pregnancy.
- Rest
- Physical therapy
- Nonsteroidal anti-inflammatory agents
- Cold and heat therapy
- Education on diagnosis and potential treatment options
- Intra-articular corticosteroids if DMARDS are ineffective

- Gold salts: Orally or intramuscular
- Corticosteroids (no more than 0 mg of prednisone daily) for short-term use
- Tumor necrosis factor (TNF) inhibitors:
  - Etanercept, infliximab, adalimumab—modifying treatment for RA—at higher risk for infections while on these drugs.

Plantar Fasciitis

Description of Disease: Plantar fascia is the thick tissue on the bottom of the foot. It connects the heel bone to the toes and creates the arch of the foot. When this tissue becomes swollen or inflamed, it is called plantar fasciitis.

Epidemiology:
- Acute or recurrent pain in the bottom of the feet aggravated by walking.

Etiology:
- Tightness in the Achilles tendon causes tears in the plantar fascia.

Risk Factors:
- Obesity
- Diabetes
- Aerobic exercise
- Prolonged standing
- Flat feet

Signs and Symptoms:
- Heel pain when you take your first steps after getting out of bed or after sitting for a long period of time
- Stiffness and pain in the morning or after resting that gets better after a few steps but gets worse as the day progresses
- Pain that gets worse when you climb stairs or stand on your toes
- Pain after you stand for long periods
- Pain at the beginning of exercise that gets better or goes away as exercise continues but returns when exercise is completed

Differential Diagnoses:
- Arthritis
- Tarsal tunnel syndrome
- Heel spur
- Stress fracture

Diagnostic Studies:
- None. Diagnosis is completed by history and physical examination

Treatment:
- Nonsteroidal anti-inflammatory drugs: Naproxen (Aleve) p.o. b.i.d., ibuprofen (Advil) p.o. every 4 to 6 hours.
  - Use orthotic foot appliance at night for a few weeks. Ice to affected foot
  - Foot stretches and massaging
  - Weight loss
  - Consider X-ray to rule out fracture and refer to orthopedics and podiatry as needed.

Joint Sprains

Description of Disease: An overstrain of the ligaments of an ankle, wrist, or other joint so as to injure without fracture or dislocation

Epidemiology:
- A sprain is an injury to the ligaments around a joint. Ligaments are strong, flexible fibers that hold bones together. When a ligament is stretched too far or tears, the joint will become painful and swell.

Etiology:
- Sprains are caused when a joint is forced to move into an unnatural position.

Risk Factors:
- Running
- Exercising
- Overall physical activity

Signs and Symptoms:
- Pain, inability to apply weight to the affected joint, edema, bruising

Degrees of Sprains:
- Ottawa rules—A mild sprain (**first degree**) is the least severe. It is the result of some minor stretching of the ligaments, and is accompanied by mild pain, some swelling, and joint stiffness. There is usually very little loss of joint stability as a result and patient is able to bear weight.
- A moderate sprain (**second degree**) is the result of both stretching and some tearing of the ligaments. There is increased swelling and pain associated with a second-degree sprain, and a moderate loss of stability at the ankle joint. Ambulation and weight-bearing are painful.
- A complete rupture of ligaments (**third degree**) is the most severe of the three. A third-degree sprain is the result of a complete tear or rupture of one or more of the ligaments that make up the ankle joint. A third-degree sprain will result in massive swelling, severe pain, and gross instability.

Differential Diagnoses:
- Fracture
- Arthritis
- Tendinitis
- Gout

Diagnostic Studies:
- X-rays, MRI

Knee Stability Tests:
Gold standard test for joint instability is the MRI.
- Drawer sign: Test for knee stability. The drawer sign is a diagnostic sign of a torn anterior cruciate ligament (ACL). This test can be completed for both anterior and posterior cruciate ligaments (PCL).
- McMurray test: Test for tearing of the medial meniscus. Knee pain followed by a "clicking" sound are indicative of a positive test.
- Lachman test: Suggestive of ACL damage within the knee. Knee joint instability or laxity of the ligament is indicative of a positive Lachman test.
- Valgus and varus stress tests of the knee: Test for medial or collateral ligament damage within the knee

Treatment:
- RICE (Rest, Ice, Compression, Elevation)
  - Cold is best for injury during the initial 48 hours.
  - 20 minutes on/20 minutes off
  - Compress joints as needed to minimize swelling and pain.
  - NSAIDS (Aleve or Naproxen b.i.d., ibuprofen q.i.d.) for swelling and joint pain

Carpal Tunnel Syndrome

Description of Disease: Carpal tunnel syndrome is a median entrapment neuropathy that causes paresthesia, pain, numbness, and other symptoms in the distribution of the median nerve due to its compression at the wrist beneath the transverse carpal ligament.

Epidemiology:
- There is a higher incidence in women than men for carpal tunnel syndrome. Age and weight play a part in the epidemiology. As aging occurs the incidence increases, and an increased weight has a higher incidence of carpal tunnel syndrome overall.

Etiology:
- Formed by the transverse carpal ligament superiorly with the carpal bones inferiorly. The median nerve must pass through this anatomic tunnel. When compression occurs, ischemia of the nerve occurs.

Risk Factors:
- Anatomic factors: A wrist fracture or dislocation that alters the space within the carpal tunnel can create extraneous pressure on the median nerve.
- Sex: Carpal tunnel syndrome is generally more common in women. This may be because the carpal tunnel area is relatively smaller than in men, and there may be less room for error.
- Nerve-damaging conditions: Chronic illnesses, such as diabetes, increase risk of nerve damage, including damage to your median nerve.
- Inflammatory conditions: Illnesses such as RA can affect the tendons in the wrist, exerting pressure on the median nerve.
- Alterations in the balance of body fluids: Fluid retention, common during pregnancy or menopause, may increase the pressure within the carpal tunnel, irritating the median nerve.
- Other medical conditions: Certain conditions, such as menopause, obesity, thyroid disorders, and kidney failure, may increase chances of carpal tunnel syndrome.
- Workplace factors: Working with vibrating tools or on an assembly line that requires prolonged or repetitive flexing of the wrist may create harmful pressure on the median nerve or worsen existing nerve damage.

Signs and Symptoms:
- Numbness or pain in your hand, forearm, or wrist that awakens you at night.
- Occasional tingling, numbness, "pins-and-needles" sensation, or pain
- Numbness or pain that gets worse while you are using your hand or wrist
- Stiffness in your fingers when you get up in the morning

Differential Diagnoses:
- Arthritis
- Sprains
- Diabetic neuropathy
- Compartment syndrome

Diagnostic Studies:
- Nerve studies
- X-rays
- MRI

Physical Examination:

Tinel Sign Test
- Tap on the inside of the wrist over the median nerve. Tingling, numbness, pins-and-needles, or a mild "electrical shock" sensation in the hand when tapped on the wrist may be indicative of carpal tunnel syndrome.

Phalen Sign Test
- Hold arms out in front and then flex wrists, let hands hang down for about 60 seconds. Tingling, numbness, or pain in the fingers within 60 seconds may be indicative of carpal tunnel syndrome.

Two-point Discrimination Test
- Used if severe carpal tunnel syndrome is suspected. Not very accurate for mild carpal tunnel syndrome. Close eyes and then use small instruments, such as the tips of two opened paper clips, to touch two points (fairly close together) on the hand or finger. Separate touches should be felt if the two points are at least 0.5 cm apart.

Treatment:
- Physical therapy
- Ice
- Rest
- Elevation
- Splinting of affected wrist
- Surgery

Low Back Pain

Description of Disease: A common musculoskeletal symptom that may be either acute or chronic, caused by a variety of diseases and disorders that affect the lumbar spine. Low back pain is often accompanied by sciatica, which is pain that involves the sciatic nerve and is felt in the lower back, the buttocks, and the backs of the thighs.

Epidemiology:
- Low back pain is often caused by sprains, muscle spasm or weakness, sciatica, soft tissue inflammation, or herniated disks (usually L5–S1).

Etiology:
- Role of physical demands at work as well as history of low back pain provide great incidence of low back pain. Rule out fracture and primary etiology is key. Some primary etiologies are metastatic cancer, spinal stenosis (ankylosing spondylitis), infection, trauma or contusion, and herniated disks.

Risk Factors:
- Overweight
- Age
- Arthritis history
- Physical demands with work

Signs and Symptoms:
- Pain
- Inflammation
- Decreased range of motion
- Persistent ache or stiffness along spine
- Muscle spasms
- Inability to stand straight without pain

Differential Diagnoses:
- Sciatica
- Spinal stenosis
- Bone cancer

Diagnostic Studies:
- MRI is gold standard for diagnosing differences between causality of back pain (i.e., sprain/strain versus disk herniation).

Treatment:
- Treatment depends on primary etiology.
- Physical therapy for muscle strengthening
- NSAIDS for uncomplicated back pain
- Muscle relaxants if muscle spasms occur
- Ice or moist heat for uncomplicated pain

Complications of Low Back Pain:
- **Cauda equina syndrome:** Considered a surgical emergency—is a serious neurologic condition in which damage to the cauda equina causes loss of function of the lumbar plexus, (nerve roots) of the spinal canal below the termination (conus medullaris) of the spinal cord.
  - Severe back pain, saddle anesthesia, incontinence, and sexual dysfunction are considered "red flags."
  - The management of true cauda equina syndrome frequently involves surgical decompression. When cauda equina syndrome is caused by a herniated disk, early surgical decompression is recommended.

Bursitis

Description of Disease: Bursitis (Ruptured Baker Cyst)—inflammation of the synovial membrane lining of the bursal sac. Humans have approximately 160 bursae. These are saclike structures between skin and bone or between tendons, ligaments, and bone. The bursae are lined by synovial tissue, which produces fluid that lubricates and reduces friction between these structures.

Epidemiology:
- The most common locations of bursitis are the subdeltoid, olecranon, ischial, trochanteric, and prepatellar bursae. The incidence of bursitis is higher in athletes, reaching highest levels in runners. Highest percentage of cases of septic superficial bursitis occurs in men. Mortality in patients with bursitis is very low. The prognosis is good, with the vast majority of patients receiving outpatient follow-up and treatment.

Etiology:
- Occurs most commonly in middle and old age, usually following a traumatic event or repetitive use of a joint unaccustomed to frequent usage.
  - It most commonly affects the subacromial, olecranon, trochanteric, prepatellar, and infrapatellar bursae.
  - Bursitis occurs when the synovial lining becomes thickened and produces excessive fluid, leading to localized swelling and pain.

Risk Factors:
- Age
- Overuse injuries
- Arthritis

Signs and Symptoms:
- Localized tenderness
- Pain: Aggravated by movement of the specific joint, tendon, or both
- Edema
- Erythema
- Reduced movement

Differential Diagnoses:
- Cellulitis
- Gout and pseudogout
- RA
- Soft tissue knee injury
- Tendonitis

Diagnostic Studies:
- None indicated in chronic, painless, stable bursitis
- Traumatic bursitis: Red blood cell count
- Joint aspiration: Aspiration and analysis of bursal fluid should be done to rule out infectious or rheumatic causes; they may also be therapeutic. Bursal fluid should be drawn for monosodium urate crystal determination, cell count with differential, Gram stain, and culture.

Treatment:
- Conservative treatment is treatment of choice.
- Rest
- Cold and heat treatments
- Elevation
- Administration of NSAIDs
- Bursal aspiration: Intrabursal steroid injections (with or without local anesthetic agents)

Gout

Description of Disease: Gout is a rheumatic disease resulting from deposition of uric acid crystals (monosodium urate) in tissues and fluids within the body. This process is caused by an overproduction or underexcretion of uric acid.

Epidemiology:
- Gout is the most common form of inflammatory arthritis in men >40 years of age, often presenting initially in the form of podagra (acute onset of pain, erythema, and swelling of the first metatarsophalangeal joint).
- Women may develop gout later in life, and in women it is more likely to involve the upper extremities. The lifetime prevalence of gout in the United States has been estimated at 6.1 million.

Etiology:
Gout and pseudogout are the two most common crystal-induced arthropathies. Gout is caused by monosodium urate monohydrate crystals; pseudogout is caused by calcium pyrophosphate crystals and is more accurately termed calcium pyrophosphate disease.

Risk Factors:
- Overweight or obese
- Hypertension
- Alcohol intake (beer and spirits more than wine)

- Diuretic use
- A diet rich in meat and seafood
- Poor kidney function

Signs and Symptoms:

- Podagra (initial joint manifestation in 50% of gout cases and eventually involved in 90%; also observed in patients with pseudogout and other conditions)
- Arthritis in other sites—the instep, ankle, wrist, finger joints, and knee; in pseudogout, large joints (e.g., the knee, wrist, elbow, or ankle)
- Monoarticular involvement most commonly—many different joints may be involved simultaneously or in rapid succession.
- Attacks that begin abruptly typically reach maximum intensity within 8 to 12 hours; in pseudogout, attacks resembling those of acute gout or a more insidious onset that occurs over several days
- Without treatment, symptom patterns change over time; attacks can become more polyarticular, involve more proximal and upper extremity joints, occur more often, and last longer.
- In some cases, eventual development of chronic polyarticular arthritis that can resemble RA occurs.
- Signs of inflammation: Swelling, warmth, erythema (sometimes resembling cellulitis), and tenderness
- Fever (also consider infectious arthritis)
- Migratory polyarthritis (rare)
- Posterior interosseous nerve syndrome (rare)
- Tophi in soft tissues (helix of the ear, fingers, toes, prepatellar bursa, olecranon)
- Eye involvement: Tophi, crystal-containing conjunctival nodules, band keratopathy, blurred vision, anterior uveitis (rare), scleritis

Differential Diagnoses:

- Arthritis as a manifestation of systemic disease
- Cellulitis
- Nephrolithiasis
- RA
- Septic arthritis

Diagnostic Studies:

- Aspirate synovial fluid for monosodium urate crystals.
- In advanced stages: Radiographs or MRIs may show bone demineralization.
- ESR may be elevated.
- White blood cell count elevated
- Uric acid levels elevated
- Hyperuricemia: Serum urate >7.5mg/dL

Treatment:

- Drugs used to treat acute attacks and prevent future attacks include the following:
  - *NSAIDs:* NSAIDs include over-the-counter options such as ibuprofen (Advil, Motrin IB, and others) and naproxen sodium (Aleve and others), as well as more powerful prescription NSAIDs such as indomethacin (Indocin) or celecoxib (Celebrex). Your doctor may prescribe a higher dose to stop an acute attack, followed by a lower daily dose to prevent future attacks. NSAIDs carry risks of stomach pain, bleeding, and ulcers.
  - *Colchicine:* Your doctor may recommend colchicine (Colcrys, Mitigare), a type of pain reliever that effectively reduces gout pain. The drug's effectiveness is offset in most cases, however, by intolerable side effects, such as nausea, vomiting and diarrhea. After an acute gout attack resolves, your doctor may prescribe a low daily dose of colchicine to prevent future attacks.
  - *Corticosteroids:* Corticosteroid medications, such prednisone, may control gout inflammation and pain. Corticosteroids may be administered in pill form, or they can be injected into your joint. Corticosteroids are generally reserved for those who cannot take either NSAIDs or colchicine. Side effects of corticosteroids include mood changes, increased blood sugar levels, and elevated blood pressure.
  - *Bed rest:* At least 24 hours after acute attack subsides
- Chronic gout management:
  - Support is needed to maintain medical regime.
  - Prophylactic medication
    - Xanthine oxidase inhibitors: Begin 40 mg daily, may increase to 80 mg daily if no effect within 20 weeks.
    - Allopurinol (Lopurin, Zyloprim). It blocks production of uric acid.
    - Febuxostat (Uloric), also acts by blocking uric acid production

○ Probenecid (Benemid) helps the kidneys remove uric acid. Only patients with good kidney function who do not overproduce uric acid should take probenecid.
○ Pegloticase (Krystexxa) is given by injection and breaks down uric acid. This drug is for patients who do not respond to other treatments or cannot tolerate them.
● Educate on food choices and dietary management.
○ Avoid foods high in uric acid (e.g., steak, seafood, beer).

Ankylosing Spondylitis

Description of Disease: Chronic inflammatory condition that mainly affects the joints of the spine and the sacroiliac joint in the pelvis.

Epidemiology:
● It occurs in 1 in 200 people and is most prevalent in Northern European countries.

Etiology:
● Average age of onset is early 20s. More common in males than females

Risk Factors:
● Gender
● Age
● Heredity

Signs and Symptoms:
● Chronic back pain: Worse in the upper back
● Low-grade fever
● Fatigue
● Chest pain with respiration (costochondritis)
● Joint stiffness that improves with activity
● Uveitis: Eye irritation, photosensitivity, eye pain
● Injected sclera and blurred vision

Differential Diagnoses:
● Arthritis
● Sprain/strain

Diagnostic Studies:
● X-ray
● MRI

Treatment:
● Referral to a rheumatologist
● First-line med treatment is NSAIDS.
● Cox-2 inhibitor can be used in those who are at high risk for bleeding.
● In severe cases of ankylosing spondylitis, surgery can be an option in the form of joint replacements.
● Physical therapy can be used to help manage pain (TENS units can be instituted).

Review Section

Review Questions

1. The Lachman maneuver is used to detect which of the following joint concerns?

   a. Knee instability
   b. Nerve damage of the knee due to past knee injuries
   c. The integrity of the patellar tendon
   d. Tears on the meniscus of the knee

2. Which of the following drugs is usually the first line of treatment in the early phases of rheumatoid arthritis?

   a. Ibuprofen
   b. Gold salts
   c. Methotrexate
   d. Cox-2 inhibitors

3. A nurse practitioner is working at the office and is returning calls to patients. Which of the following calls should she return first?

   a. A home health patient reports, "I am starting to have skin breakdown on my heels."
   b. A young male reports, "I think I sprained my ankle 2 weeks ago and it's not getting better."
   c. A 65-year-old patient reports, "My knee is still hurting from my ACL surgery last week."
   d. A patient who was just casted in your office yesterday states, "I can't feel my fingers in my hand that was just casted."

4. John, a 19-year-old male college soccer athlete, limps off the field with pain in his left knee. He tells you that he pivoted abruptly and felt a sharp severe pain in his right knee. He can no longer bear weight on it and the swelling continues to develop. On examination, you find that he has a right knee effusion, medial joint-line tenderness, and is unable to deep knee bend and has a positive McMurray sign. He states he feels a "locking" sensation when he tries to walk. The history and physical findings are suggestive that John may have:

   a. posterior cruciate ligament tear.
   b. anterior cruciate ligament tear.
   c. medial meniscus tear.
   d. medial collateral ligament tear.

5. Which of the following diagnosis has a higher incidence of occurrence in golfers?

   a. Elbow fracture
   b. Tendonitis
   c. Medial epicondylitis
   d. Arthritis

6. Initial pharmacologic treatment for an episode of gouty arthritis would include:

   a. colchicine
   b. aspirin
   c. allopurinal
   d. probenecid

7. The initial treatment for plantar fasciitis is:

   a. cortisone injections now and then every 3 months as needed.
   b. heel pad, NSAID, and exercises.
   c. hot and cold packs, heel pad, and exercise.
   d. heel pad, cortisone injection, and hot and cold packs.

8. Which of the following radiographic joint changes might be expected to be seen in rheumatoid arthritis?

   a. Soft tissue swelling, osteoporosis, and joint narrowing
   b. Erosion and sclerosis of the sacroiliac joints
   c. Narrowing of joint spaces caused by osteophyte formation
   d. Hairline fractures within the bone shaft

9. Which of the following types of arthritis is HLA-B27 positive?

   a. Osteoarthritis
   b. Ankylosing spondylitis
   c. Rheumatoid arthritis
   d. Gouty arthritis

10. Which of the following tests is most sensitive for systemic lupus erythematous (SLE)?

    a. Antinuclear antibody (ANA)
    b. HLA-B27
    c. Erythrocyte sedimentation rate
    d. Antinative DNA

Answers with Rationales

1. (a) Knee instability

   Rationale: The Lachman test is suggestive of ACL damage within the knee. Knee joint instability or laxity of the ligament is indicative of a positive Lachman test.

2. (a) Ibuprofen

   Rationale: NSAIDS are the first line of treatment for rheumatoid arthritis unless otherwise contraindicated. They act as an anti-inflammatory and analgesic to block the inflammatory cascade caused by prostaglandins.

3. (d) A patient who was just casted in your office yesterday states, "I can't feel my fingers in my hand that was just casted."

   Rationale: The patient experiencing neurovascular changes will have the highest priority. Pain after ACL surgery and skin breakdown is a gradual pain that can be addressed later today. The ankle sprain is never an emergent situation.

4. (c) medial meniscus tear.

   Rationale: Meniscal tears and injuries often occur with a twisting or pivoting motion and are often associated with sudden pain, gradual swelling, a "locking" or catching, and a positive McMurray sign.

5. (c) Medial epicondylitis

    Rationale: Medial epicondylitis is caused by excess or overuse of a specific joint such as the elbow. Golfers and baseball players are at highest risk for such injuries.

6. (a) colchicine.

    Rationale: Colchicine is effective in the initial treatment of gouty arthritis.

7. (b) heel pad, NSAID, and exercises.

    Rationale: NSAIDS decrease the inflammation and exercises help minimize re-occurrence of flare-ups.

8. (a) Soft tissue swelling, osteoporosis, and joint narrowing

    Rationale: Soft tissue swelling is a common finding with rheumatoid arthritis. Narrowing of joint spaces and osteophyte formation is common in osteoarthritis.

9. (b) Ankylosing spondylitis

    Rationale: HLA-B27 is positive in 90% of patients with ankylosing spondylitis. The remaining arthritis conditions are HLA-B27 negative.

10. (a) Antinuclear antibody (ANA)

    Rationale: These are the most sensitive test for SLE. Ninety-five percent of cases will also have a positive serum ANA.

Suggested Readings

Agency for Healthcare Research & Quality. (2010–2011). *The guide to clinical preventive services: Recommendations of the U.S. Preventive Services Task Force*. Rockville, MD: AHRQ. AHRQ Publication No 10-05145.

Anderson, B. B. (2006). *Office orthopedics for primary care* (3rd ed.). Philadelphia, PA: Saunders.

Cash, J. C., & Glass, C. A. (2012). *Family Practice Guidelines*. Philadelphia, PA: Lippincott.

Collins-Bride, G. M., & Saxe, J. M. (2013). *Clinical guidelines for advanced practice nursing: An interdisciplinary approach*. Burlington, MA: Jones & Barlett Learning.

Dunphy, L. M., Winland-Brown, J. E., Porter, B. O., & Thomas, D. J. (2015). *Primary care: The art and science of advanced practice nursing* (4th ed.). Philadelphia, PA: FA Davis.

Jameson, J. L., & Loscalzo, J. (Eds.). (2012). *Harrison's principles of internal medicine* (18th ed.). New York, NY: McGraw Hill. Retrieved from http://accessmedicine.com/resourceTOC.aspx?resourceID=4

Kane, R., Ouslander, J., Abrass, I., & Resnick, B. (2013). *Essentials of Clinical Geriatrics* (7th ed.). New York, NY: McGraw-Hill Education.

Longo, D. Fauci, A. S., Kasper, D. L., Hauser, S. L., McPhee, S., & Papadakis, M. (Eds.). (2014). *Current medical diagnosis and treatment* (53rd ed.). New York, NY: McGraw-Hill.

Chapter 9

Common Neuropsychiatric Disorders

William J. Lorman

Case Presentation

Directions: Carefully review the case study presented below. At the end of the chapter, answer the review questions. Compare your answers to the correct answers listed in the Review Section.

Arlene Forest is a 69-year-old woman who has been your patient for many years. You have been treating her for chronic back and joint pain, which has been managed fairly well with NSAIDs and Neurontin. She has been prone, over the last 10 years, to severe upper respiratory infections, which she would acquire two or three times a year. Antibiotics had always been the main course of treatment, but occasionally she would require steroids for severe bronchial inflammation and irritation. However, the steroid use had to be strictly monitored because they tended to induce manic behaviors.

Arlene came from a well-to-do family and wanted for nothing. However, her family were always busy with family businesses and rarely gave Arlene any attention. She was raised by a domestic servant, Mary, whom she loved dearly. When Arlene was 17 years old, Mary died. Arlene never really resolved the grief she experienced from the loss of Mary and her family, who never had a connection with any of the domestic staff, told Arlene that she was overreacting and needed to "grow up." Arlene eventually met a group of people whom she felt comfortable with and she, with her friends, began using drugs and alcohol. Within a year, Arlene was addicted to methamphetamine and took benzodiazepines to control the mania that the methamphetamine produced. She also found that using alcohol regularly, in increasing amounts, helped her feel more stable and she soon forgot her grief and her family. It was not until her father died 15 years later from Alzheimer disease that she decided to seek treatment for her addiction. Once stably sober, she found support from others in recovery and also from her three brothers with whom she ultimately developed a close relationship. She eventually finished graduate school with a degree in counseling and decided she wanted to work with addicted populations as her way of "giving back." She enjoyed her work very much and soon thereafter married. Her husband loved her dearly and they were very happy together. They had similar likes and dislikes, travelled extensively whenever they could, and finally Arlene believed she found her ultimate happiness. Arlene also loved working in the field of addictions and over time had been promoted and was ultimately a program director. Her brothers, who were all more than 20 years older than she, each became sickly—her oldest brother developed Parkinson disease, and the other two began having cognitive decline and were later diagnosed with Alzheimer disease. All three brothers died within the next 10 years and Arlene then realized that she may suffer a similar fate as her brothers. This remained on her mind, becoming an obsession.

Arlene's direct reports found her to be very sociable but becoming more and more eccentric in her behaviors. Her respiratory infections increased in frequency and severity and with each regimen of steroids, her mania increased in severity and duration making it very difficult for her to perform her duties at work. Over the last

2 years, her obsession with developing Alzheimer disease was beginning to also interfere with her work. As noted in your progress notes, you began to see subtle cognitive changes. You began to assess her with each visit using the Folstein mini mental status examination (MMSE) tool. Although her husband reported some problems with memory, the results of your assessment showed no major change in her MMSE scores until about a year ago. At that time, Arlene's assessment scores were progressively falling. When you discussed this with her, she was most concerned. Over the next few months, Arlene became more anxious and eventually depressed. You started her on Paxil 20 mg daily, which she tolerated well and seemed to show slow-but-steady improvement. However, her recent memory was worsening and she began arguing with her direct reports. Her staff asked for a meeting with the Human Resources Department because they were more and more concerned that Arlene was often unprofessional with staff and patients. After many meetings that also involved Arlene's husband and you, it was decided that the best alternative was for Arlene to take a leave of absence. For the past 6 months you have been seeing Arlene either weekly or biweekly to assess her current functioning and manage her growing physical complaints. Her husband called you and stated that Arlene has become frequently agitated and even aggressive—often striking him on the upper torso, a behavior she has never in the past engaged in. Although over a year ago you referred her to a neurologist for evaluation which showed no neurologic deficits, you again referred her back to the neurologist. Within a very short time, Arlene began to significantly decompensate. At one point, she was hospitalized because new symptoms were evolving. She had, over a period of 2 weeks, became incoherent, ataxic, and very disoriented. She was diagnosed with a urinary tract infection. After treatment, she began to stabilize, but her cognitive and other physical functions continued to exacerbate.

Her neurologist was stumped as to what was causing the variable symptoms. Eventually, after a conference with the medical team in which you provided an extensive and thorough history of her progression, more studies were conducted. Arlene was finally diagnosed with Alzheimer disease, Parkinson disease, and amyotrophic lateral sclerosis (Lou Gehrig disease). Within a very short time, Arlene became bed-ridden, unable to swallow, was in constant pain and seemed to have lost all her cognitive functions and memories. Two weeks later, her loving soul mate of 35 years called to tell you she died peacefully.

This case study will be discussed further at the end of the chapter.

Delirium

Description of the Disease

The essential feature of delirium is a disturbance of fluctuating attention or awareness that is accompanied by a change in baseline cognition. Symptoms develop over a short period of time, usually hours, but can progress over a few days. The symptoms tend to fluctuate during the course of the day, and usually worsen in the evening and night when external orienting stimuli decrease. The symptom presentation is not the result of a preexisting or evolving neurocognitive disorder (NCD).

Epidemiology

In the general population, the prevalence of delirium overall is low (1% to 2%) and increases with age, rising to 14% among individuals older than 85 years. The prevalence of delirium is highest among hospitalized older individuals. In those presenting to emergency departments, the prevalence is 10% to 30%; in the postoperative older population, the rate is from 15% to 53%; and in critical care areas, the rate is 70% to 87%. Delirium occurs in up to 60% of patients in nursing homes or postacute settings and in up to 83% of all individuals at the end of life.

Delirium is frequently underrecognized by health-care professionals. One of the problems is the variety of other diagnoses that are given, which confuse proper identification and treatment. Some of the misnomers include ICU psychosis, acute confusional state, encephalopathy, sundowning, cerebral insufficiency, and organic brain syndrome.

Etiology

Delirium is often unrecognized by health-care professionals and has many causes, all of which result in a similar pattern of signs and symptoms relating to the patient's level of consciousness and level of cognitive impairment. The major causes of delirium are either intoxication or withdrawal from pharmacologic or toxic agents but can also include other central nervous system or systemic disease. When evaluating the patient with a delirium presentation, the nurse should assume that any drug that the patient has taken may be etiologically relevant.

Some of the more common causes of delirium are as follows:
- Medications such as opioid pain medications, antibiotics, steroids, anesthesia, antihypertensives, anticholinergic agents, excessive dopamine-blocking agents (neuroleptic malignant syndrome), and excessive serotonin-increasing agents (serotonin syndrome)
- Central nervous system disorders such as seizure, migraine, head trauma, brain tumor, subdural hematoma, stroke, and transient ischemia
- Metabolic changes such as electrolyte abnormalities, hypo- and hyperglycemia
- Systemic disease such as infections, changes in fluid status, nutritional deficiencies, burns, heat stroke
- Over-the-counter preparations and botanicals
- Drugs of abuse
- Environmental toxins such as heavy metals and pesticides

Risk Factors

The older the patient and the longer the patient has been delirious, the longer the delirium takes to resolve. Risks for delirium increase in the presence of other functional impairments such as dementia, immobility, a history of falls, low levels of activity, and the use of drugs and medications with psychoactive properties, particularly alcohol and anticholinergics.

Signs and Symptoms

The core features of delirium include alterations in consciousness and attention (usually with a diminished ability to focus), disorientation (especially to time and place), and varying levels of amnesia. Onset is relatively rapid (usually hours). Associated features are often present and can include disorganization of thought processes such as incoherence, perceptual disturbances such as hallucinations, mood changes, and psychomotor hyperactivity or slowness. In older populations, psychomotor slowness is more common.

Differential Diagnoses

The most common differential diagnostic issue when evaluating confusion in older adults is teasing away symptoms of dementia from delirium. The nurse must determine whether the patient has delirium, delirium along with a preexisting dementia, or a type of dementia without delirium. Generally, we use the acuteness of onset as the main indicator; however, this method is difficult in the presence of a prior NCD that had not been previously recognized or those patients who develop a persistent cognitive impairment following an episode of delirium.

Other disorders in the differential include the following:
- Psychotic syndromes including mood disorders with psychotic features: Delirium that is characterized by hallucinations, delusions, language disturbances, and agitation must be distinguished from the presence of a psychotic disorder such as brief psychotic disorder, schizophreniform disorder, or schizophrenia as well as bipolar or depressive disorders with psychotic features. However, new-onset symptoms of psychosis in older patients with no history of psychiatric illness are extremely rare and a medical etiology should be primarily considered.
- Acute stress disorder: If the symptom presentation consists of fear, anxiety, and dissociative symptoms, consider acute stress disorder if there was a previous exposure to a severely traumatic event.
- Malingering or factitious disorder: Consider one of these disorders if there is an atypical presentation and in the absence of another medical condition or indication of the presence or use of a substance that is etiologically related to the cognitive disturbance.

Diagnostic Studies

The laboratory workup should include standard tests which would demonstrate findings characteristic of underlying medical conditions (or intoxication or withdrawal states); electroencephalography (EEG) shows a generalized slowing of activity. However, EEG is insufficiently sensitive and specific for diagnostic use.

Treatment

The primary goal in the treatment of delirium is to treat the underlying cause which should be pursued aggressively. For instance, if the underlying cause is cholinergic blockade causing toxicity, the use of a cholinergic agonist such as physostigmine, 1 to 2 mg intravenously or intramuscularly, with repeated doses in 15 to 30 minutes is usually indicated.

In patients with Parkinson disease, the antiparkinsonian agents used commonly cause delirium. Decreasing the dosage of the antiparkinsonian drugs is obviously the treatment of choice, but this must be weighed against the worsening of motor symptoms. If decreasing these medications is not an option, then the use of a dopamine antagonist (such as a second-generation antipsychotic medication such as risperidone, clozapine, quetiapine, and aripiprazole) may be considered. However, there are few clinical trials for use of these agents.

In addition to the use of pharmacologic agents, other environmental considerations include the provision of physical and sensory support. There should be a balance between sensory deprivation and overstimulation. Having familiar photographs, a calendar, a clock, and the presence of a friend, relative, or companion surrounding the patient can sometimes make the patient more comfortable.

Major Neurocognitive Disorder (Previously Called Dementia)

Description of the Disease

The essential features of major NCD are, first, a concern—either by the individual himself or herself, a knowledgeable informant or the clinician—that there has been a significant decline in cognitive function (including complex attention, executive function, learning and memory, language, perceptual–motor or social cognition) and, second, a substantial impairment in cognitive performance. Additionally, the cognitive deficits interfere with independence in everyday activities.

Epidemiology

The prevalence of NCD varies widely by age and by etiology (discussed later). Among individuals older than 60 years, prevalence increases steeply with age. Overall prevalence estimates are approximately 1% to 2% at age 65 years and as high as 30% by age 85 years.

Individuals and families' level of awareness regarding neurocognitive symptoms generally vary across ethnic and occupational groups and are more likely to be noticed in individuals who engage in complex occupational, domestic, or recreational activities.

Like age, culture, and occupation, gender may affect the level of concern and awareness of symptoms. Females are likely to be older, to have more medical comorbidity, and to live alone, which complicates evaluation and treatment.

Etiology

There are many etiologic subtypes of NCD which are distinguished on the basis of a combination of time course, characteristic domains affected, and associated symptoms. For instance, some subtypes depend on the presence of a potentially causative entity such as Parkinson or Huntington disease, traumatic brain injury, or vascular disease such as stroke. For other subtypes, the diagnosis is based primarily on the cognitive, behavioral, and functional symptoms found generally in the neurodegenerative diseases like Alzheimer disease, frontotemporal lobar degeneration, and Lewy body disease. Other subtypes include substance/medication induced, HIV infection, or due to another medical condition.

Risk Factors

Risk factors vary not only by etiology but also by age at onset within the specific etiologic subtypes. Although many subtypes occur exclusively or primarily in late life, some can occur throughout the life span. The strongest risk factor is age, since it is age that increases the risk of neurodegenerative and cerebrovascular disease. Female gender is also a major risk factor, but this has been attributed largely to greater longevity in females.

Signs and Symptoms

The core presentation includes both a concern about cognitive decline and performance that falls below the expected level or that has been observed to decline over time. The nurse must utilize specific questioning about specific symptoms that commonly occur in patients with cognitive deficits, for example, difficulty remembering to sort a grocery list or difficulty resuming a task when interrupted, or even planning a meal. The difficulties experienced must represent changes rather than lifelong patterns. In other words, do not be concerned when told, "my mother hasn't been able to remember her children's or grandchildren's birthdays in decades."

Differential Diagnoses

- Delirium: It may be difficult to distinguish NCD from a persistent delirium which can also co-occur with NCD. Careful assessment of attention and arousal will help to make the distinction.
- Major depressive disorder: With NCD, there are consistent memory and executive function deficits as opposed to the more nonspecific and variable performance presentations seen in major depressive disorder. However, it is possible that the only way to differentiate these two disorders is improvement through treatment with antidepressants. Sometimes, the symptom of apathy present is part of the NCD syndrome and is often confused as symptomatic of the onset of major depression. In these cases, a psychostimulant is added to the NCD treatment regimen.
- Malingering: Patients who attempt to feign memory loss do so in an erratic and inconsistent manner. In NCD, memory for time and place is lost before memory for person and recent memory is lost before remote memory.

Diagnostic Studies

Diagnosis is based on the clinical examination including a mental status examination and from collateral information from family, friends, employers, and others. Complaints of personality changes in a patient older than age 40 may suggest NCD, and this should be considered. Other neurocognitive testing is available but must not be used exclusively. Interviews with the family members are most important to determine a benchmark for further decline or response to treatment.

Treatment

The two classifications of medication used in the treatment of NCD are the cholinesterase inhibitors and the glutamate antagonists. The cholinesterase inhibitors are indicated for use in mild to moderate NCD. Currently, these medications are donepezil (Aricept), rivastigmine (Exelon), and galantamine (Reminyl, Razadyne). They have proven efficacy on cognitive function. However, there has been no cognitive benefit in the presence of vascular dementia. These medications have also been shown to ameliorate behavioral disturbances such as anxiety, disinhibition, and aberrant motor behavior as well as enhance cognition. Benefits are lost after drug withdrawal and therapeutic response following resumption of therapy has been shown to be less than that obtained with initial therapy. Therefore, it is most important not to stop these medications. In response failure to one agent, it is recommended that another agent be used. Approximately 50% of patients experiencing loss of efficacy with one drug respond to subsequent treatment with another agent. One of the more common side effects of the cholinesterase inhibitors is lucid dreaming and depersonalization (out-of-body experiences). Other common side effects—occurring more often in patients over 85 years of age and in females—include gastrointestinal symptoms such as cramping, nausea, vomiting, and diarrhea. These symptoms are dose dependent and occur more often during dose escalation and tend to resolve with time. Obviously, the use of any anticholinergic agents, including over-the-counter drugs, will reduce the effects of these drugs and should be avoided.

The glutamate antagonists (currently only memantine (Namenda) is available) are indicated for use in severe dementia. This medication has been found to be beneficial in improving cognitive functioning in vascular dementia. Memantine has been found to have additive effects with cholinesterase inhibitors and many prescribers initiate treatment using both classes of medication. The most common side effects of memantine include confusion, agitation, insomnia, paranoia, mild to moderate dizziness, and headaches. If memantine is prescribed, the patient's use of antacids should be minimized, since alkalinization of urine will reduce elimination and increase the effects of the drug.

Recent memory is lost before remote memory in NCD, and patients are generally distressed by remembering how they used to function and now experiencing their present level of functioning and deterioration. Patients will often benefit from a supportive and educational psychotherapy in which the nature and course of their illness are clearly explained. Other support includes assistance in grieving and accepting the extent of their disability. Assisting with cognitive functioning is also recommended such as keeping calendars, making schedules to help structure activities, and note-taking for memory problems. The patient's caretakers are also in need of support and possibly psychotherapy. Those who take care of patients with dementia struggle with feelings of guilt, grief, anger, and exhaustion as they watch the patient deteriorate.

Major Depressive Disorder

Description of the Disease

Depression is characterized by a feeling of loss of control of one's mood along with a subjective experience of great distress. The patient may experience a loss of energy and interest, feelings of guilt, difficulty concentrating, sleep and appetite problems, and possibly, thoughts of death or suicide. These symptoms ultimately result in impairments in interpersonal, social, and occupational functioning.

Epidemiology

Depressive symptoms are present in about 15% of all older adults. Females have a twofold greater prevalence of depression than males. The reasons hypothesized for this involves differing psychosocial stressors for women and behavioral models of learned helplessness. Another correlative is the person without close interpersonal relationships. The presence of close relationships seems to be a protective factor.

Etiology

The etiology of depression is complex and involves biologic, genetic, and psychosocial factors. Biologic factors include disturbances in specific neurotransmitters and receptors in the brain such as serotonin, norepinephrine, and dopamine. Additionally, other neurotransmitter–receptor systems have also been implicated such as acetylcholine, GABA, and glutamate. Alterations of hormonal regulation seem to also play a part in depressive symptoms.

There have been numerous family, adoption, and twin studies that have demonstrated the heritability of mood disorders like depression. However, it has been shown that gene mutations only make the individual susceptible to depression and are not the clear cause for depression's presentation.

Psychosocial factors have long been identified in causing depressive presentations. Factors include life events, environmental stress, and personality factors. Stressors in which the patient experiences subsequent low self-esteem are more likely than not to produce depression.

Risk Factors

Age itself is not a risk factor, but being widowed and having a chronic medical illness have been associated with the development of depressive symptoms. A higher risk of suicide has been found in the elderly as compared to the general population.

Signs and Symptoms

The most common symptoms of depressive disorders include reduced energy and problems with focus and concentration, sleep problems—usually early morning awakening and multiple nocturnal awakenings, decreased appetite, weight loss, and somatic complaints. Generally, in older populations, the presentation is one of physical symptoms rather than psychological symptoms. Geriatric depression scales are available to measure the presence of depressive disorder.

Differential Diagnoses

- Neurocognitive Disorder: The cognitive impairment of depressed geriatric patients is often confused with NCD or dementia. In fact, in geriatric patients whose main symptom is cognitive impairment, the name *pseudodementia* is applied. It is important to be able to differentiate dementia from pseudodementia. In dementia, intellectual performance is generally global in nature and levels of impairment are consistently poor. In pseudodementia, deficits are variable. In dementia, patients tend to confabulate: make up an answer to a question they do not know; in pseudodementia, the patient will usually respond, "I don't know."
- Depression due to another medical condition: If the symptoms of depression are, based on physical examination and laboratory findings, found to be the direct pathophysiologic consequence of a specific medical condition (such as multiple sclerosis, stroke, or hypothyroidism), then treating the underlying disease process should alleviate the depressive symptoms.
- Substance-/medication-induced depressive disorder: Here, a drug of abuse, a medication, or a toxin appears to be etiologically related to the depressive symptoms. Once the body has cleared the substance, the depressive symptoms should also disappear.
- Sadness: Periods of sadness are a part of human experience. Do not be tempted to provide medication but rather understand the basis for the sadness and determine whether it is transitory or permanent, impairing or nonimpairing, distressing or not distressing. Also, before a depressive disorder can be properly diagnosed, the patient must meet *DSM-5* (*Diagnostic and Statistical Manual of Mental Disorders*, fifth edition) criteria.

Diagnostic Studies

There are no laboratory studies that are conclusive for a major depressive episode (MDE). Instead, the nurse must rely on a complete history and physical examination along with a mental status examination.

Treatment

Treatment for the patient with depression should first guarantee the patient's safety and then a plan that addresses the patient's symptoms but also any stressful life events which are associated with relapses of symptoms. A combination of psychopharmacologic and psychotherapeutic interventions have been found to be more effective than either modality separately. The medications that have demonstrated improved efficacy and safety are the SSRIs (selective rerotonin reuptake inhibitors). The medications in this class include citalopram (Celexa), fluoxetine (Prozac), paroxetine (Paxil), escitalopram (Lexapro), sertraline (Zoloft), and vorteoxetine (Brintellex). This class of medications generally has a low risk of central nervous system, anticholinergic and cardiovascular effects. Improvement in cognitive functioning has been noted with use of SSRIs. The most common clinical mistake leading to an unsuccessful trial of a specific antidepressant is the use of too low a dosage for too short a period. Although it is important to "start low and go slow," dosages should be increased, albeit slowly, to attain therapeutic effect. Elderly patients may take longer to respond and may need trials of at least 12 weeks before treatment response is noted. Although citalopram and escitalopram have demonstrated efficacy, recent studies have shown there is a risk of QT prolongation with increased dosages, and therefore, citalopram dose should not exceed 20 mg/day and escitalopram dose should not exceed 10 mg/day. Also, hyponatremia has been reported with all SSRIs. Therefore, monitor serum electrolytes. The most common side effects from SSRI use are gastrointestinal such as nausea, vomiting, and diarrhea. Also, diaphoresis and headache are common. Side effects from the SSRIs are transient, and the patient should be told to treat any transient symptom as necessary. For example, for a headache, use whatever over-the-counter (OTC) medication the patient normally would take (acetaminophen, ibuprofen, etc.).

Use of SSRIs with other serotonergic agents may result in serotonin syndrome, a hypermetabolic state usually occurring within 24 hours of medication initiation, overdose, or change in dose. Symptoms include nausea, diarrhea, chills, sweating, dizziness, hyperpyrosis, hypertension, tremor, myoclonic jerks, hyperreflexia, agitation, disorientation, confusion, and ultimately, rhabdomyolysis, coma, and death. Treatment for serotonin syndrome includes stopping all serotonergic medications and administering cyproheptadine (Periactin) 4 to 16 mg. Residual symptoms such as muscle aches may last for up to 8 weeks.

Bereavement

Description of the Disease

Bereavement is a term that applies to the psychological reactions of those who survive a significant loss. Synonyms include grief and mourning. However, mourning is technically the process of resolving grief.

Epidemiology

The elderly face more losses than individuals at other phases across the life span. Only when bereavement does not remit or if it worsens does psychopathology occur and prevalence statistics for depression are used.

Etiology

The process of bereavement follows a predictable course with its own signs, symptoms, and expected resolution. The process begins when a significant loss occurs in the person's life. Additionally, so called anniversary reactions occur when the trigger is a special occasion such as a holiday or birthday. It is not unusual for these reactions to occur each year on the same day the person died.

Risk Factors

Comorbid medical or psychiatric illnesses increase the risk for progression to complicated/extended grief reactions which may lead to a depressive episode.

Signs and Symptoms

Response to a significant loss may include the feelings of intense sadness, rumination about the loss, insomnia, poor appetite, and weight loss, which may resemble a depressive episode. Although such symptoms may be understandable or considered appropriate to the loss, the presence of a MDR in addition to the normal response to a significant loss should also be carefully considered.

Elisabeth Kubler-Ross, a renowned psychiatrist who specialized in death and dying, identified five stages of the bereavement process:
- Denial (this isn't happening to me!)
- Anger (why is this happening to me?)
- Bargaining (I promise I'll be a better person if . . .)
- Depression (I don't care anymore)
- Acceptance (I'm ready to go on with life)

Not everyone experiences all five stages, nor necessarily in the same order. Following the death of a loved one, anger and denial may not always be apparent, but this is not an indication that it is not there and that it has no impact on the health and quality of life of the patient.

The elderly often experience grief much differently from others. An older adult may think more about dying than living and has been doing so for many years. Increasing frailty, illness, loss of independence, and the resulting reliance on others can often intensify the loneliness and fear at losing a loved one.

Differential Diagnoses

Major Depressive Episode: In distinguishing bereavement from MDE, bereavement's predominant affect is feelings of emptiness and loss; in MDE, there is a persistent depressed mood and inability to feel motivation or happiness. The dysphoria from bereavement tends to be associated with thoughts and reminders of the deceased while the depressed mood of MDE is more persistent and not tied to any specific thoughts or preoccupations.

Diagnostic Studies

Complete history delineating the loss and subsequent symptom presentation.

Treatment

Although various classes of medication have been used to minimize the symptom presentation such as benzodiazepines and SSRIs, before any medication is prescribed, there must be evidence of progressive distress or impairment in functionality. Ideally, the patient will be referred to a support group or psychotherapy (grief counseling).

Generalized Anxiety Disorder

Description of the Disease

Although anxiety is a common normal response, if it becomes distressing or impairing because of its excessive nature, then it becomes problematic. The essential feature of generalized anxiety disorder (GAD) is excessive anxiety or worrying about a multitude of actions, events, or activities. Evaluation of duration, intensity, and frequency of anxiety will be found to be out of proportion to normal worrying. Additionally, the patient finds it difficult to control the worrying and its pervasiveness becomes quite impairing so that the patient can do little else but be preoccupied with worrying.

Epidemiology

An anxiety disorder usually begins in early or middle adulthood but can appear for the first time after age 60. The 1-month prevalence of anxiety disorders in persons aged 65 and older is 5.5%. Females are twice as likely as males to experience GAD.

Etiology

The cause is not known and many patients will report that they have felt anxious and nervous all their lives and symptoms tend to exacerbate and remit across the life span, but rates of full remission are very low. Biologic and psychological factors have been identified and probably work together. Research has focused on deficits with the GABA and serotonin neurotransmitter and receptor systems. Another area of study is a finding that adrenergic receptors are hypersensitive and even normal stimulation will produce excessive nervousness and anxiety. From a psychological point of view, it appears that patients incorrectly and inaccurately respond to perceived dangers and selective attention to negative details create distortions in the processing of information. The psychoanalytic school of thought is that the patient's anxiety is a response to the unresolved, unconscious conflicts of childhood.

Risk Factors

Personality style has been identified as a risk factor. Traits of inhibition, neuroticism, and excessive avoidance have been noted. Genetics has also been identified and about one-third of the risk of developing GAD is genetic. Environmental factors, although widely studied, have not been found to correlate with the development and maintenance of GAD.

Signs and Symptoms

The essential clinical features of GAD are excessive anxiety and worry of sustained duration and accompanied by a number of physiologic symptoms such as restlessness, difficulty concentrating, irritability, muscle tension, and sleep disturbances. Additionally, the anxiety interferes with the patient's activities of daily living. The symptoms must be present, on more days than not, for at least 6 months.

Differential Diagnoses

- Anxiety disorder due to another medical condition: History, laboratory studies, and physical examination will help identify the source of the anxiety. A common example is hyperthyroidism. Once the hyperthyroidism is properly treated, the anxiety should resolve.

- Substance-/medication-induced anxiety disorder: History of substance use, which includes illicit substances, alcohol, medications, and environmental toxins, can be demonstrated. Removing the offending substance will resolve the anxiety.
- Social anxiety disorder: This is differentiated from GAD in that the anxiety is the result of and is focused on an upcoming situation in which the patient must perform or be evaluated by others (perceived or real) as opposed to a generalized feeling of anxiety.

Diagnostic Studies

Anxiety itself is a symptom found in many psychiatric and other medical disorders, and the cause must be carefully determined. Laboratory studies are used to rule out GAD, not prove it. Diagnosis relies solely on history and presentation.

Treatment

The most effective treatment of GAD involves a combination of psychopharmacologic, psychotherapeutic, and supportive approaches. Psychotherapy is focused on identifying cognitive distortions. Biofeedback and relaxation are also utilized. Many classes of medications are used (on-label and off-label) in the treatment of anxiety disorders. The four main classes are SSRIs, serotonin–norepinephrine reuptake inhibitors (SNRIs), buspirone (BuSpar), and the benzodiazepines. Other medications used include tricyclic antidepressants (TCAs), antihistamines, and β-adrenergic blocking agents.

The SSRIs are the first-line choice for the treatment of anxiety. The downside of the SSRIs in the treatment of anxiety is the initial, transitory anxiety that these medications cause in a significant percentage of patients. Inform the patient that in some patients, they initially experience an increase in anxiety, but the level of anxiety will begin to decrease after about a week. Also, in order to minimize the level of increased anxiety, start with a subtherapeutic dose (usually one-half of the starting therapeutic dose) and titrate up over a week or two. Another disadvantage is the time necessary for the SSRI to be effective—usually 4 to 6 weeks. Many prescribers will also prescribe a benzodiazepine (most commonly, clonazepam (Klonopin)) until the SSRI becomes effective. It is important to be sure to stop the benzodiazepine after 3 or 4 weeks. If refills are permitted, the patient will identify the benzodiazepine as the more efficacious drug and will often stop the SSRI and request on the benzodiazepine. The SNRIs are also very effective medications. They include venlafaxine (Effexor XR), duloxetine (Cymbalta), and desvenlafaxine (Pristiq). Again, it is important to "start low and go slow" for optimal effectiveness. Buspirone, a partial agonist at the 5-HT1A receptor, is indicated for the treatment of GAD. This medication is effective in 40% to 60% of patients with GAD. The main disadvantages are the long length of time to reach remission of symptoms and the high doses required to be effective. Apparently, the dosing initially identified in the literature is too low and most practitioners are hesitant to prescribe higher doses.

The benzodiazepines should be a medication of last resort. Generally, we are not very concerned with the patient abusing the medication (although substance use disorders [SUDs] are identified more readily in this population), but because of the active and passive diversion that occurs. The elderly have been found to freely share their medication with those they believe need it more, and younger adults (usually grandchildren or children) may avail themselves of the medication. If this class of medication is prescribed, the practitioner should educate the patient on the need to keep the prescription safe and secure and also the problems with sharing their medications.

The TCAs, themselves being SNRIs but with serious side effects, have been found to be effective in treating anxiety. Caution is required because of their cardiac side effects.

The β-blockers have also been used to effectively treat anxiety. As mentioned above, there is research demonstrating the hypersensitivity of adrenergic receptors, and by blocking these receptors (by using β-adrenergic antagonists), the anxiety is abated. The most common medication in this class used to treat anxiety is propranolol (Inderal). Propranolol is preferred over the other β-blockers because it is the most lipid soluble and therefore works more effectively centrally. The peripheral effects of hypotension are minimal when given in a dose of 10 mg twice a day.

Antihistamines are often found to be used by this population because of their easy over-the-counter availability and their main side effect of sedation. The most common medication used for this purpose is diphenhydramine (Benadryl). Antihistamines do not directly relieve anxiety, but the sedation they cause make the patient forget about the worrying. Because of their side effects, this class of medication should be avoided.

Alcohol and Other Substance Use Disorders

Description of the Disease

The essential feature of an SUD is a cluster of cognitive, behavioral, and physiologic symptoms. Symptom presentations will vary depending on the particular substance or substances used, whether the patient is intoxicated or in withdrawal, or engaged in the behavioral manifestations of craving—the need to find and use a particular substance. Although many textbooks will point to the amount, frequency, and duration of use, the diagnosis of an SUD has nothing to do with these parameters. Instead, diagnosis is based on the pathologic pattern of behaviors related to the use/misuse of the substance or substances.

Epidemiology

It is not clear whether abuse of alcohol and other drugs in older people represents a pattern of continued use, a return to use after a period of abstinence, new onset of use, or a combination of all these patterns. Older adults with alcohol use disorder will usually give a history of excessive drinking that began earlier in life. They usually have comorbid conditions such as liver disease and are single either through divorce, widowhood, or never married. Of nursing home patients, about 20% can be diagnosed with alcohol use disorder. About 10% of all behavioral and emotional problems in the elderly are the result of an SUD.

Etiology

Older people use and misuse a variety of substances. For instance, a vast majority of the elderly take prescribed medications (sometimes not as prescribed) for physical and psychiatric ailments; they buy over-the-counter medications (which they may not always take according to instructions); they drink alcohol, smoke cigarettes, and use illicit drugs such as marijuana, and there are a growing number of elderly using heroin and cocaine. Another problematic use of prescribed medications involves "borrowing" a medication from a friend or relative instead of seeking medical advice. The primary problem here is that all medications and drugs of abuse may also produce toxicity, cause withdrawal symptoms, cause physical and/or psychological harm after short- or long-term use, and they may (and generally do) interact with each other. In the end, there are further adverse effects which usually cause the person to take even more medication to neutralize these nasty side effects. The misuse of prescribed or over-the-counter drugs may involve deliberately using higher than recommended doses, using for extended periods, hoarding medications, and using medications together with alcohol.

Risk Factors

Aging itself is often associated with an increased risk of painful medical conditions. Various substances (including alcohol) are used to cope with pain. Older adults with substance use problems and who use alcohol or drugs to manage pain have poorer health outcomes.

Alcohol withdrawal in hospitalized patients is a common cause of delirium (discussed earlier), and older patients presenting with chronic gastrointestinal problems may also be misusing alcohol.

SUDs run in families, and the risk is three to four times higher in close relatives with an SUD. A strong correlate for development of an SUD is the higher number of affected relatives, the greater the risk for the patient developing an SUD.

Other risk factors include the following:
- Cultural attitudes toward drinking and intoxication
- The availability of alcohol or other drugs (including price)
- Acquired personal experiences with substances
- Stress levels
- Heavier peer substance use
- Exaggerated positive expectations of the effects of alcohol and other drugs
- Suboptimal ways of coping with stress

Signs and Symptoms

The clinical presentation of older adults with an SUD is variable and is often confused with other diagnoses since the older adult may present with poor personal hygiene, depression, malnutrition, confusion, and sequelae from environmental exposure and falls.

Unexplained gastrointestinal, metabolic, and even psychosocial problems may indicate a concurrent SUD.

Differential Diagnoses

- Personality disorder: Inappropriate behaviors associated with personality disorders are generally pervasive, inflexible in nature, and stable in their presentation, whereas behaviors related to substance use are variable, episodic, and related generally to intoxication or withdrawal from the substance.
- Delirium or neurocognitive disorder: Discussed earlier
- Nonpathological use of alcohol or other substances: The key element in diagnosing an SUD is the repeated significant distress or impaired functioning. While most alcohol or other drug users may use enough to feel intoxicated, only a minority ever develop an SUD. Therefore, using alcohol or other drugs, even on a daily basis, in low doses and occasional intoxication do not by themselves demonstrate the pathology of an SUD.

Diagnostic Studies

Drug screening, most commonly urine or blood. However, hair and nail clippings can also be used to determine past use of substances.

Other laboratory tests measure changes in target-organ function, and often the treatment of the medical problem becomes primary without consideration of the possible substance use as the cause.

Treatment

SUDs among older people are often missed or misdiagnosed, and many such problems may be confused with other difficulties of aging and are thus ignored.

In the presence of acute intoxication, the patient should be admitted to an inpatient facility for withdrawal management services (previously called detoxification). Following a short period (usually 3 to 6 days), the patient should enter an inpatient rehabilitation program for both cognitive and experiential learning related to the recovery process and relapse prevention. Once stabilized, the patient should attend and outpatient program along with support groups and meetings to help maintain sobriety.

As far as medication-assisted treatment is concerned, there are many medications available for the patient. Currently, pharmacologic treatments for opiate and alcohol use disorders are available. For alcohol use disorder, the patient might be prescribed naltrexone, a dopamine antagonist, 25 to 50 mg/day. However, there are multiple side effects along with a black box warning for liver damage—and many alcoholic adults suffer from liver problems caused from the alcohol use. An acceptable alternative is the use of the parenteral depot formulation of naltrexone (Vivitrol), which is administered once a month as a 380-mg intramuscular injection. Another medication available is acamprosate (Campral), which, although very successful in Europe, has not fared so well in the United States. This medication is a glutamate antagonist thought to resolve the anxiety associated with alcohol cravings. However, administration requires a three-times-a-day dosing of two very large tablets. Although the side-effect profile is low, adherence is a problem due to frequency and size of the tablet.

For those patients suffering from an opiate use disorder, there are two substitution therapy and one antagonist therapy options. Substitution therapy utilizes either methadone or buprenorphine. Methadone can only be prescribed by physicians so authorized by the Drug Enforcement Agency (DEA), and the patient is required to access a methadone treatment clinic on a daily basis. Buprenorphine can also only be prescribed (currently) by a waivered physician who has been trained to prescribe this medication. Patients may prefer the use of buprenorphine because their primary care physician may be able to prescribe it for them, and this medication is managed in the same way any other medication is managed and the patient may receive a monthly supply. The antagonist therapy is naltrexone—which is also used for opiate use disorder and was described above.

Sleep Disorders

Description of the Disease

The single most common factor associated with increased prevalence of sleep problems is advanced age. Older adults commonly report to the primary care providers that they have problems falling asleep, staying asleep, daytime sleepiness, daytime napping, and the use of drugs to help them sleep. These patients will usually present complaints of dissatisfaction regarding the quality, timing, and amount of sleep. In order for pathology to be assigned and a sleep disorder diagnosis made, the patient must be able to demonstrate daytime distress and impairment in functioning as a result of the sleep problem. Although sleep problems can be an independent disorder, it most frequently occurs as a symptom of another disorder since sleep problems are symptoms found in multiple psychiatric disorders.

Epidemiology

The prevalence rate for sleep problems in the general population is about 30% to 45% in adults and believed to be much higher in patients over the age of 65.

Etiology

Sleep disorders are most commonly the result of a preexisting medical condition, a psychiatric condition or an environmental condition.

The most common medical conditions associated with sleep problems include any painful or uncomfortable condition, sleep apnea syndromes, restless legs syndrome, nocturia, dyspnea, heartburn, direct substance effects, and substance withdrawal effects (especially alcohol—even in modest amounts).

The more common psychiatric and environmental conditions associated with sleep problems include anxiety, muscle tension, environmental changes, depression, and posttraumatic stress.

Risk Factors

Predisposed individuals who are exposed to precipitating events such as major life changes such as loss, separation, or illness are at high risk for sleep disturbances.

Chronic environmental factors that increase vulnerability include noise, light, and significant changes in temperature (up or down).

Genetic/physiologic factors include female gender and advancing age. There also seems to be a familial disposition toward sleep disturbances.

Signs and Symptoms

Although there are many types of sleep disturbances, insomnia is the most common. The essential feature is dissatisfaction with sleep quality or quantity and complaints of either falling asleep, staying asleep, or both. The symptoms are accompanied by clinically significant distress or impairment in social, occupational, or other important areas of functioning. More commonly, the sleep problem occurs during the course of another psychiatric or medical condition, but it may (rarely) occur independently of any other cause. The sleep problem must be present for at least 3 months on more nights than not before pathology can be assigned.

Differential Diagnoses

Always first consider the sleep disturbance as a manifestation of another psychiatric or medical illness or as a normal variant.
  - Normal sleep variant: Normal sleep duration varies among individuals. "Short sleepers"—those who require only a small amount of sleep—may be concerned about their duration. However, they rarely will complain of difficulty falling asleep or staying asleep. Instead, they awaken feeling refreshed.

- Situational sleep problems: This is a case whereby the individual identifies sleep problems lasting a few days to a few weeks, often associated with life events or changes in sleep schedules. If distress or impairment is identified, then intervention is necessary.
- Sleep deprivation: This occurs as a result of inadequate opportunities or circumstances allowing sleep. The usual cause in the older adult is from an emergency or family obligation forcing the individual to stay awake.
- Restless leg syndrome: This often produces difficulties falling asleep and/or staying asleep. In this case, treatment of the restless leg syndrome should resolve the sleep problem.
- Breathing-related sleep disorders: These individuals have a history of loud snoring, breathing pauses during sleep, and excessive daytime sleepiness.
- Substance-/medication-induced sleep disorder: The cause of the sleep problem is either a drug of abuse, a medication, or an environmental toxin. Heavy coffee consumption is a common cause of sleep problems.

Diagnostic Studies

- Polysomnography—usually shows impairments of sleep continuity
- Electroencephalography—may show high-frequency power and increased cortical arousal
- Cortisol levels may be increased along with heart rate variability.
- There are no consistent or characteristic abnormalities on physical examination.

Treatment

Insomnia is commonly treated with benzodiazepines, the Z-drugs (zolpidem (Ambien), zaleplon (Sonata), and (es)zopiclone (Lunesta)), antihistamines (diphenhydramine [Benadryl and other over-the-counter medications]), L-tryptophan (a nutriceutical preparation found in health food stores), sedating antidepressants, and ramelteon (Rozerem).

Benzodiazepines and the Z-drugs should be used with care. The over-the-counter sleep aids have limited effectiveness. Short-acting medications (Z-drugs) are useful for persons who have difficulty falling asleep. For those patients having difficulty staying asleep, a longer-acting medication will be helpful.

Caution when combined with other drugs that have central nervous system properties. Additive effects can cause confusion, disorientation, and anterograde amnesia. Also, assess whether other medications or substances such as nicotine, stimulants, or alcohol may be contributing to the sleep disturbance.

Suggest alternative methods of treating sleep problems such as cognitive–behavioral therapy, relaxation techniques, avoiding daytime naps, and avoiding caffeine or other caffeinated beverages 4 to 6 hours before bedtime. Also, recommend that when the patient goes to bed it is for the purpose of sleeping and not watching television. Additionally, ensure that the patient is in darkness when retiring since lights prevent release of melatonin.

Ramelteon is a newer medication classified as a selective melatonin agonist. Melatonin levels typically peak between 2 AM and 4 AM, and release of melatonin is stimulated by darkness and inhibited by light. Patients with sleep problems have been found to have decreased amounts of melatonin and ramelteon increases the release of melatonin.

Aggression and Agitation

Description of the Disease

Often in late-life psychosis or major NCD (dementia), patients will exhibit severe agitation and aggression with symptoms of screaming, restlessness, sexual acting out, and assaultiveness.

Epidemiology

Aggression and agitation rates are particularly high in nursing homes, and the patient is more likely than not to target persons they know, usually family members. This seems to point to the fact that aggression in this population is not directed indiscriminately.

Etiology

Etiology is unknown, although environmental factors such as changes in living space and biologic factors such as genetic predisposition may play a role. Other correlates seem to be comorbid medical illness including pain syndromes, drug toxicity such as anticholinergic effects, changes in nutritional status, and infection, along with psychological issues such as frustration, loneliness, and reduced sensory stimuli.

Risk Factors

Several psychiatric disorders are associated with the development of aggression in the elderly and, in addition to those listed above, include mental retardation, mood disorders (including substance-induced mood disorder), intermittent explosive disorder, and personality disorders.

The probability of aggressive behaviors increases when patients begin to decompensate from either the progression of a medical condition or psychiatric condition.

When assessing the presence, severity or potential for aggressive behaviors, the nurse should evaluate the presence of physical abuse or verbal taunts from others, which creates a "stimulus–response" effect. Even ongoing mildly verbal slurs or glances might cause a spiraling escalation of agitation and ultimately aggression.

Signs and Symptoms

Always consider the behavioral manifestations of agitation and aggression as the result of an underlying problem which must be identified and resolved.

Differential Diagnoses

Same as for Delirium and Major Neurocognitive Disorder.

Diagnostic Studies

As identified under Delirium and Neurocognitive Disorder.

Treatment

Pharmacologic treatments focus on the use of dopamine antagonists such as the atypical antipsychotic medications as primary treatment. However, there has been some success with the use of antidepressants and mood stabilizers. There have been many mixed reviews on the use of antipsychotics in patients with dementia, and so care must be taken when prescribing these medications. There are few pharmacokinetic studies on the use of antipsychotics in the elderly. However, studies on the use of risperidone (Risperdal) indicate that clearance of this medication does not decline with increasing age and therefore should be a useful medication. Other medications that have been found to be helpful in the management of aggression and agitation are the use of β-blockers, SSRIs, anticonvulsants, and lithium. For the treatment of sexual acting out behaviors, the use of medroxyprogesterone has been studied and found to rapidly and safely treat these behaviors. The use of cholinesterase inhibitors (described earlier) has also been found to reduce restlessness.

From a psychosocial point of view, cognitive training includes basic social skills training, effective communication tools, identifying appropriate ways for self-expression, and improved self-esteem.

Review Section

Review of Case Presentation

This is a very complex case and a difficult one to properly diagnose and manage. From a psychiatric point of view, you must first identify pertinent symptoms. In psychiatry, we generally treat symptoms, not disorders. First, we have her manic symptoms, but we are already aware of the cause—the steroids. Exogenous steroid use often causes manic behaviors. This is in contrast to patients who have excessive endogenous steroids, which generally causes depressive symptoms. Since we know the cause of Arlene's mania, we simply treat the cause—and ultimately stop the steroids. And when using steroids is unavoidable, monitor closely. This is a risk–benefit situation. If the manic symptoms are minimal, they may be able to be tolerated for a short time. However, if intolerable or the symptoms create impairment, then the decision has to be made to either stop the steroids or attempt to control the mania. Sometimes, the use of concurrent benzodiazepines may be helpful. However, Arlene has a long history of abusing benzodiazepines and starting Arlene on such a medication may cause a relapse into an active addiction. Again, risk–benefit. The use of mood stabilizers would be intuitive, but by the time these medications become effective, it will probably be time for Arlene to be off the steroids.

Arlene has also developed anxiety regarding the probability of her strong predisposition for Alzheimer disease, so much so that she has been excessively obsessed with this fear. Obsessions (recurrent, intrusive thoughts) without a compulsive act to alleviate the anxiety are not indicative of obsessive–compulsive disorder. Instead, we are seeing worrying and anxiety at its extreme. The use of a SSRI is probably the best intervention at this time along with suggesting psychotherapy to address her ongoing fears. Again, we must avoid the use of benzodiazepines in this patient unless absolutely necessary. With time, and further physical and cognitive symptom development, Arlene becomes depressed. Is the anxiety fueling the depression or could it be caused by her realization that she is having symptoms of early Alzheimer disease? Or could the depressive symptoms be part of subclinical Parkinson syndrome? It doesn't matter—we need to treat the depression. First, we would increase whatever SSRI she is taking. Let us say she is taking Paxil 20 mg, which has produced partial remission of her anxiety. We would initially increase the Paxil to 30 mg, then 40 mg after a week. However, knowing she has chronic pain syndrome, a better medication would be one that also increases norepinephrine. Excellent medications that are effective in the treatment of

anxiety, depression, and pain are venlafaxine (Effexor) and duloxetine (Cymbalta). Titrating either of these medications upward should result in improvement of Arlene's anxiety, depression, and pain. In the event Arlene has any hepatic problems, then the use of desvenlafaxine (Pristiq) would be indicated. Pristiq is the active metabolite of Effexor and is excreted unchanged by the kidney without need for further metabolism by the liver.

For Arlene's progressive symptoms of Alzheimer disease, we would start a combination of a cholinesterase inhibitor (such as donepezil) and a glutamate antagonist such as memantine. The cholinesterase inhibitors are indicated for the treatment of mild to moderate NCDs and the glutamate inhibitors are indicated for the treatment of severe NCDs. Since Arlene's condition seems to be progressing relatively quickly, many clinicians will start both medications since there are studies demonstrating the synergistic efficacy of the combination therapy.

Arlene also has been becoming more aggressive and assaultive. There are many categories of medications used in the treatment of aggressive behaviors as discussed earlier. We would avoid the atypical antipsychotics since they are all dopamine antagonists and would most likely worsen the Parkinson symptoms. Lithium would most likely cause unbearable side effects. The best addition would probably be a β-blocker such as propranolol. Propranolol is also used successfully in the treatment of anxiety, so this medication at 10 mg b.i.d. or t.i.d. would be useful to control Arlene's agitation and aggressive behaviors.

We should always be concerned, when utilizing a polypharmacy model, to be watchful for drug–drug interactions. There are multiple free-of-charge databases found on the Internet that will check for any interactions among all the medications that the patient may be taking. Sometimes, because of risk–benefit situations, we may be forced to accept and deal with drug–drug interactions. By understanding the pharmacokinetic and pharmacodynamic interactions, you will be in a much better position to properly manage the patient.

It is unfortunate that Arlene's progressive diseases ultimately caused her death. In retrospect, what we have done for Arlene was assist her at every turn in her disease process with the ultimate goal of improving her quality of life for as long as possible.

Review Questions

1. As part of the aging process, physiologic changes alter pharmacokinetics and increase the risk of adverse effects from medications. Which of the following does not occur as part of the aging process?

   a. Decreased hepatic circulation
   b. Decreased glomerular filtration rate
   c. Increased splanchnic blood flow
   d. Reduced first-pass metabolism
   e. Decreased protein-binding capacity

2. Which of the following is true about depression in the elderly?

   a. Elderly persons may deny their symptoms.
   b. The elderly find it easier to express feelings than the young.
   c. Suicidal plans are rare.
   d. Anxiety features are common.
   e. Wishing to die always indicates depression.

3. All of the following suggest a diagnosis of neurocognitive disorder except:

   a. impaired memory.
   b. fluctuating level of consciousness.
   c. difficulty dressing.
   d. difficulty in finding the way home.

4. Which of the following is not associated with suicide in the elderly?

   a. Living alone
   b. Bereavement
   c. Frequent suicidal thoughts
   d. Financial worries
   e. Previous suicide attempts

5. Which of the following is a definite risk factor for Alzheimer disease?

   a. Traumatic brain injury
   b. Age
   c. Male gender
   d. Aluminum
   e. Cigarette smoking

6. A 62-year-old female is referred for assessment of her mental state. Which of the following symptoms is most suggestive of pseudodementia?

   a. Aphasia
   b. Agnosia
   c. Rapid onset and progression
   d. Apraxia
   e. Loss of short-term memory

7. A 63-year-old male with HIV on protease inhibitors therapy presents with severe depressive and anxiety symptoms. You confirm a diagnosis of major depressive disorder and decide to start him on citalopram (Celexa) and alprazolam (Xanax). When you check your drug–drug interaction program, you are alerted that there is a potential interaction between alprazolam and its protease inhibitor in which the protease inhibitor has been found to inhibit metabolism of alprazolam. Which of the following would have the greatest likelihood of minimizing the drug–drug interaction and ensure therapeutic drug levels?

   a. Prescribe a lower-than-usual starting dose of alprazolam.
   b. Prescribe a higher-than-usual starting dose of alprazolam.
   c. Prescribe the usual starting dose of alprazolam.
   d. Increase the dosage of his protease inhibitor and prescribe the usual starting dose of alprazolam.
   e. Decrease the dosage of his protease inhibitor and prescribe the usual starting dose of alprazolam.

8. There have been concerns about the widespread use of antipsychotics in nursing homes. Which of the following strategies is least beneficial in ensuring appropriate use of antipsychotics among nursing home patients with NCD-related behavioral problems?

   a. Carefully document specific behaviors warranting antipsychotic use.
   b. Rule out preventable causes of disruptive behavior.
   c. Utilize antipsychotic medications as a p.r.n. order instead of a scheduled order.
   d. Attempt dose reduction following stabilization of disruptive behavior.
   e. Closely monitor for antipsychotic-induced adverse effects.

9. In which of the following coexisting conditions are the use of SSRIs not recommended for active and maintenance treatment of major depressive disorder?

   a. Cerebrovascular disease
   b. Cardiovascular disease
   c. Mild neurocognitive impairment
   d. Major neurocognitive impairment
   e. None of the above

10. An 85-year-old man is brought to your office by his son who raised concerns that his father stopped

caring for himself. He is usually a clean and active person, and it is surprising to see him unshaven. On further questioning, the patient denies any depression and he scored a "2" on the geriatric depression scale. He was diagnosed with NCD, Alzheimer's type and is currently on donepezil 5 mg hs. He has prominent apathy. Which of the following would be an appropriate treatment for his apathy?

a. Fluoxetine
b. Bupropion
c. Methylphenidate
d. Aripiprazole
e. Desipramine

Answers with Rationales

1. (c) Increased splanchnic blood flow

   Rationale: Physiologic changes associated with aging can alter drug pharmacokinetics and pharmacodynamics. Aging causes decreased efficiency of all organ systems. As part of the overall decreased efficiency, splanchnic blood flow is decreased, not increased, with aging. This reduces drug absorption.

2. (a) Elderly persons may deny their symptoms.

   Rationale: The older adult may deny symptoms of depression and may somatize instead, presenting with physical symptoms—usually for which a cause cannot be ascertained. They find it more difficult to express their feelings than the younger population. Wishing to die may not be a sign of depression. Further exploration is needed.

3. (b) fluctuating level of consciousness.

   Rationale: Fluctuating level of consciousness is indicative of delirium rather than NCD. Progressive impairments and difficulties in activities of daily living (the other choices) are indicative of NCD.

4. (d) Financial worries

   Rationale: Financial worries are not associated with suicide in the elderly. All the other choices are.

5. (b) Age

   Rationale: Age is the only definitive risk factor for NCD, Alzheimer type. Other possible but not definite risk factors include family history in first-degree relatives, Down syndrome, head injury, aluminum, advanced age of mother at birth, and thyroid disease.

6. (c) Rapid onset and progression

   Rationale: Pseudodementia refers to the cognitive changes occurring in depression—usually in the elderly. It can be differentiated from depression by rapid onset and progression. The cognitive functions usually return to normal with successful treatment of depression. The other choices all point to a diagnostic presentation of NCD (dementia).

7. (a) Prescribe a lower-than-usual starting dose of alprazolam.

   Rationale: Protease inhibitors are metabolized by the liver's isoenzyme P450 system, specifically the CYP3A isoenzyme. All protease inhibitors increase the concentrations of all psychotropic drugs that are metabolized by the same isoenzyme. As a result, normal starting doses of alprazolam would result in increased serum concentrations and cause oversedation.

8. (c) Utilize antipsychotic medications as a p.r.n. order instead of a scheduled order.

   Rationale: PRN use of antipsychotic medications in nursing homes is discouraged because in many cases they are clear indications of use of a chemical restraint. PRN use of antipsychotics can be considered only when the patient is in imminent danger of harming self or others.

9. (e) None of the above

   Rationale: SSRIs are safe and are well tolerated by the elderly with all the conditions identified in this question.

10. (c) Methylphenidate

    Rationale: Methylphenidate has good evidence in managing geriatric patients with apathy.

Suggested Readings

Aichhorn, W., Whitworth, A., Weiss, E., & Marksteiner, J. (2006). Second-generation antipsychotics: Is there evidence for sex differences in pharmacokinetics and adverse effect profiles? *Drug Safety, 29*(7), 581–587.

Allgulander, C. (2010). Novel approaches to treatment of generalized anxiety disorder. *Current Opinions in Psychiatry, 23*(1), 37–42.

American Psychiatric Association. (2013). *Diagnostic and statistical manual of mental disorders* (5th ed.). Washington, DC: American Psychiatric Assiciation.

American Psychiatric Association. (2007). *Practice guideline for the treatment of patients with obsessive-compulsive disorder.* Washington, DC: American Psychiatric Association. Retrieved from http://www.psychiatryonline.com/pracguide/pracguidetopic_10.aspx.

Baldwin, D., Anderson, I., Nutt, D., Bandelow, B., Bond, A., Davidson, J. R., . . . Wittchen, H. U. (2005). Evidenced-based guidelines for the pharmacological treatment of anxiety disorders: Recommendations from the British Association for Psychopharmacology. *Journal of Psychopharmacology, 19*(6), 567–596. Retrieved from http://www.bap.org.uk/pdfs/anxiety_disorder_guidelines.pdf

Bezchlibnyk-Butler, K., Jeffries, J., & Virani, A. (Eds.). (2014). *Clinical handbook of psychotropic drugs* (20th ed.). Boston, MA; Hogrefe Publishing.

Blier, P., Gobbi, G., Turcotte, J., de Montigny, C., Boucher, N., Hébert, C., Debonnel, G. (2009). Mirtazapine and paroxetine in major depression: A comparison of monotherapy versus their combination from treatment initiation. *European Neuropsychopharmacology, 19*(7), 457–465.

Chouinard, G., Chouinard, V. (2008). Atypical antipsychotics: CATIE study, drug-induced movement disorder and resulting iatrogenic psychiatric-like symptoms, supersensitivity rebound psychosis and withdrawal discontinuation syndromes. *Psychotherapy and Psychosomatics, 77*, 69–77.

Cipriani, A., Furukawa, T., Salanti, G., Geddes, J. R., Higgins, J. P., Churchill, R., . . . Barbui, C. (2009). Comparative efficacy and acceptability of 12 new-generation antidepressants: A multiple treatments meta-analysis. *Lancet, 373*(9665), 746–758.

Dailly, E., & Bourin, M. (2008). The use of benzodiazepines in the aged patient: Clinical and pharmacological considerations. *Pakistan Journal of Pharmaceutical Sciences, 21*(2), 144–150.

Davidson, J. (2010). Major depressive disorder treatment guidelines in America and Europe. *Journal of Clinical Psychiatry, 71* (Suppl E1), e04.

Dell'Osso, B., Buioli, M., Baldwin, D., & Altamura, A. C. (2010). Serotonin norepinephrine reuptake inhibitors (SNRIs) in anxiety disorders: A comprehensive review of their clinical efficacy. *Human Psychopharmacology, 25*(1), 17–29.

Donoghue, J., & Lader, M. (2010). Usage of benzodiazepines: A review. *International Journal of Psychiatry in Clinical Practice, 14*(2), 78–87.

Haddad, P., & Sharma, S. (2007). Adverse effects of atypical antipsychotics: Differential risk and clinical implications. *CNS Drugs, 21*(11), 911–936.

Lam, R., Kennedy, S., Grigoriadis, S., McIntyre, R. S., Milev, R., Ramasubbu, R., . . . Ravindran, A. V. (2009). Canadian network for mood and anxiety treatments (CANMET) clinical guidelines for the management of major depressive disorder in adults. *Journal of Affective Disorders, 117* (Suppl 1), S26–S43.

Marder, S. (2006). A review of agitation in mental illness: Treatment guidelines and current therapies. *Journal of Clinical Psychiatry, 67*(Suppl 10), 13–21.

National Institute for Health and Clinical Excellence. (2010). *Depression: The NICE guideline on the treatment and management of depression in adults.* London, England: NICE. Retrieved from http://www.nice.org.uk/nicemedia/live/12329/45896.pdf.

Pricchione, G. (2004). Clinical practice. Generalized anxiety disorder. *New England Journal of Medicine, 351*(7), 675–682.

Sadock, B. J., & Sadock, V. A. (2007). *Kaplan & Sadock's synopsis of psychiatry* (10th ed.).Philadelphia, PA: Wolters Kluwer.

Scahill, L, Carroll, D., & Burke, K. (2004). Methylphenidate: Mechanism of action and clinical update. *Journal of Child and Adolescent Psychiatric Nursing, 17*(2), 85–86.

Serretti, A., & Mandelli, L. (2010). Antidepressants and body weight: A comprehensive review and meta-analysis. *Journal of Clinical Psychiatry, 71*(10), 1259–1272.

Stahl, S. (2004). Psychopharmacology of anticonvulsants: Do all anticonvulsants have the same mechanism of action? *Journal of Clinical Psychiatry, 65*(2), 149–150.

Zemrak, W., & Kenna, G. (2008). Association of antipsychotic and antidepressant drugs with Q-T interval prolongation. *American Journal of Health System Pharmacy, 65*(11), 1029–1038.

Chapter 10

Endocrine

Ann S. McQueen

Case Presentation

Directions: Carefully review the case study presented below. At the end of the chapter, answer the review questions. Compare your answers to the correct answers listed in the Review Section.

History of Present Illness:
M.L. is a 63-year-old Caucasian female seeking evaluation in your office for increased fatigue and muscle weakness and weight gain. She reports even her face looks fuller and she cannot understand the changes in her body. She reports she is 5 ft 4 inches and weighs 140 lbs. Reports a weight gain of 15 lbs in the last 6 months.

Patient takes no medications other than vitamins: B complex, calcium 600 mg, and multivitamin.

Family History:
Mother: Deceased age 75, osteoporosis, smoker, alcoholic.
Father: Deceased age 78, lung disease from environmental exposure.
Sister: 67 years old, no health issues

Past Medical History:
Surgery: None other than wisdom teeth and C-section in 1974.
Fractures: Fingers × 2, toes × 3, R wrist fracture (FX) age 48, irritable bowel syndrome (IBS), and bouts of gastroentero reflux disease (GERD)—no medications for it currently.
Allergies: Penicillin (PCN) and Sulfa Natural Menopause age 51; took estrogen replacement for 2 years (estrogen patch) and then discontinued due to health scare of a friend.

Social History: Drinks red wine one glass daily, no cigarettes, walks 3 miles daily, yoga twice a week, and lifts weights twice a week; she is a retired Sales Executive. Lives with husband; one grown daughter lives nearby with her husband and two children. Diet: Healthy fruit and veggies with low-fat meats and whole grains, three meals a day; rare snacks are fruit only or yogurt. Drinks four to six glasses of water daily.

Health Maintenance: Mammogram: 2 years ago; Pap smear: 5 years ago; colonoscopy: 5 years ago; wears seat belt; uses sunscreen

Immunizations: Up to date; TDaP: 3 years ago when granddaughter born; Pneumo: This year flu shot yearly

Review of Systems:
Head: Denies headaches, dizziness, or balance issues
Skin: Denies rashes, new lesions, or any skin irritation
Eyes: Wears reading glasses only, denies eye pain or vision issues, last examination 18 months ago
Nose: Denies any change in smell, nasal congestion, or rhinitis
Ears: No hearing issue, no ear pain, ears itch during allergy season.
Throat: Denies sore throat, postnasal drip, or bad taste in her mouth
Respiratory: Mild SOB on exertion, denies cough or chest discomfort

Cardiac: Denies chest pain, occasional heart palpitation now but was more frequent in her 30s

Peripheral Vascular: Denies any cold feet or hands, leg pains, or change in hair growth patterns on legs

Musculoskeletal: Denies joint pain, is active in yoga for range of motion, reports legs and arms feel weak

Neurologic: Denies issues with balance, dizziness, or trouble walking or dancing

Gastrointestinal: Denies any change in bowels, abdominal pain or bloating, no current heart burn complaints

Gyno/urologic: Denies any urinary incontinence, urinary frequency, or vaginal discharge

Psych: Denies depression, trouble sleeping, or memory issues

Physical Examination:

Vital Signs: BP = 106/72   Respiration = 16   Temperature = 97.9   Pulse = 78   Pulse Ox = 98%
    Height = 63.5 inches   Weight = 144 lbs   BMI = 25.3

General Survey: Well groomed, appears younger than stated age, good eye contact and communication style, dressed appropriately for the weather, seems engaged by body language of leaning forward to engage examiner in the point of her appointment

Skin: Overall tan noted on face, arms, and legs, no rashes noted, scar on abdomen from c/s, area of dryness on back and shoulders, recent sun burn in these areas indicated by peeling skin

HEENT: Head: Without lumps or deviations, facial structures symmetrical, hair honey blond, even distribution and thickness

Eyes: 20/30 OU uncorrected, PERLA, pupils 3 mm in size, conjunctiva pink, sclera clear, extraocular movements intact(Cranial Nerves [CN] 3, 4, 6)

Ears: Tympanic membranes visualized bilaterally with dullness, no cerumen or discharge, hearing within normal range (CN 8), no pain on movement with external tragus, normal pinna

Nose: Nasal mucosa pink, septum midline, no sinus pain or tenderness, normal sense of smell, and differentiation (CN 1).

Throat: Oral mucosa pink, dentition good, no obvious caries, pharynx without exudates

Neck: Trachea midline, neck supple, thyroid lobes palpable uniform size and shape, no nodules, neck with full ROM, and good muscle strength

Lymph Nodes: No cervical, axillary, submandibular, or inguinal adenopathy

Thoracic: Lungs clear anterior to posterior, normal lung expansion bilateral, no wheeze noted, no tenderness on anterior chest palpation

Heart: Regular S1, S2 slight mitral valve prolapse heard as midsystolic click, heard at apex. No jugular vein distension or carotid bruits

Peripheral Vascular: Warm, dry, no edema, good pulses, +2 BUE and BLE, spider veins noted bilateral upper thighs and one varicose vein L lower leg, no ulcerations

Breasts: Pendulous, symmetric, no masses, nipple discharge, or dimpling noted

Abdomen: Obese, soft, some discomfort on palpation over epigastric area otherwise nontender with normal bowel sounds all quadrants, no masses or organomegaly, no CVA tenderness bil.

Genitalia: Deferred

Rectal: Deferred

Musculoskeletal: Full ROM in upper extremities, crepitus noted in bil shoulder joints, negative phalen and tinel test. Full ROM in lower extremities, L ankle slightly tender during inversion and eversion rotation, no swelling or deformity noted. Muscle strength good in overall upper and lower extremities.

Neurologic: Alert and orientated, CN intact 1 to 12, balance good, gait even with good arm swing, rapid alternate movement and point-to-point orientation normal, negative Rhomberg, reflexes +2 upper and lower extremities.

Assessment

- Fatigue
- Obesity
- Mitral valve prolapse
- Exertional SOB

Plan

- Fasting laboratory work: TSH, CBC, CMP, HGBA1C, lipid panel
- Screening mammogram
- Bone density/DEXA scan based on family history
- Refer to Cardiology for review and testing of MVP and fatigue complaint

Case Study Review Questions

1. What other information needed in history?

   Any recent travel? Any recent change in diet? Any recent change in stress level?

2. What additional studies needed for further evaluation?

   T4, T3, antithyroid microsomal antibodies, 24 hour urine for free cortisol, Dexamethasone stimulation test.

3. Possible differential diagnoses?

   Pituitary tumor, Hypothyroidism, Type 2 Diabetes new onset, Cushing Syndrome, Unintentional weight gain due to diet.

Introduction

The endocrine system consists of eight organs that are affected by the aging process. These organs of the endocrine system are **pituitary, pineal gland, thymus, thyroid, parathyroid, adrenal glands, pancreas, and testes/ovaries**. These glands are involved with multiple body systems responsible for growth and development, metabolism, breathing, digestion, elimination, body temp regulation, blood circulation, sexual function and reproduction, and mood. One hormone can affect multiple body systems and organs while one body function may require multiple hormones in coordination. Some organs, such as the pancreas, have a nonendocrine function as well as endocrine function: the exocrine portion secretes enzymes while the endocrine portion releases hormones. With age, the biggest decline of organ function is the insulin resistance in the pancreas and thyroid gland function; this leads to the growing number of older adults with type 2 diabetes and hypothyroidism.

Effects of the endocrine system decline cause changes to muscle mass, strength, and immunity that contributes to the decline in functional status and alters living independently. Often early signs of endocrine disorder are mistaken by the general population as part of the normal aging process. Careful review of what is normal aging and endocrine function decline needs to be evaluated and patients looked at on an individual basis. Creating a healthy and safe environment as well as genetics is the key to the aging body. The Nurse Practitioner must be quite knowledgeable about the normal function of the endocrine system and the expected age-related functional decline and must recognize when unexpected adversities develop. The endocrine system holds the key to healthy living and aging.

Hypothalamus is the main gland of the endocrine system that causes release and inhibition of hormones. Located in the brain, it is a pea-sized organ that coordinates sending signals to the pituitary. Hypothalamus secretes Thyrotropin-Releasing Hormone (TRH), which will stimulate Thyroid-Stimulating Hormone (TSH); Corticotropin-Releasing Hormone (CRH), which causes the release of Adrenocorticotropin Hormone (ACTH); releases Growth Hormone–Releasing Hormone (GHRH), which causes Growth Hormone (GH); and Somatostatin, also known as Growth Hormone–Inhibiting Hormone (GHIH), which inhibits Growth Hormone (GH), Gonadotropin -releasing Hormone (GnRH) that stimulates the anterior pituitary to release Follicle-Stimulating Hormone (FSH) and Luteinizing Hormone (LH) that ensure function of the ovaries and testes, and lastly Prolactin Inhibitory Factor (PIF) that inhibits release of prolactin.

Pituitary is located in the sella turcica at the **base** of the brain. It is divided into the anterior and posterior sections. **Anterior gland** influenced by the hypothalamus produces six hormones: FSH, which produces estrogen and stimulates growth of ovarian follicles; LH, which stimulates ovulation and progesterone production in women and stimulates testicles to make testosterone in men; TSH, which stimulates the thyroid to produce hormones; GH, which stimulates growth in the body; ACTH, which stimulates adrenal glands to make cortisol and aldosterone; and lastly PROLACTIN, which affects milk production in the breasts.

Posterior gland: This part of the pituitary gland secretes and stores antidiuretic hormone (ADH), also known as vasopressin and oxytocin made by the hypothalamus. The function of ADH is to retain water in the body via the kidneys and increase peripheral vascular resistance by constricting the blood vessels that increases the blood pressure. The other hormone stored in the posterior pituitary is oxytocin, which causes the uterus to contract during birth and stimulates the release of breast milk when the infant is at the breast.

Thyroid and Parathyroid Glands: Located low in the front of the neck, the thyroid is a butterfly-shaped gland, and the parathyroid glands are small glands located behind the thyroid. The **thyroid** releases two distinct hormones, thyroxine (T4) and triiodothyronine (T3), that the thyroid requires iodine to formulate. These two are stored in the gland until release is mediated by the release of TSH from the anterior pituitary. The hormones control the body's metabolism and metabolic rate and increase protein and bone turnover. Thyroid gland produces calcitonin that causes calcium to deposit in the bones and decreases the calcium in the extracellular body fluid. The **parathyroid glands** are small little glands located by the thyroid; they produce PTH, which regulates serum calcium by absorption from the intestines and kidneys and releases from the bones.

Thymus: This spongy organ located behind the sternum has an important role in secreting humoral factor during puberty. It produces the hormone thymosin, which stimulates T cells in other lymphatic organs. These hormones allow the development of a healthy immune system for life. The thymus decreases in size after puberty and is replaced by fat in the later years.

Pineal Gland: Located deep in the center of the brain, this is a pine cone-shaped tiny gland. Referred to as the "third eye," this gland regulates sleep and circadian rhythm by the release of melatonin. Pineal gland also influences pituitary by blocking secretion of FSH and LH.

Adrenal Glands: A pair of glands located on the kidneys. The adrenal gland has two parts: medulla and cortex. The adrenal medulla secretes the catecholamines, epinephrine and norepinephrine. These two are responsible for the sympathetic nervous system response of "fight or flight." The adrenal cortex produces mineralocorticosteroids, such as aldosterone, that regulate the electrolytes—sodium absorption and potassium loss from the kidney. Formation of glucocorticoid, cortisol, in the adrenal cortex has multiple effects on metabolism of protein, carbohydrates, and fats. It also regulates blood glucose levels, has anti-inflammatory effects, and affects growth and decreases signs of stress on the body. The last hormones produced by the adrenal gland cortex are androgens, mostly dehydroepiandrosterone (DHEA) and androstenedione, which are converted to testosterone and dihydrotestosterone.

Pancreas: It is located in the abdomen behind the stomach across the back of the abdomen. The pancreas is a 6-inch long organ that has both digestive and endocrine functions. The exocrine function releases pancreatic enzymes into the small intestine essential for the breakdown of protein, fat, and sugars so they can be released into the bloodstream for energy. The endocrine function of the pancreas releases via the β-islet cells insulin and glucagon from the islet of Langerhans. Insulin regulates the blood glucose and metabolizes fat, protein, and carbohydrates. Glucagon increases the synthesis and release of glucose from the liver into the bloodstream, increasing the blood sugar. Somatostatin is also produced in the pancreas and inhibits secretion of insulin and glucagon. This hormone system is a very fine-tuned balance mechanism until alterations occur.

Testes: A pair of glands, size of large olives, that are located within the scrotum. The hypothalamus–pituitary–testes axis stimulates to produce the androgen testosterone which gives the male secondary sexual characteristics and sperm produced by spermatogenesis. Testosterone is formed in the testes by stimulation of LH produced in the anterior pituitary, which was stimulated by the hypothalamus. When in the body testosterone decreases and secretion of GnRH and LH increase.

Ovaries: A pair of glands located in the pelvis along the lateral wall of the uterus. The ovary produces ovum monthly and controls sexual hormone development of estrogen and progesterone. Estrogen controls the development of the mammary glands and stimulates the lining of the uterus during the menstrual cycle. Progesterone acts on the lining of the uterus during pregnancy. The hypothalamus triggers release of LH and FSH from the pituitary that signals the ovary to make estrogen and progesterone. In older women, the ovary is much less sensitive to FSH and LH.

Aging changes on endocrine system: Hypothalamus is the center of aging in the body; according to new research, it is speculated there may be a process in the future to slow the process. The hypothalamus has influence on all the organs in the endocrine system.

The pituitary reaches its maximum size in middle age, then begins to decrease in size.

Thyroid gland, with the aging process, begins to slow down, and the gland gets bumpy (nodular) in texture.

The parathyroid glands, with aging, increase the production of PTH, adding to the risk of osteoporosis in the geriatric years.

Pineal gland has diminished activity in the elderly, which affects the circadian rhythm and could be the link to sleep regulation and disordered sleep.

With the adrenal glands, the aging process causes decrease in aldosterone, which contributes to dizziness and orthostatic hypotension; aging is also the cause of decreased release of cortisol.

Pancreas becomes less sensitive to insulin as the body ages. Fasting blood sugar can increase 6 to 14 mg/dL for every 10 years after 50.

Testes/ovaries are affected by the drastic changes from decreased production and secretion of steroid hormones. The aging process that contributes to this causes pathophysiologic change as well as metabolic changes.

Aging Hormone Changes:

Hormones That Decrease:
- Estrogen
- Prolactin (in women)
- Testosterone
- Calcitonin
- Aldosterone
- GH
- Renin

Hormones That Decrease Slightly:
- Insulin
- Cortisol
- Epinephrine
- T3 and T4

Hormones That increase:
- FSH
- LH
- Norepinephrine
- PTH

Female Reproductive Cycle

Women begin reproductive cycling at around age 12 and continue until the average age of 51 years. This means the average women will have 30 years of ovulatory cycles and menstruation.

Etiology:
- Reproductive ovulatory cycles may be interrupted in their cyclic occurrence by pregnancy, breast-feeding, medications, perimenopausal changes, and endocrine disorders.

Epidemiology:
Puberty: Also known as menarche is the first menstruation of a girl aged 11 to 13 (average age being 12)

There are three phases of physiologic development building up to menarche:
- First is **thelarche**, the development of breasts from previous breast buds controlled by stimulation from estrogen and progesterone production from the ovaries.
- Second is **pubarche**, the development of pubic hair and axillary hair under the influence of androgens produced by the adrenal glands.
- **Menarche** is the last phase, the first menstruation is normally anovulatory.
- The journey from thelarche to menarche in girls is usually 2 to 4 years.
- Cycles become regulated usually 3 years after menarche.

In some young girls even with an intact endocrine system and gonads present, puberty may be delayed and menarche never achieved; this would be defined as primary amenorrhea (see Chapter 6: Women's Health Review)

Increased body weight and obesity seem to be related to earlier onset of puberty, just as low body weight is attributed to delayed onset of puberty.

Menstrual Cycle: Begins with day 1 of menses and completes with the next onset of bleeding which is day 1 of the next cycle.

- The average cycle length is 28 days, but normal range can be plus 7 days or minus 7 days (21 to 35 days).
- The length of flow has an average range of 5 to 7 days but can be as short as 1 day or as long as 8 days without endocrine abnormalities.
- Blood loss: 20 to 60 mL of dark, nonclotted blood

Phase 1: Menstruation and Follicular Phase

Day 1 of vaginal bleeding indicates no pregnancy has occurred; in the endocrine system the following is occurring:

- Serum concentrations are low for estrogen, progesterone, and LH but a high level of FSH.
- FSH triggers a growth of new follicles in the ovary, starting a new reproductive cycle.
- Many follicles are growing in both ovaries by this stimulation.
- About day 6 of the cycle, estrogen levels are increasing; one dominant follicle is identified and with its ability to make estrogen will go on to ovulate.
- The rise in estrogen levels seals the endometrium from further shedding and repairs the lining.
- The other follicles developing on the ovaries regress, while the primordial follicle secretes estrogen that acts as a feedback loop to the pituitary, causing the release of more LH.
- LH-induced ovulation is about 24 to 48 hours after estradiol peaks.
- The later phase of the follicular phase the LH level rises—the length of the follicular phase is about 14 days (can be shorter in women with shorter overall cycles from day 1 to day 1 of next cycle).

Phase 2: Ovulation:

LH surge occurs around day 11 to 13 of the cycle and the dominant follicle ovulates:

- It is noted that 30 to 36 hours before ovulation the LH surge begins with the peak level of LH 10 to 12 hours before ovulation (this has been caught by technology in the ovulation predictor urine testing kit).
- Women experience slight discomfort to burning pain, known as mittelschmerz, at ovulation with the release of a small amount of fluid into the peritoneal cavity when the oocyte is released from the follicle.
- The oocyte or ovum is picked up from the ovary by the fimbriated ends of the fallopian tubes that transport it to the uterus—at which time if spermatozoa are present in the next 24 hours of the journey, penetration of the oocyte can occur and conception takes place.
- After this event of ovulation, the body begins the Luteal phase of the cycle leaving the ovarian cycle behind.

Phase 3: Luteal Phase:

Begins after the LH surge when the dominance of estrogen ends and progesterone is the primary sex steroid produced:

- The granulosa and theca cells of the follicle lining form the corpus luteum, and these cells can produce progesterone and estrogen during this phase.
- Progesterone feeds back to the pituitary in a negative feedback loop, suppressing further release of FSH and LH.
- Production of progesterone begins 24 hours after ovulation and continues to climb, supporting the corpus luteum for 9 to 11 days if no conception the level regresses.
- If no conception, the corpus luteum begins to regress and decrease in size and progesterone levels drop off quickly.
- This event of decreased progesterone production in the ovary causes the feedback cycle to the pituitary to release FSH.
- FSH gets ready to initiate a new cycle with day 1 of bleeding.

Uterine Cycle:

Based on the hormonal influences of estrogen and progesterone the lining of the uterus follows a cycle of phases as well:

- During menses the lining is completely shed, leaving a thin basal layer.
- In the follicular phase under the influence of estrogen, the layer begins to grow rapidly in thickness, known as the proliferative endometrium.
- The endometrium will reach maximum thickness right at the time of ovulation.
- As endometrium proliferates FSH/LH/progesterone receptors form.
- At ovulation with the switch to progesterone and estrogen from the corpus luteum influence, the lining becomes vascular and slightly swollen, giving the appearance of edematous lining.
- This phase of growth is referred to as the luteal phase or secretory phase.
- When the corpus luteum begins to regress after 9 to 14 days the linin begins to shed ending the cycle.

- If ovulation does not occur, **anovulation**, there is no formation of the corpus luteum nor influence of progesterone on the lining of the uterus.
- Estrogen continues to stimulate the lining, and it becomes thicker in composition.
- Proliferative lining becomes thick enough that it outgrows its blood cycle; this causes random endometrial sloughing.
- The menstrual flow can be scanty flow to heavy flow and usually occurs at less than 28 days from last cycle.

Pituitary Tumor

Description of the Disease: An abnormal growth within the pituitary gland that grows and causes symptoms or can be classified as nonfunctional found in an incidental way.

Epidemiology:
- These tumors can exist without symptoms or nonspecific symptoms or they can cause excessive hormone levels. The tumor itself can cause restriction that affects the normal function of the gland.
- The sella turcica has little room for growth and tumor expansion.
- Tumors can start growing at any age.
- Some genetic component in those carrying MEN1
- Vast majority of these tumors are adenomas and noncancerous.

Etiology:
- Prolactinomas comprise 40% to 57% all adenomas. Nonfunctional 28% to 37%. ACTH-secreting tumors are 1% to 2% and FSH-/LH-/TSH-secreting tumors are rare.
- **Pituitary microadenoma** is a tumor less than 10 mm in size; it does not damage the pituitary or surrounding tissues. Microadenomas are slightly more common than macroadenomas. Can cause hormone changes such as Cushing syndrome
- **Pituitary macroadenoma** is a tumor greater than 1 cm in size, puts pressure on the pituitary gland and surrounding structures. Can cause diabetes insipidus from tumor structure

Signs and Symptoms:
- Vision loss, particularly loss of peripheral vision
- Headache
- Nausea and vomiting
- Symptoms of pituitary hormone deficiency
- Weakness
- Less frequent or no menstrual periods
- Body hair loss
- Sexual dysfunction and decreased libido
- Increased frequency and amount of urination
- Unintended weight loss or gain
- Galactorrhea

ACTH SECRETING PITUITARY TUMOR

Description of the Disease: Stimulates adrenals to make increased cortisol, causing Cushing syndrome

Signs and Symptoms:
- Labile mood, depression
- Proximal muscle weakness
- Skin changes: Striae/bruising, skin thinning
- Changes in facial features: Moon facies, acne, weight gain
- Menstrual changes: Irregular menses, hirsutism, decrease in libido
- Central obesity, hypertension
- Glucose intolerance, neutrophilia, lymphocytopenia, eosinopenia
- Can lead to diabetes mellitus, cardiac disease, osteoporosis

Diagnostic Tests:
- 24-hour urine collection for free cortisol
- Midnight salivary cortisol level
- Dexamethasone stimulation test

Treatment:
- Surgery: Transsphenoidal to remove tumor, with or without radiation
- Radiation: Alone or before or after surgery
- Drug therapy: To suppress tumor from making ACTH

GH-SECRETING PITUITARY TUMOR

Description of the Disease: Effects of increased growth hormone can lead to acromegaly

Signs and Symptoms:
- Increase in hand and foot size
- Change in facial features (large mandible), coarse facial features
- Change in hands: Carpal tunnel symptoms, hyperhidrosis
- Fatigue, proximal muscle weakness
- Decrease in libido, menstrual changes
- Hypertension, left ventricular hypertrophy, cardiomyopathy
- Enlargement of internal organs: Spleen, liver, kidney, pancreas, stomach

Risks:
- Cardiac disease
- Diabetes
- Sleep apnea
- Increased risk of colon cancer
- Osteoporosis

Diagnostic Tests:
- Oral glucose suppression testing with 75 g glucose load and watching GH levels after 2 hours
- Serum insulin like growth factor 1 level

Treatment:
- Surgery (usually transsphenoidal or endoscopic transsphenoidal surgery) to remove the tumor, with or without radiation treatment
- Drug therapy to stop the tumor from making GH

PROLACTIN-SECRETING TUMOR

Description of the Disease: Prolactinoma causes decrease in **estrogen** level (in women) or decreased **testosterone** level (in men).

Signs and Symptoms:
- Galactorrhea, decrease in libido, infertility
- Men: Gynecomastia, impotence, hypogonadism, testicular atrophy
- Premenopausal women: Oligomenorrhea or amenorrhea

Risk:
- Osteoporosis

Diagnostic Studies:
- Serum LH/FSH/TSH/hCG levels

Treatment:
- Surgery: Transsphenoidal to remove tumor with or without radiation therapy
- Medication: Dopamine agonists for prolactin-secreting tumors either instead of surgery or afterward to suppress levels
- Bromocriptine (Parlodel)
- Cabergoline (Dostinex)

GONADOTROPIN-SECRETING ADENOMA

Description of the Disease: Also known as nonfunctioning pituitary tumors, it has **no symptoms** unless they grow to macroadenomas
- 15% to 40% of pituitary tumors, half of all macroadenomas are this type.

Signs and Symptoms:
- If large tumor
  - Men: Low testosterone, high FSH, LH
  - Women: FSH markedly elevated, LH suppression, Estradiol 80 if greater than normal

Diagnostic Studies:
- LH/FSH/ HCG serum levels

Source: McQueen, A.S. (2014) Adult-Gero. Review Book/Endocrine System.

TSH-SECRETING TUMOR

Description of the Disease: Pituitary overproduces TSH, making hyperthyroid symptoms

Signs and Symptoms:
- Increased weight loss
- Increased heart rate
- Frequent moving bowels
- Nervous/irritable
- Feeling warm or hot
- Visual disturbance
- Enlarged thyroid (goiter)

Diagnostic Testing:
- TSH serum level
- Thyroxine level (T4)

Treatment:
- Drug therapy: Stops tumor growth and stops tumor from making prolactin
- Surgery: To remove tumor (transsphenoidal or γ-knife or craniotomy) when tumor does not respond to medication or when patients cannot take medications
- Radiation Therapy: After surgery or if surgery not possible:
- Radioiodine
- Medications: To suppress TSH production
- Methimazole (Tapazole)
- Propylthiouracil (PTU)

Hypothyroidism

Description of the Disease: A deficiency in thyroid hormones T4 (thyroxine) and T3 (triiodothyronine) that affect the metabolism that maintains the rate the body uses fats and carbohydrates, produces protein, and regulates body temperature and heart rate. With a deficiency it causes an array of symptoms. In the elderly these symptoms seem similar to the aging process and can be insidious.

Epidemiology:
- Mostly affects women aged 30 to 60. In men 10 times less common but possible. Accounts for 80% of autoimmune disease. Aging causes the atrophy, fibrosis, and inflammation of the thyroid gland, causing decreased T4 and T3 and decreased TSH.

Etiology:
- Primary hypothyroidism: 99% of cases are autoimmune or iatrogenic. Some of the iatrogenic causes are as follows:
  - Surgical removal or irradiation of thyroid tissue
  - Medication side effect especially with lithium, amiodarone, and antithyroid preparations
  - Postpartum thyroiditis
  - Inadequate diet missing iodine and tyrosine
  - Subacute granulomatous thyroiditis
  - Hashimoto disease or autoimmune thyroiditis: Most commonly affects 14 million Americans (2 million male, 12 million female)
- Secondary hypothyroidism: Insufficient stimulation of the thyroid either from pituitary or hypothalamus

Risk Factors:
- Autoimmune disease
- Close relative with history of autoimmune disease
- History of radiation to neck and upper chest

Signs and Symptoms:
- Symptoms can arise slowly and develop over time without patient being aware.
- Decreased metabolic rate, low temp <97.8
- Weight gain and unable to lose weight
- Nonpitting edema (myxedema) can also be around eyes, hands and feet, and between scapulas.
- Tongue may appear enlarged and voice become huskier.
- Sleepy and easily fatigued and sluggish
- Cold hands and feet
- Seasonal affective disorder
- Poor digestion, constipation
- Hormonal imbalance
- Hair loss, dry hair, and skin

Note: Life-threatening myxedema coma: In women usually during winter months, from un diagnosed or untreated hypothyroidism can cause bradycardia, hypotension, hypoventilation, hypoglycemia, hyponatremia, and deterioration of neurologic status into coma, respiratory collapse then shock, and cardiac collapse. Treatment is an emergency care with mechanical ventilation, thyroid replacement therapy, IV fluids with dextrose, vasopressor, and passive rewarming.

Differential Diagnoses:
- Hypoglycemia
- Chronic fatigue syndrome

Diagnostic Studies:
- Blood testing:
  - T3 normal 80 to 180 ng/dL
  - T4 normal 4.6 to 12 μg/dL
  - TSH normal 0.4 to 6.0 IU/mL
  - Antithyroid microsomal antibodies (Anti-TPO), normal <9.0
  - If testing for Hashimoto thyroiditis, add TgAb (antithyroglobulin antibody) level as well.
  - Ultrasound: Evaluate for nodules and gland size.

Treatment
Pharmacologic:
- Synthroid, Levothyroxine, Levoxyl, all three synthetic brands of T4, available in a variety of oral doses, titrated up slowly to correct to a euthyroid state.
- Cytomel: Synthetic brand of T3 also known as liothyronine
- Diet: Must avoid soy products and high-protein diet when taking these supplements as well as taking on empty stomach to avoid tampering with absorption that is caused by iron supplements, calcium supplements, aluminum hydroxide antacids, and cholestyramine
- Natural thyroid extracts: Many on the market made from pig thyroid used in extracts and powders

Nonpharmacologic:
- Many feel looking at diet, gut, and lifestyle to treat hypothyroidism without medications. Plans include eliminate sugar and caffeine from diet, skip goitrogens vegetables, such as broccoli, kale, cabbage, cauliflower, switch to gluten-free diet, multivitamin supplements, healthy intake of fats, meditation and relaxation, decrease stress.

Hyperthyroidism

Description of the Disease: Metabolic imbalance in the body over the excess production circulating thyroid hormone causing metabolism and electrolyte shifts.

Epidemiology:
- Most common in women versus men, especially after age 70. The body reacts in a state of flight or fight mechanism. In elderly two-third will present the same as younger patients and one-third present with apathetic

hyperthyroidism. Atrial fibrillation occurs with age independent of onset of hyperthyroidism; comortality exists from hyperthyroid being untreated. In osteoporosis, hyperthyroidism leads to low bone mineral density.

Etiology:

- This condition can be acute or chronic depending on cause. The term thyrotoxicosis describes effects of overproduction of thyroid hormone. There are many suggested causes such as ingestion of excess thyroid hormone dose (geriatric poly pharmacy) or amiodarone use, thyrotoxicosis from radiation exposure, pituitary tumor, toxic multinodular goiter (caused by multiple thyroid nodules).
- Graves disease, an autoimmune disease, is the most common cause as it overstimulates the thyroid gland, causing the increase of T3 and T4, which secreted through a negative feedback loop to the hypothalamus, pituitary, and thyroid glands. Graves disease is most common.

Risk Factors:

- Comorbidities

Signs and Symptoms:

- Increased sweating, thin, silky skin, and hair
- Increased tremors and twitching
- Tachycardia and heart palpitations (in those without heart disease)
- Restless, irritable, anxiety, difficulty concentrating
- Dyspnea on exertion
- Weight loss and heat intolerance
- Increased appetite but also diarrhea from increased GI motility
- Muscle weakness, fatigue
- Eye lid lag and exophthalmos (in Graves disease)
- Oligomenorrhea or amenorrhea

Differential Diagnoses:

- Anorexia
- Depression
- Stress

Diagnostic Studies:

- Lab evaluation of blood work
  - T3 normal 80 to 180 ng/dL
  - T4 normal 4.6 to 12 μg/dL
  - TSH normal 0.4 to 6.0 IU/mL
  - T3 uptake normal range male 27% to 37%, female 20% to 37%
  - Thyroid-stimulating immunoglobulin/microsomal thyroid antibodies 0.0 to 0.5 IU/mL
  - Radioiodine uptake and thyroid scan: To evaluate size of thyroid, position, and function
  - Thyroid ultrasound to rule out nodules as cause of increase in size

Treatment

Pharmacologic:

- Antithyroid drugs: Tapazole (Methimazole) or PTU (propylthiouracil) taken orally daily may improve symptoms in 6 to 12 weeks. Elderly may have more side effects than younger patients.
- β-Androgenic blockers: Atenolol, nadolol, metoprolol, acebutolol, etc. Symptomatic relief seen as decrease in heart rate and systolic blood pressure but do not decrease thyroid levels, helps with tremor, irritability, exercise intolerance. Adjunct therapy to antithyroid medication and radioactive iodine.
- Radioiodine ablation: Safe, efficacy, cost effective. Dose calculated by thyroid uptake scan results. Taken by mouth gland shrinks and symptoms decrease in 3 to 6 months. Eighty percent of patients will develop hypothyroidism as a consequence of treatment requiring supplementation.

Nonpharmacologic:

- Surgery: Subtotal or near-total thyroidectomy to decrease thyroid gland's ability to produce hormone. Less common approach in elderly due to comorbidities.

Hyperparathyroidism

Description of the Disease: When the parathyroid glands produce too much PTH putting the body at risk for fractures, osteoporosis, and kidney stones

Epidemiology:
- Normally over age 60 but can occur in young adults also, women more inclined than men, rare is the cause parathyroid carcinoma. Parathyroid levels increase with age and may contribute to osteoporosis.

Etiology:
- Parathyroid glands are on back of the thyroid gland: there are four but sometimes three or six in number located to right, left, inferior, and superior; sometimes inferior gland can migrate to embryonic site in the thymus.
- Parathyroid glands produce PTH which controls the calcium, phosphorous, and vitamin D in the body. One or more parathyroid gland can grow larger, producing too much PTH. In 85% of cases it is a single adenoma causing parathyroid hyperplasia. In 15% it is caused by diffuse hyperplastic tissue.
- When the calcium level in the blood is too low, increased PTH causes calcium levels to elevate by robbing it from the bones and resorbing from the kidney and small intestines.

Primary Hyperparathyroidism:
- Accounts for most hyperparathyroidism resulting from excess release of PTH that manifests in hypercalcemia, no malignancies but hyperplasia of any of the parathyroid glands. Cancer would be diagnosed in <0.5% of cases. There also can be an inherited gene to hyperparathyroidism. There is also asymptomatic primary hyperparathyroidism. If there is a fracture is most likely distal third of radius where cortical bone is vulnerable to catabolic action of PTH. In menopause cancellous bone in the lumber spine is lost first.

Secondary Hyperparathyroidism:
- Parathyroid glands become hyperplastic from long-term hyperstimulation and release of PTH and response with hypocalcemia because of chronic renal failure. The kidneys must be able to convert vitamin D into a form the body can use. Two other causes for secondary hyperparathyroidism can be the body's overcompensation from severe vitamin D deficiency or severe calcium deficiency.

Risk Factors:
- Radiation to head and neck predisposes patient to potential hyperparathyroidism in the future

Signs and Symptoms:
- Often diagnosed before symptoms
- Known as "bones, kidney stones, abdominal groans and psychic moans"
- Nausea and loss of appetite
- Kidney stones
- Increased amount of urine production
- Fragile bones of limbs and spine
- Feeling tired, weak, and ill
- Depression and forgetfulness
- Bone pain and tenderness

Differential Diagnoses:
- Osteoporosis
- Multiple myeloma
- Kidney stones from dietary sources
- Sarcoidosis

Diagnostic Studies:
- Blood testing: PTH, calcium, alkaline phosphate
- PTH: Normal 10 to 65 pg/mL
- Calcium: Normal 8.4 to 10.2 mg/dL
- Alkaline phosphate: Normal 44 to 147 IU/L
- 24-hour urine test to determine how much calcium is being removed from the body
- X-rays and DEXA Scan: To determine bone loss/bone softening and rule out fractures
- X-ray/ultrasound/CT scan of kidneys and urinary tract to show calcium deposits or blockage

Treatment
Pharmacologic:
- Extra calcium and vitamin daily
- Avoid phosphates in diet (high-protein foods)
- Sensipar (Cinacalcet) oral tablets taken daily for one of three situations
  - Primary hyperparathyroidism where surgical resection not possible

- Secondary hyperparathyroidism in adult with chronic kidney disease and dialysis
- Treatment for those with parathyroid carcinoma
- Dose must be titrated based on frequent serum calcium levels

Nonpharmacologic:
- Drink lot of water to prevent kidney stone formation
- Exercise to build bone strength
- Avoid thiazide diuretics
- Surgery: To remove overactive glands (in those over age 50) minimally invasive parathyroidectomy
- Risk: Injury to laryngeal nerve and hypoparathyroidism.
- Follow laboratory levels after surgery to see the expected drop in PTH and monitor it does not increase.

Hypoparathyroidism

Description of the Disease: Uncommon endocrine disorder where the body secretes low levels of PTH, causing low calcium levels and increased serum phosphorus (hyperphosphatemia).

Epidemiology:
Transient hypoparathyroidism after thyroidectomy and parathyroidectomy surgery is in 10% to 46% of patients. Permanent hypoparathyroidism is in 0% to 43% of patients.
- Primary hypoparathyroidism: Low-concentration PTH with low calcium level
- Secondary hypoparathyroidism: Serum PTH concentration is low and serum calcium is elevated.
- Pseudohypoparathyroidism: Serum PTH concentration is elevated as result of resistance to PTH caused by mutations in the PTH receptor.

Etiology:
PTH regulates phosphorus and calcium in the body with decreased level; it causes low ionized calcium in blood and bones.
- Acquired hypoparathyroidism: After surgery and other damage from head and neck surgery
- Autoimmune: Antibodies created against parathyroid tissue, parathyroid stops producing PTH
- Hereditary: Parathyroid gland not present or not functioning
- Low levels of magnesium in the blood can effect formation of parathyroid hormone

Risk Factors:
- Head and neck surgery
- Family history of hypoparathyroidism
- Autoimmune or endocrine condition such as Addison disease with deficit of hormones

Signs and Symptoms:
- Tingling and burning in toes, fingertips, and lips
- Muscle aches and cramps in legs, feet, abdomen, or face
- Twitching/tetany cramp like spasm of muscle around mouth, throat, hands, and arms
- Patch hair loss, thinning eye brows
- Dry/coarse skin, brittle nails
- Headaches
- Depression, mood swings and memory issues

Differential Diagnoses:
- Hypocalcemia
- Pseudohypoparathyroidism

Diagnostic Studies:
- Check serum blood levels
- Calcium normal 8.4 to 10.2 mg/dL
- PTH normal 15 to 65 pg/mL
- Phosphorus normal 2.4 to 4.5 mg/dL
- Magnesium normal 1.5 to 2.5 mg/dL
- Urine: Check for loss of calcium in the urine.

Treatment

Pharmacologic: Supplements
- Calcium carbonate 500 mg three times a day, watch GI upset and constipation

- Vitamin D: In high doses in the form of calcitriol 0.25 mcg daily or double dose as needed
- Intravenous calcium gluconate: If positive Chvostek or Trousseau signs when tapping on side of cheek over facial nerve, indicating latent tetany

Nonpharmacologic:
- Diet rich in calcium: Green leafy vegetables, dairy, breakfast cereals, fortified OJ
- Low-phosphorous diet: Avoid carbonated beverages, limit eggs and meats

Andropause

Description of the Disease: The age-related hormone changes in men from the gradual drop in testosterone. The syndrome has symptoms that effect the physical, emotional, and psychological functioning of men.

Epidemiology:
- With the aging process the testes decrease in size and weight and soften from atrophy, seminiferous tubules thicken, and there is decreased spermatogenic capacity. Ejaculation is slower and more stimuli are needed to achieve erection. After age 30, there is a 1% decrease in testosterone per year. By age 70 the testosterone is 50% of what it once was, with a normal testosterone level being 300 to 1,200 ng/dL. There is also an increase in FSH and LH with aging.

Etiology:
- Also known as hypogonadism, hypoandrogenism, testosterone deficiency

Risk Factors:
- Hypotestosteronemia is linked to coronary arteriosclerosis, risk factor for heart failure and osteoporosis

Signs and Symptoms:
- Physical symptoms: Increased fat mass, decreased lean muscle, osteoporosis, alopecia, anemia, weakness, hot flashes
- Sexual symptoms: Erectile dysfunction, loss of libido, infertility
- Psychological symptoms: Fatigue, depression

Differential Diagnoses:
- Somatopause, pituitary tumors, diabetes mellitus, hyperthyroidism, medication use side effects, primary testicular hypogonadism, secondary hypothalamic–pituitary hypogonadism

Diagnostic Studies:
- Laboratory panel: Check the following serum blood work.
  - Total testosterone (range 300 to 1,000 ng/dL)
  - Free testosterone (range 9 to 30 ng/dL)
  - Bioavailable testosterone (75 to 235 ng/dL)
  - LH (1.2 to 8.6 mIU/mL)
  - FSH (1.3 to 9.9 mIU/mL)
  - Prolactin (1.6 to 18.8 ng/mL)

Treatment:
Pharmacologic:
- Testosterone supplementation benefits: Improved libido, increased muscle mass, improved sexual function, increased bone density, decreased body fat mass. There are many contraindications to testosterone supplementation; a complete health history needs to be performed to evaluate for untreated prostate cancer, lower urinary tract obstruction, BPH, high hematocrit above 52%, untreated sleep apnea, history of elevated PSA, or history of congestive heart failure
- Testosterone gel/patch: Easier use but more expensive, better maintains the circadian rhythm of testosterone; application can cause skin irritation, must wash hands carefully after application of gel or patch to avoid transmission to women or children.
- Pellets: Number of pellets placed is based on T level, placed under the skin in the buttocks in 100 to 200 mg pellets needed to be replaced every 4 to 6 months
- Long-acting testosterone injections: Enanthate or cypionate is effective testosterone products, safe, inexpensive but unable to regulate testosterone levels, peak 2 to 3 days after injection, treat every 2 to 3 weeks. These injections can cause site irritation and pain, loss of circadian rhythm of testosterone, and possible infertility.

Nonpharmacologic:
- Chinese Herbs: Balance for individual patient the yin and yang through herbal supplements
- Exercise, yoga, and others to release stress
- Diet: Low fat, high fiber, limit caffeine and alcohol
- Drink lots of water
- Plenty of sleep

Menopause

See Chapter 6: Women's Health Review.

Somatopause

Description of the Disease: The change of state of the body after the gradual decline in triad of GHRH, GH, and insulin-like growth factor (IGF). IGF-1 is also known as somatomedin C decline. The results of somatopause are the increase in adipose tissue, loss of vitality, cardiovascular complications, and the decline in lean muscle mass. This is often referred to as the middle-age spread.

Epidemiology:
- The amount of visceral body fat is inversely related to the GH secretion. The GH secretion is proportionally related to the testosterone level. Exercise has been shown to increase the GH pulsatility. Neuroendocrine suppression of growth and regulation of energy. Decreased GH secretion will increase body fat.

Etiology:
- There is a 14% decrease in GH every decade of life. Somatopause contributes to functional decline in elderly but little is known of the biologic effects of this condition. Decrease in GH has been correlated with decreased energy levels.

Risk Factors:
- 1% to 3% per year bone mineral density decline
- 30% to 50% loss of lean body mass
- 80 million baby boomers now starting into somatopause in their mid-30s

Signs and Symptoms:
- Weight gain
- Lack of energy
- Sleep disturbance
- Reduced immune function
- Decreased muscle mass and bone density
- Increased homocysteine level
- Abnormal blood lipids
- Impaired glucose level

Differential Diagnoses:
- Menopause
- Andropause

Diagnostic Studies:
- GH stimulation test
- ICF-1 level in blood test
- Measurement of somatomedin C

Treatment
Pharmacologic:
- GH injections: Tesamorelin (Egrifta): Stimulates the pituitary gland to release GH, very costly, $1,500/month in injections
- Side effects: Difficult moving, muscle pain and stiffness, pain in joints, water retention, swelling of hands, ankles and feet, headache, pounding in ears, hypertension and cardiac effects, gynecomastia, GI intolerance, and insulin resistance

- Benefit: Puts on muscle like steroids, pulls off body fat, but no positive effect on oxygen consumption or muscle strength. Improved quality of life and restored physical capacity has been reported.
- Example: 28 lbs of fat lost off a 200 lbs frame
- After 6 months of GH treatment the effect is like reversal of 10 to 20 years of aging on lean muscle and adipose tissue.

Nonpharmacologic:
- Exercise regime with quick intense bursts of anaerobic exercise
- Example: Work muscles hard for 30 seconds, recover for 90 seconds, then repeat (eight cycles) in patterns like jump rope, stair climb, wind sprints.
- Must start program slow and build up endurance.

Acromegaly

Description of the Disease: A condition from pituitary producing too much growth hormone causing an increase in bone size and a range of other symptoms that develops gradually. This can be life threatening if not treated.

Epidemiology:
- Also known as hyperpituitarism. The condition can cause health issues such as hypertension, osteoarthritis, diabetes mellitus, precancerous growth of polyps in colon, carpal tunnel, sleep apnea, vision loss, uterine fibroids, and spinal cord compression.

Etiology:
- Over production of GH by pituitary triggers IGF-1 to stimulate bone and tissue growth. In adults usually tumor is a reason for increased GH release. It can be a nonpituitary tumor also lung, pancreas, or adrenal.

Risk Factors:
- Benign pituitary tumor (pituitary adenoma)
- Hyperplasia from excessive GHRH secretion from hypothalamus

Signs and Symptoms:
- Enlarged feet and hands (rings do not fit and shoe size is increasing)
- Deepened husky voice
- Coarsened enlarged facial features
- Shape of face changes over time: Jaw protruding (prognathism), thickened lips, wider spacing between teeth, enlarged tongue (macroglossia), prominent brow
- Excessive sweating and body odor
- Oily thickened skin and skin tags
- Snoring due to obstructed upper airway
- Increased chest size (barrel chest)
- Vision changes: Loss of vision acuity, peripheral vision, and blindness
- Headaches: Severe and central in focus
- Menstrual irregularities
- Excessive hair growth in women
- Unintentional weight gain
- Enlargement of liver, heart, kidneys, spleen
- Joint pain, limited movement, swelling of boney areas

Differential Diagnoses:
- Pituitary tumor
- Endocrine overactivity
- Thyroid hyperplasia

Diagnostic Studies:
- GH and IGF-1 Levels in fasting blood work (random GH level alone not recommended)
- Fasting glucose level and prolactin level
- GH suppression test: Checking blood levels before and after drinking glucose preparation
- MRI of brain: To view pituitary and also look at nonpituitary site
- Echocardiogram
- Colonoscopy to screen colon for neoplasia (after diagnosis confirmed)

Treatment
Nonpharmacologic:
- Surgery: Primary therapy for acromegaly, transsphenoidal approach to remove antipituitary tumors
- Imaging and blood levels 12 weeks post-op to confirm improvement
- Radiation: When tumor cells present after surgery, this treatment will decrease GH level from remaining cells and takes years for this treatment to noticeably improve the acromegaly
  - Conventional Radiation: Daily treatment for 4 to 6 weeks results may take up to 10 years to be fully effective
  - Stereotactic Radiosurgery (γ-knife) high-dose therapy and tumor cells limiting treatment not affecting surrounding tissues, brings GH levels back to normal in 3 to 5 years

Pharmacologic:
- If surgery not an option
  - Somatostatin analog: Synthetic versions of brain hormone somatostatin
    - Octreotide (Sandostatin)
    - Lanreotide (Somatuline Depot)
    - Action: Decreases GH level rapidly by suppressing GH secretion in the pituitary
    - Given SQ three times a day, if tolerated use long-acting form IM monthly in the office
  - Dopamine agonist: Oral medication
    - Cabergoline
    - Bromocriptine (Parlodel)
    - Action: This class may decrease GH and IGF-1 levels, may also decrease tumor size
    - Side effects: Compulsive behavior like gambling
  - GH antagonist
    - Pegvisomant (Somavert)
    - GH antagonist, blocks effects of GH on body tissue
    - Self-administer via SQ injection daily after loading dose at physician's Office
  - Signifor LAR if surgery in adequate response or surgery not possible
    - IM injection every 4 weeks in physician's office

Addison Disease

Description of the Disease: Chronic disorder that occurs when body produces insufficient amounts of adrenal gland hormones cortisol and aldosterone. This disorder is also known as primary adrenal insufficiency or hypocortisolism or hypoadrenalism.

Epidemiology:
- Occurs from destruction from autoimmune disease in 80% of cases. Age range seems to be 30 to 50 years old. Symptoms are slowly progressing in Addison disease.

Etiology:
- Occurs in all age groups of male and female, can be life threatening in Addison crisis that untreated can cause death. This disorder can be primary or secondary adrenal insufficiency.
- Primary adrenal insufficiency is caused within the adrenal gland. The gland is damaged and cannot produce enough cortisol and the adrenal hormone aldosterone is also missing. Autoimmune disease can cause this also.
- Secondary adrenal insufficiency is caused outside the gland like a pituitary tumor. The pituitary fails to produce enough ACTH that stimulates the adrenals to produce cortisol. Some of the causes of this can be a pituitary tumor causing pressure on the pituitary gland, severe infection, or severe head injury traumatizing the pituitary.
- APS Type 2: An autoimmune disorder that affects those age 18 to 30 that has conditions that include Addison disease, celiac disease, vitiligo, and diabetes.

Risk Factors:
- Autoimmune diseases:
  - Hypopituitarism, hypoparathyroidism, chronic thyroiditis, Type1 DM, vitiligo

Signs and Symptoms:
- Muscle weakness and fatigue
- Weight loss and decreased appetite
- Darkening of skin (hyperpigmentation)—classic finding

- Seen on distal portion of extremities and sun-exposed areas
- Low BP, even fainting—classic finding
- Salt craving
- Low blood glucose
- Nausea/vomiting/diarrhea
- Anorexia and weight loss
- Irritability
- Postural dizziness
- Headache
- Dehydration
- Depression
- Loss of body hair
- Sexual dysfunction in women
- Irregular menses

Differential Diagnoses:
- Adrenal crisis, adrenal hemorrhage, TB, eosinophilia, sarcoidosis, hyperkalemia, histoplasmosis

Diagnostic Studies:
- 24-hour urine cortisol collection
- Ultrasound to evaluate adrenal and pituitary for tumors or trauma
- ACTH-stimulation test: After dose of synthetic ACTH blood draws. Normal response would be increased in cortisol levels, in Addison disease due to secondary adrenal insufficiency or little response in cortisol levels.
- CRH stimulation test: If abnormal ACTH-stimulation test this is run to help determine a cause of insufficiency. CRH in a synthetic version is given and blood tested 30, 60, 90, and 120 minutes after. CRH will not stimulate ACTH secretion if the pituitary is damaged. No ACTH detected after the bolus indicates pituitary as the source. A delayed ACTH response shows hypothalamus as the cause of the problem.
- TB testing with a PPD skin test rules out the adrenal insufficiency is related to a tuberculosis infection in the body.

Treatment
Pharmacologic: Maintenance versus Crisis Treatment
- Maintenance therapy: Life long
  - **Replacement** of the missing cortisol with hydrocortisone tablets or prednisone tablets to mimic missing concentration; if aldosterone also missing, try supplement with fludrocortisone (Florinef). One-quarter of prednisolone dose equals hydrocortisone dose.
  - Avoid ketoconazole, P450 inducers such as rifampin, phenytoin, and barbiturates.
- Crisis treatment: IV injection of glucocorticoids in large amounts of saline with dextrose. Then when stable switch to oral glucocorticoids and possible fludrocortisone dose if an aldosterone deficiency.
  - For crisis, patient to carry an emergency corticosteroid injection

Nonpharmacologic: None
- Wear Medi-Alert bracelet to notify others in case of emergency.

Make emergency medical plan if any of the following situations:
- Pregnancy
- Infections
- Stress
- Injury
- Surgery

Cushing Syndrome

Description of the Disease: A condition that affects the body with a group of signs and symptoms after prolonged exposure to high cortisol levels.

Epidemiology:
- Pituitary adenoma can cause high cortisol, corticotropin produced elsewhere in the body such as a pancreatic cancer or lung cancer tumor, adrenal tumor causing increased cortisol or overuse of steroids in chronic disease states such as asthma and rheumatoid arthritis; if something is wrong with the adrenal gland the feedback to the pituitary or hypothalamus blocks the switch to turn off cortisol production so it continues.

Etiology:

- Occurs often in the 40s, age range from 20 to 50, females to males 3:1, those with chronic health issues requiring steroids are at greater risk. Overproduction of cortisol exists in patients with any of the following alcoholism, malnutrition, panic disorders, or depression.

Risk Factors:

- Corticosteroid long-term use with chronic disease

Signs and Symptoms:

- Dorsocervical hump (buffalo hump)
- Simple obesity/moon facies
- Obesity/weight gain (hallmark classic sign)
- Ecchymosis
- Headache/backache
- Abdominal pain
- Female balding but excessive facial hair
- Irregular menstrual cycles, or amenorrhea
- Hypertension
- Hyperglycemia
- Purple striae/stretch marks on abdomen, thighs, buttocks, arms, and breasts
- Males with impotence and decreased libido
- Severe fatigue
- Irritability and anxiety
- Thinning arms and legs
- Bone and muscle weakness

Differential Diagnoses:

- Diabetes type 2
- PCOS
- Adolescent weight gain
- Metabolic syndrome

Diagnostic Studies:

- DEXA Suppression test: Dexamethasone (a synthetic glucocorticoid) is given at night then blood level draws next morning, level is normal if 1.8 μg/dL
- If abnormal result with high cortisol and high ACTH this test points to pituitary tumor as the cause of Cushingoid symptoms. If test results show low ACTH and high cortisol an adrenal tumor is suspected.
- Salivary F. RIA: Cortisol tested when it is lowest when sleeping level done at night, watch sleep pattern to time correctly, normal (ELISA) < 4 nm/dL
- 24-hour Urine Free Cortisol: A urine collection of 24 hours' level
- CRH Stimulation Test: Baseline laboratory samples are drawn for ACTH and cortisol then after CRH bolus levels are monitored to differentiate tumor type: **Adrenal** causes low ACTH and high cortisol after the test, **pituitary** causes rise in ACTH and cortisol, **ectopic** tumors lung or oat cell cause high ACTH and high cortisol pretest and no change in levels after the bolus.
- CT scan or MRI of abdomen/chest/pelvis to rule out endocrine tumor
- CT scan to evaluate the adrenals and pituitary for tumors

Treatment:

Nonpharmacologic

- Surgery: Most common pituitary tumor (ACTH secreting pituitary adenoma) removed via transsphenoidal approach or adrenal tumor surgery, or post-op may require hormone replacement therapy
- Radiation: If surgery not possible or surgery fails to depress hormone level, 6-week course usually given

Pharmacologic

- Chemotherapy: If tumor exists such as in lung cancer
- Medications used alone or in combo: Ketoconazole (Nizoral), mitotane (Lysodren), or metyrapone (Metopirone) can be given to inhibit steroidogenesis, also known as medical adrenalectomy
- Mitotane (Lysodren) suppresses cortisol production
- After surgery replacement needed for ACTH that drops below normal, so replacement required.

Endocrine Cancers

MEN is a hereditary disorder of over activity and enlargement of endocrine glands. The glands affected are pituitary, thyroid, parathyroid, adrenal and pancreas. This overactivity causes neoplasia of both benign and malignant tumors. One generation seems to pass disorder to the next generation. Diagnosis: genetic blood tests, blood & urine hormone levels and CT/ultrasound to determine location of tumors.

Treatment: Tumor removal, thyroid gland removal or medication to suppress glands if surgery not possible. Currently there is no cure for MEN.

There are three types:
- **MEN 1:** Pituitary tumors, parathyroid tumors and pancreatic tumors
- **MEN 2a**: Medullary thyroid cancers, pheochromocytoma, parathyroid tumors
- **MEN 2b**: Medullary thyroid cancer, neuromas, pheochromocytoma

Parathyroid Carcinomas are very rare. PTH hormone levels are extremely high in the thousands versus the hundreds in hyperparathyroidism condition. Often a mild cancer, it is not aggressive, does not cause patient's death. Cure rate is best if treated early. Prognosis is based on if the carcinoma is in the glands or metastasized to lymph nodes or lung area. Because this form of cancer can reoccur up to 30 years later, yearly blood levels of PTH and calcium are suggested.

Polycystic Ovarian Syndrome

Description of the Disease: An endocrine, hormonal, disorder of reproductive-age women. Symptoms first appear in adolescence, around the start of menstruation. In some women they do not develop symptoms until their early to mid-20s and can persists through and beyond the reproductive years.

Epidemiology:
- Common disorder 4% to 18% of reproductive-age women
- Up to 20% of women overall have some androgen excess.
- Genetic component from inheritance
- Environmental exposure and weight gain
- Ovary produces excess levels of testosterone and androgen excess.
- Long-term risk of heart disease, diabetes from lipid imbalance of increased total cholesterol, increased triglycerides, and low HDL

Etiology:
- Also known as Stein–Leventhal syndrome, PCO, POD
- Ovaries are enlarged and contain small collections of fluid.
- Can develop in the response to gaining weight
- Less than eight menstrual cycles a year
- Hyperandrogenemia (high normal or slightly increased testosterone) OR
- Hyperandrogenism (hirsutism, acne, male pattern baldness)

Risk Factors:
- Infertility
- Nonalcoholic fatty liver (steatohepatitis)
- Sleep apnea
- Endometrial cancer (from long-term unopposed estrogen exposure)

Signs and Symptoms:
- Infrequent menses: >35 days between, fewer than eight times a year
- Prolonged menses: Light or heavy
- Excess hair growth (hirsutism face and body)
- Male pattern baldness
- Acne and oily skin
- Skin changes: Dark or thick skin markings in arm pits, groin, neck, and breasts
- Obesity
- Deepened voice
- Decreased breast size
- Enlarged clitoris

Differential Diagnoses:
- PCOS is a diagnosis of exclusion.
  - Secondary amenorrhea
  - Hypothyroidism
  - Congenital adrenal hyperplasia
  - Acromegaly
  - Cushing syndrome

Diagnostic Studies:
- Laboratory testing: Serum BHCG
  - Estrogen level
  - FSH (low or normal)
  - LH (elevated)
  - LH/FSH ratio (>3)
  - 17 Hydroxyprogesterone (17OHPG)
  - Testosterone level (free T normal 100 to 200 pg/dL)
  - Free testosterone level
  - Fasting blood glucose and fasting insulin level
  - Glucose tolerance test (GTT; 3 hour)
  - DHEAS-S level
  - Dexamethasone-stimulation test
  - Urinary free cortisol level
  - ACTH-stimulation test
  - Lipid panel
  - Thyroid function studies
  - Prolactin level
  - BUN/CR level
- Ultrasound: Vaginal/abdominal to view ovaries: Looking for 12 or more follicles per ovary confirms dx. With PCO (otherwise known as PCOS) the increased number of follicles seen on ultrasound can help confirm diagnosis.
- CAT scan or MRI to view adrenals and ovaries
- Pelvic laparoscopy

Treatment

Pharmacologic:
- Metformin 1,500 mg to 2,250 mg to help with weight loss and regulate menses, prevent Type 2 diabetes and gestational diabetes
- Clomid (clomiphene citrate) 50 to 100 mg × 5 days each cycle if attempting to conceive
- Spirolactone for acne and excess body hair
- Oral contraceptive pill (OCP) to help regulate cycle and slough endometrial lining
- Benzol peroxide for acne or clindamycin gel
- Prometrium (progesterone) to stabilize the endometrial lining
- Eflornithine topical gel for facial hair control
- Statin to control hyperlipidemia

Nonpharmacologic:
- Weight loss
- Exercise program
- Laser hair removal/electrolysis
- Surgery: Small portion of ovary destroyed via electric current or drilling process to ovary to hopefully restore ovulation

Diabetes

The disease of Diabetes has **four main types** from different causes and some **subsets** when diagnosing.
- Type 1: Selective β-cell destruction causes severe or absolute insulin deficiency, may have immune or idiopathic cause. Treated with insulin.

- Type 2: The tissue resistance to the action of insulin combined with a relative deficiency in insulin secretion. Treated with oral meds and diet and sometimes expands into insulin use.
- Latent autoimmune diabetes mellitus (LADA), also called type 1.5, a slowly progressing type 1 DM often misdiagnosed as type 2 in those 35 and older with autoimmune disorder and/or a family history of type 1 DM. Treated with insulin or metformin
- Type 3: Multiple other specific causes of the diabetes to develop including surgery, pancreatectomy, pancreatitis or from medication use interferon, glucocorticoids, dilantin, thiazides, and others and also from nonpancreatic disease
- Type 4: Gestational diabetes from placenta and placental hormones cause insulin resistance, most pronounced in third trimester of pregnancy
- Secondary diabetes: This is diabetes that develops from a secondary syndrome called endocrinopathies. Causes: acromegaly, Cushing syndrome, glucagonoma, somatostatinoma, pheochromocytoma, hyperthyroidism
- MODY (Maturity-Onset Diabetes of the Young) can display symptoms of both type 1 and type 2 diabetes, caused from mutations to multiple genes or a single gene, starts before age 25 in nonobese patients, requires blood testing to accurately diagnose.

Type 1 Diabetes

Description of the Disease: It is defined as selective β-cell destruction that leads to severe or absolute insulin deficiency

Epidemiology:
- 5% of all diabetic patients have Type 1 Diabetes

Etiology:
- This type of diabetes can be caused by autoimmune or idiopathic factors, 10 to 155 of these are family history, need to inherit risk factors from both parents. Autoantibodies are detectable in the blood years before symptoms develop.

Risk Factors:
- Attack of autoimmune disease
- Genetic disorder
- Family history
- Geography: Further away for the equator higher incidence of type 1 diabetes

Signs and Symptoms:
- Very hungry
- Increased urination
- Extreme thirst
- Sleepy
- Rapid weight loss
- Extreme fatigue and weakness
- Nausea/vomiting/irritability

Diagnostic Studies:
- Random blood glucose
- Hemoglobin A1C
- CBC (to look at WBC to rule out infections)
- Urine dip for ketones
- Measure Insulin levels
- Fructosamine level
- C peptide level and immune markers (if level of c peptide <0.6 mg/mL type 1 DM)

Treatment
  Nonpharmacologic:
- Carbohydrate counting
- Frequent blood glucose monitoring
- Eat healthy diet
- Exercise program

Pharmacologic:
- Insulin: Both human and human analog

Basal Insulin	Prandial Insulin
NPH (Humulin N, Novolin N)	Regular (Humulin R, Novolin) Short duration, slower acting
	Lispro (Humalog) Short duration, rapid acting
Glargine (Lantus)—long-duration	Aspart (Novolog) Short duration, rapid acting
Detemir (Levemir)—intermediate	Glulisine (Apidra) Short duration, rapid acting

Source: Blair, E. (2016). *Insulin a to z: A guide on different types of insulin.* Joslin Diabetes Center. www.joslin.org/info/insulin_a_to_zguide_on_different_types_of_insulin.html

- General: Therapy should consist of a basal insulin plus a bolus insulin that is given 15 minutes before each meal.
- Dose:
  - A minimum of two daily injections should be considered.
  - Many patients need three to four injections per day.
  - Normal starting dose is 10 units or empiric weight-based dosing can be used
  - Sliding scale can be used
  - Doses should be individualized according to the patient, and adjusted regularly, in 1 to 2 unit increments, based on blood glucose levels.
- Adverse Reactions: Hypoglycemia, hypokalemia, lipodystrophy, local reaction
  - Somogyi effect—may be mistaken for inadequate control
    - A rebound of hyperglycemia that occurs after an early morning episode of insulin-induced hypoglycemia
    - Happens at approximately 3:00 AM, the body overcompensates resulting in a high blood sugar.

Type 2 Diabetes

Description of the Disease: In this type of diabetes the body shows insulin resistance and is unable to produce enough insulin to keep the blood glucose level stable.

Epidemiology:
- 95% of all diabetic patients have Type 2 Diabetes
- 9.3% or 29.1 million of US population have type 2 diabetes: 21 million are diagnosed, 8.1 million are undiagnosed, 51% are older than age 65.
- There is an increase of 10 mg/dL in blood glucose per decade
- Decrease in β-cell function with aging at 1% per year
- Type 2: 90% of elderly with diabetes have type 2.
- Onset of symptoms of type 2 diabetes takes years to show.
- Inherited risk factor from both parents can lead to type 2 diabetes, environment, autoimmune, and idiopathic, other possible causes.

Etiology:
- Glucose builds up in the blood instead of going into the cells
- Insulin from the pancreas stimulates blood glucose to be removed from the blood and uptake into the muscle/fat cells/liver in type 2 diabetes this mechanism does not work
- Autoimmune destruction of β-cells can be a cause.

Source: McQueen, A.S. (2014) Adult-Gero. Review Book/Endocrine System.

Risk Factors:
- Overweight or obesity
- Sedentary lifestyle
- Age 45 years or older

- Family history (first-degree relative)
- Genetic predisposition
- Impaired fasting glucose
- Waist circumference: Men >40 inches women >35 inches
- Gestational diabetes (35% to 60% chance of developing diabetes type 2 in 10 years)
- Macrosomia (delivery of baby >9 pounds)
- Women with PCOS
- Hypertension
- Ethnicity/racial groups: African Americans, Hispanic/Latino Americans, American Indians, and some Pacific Islanders and Asian Americans

Signs and Symptoms:

- Very thirsty
- Frequent urinating
- Rapid weight loss
- Feeling very hungry
- Nausea/vomiting/irritable
- Extreme fatigue/weakness
- Skin infections that do not heal
- In women frequent yeast infections
- Excessive itching
- Dry itchy skin
- Velvety dark skin in areas
- Pins/needles feeling in the feet
- Blurred vision

Source: McQueen, A.S. (2014) Adult-Gero. Review Book/Endocrine System.

Signs and Symptoms in the Elderly:

- Classic signs of polydipsia, polyphagia, and polyuria when plasma glucose greater than 200. Presentation of new onset diabetes in elderly often include the following: dehydration, new urinary incontinence (polyuria), recurrent candidiasis in females, paresthesias, anorexia, confusion, delirium, vision change, slow wound healing

Differential Diagnoses:

- Type 1 diabetes
  - LADA
  - MODY

Diagnostic Studies:

- A1C (Hbg AIc) test to see the average of blood glucose levels in past 3 months
- Random glucose test for screening
- Fasting blood glucose to see effect after fasting
- Oral Glucose Tolerance Test (OGTT): Can diagnose prediabetes and diabetes by drawing fasting blood glucose, then give 75 mg glucose bolus followed by glucose blood levels drawn at 1, 2, and 3 hours.
- C-peptide level to differentiate from type 1 diabetes

Treatment
Pharmacologic:

- Initiation of therapy:
  - Asymptomatic patients with type 2 diabetes with blood glucose levels >126 mg/dL and <250 mg/dL should be started on oral diabetic agents.
  - Blood glucose levels >250 mg/dL, or with signs of hyperglycemia or ketosis, should be started on insulin therapy.
- Seven Classes of Oral Antidiabetic agents in USA
  - Insulin secretagogues (sulfonylureas, meglitinides, D-phenylalanine derivatives)
  - Biguanides
  - Thiazolidinediones
  - α-Glucosidase inhibitors
  - Incretin-based therapies
  - Amylin analog
  - Bile acid-binding sequestrants

- Most common start of oral medication is biguanides like metformin
- Metformin is inexpensive, has an excellent glycemic response, is weight-neutral, and has demonstrated a beneficial effect on cardiovascular outcomes
- Much more controversial is the choice of a second agent.
- Sulfonylureas—inexpensive and generally as effective as metformin
- Thiazolidinediones (glitazones)—when used with metformin will not result in hypoglycemia
- Insulin—which may be the most effective
- In patients with high levels of hyperglycemia (e.g., A1C > 8.5%), utilizing drug classes with greater and more rapid glucose-lowering effectiveness
  - Or in the alternative the earlier initiation of combination therapy is recommended.
- In patients with more modest hyperglycemia (e.g., A1C < 7.5%), medications with lesser potential to lower hyperglycemia and/or those drugs with a slower onset of action may be considered.
- If multiple agents no longer able to control HgBA1C consider starting insulin
  - Individualized drug therapy is important—knowledge of the patient's quantitative and qualitative meal patterns, activity levels, pharmacokinetics of insulin preparations, and pharmacology of oral antihyperglycemic agents are essential to individualize the treatment plan while optimizing the blood glucose control and minimizing risks for adverse effects.
  - All patients with DM should be on aspirin 81 mg daily, unless contraindicated.

Nonpharmacologic:
- Weight loss
- Diet modifications: Control of carbohydrates and healthy eating
- Cinnamon added to diet
- Blood glucose monitoring daily and recorded
- Regular exercise
- Careful monitoring of BP and lipid panel
- Foot check daily

Gestational Diabetes Mellitus

Description of the Disease: Glucose resistance that develops during pregnancy from placental hormone influence. Fetal pancreas responds to maternal elevated glucose by producing more insulin.

Epidemiology:
In most patients, resorts back to normal glucose tolerance postpartum
- 9.2% of pregnancy gestational diabetes mellitus (GDM) develops in third trimester.
- Increasing numbers as population is getting more obesity during reproductive years.
- 10% to 20% GDM patients will require insulin to reach glucose goal.

Etiology:
- Extra glucose in fetus is stored as fat, making baby grow larger (macrosomia).
- Risk of fetal size increases at delivery for complications such as shoulder dystocia

Risk Factors:
- Age
- + Family history
- BMI > 30
- Over age 35 years old
- Hypertension
- Unexplained stillborn or miscarriages
- Two out of three chances of repeat GDM with subsequent pregnancies
- Previous pregnancy with elevated BS

Signs and Symptoms:
- Usually none but if present
  - Nausea and vomiting
  - Increased urinating
  - Fatigue
  - Blurred vision
  - Increased thirst
  - Weight despite increased appetite

Diagnostic Studies:
- Glucose tolerance (1 hour 50 g) test at 24 to 28 weeks If >130 to 140 mg/dL abnormal
- Then 3 hours GTT: Four glucose samples drawn over 3 hours
- If two out of four levels abnormal diagnosed as GDM

Treatment:

Nonpharmacologic
- Blood glucose monitoring
- Diet monitoring with GDM diet: 35% fat, 45% carbohydrate, 20% protein 2,200 to 2,500 cal/d
- Monitoring fetal movement and growth and well-being

Pharmacologic:
- Glyburide (oral agent): Does not cross the placenta so is safe if diet not managing BS
- Metformin not recommended beyond first trimester (type 2 DM pregnant patient)
- Insulin: If oral medication not helping glucose to reach goal, frequently a combination of I intermediate-acting and fast-acting insulin

Diabetes Insipidus

Description of the Disease: Excessive urination and extreme thirst from inadequate output of the pituitary hormone ADH (vasopressin) or lack of kidney response to ADH

Epidemiology:

Three types of diabetes insipidus:
- Central: Caused by damage to the pituitary gland or hypothalamus vasopressin producing cells from:
  - Illness: Such as meningitis
  - Surgery
  - Brain tumor such as pituitary adenoma or craniopharyngioma
  - Inflammation or intracerebral occlusion
  - Head injury
- Nephrogenic: Kidneys unable to regulate ADH in the kidney tubules from the following:
  - Chronic kidney disorder
  - Polycystic kidney disease
  - Inherited disorder of gene AVP-NP11
  - Drugs can cause this also: Lithium (used in bipolar), demeclocycline (TCN antibiotic)
- Gestational diabetes: During pregnancy in some women with GD the placenta can destroy the ADH utilization in the patient.
  - Blood vessel supply to hypothalamus and pituitary gland may be compromised.

Etiology:
- ADP is manufactured in the hypothalamus and stored in the pituitary.
- ADP functions to keep body from excreting all body fluids and prevents dehydration.
- Can occur from syndromes such as Sheehan and Wolfram
- Also can occur in chronic conditions like hemochromatosis

Risk Factors:
- Illness: Encephalitis and meningitis
- Medication use
- Head trauma especially basal skull fracture
- Infection
- Stroke and lose of oxygen to the brain
- Surgery to brain

Signs and Symptoms:
- Thirst (polydipsia)
- Large amounts of urine produced (polyuria)
- Urine output up to 2 L/d
- Nocturia (in children/teens bedwetting)
- Poor tissue turgor
- Dry mucous membranes
- Constipation

- Anorexia and epigastric fullness
- Dizziness
- Muscle weakness
- Difficulty sleeping due to frequent risings with nocturia
- Disruption of daily activity such as work
- Irritability and difficulty concentrating

Differential Diagnoses:
- Bladder infection
- Urinary incontinence

Diagnostic Studies:
- Urinalysis: Findings of low Sp. Gr. less than 1.005 g, low osmolality 50 to 200 mOsm/kg
- MRI of the head: To look at abnormality of the pituitary
- Water Deprivation Test: Measure ADH during test of hydrating patient after fluid deprivation.

Treatment
Pharmacologic:
- Central diabetes insipidus:
  - Treated with desmopressin (DDAVP), a synthetic analog of natural pituitary ADH
  - Given as nasal spray, tablets, or injection
  - Body can be abnormal in ADH release, so dose may need to be regulated daily.
  - Signs of overdose: Lethargy, confusion, headache, sudden weight gain, difficulty urinating
- Gestational diabetes insipidus:
  - Treated with desmopressin (DDAVP) as nasal spray or tablets
  - Pregnancy category B so safe to use
  - Watch for signs of overdose of medication

Nonpharmacologic:
- Conserve patient's energy, short naps
- Nephrogenic diabetes insipidus:
  - Not treated with medications because kidneys do not responding to ADH
  - Low-salt diet to limit amount of urine produced
  - Hydrochlorothiazide can be useful for these patients to reverse urine

Review Section

Review Questions

1. In January, G.J., a 52year-old male, presents at an Urgent Care with main complaint of fatigue after 3-day history of URI: Congestion, cough, and resolved pharyngitis. Patient is a type 2 diabetic since age 45—taking Metformin 500 mg t.i.d. and Lantus 15 units every night. G.J. reports not as strict on his diet over the holidays but weight loss of 10 lbs. Baseline BP at Urgent Care was 96/70.

   Which diagnosis would NOT be in your differential?

   a. Addison disease
   b. Hypothyroidism
   c. Uncontrolled type 2 diabetes
   d. Hyperthyroidism

2. A 79-year-old woman is admitted to the ER with an asthma flare and corticosteroids are administered.

   Her BS is 229 in the hospital but next day after discharge at home her FBS is 121.

   What is the likely cause of the elevation of glucose?

   a. Age-related increase in nonfasting glucose
   b. New-onset type 2 diabetes
   c. Normal FBS increase to glucose level with stress
   d. Steroid medication induced hyperglycemia

3. J.L. is a 44-year-old female; all EXCEPT which of the following conditions could lead to developing Cushing syndrome in this patient?

   a. Ectopic hormone production by a neoplasm
   b. Atrophy of the adrenal gland
   c. An adrenal adenoma
   d. Hypothalamic–pituitary hyperfunction

4. Which of the following is NOT a characteristic of a newly diagnosed 35-year-old patient with type 2 diabetes?

    a. Relatively insensitive to insulin
    b. Likely to have an elevated BMI
    c. Prone to diabetic ketoacidosis
    d. Abnormal lipid profile with elevated cholesterol, LDL, and triglycerides but decreased HDL

5. In relation to MEN (Multiple Endocrine Syndrome) all of the following are true EXCEPT:

    a. parathyroid cancer, although rarely runs in families.
    b. medullary familial thyroid cancer in 5- to 18-year-olds is directly related.
    c. genetic testing is not available yet for diagnosis of MEN.
    d. pancreatic cancer can be linked to MEN1.

6. As a Nurse Practitioner you overhear a 50-year-old women complain to her hairdresser about changes in her hair, both on her scalp and body hair as well. Which disorder would be the LEAST of your differential diagnoses for this woman?

    a. Menopausal hypogonadism
    b. Hypothyroidism
    c. Cushing syndrome
    d. Hyperthyroidism

7. J.M. is a 57-year-old male with history of asthma reports increased thirst and urinary frequency in the past month. Before laboratory studies or other assessments, which disorder would NOT be in your differential diagnosis?

    a. Type 2 diabetes
    b. GH-secreting tumor
    c. ACTH-secreting tumor
    d. Prolactin-secreting tumor

8. B.N. is a 38-year-old African American male who works for a chemical company. He comes to the office complaining of fatigue and abdominal and back pain. Which is NOT a risk factor for having pancreatic CA?

    a. Chemical exposure at employment
    b. Age <40
    c. Weight gain/obesity
    d. Tobacco use

9. The mother of an 11-year-old girl brings her daughter for annual physical examination. The mother is concerned by her daughter's breast buds and wants to know when she might reach menarche. The correct answer would be:

    a. 1 year
    b. 2 years
    c. 3 years
    d. 4 years

10. G. S. was newly diagnosed by her GYN with Polycystic Ovarian Syndrome (PCOS). What is NOT a risk factor she needs to worry about with this diagnosis?

    a. Diabetes
    b. Hyperlipidemia
    c. Heart disease
    d. Increased breast size

Answers with Rationales

1. (b) Hypothyroidism

    Rationale: Hypothyroidism could definitely contribute to fatigue, and autoimmune component cannot be ruled out, BUT weight loss does not fit the description of hypothyroidism nor hypotension.

    Addison disease could contribute to the fatigue by hypotension and consider asking about skin pigmentation changes.

    Type 2 diabetes not controlled could lead to fatigue and weight loss as body attempts to rid itself of excess glucose. Patient did mention not good diet control over the holidays. Sudden onset of fatigue also is associated with hypoglycemia if diet and insulin are not consistent in delivery.

    Hyperthyroidism can cause a gradual onset of fatigue as the body is in state of constant metabolic rate. Look to onset of other symptoms and change in tolerance of activities of daily living.

2. (d) Steroid medication induced hyperglycemia

    Rationale: One elevated BS does not lead to new diagnosis of type 2 DM. With the aging process there is a 10 mg/dL/decade increase in nonfasting blood glucose. The level can correct back to normal an hour later. β-Cell function decreases with age increasing the blood sugar normally. Asthma is treated with glucocorticoids that stimulate glucose production in cells particularly in the liver, which increase the glucose level.

3. (b) Atrophy of the adrenal gland

Rationale: Atrophy of the adrenal gland would cause decreased production of cortisol and ACTH therefore not putting J.L at risk of Cushing syndrome. A neoplasm stimulates excess hormones to be produced putting her at risk. The adrenal adenoma functions by over production of cortisol. The hypothalamic–pituitary hyperfunction causes the hypothalamus to release excess ACTH.

4. (c) Prone to diabetic ketoacidosis

Rationale: Ketoacidosis is a risk with type 1 diabetes is rarely seen in type 2 diabetes without a predisposing event. Type 2 diabetes is the body's response to being insensitive to insulin. The BMI is likely elevated in someone with early onset type 2 diabetes. Abnormal lipid metabolism and high elevation are part of type 2 diabetes' presentation.

5. (c) genetic testing is not available yet for diagnosis of MEN.

Rationale: Genetic blood testing as well as measuring hormone levels in blood and urine are crucial to the diagnosis of MEN. Medullary thyroid cancer affects young patients, and early treatment with surgery is recommended. Pancreatic cancer is related to MEN1 because one-third of islet cell tumors are cancerous. Parathyroid cancers can be linked to either MEN1 or noncancerous MEN2a.

6. (c) Cushing syndrome

Rationale: Cushing syndrome. Estrogen deficit in hypogonadism leads to hair loss as hair becomes dyssynchronous in growth cycle. Hypothyroidism can cause a change to texture of hair making it coarser. Hyperthyroidism causes hair to become fine. Cushing syndrome peaks at ages 25 to 40 and causes hirsutism.

7. (d) Prolactin-secreting tumor

Rationale: Prolactin-secreting tumor does not elevate the blood glucose like type 2 diabetes. GH-secreting tumors and ACTH-secreting tumors elevate blood sugar. As an asthmatic he may be using high level of glucocorticoids also that could lead to increased glucose causing urinary symptoms.

8. (b) Age <40

Rationale: Age at diagnosis is normally over age 45, highest risk at age 60 to 80. Occupational chemical exposure is a risk factor as well as obesity or being overweight. Tobacco use is also a known risk factor.

9. (c) 3 years.

Rationale: From the development of breast buds to first menses is on average 2 to 4 years. She is 11 and the average age of menarche is 13 years old, so she is well within range.

10. (d) Increased breast size

Rationale: The condition PCOS often causes a decrease in breast tissue. The increase in lipid panel numbers makes higher risk for heart disease and diabetes complications.

Suggested Readings

Beckman, C., Ling, F., Herbert, W., Laube, D., Smith, R., . . . Weiss, P. (2014). *Obstetrics and gynecology* (7th ed.). Philadelphia, PA: WoltersKluwer Lippincott Williams & Wilkins.

Bilezikian, J. P., & Silverberg, S. J. (2004). Clinical practice. Asymptomatic primary hyperparathyroidism. *New England Journal of Medicine, 350*(17), 1746–1751.

Borawski, D., & Bluth, M. H. (2011). Reproductive function and pregnancy. In: R. A. McPherson & M. R. Pincus (Eds.). *Henry's clinical diagnosis and management by laboratory methods* (22nd ed.). Philadelphia, PA: Elsevier Saunders.

Chakrabarty, A. D. (2013). Adult primary hypoparathyroidism: A rare presentation. *Indian Journal of Endocrinology and Metabolism, 17*(Suppl. S1), 201–202.

Cooper, O., Geller, J. L., & Melmed, S. (2008). Ovarian hyperstimulation syndrome caused by an FSH-secreting pituitary adenoma. *Nature Clinical Practice. Endocrinology & Metabolism, 4*(4), 234–238. doi:10.1038/ncpendmet0758

Ezzat, S., Asa, S. L., Couldwell, W. T., Barr, C. E., Dodge, W. E., Vance, M. L., & McCutcheon, I. E. (2004). The prevalence of pituitary adenomas: A systematic review. *Cancer, 101*(3), 613–619. doi:10.1002/cncr.20412. PMID 15274075.

Hatcher, R., Trussell, J., Nelson, A., Cates, W., Stewart, F., & Kowal, D. (2011). *Contraceptive technology* (20th ed.). Atlanta, GA: Ardent Media.

Hillier, T., & Pedula, K. (2001). Characteristic of an adult population with newly diagnosed type 2 diabetes: The relation of obesity and the age of onset. *Diabetes Care, 24*(9), 1522–1527. doi:10.2337/diacare.24.9.1522

Hoffman, A., Lieberman, S. A., Butterfield, G., Thompson, J., Hintz, R. L., Ceda, G. P., & Marcus, R. (1997). Functional consequences of the somatopause and its treatment. *Endocrine, 7*(1), 73–76.

Katznelson, L., Laws, E. R., Jr., Melmed, S., Molitch, M. E., Murad, M. H., Utz, A., & Wass, J. A. (2014). Acromegaly: An endocrine society clinical practice guideline. *Journal of Clinical Endocrinology and Metabolism*, 99(11), 3933–3951.

Kepper, P. J., & Baum, N. (2014). Managing hypoandrogenism in the aging man. *Consultant. 54*(2), 102–104. Retrieved from www.consulatant 360.com.

Life Extension. *Adrenal disorders (Addison's Disease & Cushing's Syndrome)*. Retrieved from http://www.lef.org/Protocols/Metabolic-Health/Adrenal-Disorders/Page-08

Lake, M. G., Krook, L. S., & Cruz, S. (2013). Pituitary adenomas: An overview. *American Family Physician*, 88(5), 319–327.

Lamberts, S., van den Beld, A., & van der Lely, A. (1997). The endocrinology of aging. *Science*, 278(5337), 419–424. doi:10.1126/science 278.5337.419

Lee, Y. (2014). Androgen deficiency syndrome in older people. *Journal American Association of Nurse Practitioners, 26*, 179–186.

Mandal, A. (2013). *Diabetes insipidus pathophysiology*. Retrieved from http://www.news-medical.net/health/Diabetes-Insipidus-Pathophysiology.aspx

Melmed, S., Kleinberg, D., & Ho, K. (2011). Pituitary physiology and diagnostic evaluation. In S. Melmed, D. Kleinberg, & K. Ho (Eds.). *Williams' textbook of endocrinology* (12th ed.). Philadelphia, PA: Saunder Elsevier.

Moran, L. J., Hutchison, S. K., Norman, R. J., & Teede, H. J. (2011). Lifestyle changes in women with polycystic ovary syndrome. *Cochrane Database of Systematic Reviews*, (2), CD007506. doi:10.1002/14651858.CD007506.pub3

NIH. (2014, January). Information on Endocrine and Metabolic Diseases: Adrenal Insufficiency and Addison's Disease. NIH Publication No. 14–3054.

Papaleontiou, M., & Haymart, M. R. (2012). Approach to and treatment of thyroid disorders in the elderly. *Medical Clinics of North America*, 96(2), 297–310. doi:10.1016/j.mcna.2012.01.013

Radosh, L. (2009). Drug treatments for polycystic ovary syndrome. *American Family Physician*, 79(8), 671–676.

Reiter, R. J. (1995). The pineal gland and melatonin in relation to aging: A summary of the theories and of the data. *Experiential Gerontology, 30*(3–4), 199–212.

Rudman, D., Feller, A. G., Nagraj, H. S., Gergans, G. A., Lalitha, P. Y., & Goldberg, A. F. (1990). Effects of growth hormone in men over 60 years old. *New England Journal of Medicine*, 323, 1–6. doi:10.1056/NEJM199007053230101

Sattler, F. R. (2013). Growth hormone in the aging male. *Best Practice and Research. Clinical Endocrinology and Metabolism*, 27(4), 541–555. doi:10.1016/j.beem.2013.05.003. PMID 24054930.

Song, C. M., Jung, J. H., Ji, Y. B., Min, H. J., Ahn, Y. H., & Tae, K. (2014). Relationship between hypoparathyroidism and the number of parathyroid glands preserved during thyroidectomy. *World Journal of Surgical Oncology*, 12, 200.

Touchy, T., & Jett, K. (2012). *Eversoele & Hess' toward healthy aging: Human needs & nursing response* (p. 52, 8th ed.). St Louis, MO: Elsevier Mosby.

Tong, I. L. (2013). Nonpharmacological treatment of postmenopausal symptoms. *Obstetrician & Gynaecologist, 15*(1),19–25.

Zhang, G., Li, J., Purkayastha, S., Tang, Y., Zhang, H., Yin, Y., . . . Cai, D. (2013). Hypothalamic programming of systemic ageing involving IKK-β, NF-κB and GnRH. *Nature*, 497(7448), 211–216. doi:10.1038/nature12143

Chapter 11

Hematopoietic System

Mary L. Wilby

Case Presentation

Directions: Carefully review the case study presented below. At the end of the chapter, answer the review questions. Compare your answers to the correct answers listed in the Review Section.

History of Present Illness: A 76-year-old man presents to his primary care provider with a complaint of increasing fatigue over the last 2 to 3 months. He also notes shortness of breath, especially when walking up stairs or carrying groceries to his car. He has difficulty when climbing stairs, having to stop midway up a flight to catch his breath. He has previously been in good health, with mild hypertension treated with a diuretic and arthritis managed with over-the-counter nonsteroidal anti-inflammatory drugs. He has not noticed any change in the color of his stools.

Review of Systems:
He denies any chest pain, palpitations, or nausea. He has a good appetite and denies any weight loss. He denies any change in his bowel habits or abdominal pain. He has a history of intermittent constipation. He reports that his arthritis "has been acting up." He has occasional nocturia and denies any urgency, frequency, or changes in urine color. He denies numbness or tingling in hands or feet. He has had no change in sleep patterns. He denies feeling sad or hopeless.

Current Medications:
Hydrochlorothiazide 25 mg and ibuprofen 400 to 600 mg three to four times daily.

Medical and Surgical History:
The patient reports an inguinal hernia repair in 1989 and pneumonia in 1997. He has benign prostatic hypertrophy and hypertension.

Family History:
There is no family history of blood disorders. His mother died at age 78 of stroke, she had hypertension and diabetes. His father died at age 69 of emphysema, he smoked cigarettes and had hypertension. His son is 56 years old and has hypertension. His daughter is 47 and has no known health problems.

Social History:
Patient is widowed with two adult children, both living out of state. He is a retired machinist. He served in the Army for 8 years. He is a former 30-pack-year smoker who quit smoking 20 years ago. He drinks alcohol occasionally; he has no current sexual partners. He denies ever using any illicit drugs.

Health Maintenance:
Patient is up to date with immunizations, including influenza and pneumococcal vaccines; he declined the herpes zoster vaccine. Last colonoscopy was 5 years ago with no abnormalities noted.

Physical Examination:
General: Patient is well groomed and appears his stated age. He is in no acute distress.
Vital Signs: Temperature = 97.8°F   Heart rate = 76   Respiratory rate = 16   BP = 130/86

Head, Eyes, Ears, Nose, Throat (HEENT): Head is normocephalic, atraumatic. Conjunctivae are pale. Tympanic membranes are intact. No nasal discharge. Pharynx is without exudate; tonsils are +1. No cervical lymphadenopathy. Trachea is midline; thyroid not enlarged, nontender, no nodules.

Heart: regular rate and rhythm, no murmurs or gallops

Lungs: Clear to auscultation, no accessory muscle use

Abdomen/Gastrointestinal: Nondistended, normal bowel sounds, soft, nontender. No hepatosplenomegaly, no palpable masses. No stool in rectal vault

Extremities: No edema, no cyanosis or clubbing

Neurologic: Awake, alert and oriented $\times 3$, affect appropriate.

Musculoskeletal: Positive crepitus in both knees, Heberden nodes bilaterally

Skin: Diffuse pallor, no rashes, no bruising, or petechiae

Assessment

Anemia, unknown etiology

Differential Diagnoses:

- Iron deficiency associated with gastrointestinal blood loss
- Vitamin B_{12} deficiency
- Folate deficiency
- Myelodysplasia
- Multiple myeloma

Plan

Diagnostic Studies:

Complete blood count (CBC) with differential, serum ferritin, serum B_{12} and folate levels, stool for fecal occult blood (FOB), endoscopic gastroduodenoscopy (EGD), and colonoscopy.

Diagnostic studies demonstrated the following: CBC with microcytic anemia MCV 76, MCH 22 pg/cell, MCHC 28%, with hemoglobin 10.8 g/dL, hematocrit 32, WBC 5.1×10^3, serum ferritin level 28 ng/mL, B_{12} level 300 pg/mL, folate level 5.8 ng/mL. Urinalysis negative for blood or protein. EGD revealed duodenal ulcer, likely associated with NSAIDs, and colonoscopy was negative for malignancy, two benign polyps were removed. Cultures done at the time of the EGD were negative for *Helicobacter pylori* infection.

The diagnosis of iron deficiency anemia was made. Blood loss was most likely associated with use of ibuprofen taken for his arthritis.

The patient was contacted to discuss the results of his evaluation. The ibuprofen was discontinued, and a regimen of acetaminophen 1,000 mg every 8 hours as needed for pain was recommended. In addition, he was instructed to begin Lansoprazole 30 mg daily. Treatment of iron deficiency anemia was begun. The patient was instructed to begin ferrous sulfate 325 mg three times daily, taken with orange juice. Taken with ascorbic acid, iron absorption is enhanced (Teucher, Olivares, & Cori, 2004). Follow-up was scheduled for repeat laboratory evaluation to reassess the hemoglobin and hematocrit. The patient was advised to contact the office for any signs or symptoms of bleeding, including blood in stool, increased fatigue or weakness, dizziness, or shortness of breath. The patient will schedule follow-up with gastroenterology as per their recommendation for repeat colonoscopy regarding polyps.

The Hematopoietic System

Understanding the causes of anemia and other blood disorders requires understanding the hematopoietic system and hematopoiesis, blood cell development, and the functions of the hematopoietic system. Blood cells and blood components circulate by way of the cardiovascular system. Cells are suspended in a solution of protein and other materials and delivered to all parts of the body, allowing all of critical functions to take place. Blood functions to transport materials are needed for cellular metabolism, to eliminate waste products of cellular metabolism, to maintain acid–base balance, and to protect the body from microorganisms and injury

(Rote & McCance, 2010a). Mature blood cells are relatively short lived and are generated from stem cells, which are present throughout life to replace the progenitors and precursors of hematopoietic cells lines. Stem cells are capable of regeneration to create new stem cells able to produce all blood cell types (Orkin & Zon, 2008).

Blood Plasma

Plasma makes up approximately one-half of blood volume. In addition to a number of organic and inorganic elements, plasma contains a large quantity of proteins. These plasma proteins differ in structure and function and are categorized in two primary groups, globulins and albumin. The majority of plasma proteins are produced in the liver; however, immunoglobulins, or antibodies, are produced by plasma cells in lymphoid tissue (Rote & McCance, 2010a). A third type of plasma protein is fibrinogen, the inactive precursor of fibrin, which is required for blood clot formation (Kotter & Trevithick, 2013).

Albumin acts primarily to facilitate the passage of water and solutes through the vascular system. Molecules are large and unable to diffuse freely across vascular endothelium and are critical in maintaining colloidal osmotic and hydrostatic pressure. Albumin acts as a carrier molecule for drugs that are poorly soluble in water as well as for blood components (Rote & McCance, 2010a).

Other plasma proteins include clotting factors, regulatory hormone and complement proteins. Transport proteins are able to bind and carry other important molecules including iron, copper, and vitamins. Lipids, triglycerides, phospholipids, and other substances are carried in the blood as complexes when combined with plasma proteins. Proteins such as cytokines perform important functions in communication between cells. Plasma also contains charged particles important for cell function and maintaining acid–base balance (Rote & McCance, 2010a).

Cellular Components of Blood

The amount of cellular components in the blood varies with age, but hematopoietic stem cells maintain and replace all types of blood cells and are activated by the changing needs of blood in the periphery (Granick, Simon, & Borjesson, 2012). Cellular components of the blood include red blood cells (RBCs; erythrocytes), platelets (thrombocytes), and white blood cells (WBCs; leukocytes). WBCs are further divided into more specific categories based on their structure and functions.

RED BLOOD CELLS

RBCs are the most plentiful cells in the blood with normal concentration ranging from 4.2 to 6.2 million cells/mm^3. RBCs account for approximately 48% of blood volume in men and 42% in women. RBCs contain hemoglobin, which carries gases and buffers blood pH. Fully developed RBCs do not have a nucleus or cytoplasmic organelles and are unable to carry out protein synthesis. Unable to carry out mitosis, RBCs have a limited lifespan ranging from 80 to 120 days (Kotter & Trevithick, 2013). When no longer able to carry out their functions, they are removed from the circulation and replaced with new cells. The RBCs' size and shape facilitate their ability to serve as gas carriers. The RBCs' biconcave shape allows optimal gas diffusion and its ability to change shape as it passes through capillaries and sinusoids in the spleen (Rote & McCance, 2010a).

WHITE BLOOD CELLS (LEUKOCYTES)

WBCs serve to defend against infection and remove debris from dead and damaged cells. The average adult has 5,000 to 10,000 WBCs per cubic millimeter of blood (Kotter & Trevithick, 2013). WBCs are classified either as granulocytes or agranulocytes, or as phagocytes or immunocytes. Granulocytes contain granules in their cytoplasm that contain enzymes, which when activated are able to kill microorganisms and destroy debris created during phagocytosis. Additionally, granules also contain other mediators that are active during inflammation and immune functions. Granulocytes include neutrophils, basophils, and eosinophils. All are phagocytes. Agranulocytes, including monocytes, macrophages, and lymphocytes, contain few granules in the cytoplasm (Rote & McCance, 2010a).

Neutrophils are the most numerous of the granulocytes. Immature neutrophils are called bands, while mature cells are called segmented neutrophils owing to their central nucleus divided into distinct segments. Neutrophils reach maturity while in the bone marrow. Maturation typically takes 14 days, but the process may be accelerated in the presence of infection or use of colony stimulating factors (CSFs). When bacteria invade the body, neutrophils travel out of the capillaries to ingest and destroy microorganisms and the debris associated with this activity and die within a day or two. The cytoplasmic granules contain enzymes that dissolve the cellular debris and promote healing (Rote & McCance, 2010a).

Basophils contain cytoplasmic granules containing chemotactic factors, histamine, proteolytic enzymes, and heparin. Activation of basophils stimulates production of vasoactive substances including leukotrienes and cytokines, such as interleukin. While the exact functions of basophils is not well understood, they are often found at sites of allergic reactions and parasitic infection. Mast cells are very similar to basophils but are generated from a different type of precursor cell in the bone marrow. Mast cells migrate into tissue as immature forms and play an important role in inflammation and healing, especially in the submucosa of the gastrointestinal and respiratory tracts and the dermis (Rote & McCance, 2010a).

Eosinophils are also capable of phagocytosis. They are also capable of ingesting antigen–antibody complexes as well as viruses. Eosinophils can also be induced to attack parasites by chemotactic factors contained in mast cells. Eosinophil granules contain histamine and other substances involved in the inflammatory process (Rote & McCance, 2010a).

Lymphocytes are the primary blood cells involved in the immune response. Most lymphocytes circulate for a short time in the blood stream and then migrate to lymphoid tissue as mature T cells, B cells, or plasma cells. Depending on the type and subtype, the lifespan of lymphocytes can be days, weeks, or years. Natural killer (NK) cells, which appear as large granular lymphocytes, have the ability to kill certain types of tumor cells and viruses without previous exposure to these antigens unlike T cytotoxic cells, which are activated after exposure to an antigen. NK cells are also able to produce several cytokines important in immune responses (Rote & McCance, 2010a).

Monocytes and macrophages constitute the mononuclear phagocyte system, sometimes referred to as the reticuloendothelial system. These active phagocytes are involved in inflammatory and immune functions. They also ingest dead and damaged blood cells. Monocytes are formed and released by the bone marrow, then migrate to lymphoid and other tissue where they develop into tissue macrophages and myeloid dendritic cells. Macrophages typically remove old and damaged cells from the bloodstream. Macrophages also act as important antigen processing and antigen presenting cells that initiate immune responses. They are also active in wound healing and tissue remodeling and secrete a variety of active substances involved in inflammation (Rote & McCance, 2010a).

PLATELETS

Platelets are disk-shaped cytoplasmic fragments rather than true cells that are essential for blood coagulation. They are created by fragmentation of large megakaryocytes. Without a nucleus or DNA, they are unable to perform mitosis. The majority of platelets are found in the peripheral circulation while approximately one-third are held in reserve in the spleen. Cytoplasmic granules contained in platelets are activated when stimulated by damage to blood vessels with release of a number of substances necessary for coagulation. Platelets typically circulate for 10 days before being removed by macrophages (Rote & McCance, 2010a).

The lymphoid system is closely connected to the hematopoietic system. Lymphoid tissue is classified as either primary or secondary tissue. Primary lymphoid tissue includes the thymus and the bone marrow. Secondary lymphoid organs include the spleen, lymph nodes, Peyer patches in the small intestine, and tonsils. The hematopoietic and immune systems are connected by the lymphoid organs as they are the sites of activity of lymphocytes, monocytes, and macrophages (Banasik, 2013; Rote & McCance, 2010a).

The spleen is the largest of the secondary lymphoid organs. It is involved in fetal hematopoiesis. After birth, monocytes in the spleen serve to mount immune responses. It also serves as a reservoir for blood cells. Located in the left upper quadrant of the abdomen, the adult spleen is approximately the size of a fist. Compartments in the spleen contain collections of lymphoid tissue known as splenic pulp. The pulp is filled with a network of blood vessels which are capable of expanding to store blood. While not absolutely necessary for life, absence of the spleen may result in a variety of effects. These effects include leukocytosis, decreased iron levels, and impaired immune function, resulting in increased susceptibility to infection by some forms of bacteria (Banasik, 2013; Rote & McCance, 2010a).

Lymph Nodes

Lymph nodes are distributed throughout the body providing filtration of lymph fluid as it travels through the lymphatic vessels. Lymph nodes function as part of the hematologic and immune systems and are the initial site of interaction between antigens and lymphocytes. Lymphocytes enter the lymph nodes by migrating across the endothelial lining. Macrocytes contained in the lymph nodes filter debris, foreign substances, and microorganisms from the lymph fluid and act on antigens. B lymphocytes multiply in response to antigens during infection. This process may result in enlargement of lymph nodes (Banasik, 2013; Rote & McCance, 2010a).

Hematopoiesis

Blood cell production or hematopoiesis is an ongoing process, occurring in utero in the spleen and liver and in the bone marrow (medullary hematopoiesis) after birth. Extramedullary blood production in adults is typically associated with disease. The process requires stimulation of undifferentiated stem cells to undergo mitosis and development (differentiation) to differentiate into mature blood cells. Erythrocytes and granulocytes typically differentiate completely in the bone marrow before entering the peripheral blood while monocytes and lymphocytes continue to mature in the blood and secondary lymphatic organs. Hematopoiesis continues throughout life and increases as needed as to replace cells lost through hemorrhage or abnormal cell destruction, injury, or infection (Rote & McCance, 2010a).

Bone marrow is the primary site of hematopoietic blood stem cells. Active red or hematopoietic marrow is supplied with blood with the arteries of the bones. Yellow or inactive marrow consists primarily of fat which gives it its yellow color. Red marrow is found primarily in the flat bones of the pelvis, vertebrae, cranium, mandible, sternum, and ribs as well as the most proximal portions of the humeri and femurs. Yellow marrow is found in the cavities of other bones. Bone marrow mesenchymal stem cells are capable of differentiating into fibroblasts, osteoblasts, and adipocytes. Bone marrow fibroblasts secrete a variety of cytokines required for hematopoiesis to take place, including granulocyte–macrophage colony stimulating factor (GM-CSF) and macrophage colony stimulating factor (M-CSF). Bone marrow macrophages secrete cytokines that control growth of hematopoietic progenitor cells. Osteoclasts present in the bone function to remodel bone but also have the capacity to produce cytokines that influence growth of hematopoietic cells (Rote & McCance, 2010a).

All blood cells originate from common hematopoietic stem cells that grow and mature under the influence of cytokines and growth factors. This process requires that cells enter different pathways to differentiate into more differentiated stem cells before committing to a particular cell line. Stem cells are self-renewing, keeping the number of stem cells available relatively constant. A variety of cytokines including CSFs, also called hematopoietic growth factors, trigger growth of progenitor cells and their offspring and initiate the process of maturation into fully mature blood cells. CSFs are produced by a variety of cells including fibroblasts, endothelial cells, and lymphocytes (Rote & McCance, 2010a).

Erythropoiesis

Erythropoiesis or RBC production begins with proliferation of erythroid progenitor cells. These cells then differentiate into proerythroblasts, which are committed to developing into erythroid cells. Proerythroblasts are able to produce proteins and differentiate through a number of intermediate cell forms of erythroblasts while making hemoglobin and removing most intracellular structures including the cell nucleus. The maturing erythroblast is smaller and begins to assume the shape of the mature RBC. Hemoglobin content increases as the nuclear size decreases. The last immature form of the cell is the reticulocyte, which has mesh-like (reticular) network of RNA, which is visible under the microscope when stained. The reticulocyte matures into a RBC within 24 to 28 hours. During this final maturation period, the cell becomes smaller and more disk shaped. Additionally, the cells lose their ability to synthesize hemoglobin. The normal reticulocyte count is approximately 1% of the total RBC count. It can serve as an index of RBC production (Rote & McCance, 2010a).

The process of erythropoiesis is primarily under the control of a feedback loop that involves erythropoietin (EPO). EPO is secreted by the peritubular cells of the kidneys as well as the liver when tissue hypoxia is present. Increasing levels of EPO trigger proliferation and differentiation of proerythroblasts in the bone marrow. Normal erythropoiesis cannot take place without adequate amounts of essential nutrients including protein, vitamins B_{12}, folate, B_6, riboflavin, pantothenic acid, niacin, ascorbic acid, vitamin E, iron, and copper (Kotter & Trevithick, 2013; Rote & McCance, 2010a).

When removed from the circulation via the spleen, they are replaced by new cells (Rote & McCance, 2010a). Blood cell production or hematopoiesis is typically a continuous process in the bone marrow, with production of new cells in response to the need for replacement cells as cells are removed from the circulation. All blood cells originate from hematopoietic stem cells and differentiate into various forms under the influence of cytokines and growth factors. Erythropoiesis occurs as erythroid progenitor cells differentiate into proerythroblasts. Subsequently, the proerythroblasts, which are able to produce proteins, differentiate into erythroblasts and synthesize hemoglobin. During this process, much of the intracellular structures, including the nucleus, are removed. This allows the cells to assume their mature size and shape. The final stage, before reaching maturity, creates the reticulocyte. As the reticulocyte matures into the erythrocyte, it loses any remaining reproductive capacity as the mature RBC is finally formed. Reticulocytes are released into the bloodstream and migrate to the spleen as they complete the maturation process. In the absence of disease, the reticulocytes account for approximately 1% of the total RBC count. Monitoring of the reticulocyte count can be very useful as an indication of erythropoietic activity. The principle regulator of RBC production is EPO. In the presence of hypoxia in the tissues, EPO is secreted by the kidney and to some extent, the liver. This in turn stimulates the process of proerthyroblast production in the marrow (Rote & McCance, 2010a).

Hematopoiesis and development of hemoglobin requires the availability of necessary nutrients including minerals, vitamins, and protein. When any of these are lacking for an extended period of time RBC production is reduced with subsequent anemia. Lack of vitamins, including vitamin B_{12}, folate, vitamin B_6, riboflavin, pantothenic acid, niacin, ascorbic acid, and vitamin E, can interfere with hematopoiesis. The most important of these nutrients are vitamin B_{12} and folate. Absorption of vitamin B_{12} in the small intestine requires the presence of intrinsic factor produced in the parietal cells in the stomach; anemia associated with absence of intrinsic factor with resulting vitamin B_{12} deficiency is referred to as pernicious anemia. Folate is required for adequate maturation of RBCs and is absorbed from the small intestine. Folate stores in the body can be depleted quickly and anemia associated with folate deficiency typically occurs more quickly than vitamin B_{12} deficiency (Rote & McCance, 2010a).

Normal destruction of erythrocytes occurs approximately every 120 days. Cells are removed by tissue; macrophage is broken down into bilirubin in the spleen and then lysed by enzymes in the macrophages. Heme and globin dissociate, and the globin is broken down into its component amino acids. The iron present in hemoglobin is oxidized and recycled. Porphyrin, which is also produced when cells are lysed, is further broken down into bilirubin, which is transported to the liver where it is conjugated and excreted in bile. When RBC destruction is accelerated, as with hemolytic anemia, the amount of bilirubin for liver clearance is increased, which in turn increases urinary excretion of urobilinogen (Rote & McCance, 2010b).

Leukocyte Production

Most leukocytes are generated from stem cells in the bone marrow. Hematopoietic stem cells differentiate into two types of progenitor cells: (1) lymphoid progenitors and (2) myeloid progenitors. Myeloid progenitors remain in the bone marrow and differentiate into progenitors for basophils, eosinophils, mast cells, megakaryocytes, and granulocyte/monocyte progenitors. Each differentiates further ultimately developing into particular cell types. Lymphoid progenitors that remain in the bone marrow differentiate into the B-cell lineage and are then released into the circulation where they travel to secondary lymphoid tissue for further maturation. Leukocyte production accelerates in the presence of infection, steroids, and reduction of cell reserves in the bone marrow. Stresses including seizures, intense heat or exercise, pain, vomiting, and anxiety can also increase leukocyte production (Rote & McCance, 2010a).

Platelet Development and Function

Thrombocytes or platelets are produced from megakaryocytes derived from stem cells. A single megakaryocyte is then fragmented to produce thousands of platelets. The majority platelets enter the circulation while others remain in reserve in the spleen. Their life span is approximately 10 days after which they are removed from the circulation and eliminated through phagocytosis in the spleen. The normal platelet count ranges from 150,000 to 350,000.

Thrombocytopenia refers to platelet counts less than 100,000; however, significant risk for spontaneous bleeding does usually not occur until the count drops to 20,000 or less. Thrombocytosis may result in an increased risk for spontaneous clotting causing increased risk for stroke and myocardial infarction (Rote & McCance, 2010a).

Platelets circulate in an inactive state until activated by injury. Once activated, they perform several critical functions including regulation of blood flow at the site of injury, forming platelet clusters to stop bleeding, and activation of the clotting cascade, to stabilize clots, and begin the repair process with dissolution of the clot (Rote & McCance, 2010a).

Hemostasis

Control of bleeding in the presence of injury is a critical function of blood components. In addition, hemostasis is also regulated in part by the vascular system, but in discussing hemostasis in this chapter, the discussion will be limited to the functions of platelets and clotting factors present in blood.

As noted above, platelets circulate freely in plasma until they are activated. Vascular injury triggers platelet activation causing the platelets to adhere to the blood vessel wall followed by release of substances from the platelets which stimulate changes in the shape of the platelets. This is followed by aggregation of platelets, which subsequently activates the clotting system (Rote & McCance, 2010a).

The coagulation cascade that leads to hemostasis involves a complex series of processes including protease reactions involving in excess of 20 different proteins. These reactions convert fibrinogen to insoluble strands of fibrin, which, joined with platelets, form a stable clot or thrombus (Thrombosis Adviser, 2015). Coagulation can be divided into three distinct stages: (1) the initiation phase in which a small quantity of clotting factors are produced in response to injury; (2) the amplification phase, in which there is an increased in the number of clotting factors released; and (3) the propagation phase, in which clotting factors attach to platelet membranes along with fibrin to form clots. Once hemostasis has been achieved, the process is turned off and a series of inhibitors and proteolytic feedback mechanisms (Versteeg, Heemskerk, Levi, & Reitsma, 2013).

What Is Anemia?

Anemia is a common finding in clinical practice. Defined as a deficient number of RBCs, the presence of anemia suggests a decrease in the blood's oxygen-carrying ability. It is considered by some to be a sign or symptom of an underlying disease. Etiology can vary widely, depending on the client's age and other risk factors. Depending on its cause, it can be mild or carry significant morbidity and mortality. Mild anemia may be asymptomatic in otherwise-healthy adults and only become evident when an abnormal CBC is found on routine laboratory testing (Griffis, 2013; Mais, 2014).

While hemoglobin concentration is used widely as parameter to define the presence of anemia, hemoglobin concentration varies among infants and children, adult men, adult women, pregnant women, and elderly making age-related, and gender-appropriate variations important in making the diagnosis of anemia (Mais, 2014). Anemia in adults is most often defined when hematocrit is less than 41% in males, or less than 36% in females (Damon & Andreadis, 2014).

The World Health Organization (WHO) definition of anemia varies based on the age of the individual. This definition is not universally accepted but provides a guideline or assessment. The following table illustrates the WHO recommendation for diagnosis anemia.

Group	Hemoglobin Level (g/dL)
Infants and children, 6 mo–6 yr	<11.0
Children 6–14 yr	<12
Pregnant females	<11
Nonpregnant females (15 yr and older)	<12
Adult males (15 yr and older)	<13

From World Health Organization. (2011). *Haemoglobin concentrations for the diagnosis of anaemia and assessment of severity.* Geneva, Switzerland: World Health Organization.

SIGNS AND SYMPTOMS

The symptoms associated with anemia are linked to the reduced oxygen-carrying capacity of the blood, hypoxia, and mechanisms used to compensate for reduced tissue oxygenation. The degree of physiologic adaptation can be influenced by the ability of the cardiac and respiratory systems to carry out compensatory actions, the severity and duration of the anemia, the individual's oxygen demands, the underlying cause of the anemia, and the presence and severity of any comorbid medical conditions (Kotter & Trevithick, 2013; Schrier, 2010).

Recognizing anemia and providing treatment carry important implications for quality of life for many patients. Identifying anemia in the elderly can be particularly challenging as there are many potential causes, including nutritional deficiencies and chronic diseases. Even mild anemia in the elderly can be associated with impaired mobility, deceased cognitive function, depressive symptoms, and risk for falls (Wilby, 2011).

Symptoms associated with mild to moderate anemia include fatigue, generalized weakness, lack of energy, as well as exertional dyspnea and tachycardia. Symptoms are typically less apparent when the anemia has evolved slowly. Otherwise-healthy individuals may have few symptoms, even when hemoglobin levels drop to 7 or 8 g/dL, while older adults with heart or lung disease may become symptomatic when hemoglobin levels are only moderately decreased. Moderate to severe anemia may be evidenced by a hyperdynamic state, which includes dizziness, syncope, bounding pulses, palpitations, and roaring in the ears. More severe anemia can cause life-threatening consequences including congestive heart failure and myocardial ischemia. When caused by acute blood loss, anemia with hypovolemia can be associated with fatigue, lethargy, syncope, and when severe, hypotension, shock, and death (Kotter & Trevithick, 2013; Schrier, 2010). Vitamin B_{12} deficiency may also be manifested by neurologic symptoms including numbness as a result of loss of nerve fibers in the spinal cord (Rote & McCance, 2010b).

Evidence of anemia can be manifested in the physical examination by tachycardia as a result of increased oxygen demands. In the case of chronic blood loss this may be experienced with exertion. When the anemia is more acute, it may occur even at rest. Skin, nail beds, conjunctivae, and oral mucous membranes appear pale when hemoglobin concentration is decreased. When anemia is caused by hemolysis, jaundice may be evident. Chronic anemia may result in tissue hypoxia, which in turn results in impaired tissue healing and decreased skin elasticity. Gait disturbances, weakness, spasticity, and abnormal deep tendon reflexes may be observed as a result of vitamin B_{12} deficiency (Rote & McCance, 2010b).

Signs and symptoms associated with anemia may vary depending on the rate at which it has developed and its severity, and the body's oxygen demands. Symptoms are typically less apparent when the anemia has evolved slowly. Symptoms are directly linked to the decreased oxygen-carrying capacity and in the case of acute blood loss, hypovolemia (Schrier, 2010).

EPIDEMIOLOGY

The third National Health and Nutrition Examination Survey (NHANES III) reported that approximately 10% of community-dwelling older adults were anemic. Among these individuals, nearly one-third had anemia related to nutritional deficits, including iron, vitamin B_{12}, and folate. Another one-third of anemias were related to kidney and other chronic diseases while the remaining one-third had unexplained causes (Guralanik, Eisenstadt, Ferrucci, Klein, & Woodman, 2004). A number of studies have identified and increased prevalence of anemia among elderly African Americans when compared to Caucasian, non-Hispanic, and Asian Americans (Denny, Kuchibhatla, & Cohen, 2006). In adults one of the most important causes of iron deficiency is blood loss associated with gastrointestinal bleeding linked to use of aspirin and other anti-inflammatory drugs (Damon & Andreadis, 2014).

ETIOLOGY

Identifying the cause of anemia is often uncomplicated. Examination of the peripheral blood smear in the laboratory provides critical information and is described more thoroughly in the Diagnostic Studies section of this chapter. Anemia may be caused by reduced RBC production, acute or chronic blood loss, increased RBC destruction, or a combination of these factors. Anemias may be classified by pathophysiologic category: either a defect of cell production or destruction or cell size or hemoglobin content of the cells. Differences in cell size and hemoglobin are described using a variety of terms. "Chromic" as in hypochromic indicates hemoglobin content while "cytic" indicates cell size. In addition, anisocytosis refers to cells of various sizes, and poikilocytosis refers to cells of various shapes (Rote & McCance, 2010b).

Macrocytic or megaloblastic anemias are distinguished by abnormally large stem cells that mature into RBCs that are also unusually large. Hemoglobin content in these large cells is normal (normochromic). This is a result of defective RBC precursor genetic material, often as a result of vitamin deficiency. The immature forms of megaloblastic cells are less likely to reach maturity, resulting in anemia. Other cells in the body, particularly those with high turnover rates, may also be affected resulting in some of the other symptoms associated with macrocytic anemia (Rote & McCance, 2010b).

Microcytic–hypochromic anemias are typified by RBCs that are abnormally small with reduced amounts of hemoglobin. Microcytic anemias can result from disorders of iron metabolism, abnormal porphyrin or heme synthesis, and disorders of globin synthesis. Most commonly these are manifested by iron deficiency, sideroblastic anemia, and thalassemia (Rote & McCance, 2010b).

Normocytic normochromic anemias are characterized by a reduced number of RBCs that are relatively normal in size and hemoglobin content. There is no common etiology for this type of anemia. Prevalence is less than with other types of anemia. Five well-defined types of normocytic normochromic anemia include the following:
- Aplastic
- Posthemorrhagic
- Hemolytic
- Sickle cell disease
- Anemia of chronic disease or ACD (Rote & McCance, 2010b)

Treatment is dependent on the cause of normocytic anemia.

ACUTE BLOOD LOSS

Acute blood loss is typically associated with traumatic injury, surgery, gastrointestinal disease, or retroperitoneal bleeding. Signs and symptoms are frequently obvious, with tachycardia, tachypnea, and hypotension associated with acute decrease in intravascular volume. Chronic blood loss in otherwise-healthy individuals is often better tolerated and presents with iron deficiency. Acute anemia may also be associated with nonhemorrhagic causes including acute intravascular hemolysis, exposure to toxins such as snake venom, hemolytic transfusion reaction, and infection (Mais, 2014).

IRON DEFICIENCY ANEMIA

Iron deficiency is the most common form of anemia. Throughout the world, lack of iron in the diet is the primary cause of iron deficiency anemia. However, in the United States the causes of iron deficiency are most often associated with disease in the gastrointestinal tract including celiac disease. Iron deficiency in toddlers and women of childbearing age may be associated with insufficient iron intake in comparison to the body's needs. In infants and young children, the primary cause of iron deficiency is due to dietary insufficiency, often associated with excessive milk intake or prolonged breast-feeding without adequate iron supplementation. Adolescent girls are more likely to develop iron deficiency anemia primarily from acute or chronic heavy menstrual bleeding (Powers & Buchanan, 2014). The most important cause of iron deficiency in United States adults is chronic blood loss, most often via the gastrointestinal tract. The American Gastroenterology Association suggests that in men and postmenopausal women, iron deficiency should be assumed to be associated with gastrointestinal blood loss until proven otherwise. Blood loss may be associated with chronic use of anti-inflammatory drugs including aspirin. Upper gastrointestinal tract lesions include esophagitis, Cameron ulcers, gastric and duodenal ulcers, vascular lesions, and gastric cancer. Colonic lesions associated with bleeding may include malignancies, polyps, vascular lesions, and colitis (Bull-Henry & Al-Kawas, 2013; Carter, Levi, Tzur, Novis, & Avidan, 2013). Chronic hemoglobinuria may also be linked to iron deficiency but is uncommon. Menorrhagia and other uterine bleeding in women must be investigated in women with iron deficiency anemia (Damon & Andreadis, 2014; Mais, 2014). It is recommended that when there is microcytic anemia with mean corpuscular volume (MCV) of less than 95 μm^3 that serum ferritin be assessed (Short & Domagalski, 2013). Low levels of serum ferritin define iron deficiency with levels less than 12 or 30 ng/mL when accompanied by anemia.

Iron deficiency anemia advances in a series of stages, beginning with iron deficiency with anemia with normal cell size. This is followed by a decrease in cell size evidenced by decreased MCV. As MCV decreases, the blood smear reveals microcytic, hypochromic cells. As iron deficiency progresses, the appearance of the RBCs can vary greatly. The platelet cell count may be increased in severe iron deficiency anemia (Damon & Andreadis, 2014; Short & Domagalski, 2013).

Ferritin is also an acute phase reactant and may be elevated in the presence of infection or chronic inflammation. Iron deficiency anemia is possible in the presence of inflammatory disorders when serum ferritin is less than 50 ng/mL. In situations where the ferritin level is inconclusive additional studies including serum iron, total iron-binding capacity (TIBC), and transferrin saturation may be useful. Ferritin levels equal to or greater than 100 ng/mL rule out the presence of iron deficiency (Short & Domagalski, 2013).

ANEMIA OF CHRONIC DISEASE

Persistent systemic inflammation influences iron utilization on the bone marrow and hinders hematopoiesis as well as diminishing the response of EPO in the presence of anemia. ACD is one of the most common forms of anemia in the United States, with the majority of cases associated with rheumatic diseases including rheumatoid arthritis and lupus, chronic infection, and malignancies (Mais, 2014). The mechanisms by which ACD develops are unclear, but when bone marrow biopsies are performed in the presence of ACD, iron stores are normal with decreased utilization of iron by premature erythrocytes. Erythroblasts have fewer transferrin receptors, and there is decreased production of EPO in response to anemia (Mais, 2014). A key characteristic of ACD is the disruption of iron homeostasis. Increased concentrations of inflammatory cytokines, including tumor necrosis factor, interferon, and interleukins, are believed to alter ferritin synthesis and cause an increased uptake of iron by macrophages and hepatocytes restricting its availability for erythropoiesis. These same cytokines may also suppress EPO production and interfere with the response to existing EPO levels (Sabol et al., 2010).

Anemia associated with organ failure may accompany kidney disease, hepatic failure, or endocrine gland failure. EPO levels decline and RBC mass decreases. Anemia of the elderly develops as a result of RBC resistance to the effects of EPO, reduced EPO production associated with decreased nephron mass, and the influence of low levels of inflammation in older adults. Serum iron levels are typically with in normal limits (Damon & Andreadis, 2014).

Treatment of ACD is not always necessary. Management of anemia hinges on management of the underlying disease. When anemia is severe or associated with symptoms with significant impact on quality of life, RBC transfusion or use of recombinant EPO may be used. Indications for use of parenteral EPO include hemoglobin less than 10 g/dL and anemia associated with rheumatoid arthritis, hepatitis C, inflammatory bowel disease, myelosuppressive chemotherapy for cancer, and chronic kidney disease. Treatment should be individualized to achieve and maintain hemoglobin levels between 10 and 12 g/dL. Use of recombinant EPO is associated with increased risk for thromboembolism (Damon & Andreadis, 2014).

THALASSEMIAS

Genetic mutation causing decreased production of structurally normal α- and β-globin chains is associated with the thalassemias. α-Thalassemia is associated with impaired synthesis of α-globin chains while β-thalassemia is heralded by diminished production of β-globin chains. Under normal circumstance two genes regulate β-chain synthesis and four genes regulate α-chain synthesis. β-Thalassemia is most prevalent among individuals of Greek, Italian, Arabic, and Sephardic Jewish descent. α-Thalassemia is most common in Asians of Chinese, Vietnamese, and Cambodian descent. Both types may also be seen in Blacks (Kline, 2010). α- and β-thalassemias can be classified as major or minor, depending on the number of defective genes (Kline, 2010). Both α- and β-thalassemias are associated with microcytosis, decreased RBC production, abnormal hemoglobin, and hemolysis (Mais, 2014).

There are four types of α-thalassemia, including
- α-Trait, a carrier state where one alpha-chain-forming gene is defective
- α-Thalassemia minor, with two defective genes
- α-Thalassemia intermedia or hemoglobin H disease, with three defective genes
- α-Thalassemia major, in which all α-chain-forming genes are abnormal, prohibiting release of oxygen leading to cell death (Kline, 2010).

Individuals with α-trait are typically asymptomatic and may exhibit a slight microcytosis. Those with α-thalassemia minor often have symptoms similar to those with β-thalassemia major, but less severe with microcytic–hypochromic anemia, enlarged spleen and liver, and bone marrow hyperplasia. α-Thalassemia intermedia or hemoglobin H disease causes hemolytic anemia while α-thalassemia major with hemoglobin Bart's usually causes hydrops fetalis and is fatal (Kline, 2010; Muncie & Campbell, 2009).

β-Thalassemia involves the uncoupling of α- and β-chain production. Moderate depression of β-chain production is referred to as β-thalassemia minor while β-thalassemia major, sometimes referred to as Cooley's anemia, involves more severe depression of β-chain synthesis. Depression of β-chain synthesis leads to RBCs with a reduced amount of hemoglobin ad increased numbers of α-chains. Unstable α-chains result in hemolytic anemia as well as defective erythropoiesis with resulting anemia. β-Thalassemia is more common than α-thalassemia (Kline, 2010).

β-Thalassemia minor may be manifested by mild to moderate microcytic, hypochromic anemia, splenic enlargement, and brawny skin. Reticulocytosis may be present depending on the degree of anemia. Hyperplasia of the bone marrow may result in skeletal abnormalities. Hemolysis of defective cells may cause elevation of serum iron levels (Kline, 2010).

β-Thalassemia major is often associated with significant morbidity. Anemia is more severe and is linked with high-output congestive heart failure. β-Thalassemia major is associated with hemolytic anemia, skeletal malformations, and delayed growth in infancy. Children affected by β-thalassemia major require life-long RBC transfusions. β-Thalassemia intermedia is less severe, but intermediate transfusion may also be required (Kline, 2010). Frequent blood transfusion can extend life dramatically but is associated with iron overload, which can be fatal. Liver enlargement results from deposition of iron in the liver. Patients with iron overload often require chelation therapy to remove excess iron. Splenic enlargement also occurs as a result of extramedullary hematopoiesis and hemolysis. Bone marrow hyperplasia causes deformity of the skeleton (Muncie & Campbell, 2009).

Laboratory markers of the thalassemias are small, hypochromic RBCs characterized by low MCV and mean corpuscular hemoglobin (MCH), anemia, and a normal or increased number of small RBCs. α-Thalassemia may be confused with iron deficiency since RBCs are microcytic. Laboratory testing to rule out iron deficiency and to identify the presence of abnormal hemoglobin is important in making the diagnosis of thalassemia. Hemoglobin A is the primary form of hemoglobin found in the blood of adults. Patients with β-thalassemia major demonstrate elevated levels of hemoglobin F at birth and are rarely symptomatic until 6 months of age (Muncie & Campbell, 2009).

Morbidity associated with α-thalassemia is dependent on the number of α-globin chains abnormalities identified. Silent carriers are usually asymptomatic and may have normal CBC. Microcytic, hypochromic cells may be found in the peripheral smear. Genetic testing may detect silent carriers. Those with thalassemia trait may also be asymptomatic. Evidence of hypochromia, microcytosis, and target cells may be seen on the peripheral smear. Hemoglobin electrophoresis is usually normal (Cheerva et al., 2014).

Patients who are transfusion dependent become iron overloaded and require iron chelation beginning at an early age. Iron chelators bind to iron and remove it from the body. Deferoxamine has long been used as an effective chelator, but it requires subcutaneous or intravenous administration. Deferasirox, a newer agent, is administered orally (Muncie & Campbell, 2009). Preconception genetic counseling is advised for all people with thalassemia. Two parents with β-thalassemia trait have a one-in-four chance of conceiving a child with β-thalassemia major. Persons with α-thalassemia trait have a more complex pattern of inheritance (Muncie & Campbell, 2009).

FOLATE DEFICIENCY

Folate is a water-soluble B vitamin that is an important cofactor in DNA synthesis. Found in many food sources, including fresh fruits and vegetables, legumes, it may be destroyed during cooking. Deficiency of folate can result from inadequate intake, decreased absorption, altered metabolism, bariatric surgery, medications including chemotherapy and antiepileptics or chronic alcohol intake. Older adults are especially at risk for folate deficiency. While the United States and some other counties have undertaken the practice of fortifying cereals and other foods with folate as a preventive strategy, folate deficiency is a significant health problems in many countries throughout the world (Koitke et al., 2012).

Folate deficiency is associated with megaloblastic anemia. The term "megaloblastic anemia" stems from the appearance of precursor cells in the bone marrow with large, immature nuclei. Megaloblastic changes affect RBCs, granulocytes, and megakaryocytes. Cells that do mature are macrocytic with increased MCV. Folate is absorbed in the duodenum and inadequate intake, increased demand, and malabsorption are most often linked to folate deficiency (Mais, 2014).

VITAMIN B$_{12}$ DEFICIENCY

Vitamin B$_{12}$ deficiency is also associated with megaloblastic anemia. Additionally, B$_{12}$ deficiency is also manifested by a degenerative neurologic condition which presents with paresthesia, weakness, and gait abnormalities linked to demyelination and loss of nerves in the dorsal columns (Mais, 2014). Total human body content of vitamin B$_{12}$ is 2 to 5 mg. B$_{12}$ loss is estimated to be about 0.1% to 0.2% of the total content through urinary and gastrointestinal excretion. The average diet provides 5 to 15 mcg vitamin B$_{12}$ per day, but up to 80% of ingested vitamin is eliminated or metabolized by intestinal flora. Requirements vary depending based on age (Hooper, Hudson, Porter, & McCaddon, 2014).

Dietary sources of vitamin B$_{12}$ are abundant, making dietary deficiency uncommon. There are some individuals at risk for deficiency since many B$_{12}$-rich foods are of animal and bacterial origin, though other foods are fortified with vitamin B$_{12}$ (Hooper et al., 2014). When vitamin B$_{12}$ is ingested, it binds to protein carriers then is dissociated by the acidic environment present in the stomach. Intrinsic factor that is produced by the parietal and zymogenic cells in the stomach binds to B$_{12}$ in the duodenum, traveling through into the ileum where it is then absorbed. Failure in any portion of this process can lead to vitamin B$_{12}$ deficiency. Malabsorption may result from loss of the ileal receptors as a result of surgery or inflammatory bowel disease (Tweet & Polga, 2010).

Pernicious anemia is a consequence of autoimmune destruction of the parietal and zymogenic cells with subsequent loss of intrinsic factor production. Additionally, intrinsic factor antibodies may bind to available intrinsic factor rendering it inactive (Tweet & Polga, 2010).

Another factor linked vitamin B$_{12}$ deficiency is achlorhydria. The absence of acid in the stomach can also perpetuate B$_{12}$ deficiency. When acid is lacking in the stomach, the B$_{12}$ and protein carrier are unable to separate and intrinsic factor is unable to bind to vitamin B$_{12}$. Achlorhydria can be a result of use of medication that blocks gastric acid production, such as proton pump inhibitors, or can occur as a result of aging (Tweet & Polga, 2010). Surgical procedures including antrectomy and Roux-en-Y gastric bypass have also been associated with achlorhydria (Schauer, Ikramuddin, Gourash, Ramanathan, & Luketich, 2000).

LEAD POISONING

Lead serves no useful function in the human body, and its presence can lead to toxic effects, regardless of the mechanism of exposure. Toxicity can affect every organ system, including the hematopoietic system. At the molecular level, the proposed mechanisms for toxicity involve basic biochemical processes include lead's ability to inhibit or imitate the actions of calcium affecting many calcium-dependent processes and to interact with proteins, including those with sulfhydryl, amine, phosphate, and carboxyl groups (Agency for Toxic Substances and Disease Registry [ATSDR], 2007). Toxicity associated with lead, sometimes referred to as plumbism, can affect RBCs, renal epithelial tissues, and the nervous system. Exposure to lead occurs primarily through environmental exposure to lead based, paint, lead plumbing, contaminated soils, and manufacturing. When affecting the hematologic system, lead poisoning typically presents with microcytic, hypochromic anemia. Lead poisoning influences blood formation in different ways. Lead inhibits the body's ability to make hemoglobin by interfering with several enzymatic steps in the heme pathway. The Environmental Protection Agency estimated the threshold blood lead levels for a decrease in hemoglobin to be 50 μg/dL for occupationally exposed adults and approximately 40 μg/dL for children, although other studies have indicated a lower threshold for children (ATSDR, 2007).

Lead can induce two types of anemia. Acute high-level lead exposure has been associated with hemolytic anemia. Profound anemia is not typically an early manifestation of lead exposure and is evident only when lead levels are significantly elevated for prolonged periods. In chronic lead exposure, lead induces anemia by both interfering with heme biosynthesis and by decreasing RBC survival. Anemia associated with lead toxicity is hypochromic, and normo- or microcytic with reticulocytosis. The heme synthesis pathway, on which lead has an effect, is involved in many other processes in the body including neural, renal, endocrine, and hepatic pathways (ATSDR, 2007; Mais, 2014).

HEMOGLOBINOPATHIES

Structural defects in hemoglobin are referred to as hemoglobinopathies. Hemoglobinopathies are most often a result of mutations in one of the hemoglobin genes. Hemoglobin S is the most common hemoglobin abnormality in the United States. It is estimated that sickle cell disease affects 1 in 375 African Americans. It may also affect individuals of Mediterranean, Caribbean, South and Central American, Arabian, and East Indian descent. Homozygous sickle cell anemia (sickle cell disease) leads to change in the shape of the RBC under situations when hypoxia is present. The lifespan of normal RBCs is approximately one hundred and twenty days and while in the setting of sickle cell disease, it is often less than 30 days. Hemoglobin electrophoresis demonstrates that RBCs contain mostly hemoglobin S. Individuals with sickle cell disease experience chronic hemolysis and intermittent episodes of complex events referred to as vaso-occlusive crises. Chronic hemolysis with resulting chronic anemia leads to many long-term sequelae, including delayed puberty and growth retardation in the young. Decreased exercise tolerance, jaundice, and cholelithiasis associated with formation of pigmented gall stones are also common problems. Vaso-occulsive crises may result in significant pain and disability as a result of stroke, avascular necrosis of bone, and splenic infarction. An increased risk for infection is associated with impairment of splenic function. Individuals with sickle cell disease are particularly susceptible to infection with encapsulated bacterial organisms including *Haemophilus influenzae* and *Streptococcus pneumoniae*. Death in those with sickle cell disease is most often caused by infection, stroke, and thromboembolic events (Mais, 2014).

Heterozygous hemoglobin S, or sickle cell trait, is typically asymptomatic. Hemoglobin electrophoresis will demonstrate 35% to 45% hemoglobin S. In situations when hypoxia occurs individuals with sickle cell trait are at risk for infarction (Mais, 2014).

Hemoglobin E is unlikely to cause symptoms but those with this condition often have RBC indices similar to those with thalassemia (Mais, 2014).

AUTOIMMUNE HEMOLYTIC ANEMIA

Autoimmune hemolytic anemia is an acquired disorder that occurs when an IgG autoantibody binds to the RBC membrane. The autoantibody is often directed against a component of the Rh system. When the antibody is recognized by macrophages from the reticuloendothelial system, the response is to remove the RBC membrane forming a spherocytes. The spherocytes, in turn, are trapped in the spleen. Additionally, Kupffer cells in the liver contribute to the extravascular hemolysis that occurs. Onset of symptoms, including dyspnea and chest pain, is often rapid and may be life threatening. Nearly half of all cases of autoimmune hemolytic anemia are idiopathic. It is also associated with autoimmune disorders such as systemic lupus erythematosus, chronic lymphocytic leukemia, and lymphoma (Damon & Andreadis, 2014).

HEREDITARY SPHEROCYTOSIS

Hereditary spherocytosis is characterized by defects in RBC cell membranes resulting in a spherical shape rather than the biconcave RBC typically seen. These abnormally shaped cells are removed from the circulation and hemolyzed by the spleen (Damon & Andreadis, 2014). Rather than a single disorder, hereditary spherocytosis (HS) is a group of disorders varying in clinical presentation, protein defects, and mode of inheritance. Common in Caucasians, most individuals have mild or moderate symptoms associated with hemolysis, although in some cases, hemolysis may be severe. HS is the most common form of RBC membrane disorder. It most often presents in childhood and is heralded by anemia, jaundice, and enlarged spleen, but it may be diagnosed at any age. A family history of HS is almost always present. When other hematologic disorders are also present, the diagnosis can be challenging (Bolton-Maggs et al., 2004; Brill & Baumgardner, 2000).

In those with positive family history, splenic enlargement, elevated MCHC, and elevated reticulocyte count, the diagnosis is straightforward. The severity of anemia is linked to the degree of hemolysis and size of the spleen. Individuals with HS are usually categorized as having mild, moderate, or severe. Severity of disease should be determined when the patient is at baseline with a reference hemoglobin level, degree of jaundice, reticulocyte count, and activity level. Diagnosis is generally made based on clinical history, family history, and physical findings, including splenomegaly and jaundice, and laboratory data. Laboratory data most important in making the diagnosis of HS includes CBC, with RBC indices with morphology, and reticulocyte count (Bolton-Maggs et al., 2004).

GLUCOSE-6-PHOSPHATE DEHYDROGENASE DEFICIENCY

Glucose-6-phosphate dehydrogenase (G6PD) deficiency is the most common form of RBC enzyme defect. The disorder was first identified while investigating the occurrence of hemolytic anemia in individuals being treated or malaria. The gene for G6PD is located on the X chromosome and is an X-linked inherited disorder seen primarily in men. In the United States, G6PD deficiency is most common in Black men but may also be seen men of Mediterranean and Southeast Asian descent. Because RBCs lack a nucleus, they are unable to form new enzymes. As cells mature, enzymes degrade and when critical enzymes are unable to perform their functions cells die prematurely. RBCs are dependent on G6PD to produce glutathione to reduce the effects of oxidative stress on hemoglobin. There are three classes of G6PD deficiency: class 1, in which there is chronic low-level hemolysis; class 2, which is manifested by severe intravascular hemolysis in the presence of oxidative stress; and class 3, where there is mild-to-moderate hemolysis with oxidant stress. Most individuals with G6PD deficiency are asymptomatic unless exposed to excess oxidant. Exposure can occur in the presence of infection, diabetic ketoacidosis, or with ingestion of certain foods (fava beans) and medications, including nitrofurantoin, sulfa drugs, and antimalarials (Mais, 2014). The most important treatment or G6PD deficiency is the avoidance of oxidative stress. Although anemia may be severe enough to warrant RBC transfusion, this is unusual. Splenectomy is typically not needed. While folic acid and iron can potentially be beneficial in the presence of hemolysis, the hemolysis associated with G6PD deficiency is usually short-term, making such treatment unnecessary (Frank, 2005).

Drugs to Avoid with G6PD Deficiency

Class	Drugs
Antimalarials	Primaquine, Pamaquine
Sulfonamides	Sulfacetamide, Sulfanilamide, Sulfamethoxazole (e.g., Septra, Bactrim), Sulfasalazine
Analgesics	Phenacetin, Acetanilid, Phenazopyridine (Pyridium)
Antibacterials	Nitrofurantoin, Nalidixic Acid, Dapsone, Mafenide Cream (Sulfamylon)
Miscellaneous	Quinine, Flutamide (Eulexin), Methylene Blue, Rasburicase

Adapted from Pharmacology Weekly. (2014). What are common medications that should be avoided in patients with known G6PD deficiency? Retrieved from http://www.pharmacologyweekly.com/articles/G6PD-deficiency-medications-drugs-avoid

PAROXYSMAL NOCTURNAL HEMOGLOBINURIA

Paroxysmal nocturnal hemoglobinuria (PNH) stems from an acquired mutation in the PIG-A gene of the hematopoietic stem cell which leads to lysis of RBCs by complement as well as leukopenia and thrombocytopenia. Intravascular hemolysis occurs in varying degrees and is reflected in hemoglobinuria. Hemolysis may be intermittent or continuous. Urinary loss of hemoglobin results in iron deficiency anemia. Despite its name, exacerbations are not nocturnal. Development of thrombosis is also often associated with PNH. Abdominal pain often associated with splenomegaly and low back pain are common symptoms in addition to symptoms characteristic of severe anemia. Individuals with PNH are at risk for developing aplastic anemia (Mais, 2014).

MYELODYSPLASTIC SYNDROMES

Myelodysplastic syndromes (MDS) are one of five major categories of myeloid malignancies. Characterized by dysplastic and ineffective blood cell production, MDS carries the risk of transformation to acute leukemia. Incidence of MDS increases with age, and these diseases are among the most common hematologic malignancies in those over 70 years of age (Doll & Landaw, 2010; Tefferi & Vardiman, 2009).Those with MDS frequently present with anemia along with other cytopenias. Bone marrow dysplasia involving at least 10% of the cells of a specific myeloid line is the most important feature of MDS. Other conditions characterized by erythroid dysplasia must be ruled out before the diagnosis of MDS is made. Such disorders include deficiencies of vitamin B_{12}, folate, and copper, as well as viral infections including HIV infection, chronic alcohol use, lead and arsenic poisoning, and congenital disorders (Tefferi & Vardiman, 2009). Symptoms of MDS are often nonspecific. Patients may be asymptomatic and have irregularities in the CBC found during routine laboratory testing. Symptoms may include fatigue, weakness, and a decreased sense of well-being. As the disease progresses, infection, bleeding, or bruising may prompt someone to seek medical attention. A small percentage of individuals with MDS develop autoimmune manifestations such as pericardial effusion, peripheral neuropathy, iritis, and skin ulcerations (Doll & Landaw, 2010).

APLASTIC ANEMIA

Aplastic anemia is a rare hematologic disorder that was almost always fatal a few decades ago, but can now be treated and sometimes cured with the use of immunosuppressive therapy and or stem cell transplant. Found in both children and adults, the majority of cases are idiopathic. It can be associated with exposure to drugs, chemicals, radiation, viruses, and pregnancy. The exact mechanism of disease is unknown, but it is believed to be a result of assault of effector T lymphocytes on hematopoietic stem cells, which ultimately results in failure of the bone marrow with pancytopenia. Peripheral blood smears are pancytopenic without significant morphologic abnormalities in the cells that remain in the blood. Bone marrow biopsy typically shows a hypocellular marrow with reduced numbers of all cell lines. Patients who initially present with PNH may eventually develop aplastic anemia (Weinziehr & Arber, 2013).

Patients with aplastic anemia may present with bleeding and infection as well as anemia. The onset of signs and symptoms is typically acute. The physical examination may show pallor, evidence of bleeding with petechiae or purpura, though at the onset the examination may not reveal any significant changes (Griffis, 2013).

Medications Associated with Aplastic Anemia

Class	Agent
Antibiotics	Penicillin, chloramphenicol, sulfonamides
Antidepressants	Lithium, tricyclics
Anti-inflammatories	Gold salts, nonsteroidals, salicylates
Antimalarials	
Anticonvulsants	

From Griffis, K. P. (2013). Evaluation and management of hematologic disorders. In T. M. Buttaro, J. Tryulski, B. P. Bailey, & J. Sandberg-Cook (Eds.), *Primary care: A collaborative practice.* (4th ed., pp. 1139–1181). St. Louis, MO: Elsevier Mosby.

MULTIPLE MYELOMA

Multiple myeloma is characterized by production of abnormal plasma proteins. Under normal conditions plasma cells produce immune globulins; however, with multiple myeloma monoclonal plasma cells produce an excess of abnormal proteins. Immune globulin molecules normally contain two heavy chains along with one light chain attached. Myeloma cells produce abnormal light chains as well as cytokines which are capable of triggering osteoclast activity, diminishing osteoblast activity, and causing angiogenesis. The incidence of multiple myeloma increases with aging, with a median age of 70 at diagnosis. Environmental factors coupled with genetic predisposition are most likely to trigger the disease process. Exposure to radiation, pesticides used in agriculture, and petrochemicals are associated risk factors. The increased amounts of abnormal proteins are associated with a number of pathologic processes. Hyperviscosity of the blood due to the increased amount of circulating proteins is associated with abnormal bleeding, visual changes, and neurologic symptoms. Invasion of the bone marrow is associated with anemia. Bony lesions associated with osteoclastic activity are often associated with pain, fractures, and hypercalcemia. Immune dysfunction often leads to increased risk for infection. Approximately one third of individuals are asymptomatic at the time of diagnosis. Anemia is common at diagnosis and with progressive disease (Nau & Lewis, 2008)

Risk Factors for Anemia

Decreased RBC production in relation to RBC destruction results in anemia. Reduction in blood production may be a consequence of lack of nutrients, including iron, folate, or vitamin B_{12}. Such deficiencies may result from inadequate intake, malabsorption of nutrients, or blood loss. Bone marrow disorders include myelodysplasia, aplastic anemia, RBC aplasia, or infiltration of malignancy in the bone marrow. Bone marrow suppression from cancer chemotherapy or other drugs and radiation may also reduce RBC production. Low levels of hormones known to stimulate RBC production, including EPO, thyroid hormone, and testosterone, are also associated with anemia. ACD is seen in inflammatory, infectious, and malignant diseases. Reduced availability of iron, relatively low EPO levels, and reduced RBC lifespan are all characteristics of ACD (Schrier, 2010).

RBC destruction or hemolysis is defined by RBC life span of less than 100 days (Schrier, 2010). Examples of hemolytic anemia include disorders such as HS, sickle cell disease, and thalassemia major. Acquired hemolytic anemias include Coombs positive autoimmune hemolytic anemia, thrombotic thrombocytopenic purpura–hemolytic uremic syndrome, and malaria (Schrier, 2010).

Blood loss is the most common cause of iron deficiency in the United States. Obvious bleeding may manifest as melena, hematemesis, menorrhagia, or as a result of trauma. Occult bleeding is often associated with malignancy or slow bleeding from ulcerative gastrointestinal lesions. When bleeding is present in addition to loss of blood cells, the bone marrow must also replace the iron lost with bleeding. This ultimately leads to depletion of the body's iron stores. Cumulative blood loss over time of greater than 1 L in men and greater than 600 mL in women results in significant iron depletion. Up to 25% of menstruating women have inadequate iron stores resulting in anemia with any amount of bleeding (Schrier, 2010).

MDS may occur without a clear etiology but may also present after exposure to potentially mutagenic therapy including radiation or chemotherapy (Doll & Landaw, 2010).

Differential Diagnoses

- Microcytic anemia:
  - Iron deficiency
  - ACD (inflammatory)
  - Thalassemia
  - Copper deficiency
  - Hemoglobinopathy
  - Congenital of acquired sideroblastic anemia
- Macrocytic anemia:
  - Vitamin B_{12} deficiency
  - Folate deficiency
  - MDS
  - Acute leukemia
  - Alcohol abuse
  - Liver disease
  - Hypothyroidism
- Normocytic anemia:
  - ACD (renal disease)
  - Acute blood loss
  - Hypersplenism
  - Hemolytic disorders
  - Hyperthyroidism

Treatment of Anemia

IRON SUPPLEMENTATION

Effective treatment requires identifying and treating the underlying cause of the anemia. Costs associated with care of patients with anemia have been shown to be significantly higher with increased utilization of health resources than in those without anemia (McEvoy & Shander, 2013).

Treatment of iron deficiency with oral supplementation is the preferred therapy in most situations. It is cost-effective and generally well tolerated. The standard of treatment is 200 mg/day of elemental iron, available in varying concentrations through ingestion of ferrous salts. Ferrous sulfate 325 mg three times daily provides 180 mg of elemental iron daily, slightly less than the standard of 200 mg daily. Ferrous gluconate, titrated to five tablets daily, can provide up to 175 mg, while ferrous fumarate, containing 107 mg/tablet, can provide 214 mg when taken twice daily (Sabol et al., 2010). Side effects including constipation and nausea sometimes limit adherence. Tolerability may be improved by gradually increasing the dose and administering it with food.

Treatment should continue for three to 6 months to replace iron stores. Response to therapy can be seen as early as 3 weeks after initiation with a partial increase in hematocrit. Return to normal hematocrit is typically noted after 2 months. Failure to respond is often associated with nonadherence, but consideration should be given to the possibility of poor absorption (Damon & Andreadis, 2014). Excessive supplementation can be associated with toxicity from iron overload making monitoring of ferritin and transferrin saturation levels useful in determining when therapeutic goals have been reached. If symptomatic iron overload does occur, administration of deferoxamine, an iron chelating agent or therapeutic phlebotomy, may be indicated (Sabol et al., 2010).

Intake of some foods and supplements may hinder absorption of iron supplements, including soy protein, bran, dairy products, tea and coffee, antacids rich in calcium, and high-fiber vegetables. Iron is best absorbed on an empty stomach along with ascorbic acid. Patients should avoid taking multivitamins with calcium within 1 to 2 hours of taking iron supplements (Griffis, 2013).

When oral replacement is not tolerated or gastrointestinal disease prohibits the use of oral supplementation, parenteral iron preparations should be considered. Until recently, use of parenteral iron with preparations such as iron dextran was difficult with prolonged infusion times and risk for hypersensitivity reactions. Newer preparations, including iron gluconate and iron sucrose, allow for shortened infusion times and are markedly safer (Damon & Andreadis, 2014; Sabol et al., 2010)

FOLIC ACID SUPPLEMENTATION

Folic acid deficiency is treated with a daily oral dose of 1 mg although doses of 3 mg may be needed in severe deficiency. Improvement is typically noted within 1 week, with patient reports of improved well-being and an increase in the reticulocyte count. A return to normal blood indices is usually observed within 2 months (Sabol et al., 2010).

VITAMIN B$_{12}$ SUPPLEMENTATION

Treatment for vitamin B$_{12}$ deficiency has historically been with parenteral supplementation. Intramuscular or subcutaneous doses of 100 mcg are usually adequate, with daily doses given for 1 week followed by weekly doses for 1 month and then by monthly doses thereafter for life. Oral or sublingual doses of methylcobalamin of 1 mg/day may be used after correction of the original deficiency. Supplementation must be continued in definitely and intermittent monitoring of serum vitamin B$_{12}$ levels should be done to know that supplementation is sufficient. Response to therapy is rapid with improved sense of well-being within days. An increased reticulocyte count is often evident within 1 week and normalization of the hematologic profile returns in approximately 2 months after treatment is initiated. Nervous system symptoms may be reversed if they have been present for 6 months or less (Damon & Andreadis, 2014).

ERYTHROPOIESIS-STIMULATING AGENTS

Epoetin-α is classified as an erythropoiesis-stimulating agent (ESA). It is human EPO-α produced using recombinant DNA technology. Given by subcutaneous or intravenous injection, it is primarily indicated for treatment of anemia associated with chronic renal failure, anemia associated with treatment for cancer, anemia related to treatment with zidovudine for human immunodeficiency virus infection, and for individuals with anemia, scheduled to have surgery to reduce the need for perioperative transfusions. It is not indicated for immediate improvement for severe anemia, but it is effective in reducing the need for maintenance transfusions in individuals with chronic anemia (Ackerman, 2014; Sabol et al., 2010). The dose varies depending on the indication for its use. Darbepoetin is a similar preparation which is administered less frequently to achieve similar results. ESAs can precipitate sudden increases in blood pressure particularly when hypertension is poorly controlled. Both hypertension and seizures have been noted in cases where hematocrit rises quickly. A black box warning for prescribers of ESA cautions about an increased risk for thromboembolism, stroke, myocardial infarction, and risk for tumor progression in individuals being treated for cancer. The lowest possible dose should be used to achieve the desired results. Ferritin and transferrin saturation should be monitored periodically throughout treatment to monitor for iron deficiency. Adverse effects of ESAs include hypertension, including hypertensive crisis and seizures, particularly when rapid increase in hematocrit occurs. Other side effects include rashes, nausea, diarrhea, headaches, and paresthesias. Treatment with ESAs is quite costly and should be prescribed by following guidelines set forth by the manufacturer (Ackerman, 2014).

RED BLOOD CELL TRANSFUSION

RBC transfusion is the fastest means to increase hemoglobin levels, and in situations where hemoglobin levels are dangerously low, transfusion is the mainstay of treatment. However, transfusion is costly and associated with a significant number of risks. When considering transfusion the risks and benefits must be considered against those of other treatments (McEvoy & Shander, 2013; Shander, Javidroozi, Ozawa, & Hare, 2011). While very rare with the advent of widespread screening for infectious agents, there is risk for transmission of pathogens. More importantly, noninfectious complications can result as a consequence of human error in preparation and transfusion of blood products. Transfusion of RBCs has been linked to many negative outcomes, including cardiac, pulmonary, renal, and neurologic events. Given these risks, the decision to use transfusion to treat anemia should be made carefully (Shander et al., 2011).

RBC transfusion is viewed as a critical part of treatment for individuals with sickle cell disease with a majority of patients receiving multiple transfusions during their lifetimes. Transfusion is indicated for reducing risks for complications in pregnancy in women with sickle cell disease as well as for decreasing risk for stroke in children and reducing risk for perioperative complications for patients undergoing surgery. Alloimmunization, autoimmunization, iron overload, hemolysis, and hyperviscosity are the side effects of transfusion occurring most commonly.

Prevention

NUTRITIONAL DEFICIENCY

Ongoing health assessment is crucial in care of older adults to identify conditions that may pose risk for anemia associated with nutritional deficiency. Alterations in sense of taste and/or smell, dysphasia, and dental problems can pose significant problems with intake of an adequate diet (Sabol et al., 2010).

Risk for nutritional deficiency is also associated with poverty. The WHO (2001) reports that access to iron rich foods, including meat and fish and nonanimal foods including legumes and leafy green vegetables, as well as foods that enhance absorption and utilization of iron, including some fruits and vegetables, should be a priority in decreasing risk for iron deficiency anemia.

For children education about the benefits of limiting cow's milk intake and providing a varied well-balanced diet are necessary. Emphasis should be placed on limiting milk intake to 20 ounces/day, which helps to encourage diversity in the child's diet and include foods with higher iron content, including meat, fish, and beans, while continuing to provide adequate dietary calcium and vitamin D (Powers & Buchanan, 2014).

Avoiding ingestion of substances that inhibit iron absorption is an important factor when iron deficiency is present (Griffis, 2013).

GASTROINTESTINAL BLEEDING

The American College of Gastroenterology has issued guidelines for prevention of NSAID-induced gastrointestinal complications. The authors of this report note that risk for bleeding associated with NSAID use increases in individuals with increased age, previous history of bleeding, and concurrent use of certain medications, including, anticoagulants, other NSAIDS, including low-dose aspirin, and corticosteroids. *H. pylori* infection also increases risk for NSAID-induced gastrointestinal bleeding. The recommendations include *H. pylori* infection testing and treatment if positive prior to starting long-term therapy with NSAIDs. In addition, treatment with medication is effective in reducing risk for mucosal injury associated with NSAID use. Misoprostol at a dose of 800 mg/day is effective in preventing ulcers but unpleasant gastrointestinal side effects in its use. Proton pump inhibitors also significantly reduce risk for ulcers. COX-2 inhibitors have also been shown to reduce the incidence of gastric and duodenal ulcers when compared to conventional NSAIDs, but the utility of this class of drugs is limited by the associated risk for cardiovascular events (Lanza, Chan, Quigley, & Practice Parameters Committee, 2009).

Other Blood Disorders

NEUTROPENIA

Neutropenia is identified when the absolute neutrophil count is less than 1,800/μL. The presence of neutropenia typically increases risk for infection caused by gram-negative and gram-positive organisms as well as fungi. Risk for significant life-threatening infection increases as neutrophil counts drops precipitously. There is a subset of individuals, including some Blacks and Asians, who under normal circumstances have neutrophil benign chronic neutropenia are able to release adequate amounts of neutrophils when faced with infection or inflammatory stimuli (Damon & Andreadis, 2014).

A number of conditions are associated with neutropenia. While there should be concern for a bone marrow disorder, it is important to recognize that there are a number of nonmarrow disorders that can result in neutropenia. Medications, including some antiretrovirals, sulfonamides, cephalosporins, and phenytoin are associated with neutropenia. Immune disorders including HIV infection and systemic lupus erythematosus and aplastic anemia may also be linked to neutropenia. Bone marrow disorders may be congenital, such as Fanconi anemia, or dyskeratosis congenita, or acquired disorders including hairy cell leukemia and myelodysplasia (Damon & Andreadis, 2014).

MYELOPROLIFERATIVE DISORDERS

Myeloproliferative disorders occur as a result of acquired abnormalities in hematopoietic stem cells. Because stem cells generate all cell lines, abnormalities may appear in myeloid, erythroid, and platelet cells. Diseases can evolve over time from one type to another, and all myeloproliferative disorders have the potential to progress to acute myeloid leukemia. Myeloproliferative disorders are classified as (1) myeloproliferative neoplasms, including polycythemia vera (PV), primary myelofibrosis, essential thrombocytosis, and chronic myeloid leukemia (CML); (2) MDS; and (3) acute myeloid leukemia (Damon & Andreadis, 2014).

PV causes overproduction of all three of the hematopoietic cell lines, but the erythroid line is most pronounced. An elevated hematocrit is the finding most characteristic of PV, with hematocrit over 54% in men and 51% in women. Common symptoms are related to increased blood volume and can include headache, blurred vision, fatigue, and tinnitus. Epistaxis may occur as a result of engorged mucosal blood vessels and altered platelet function. Generalized itching, particularly after a warm bath, is a result of histamine release associated with increased basophils. While PV may occur in adults under 40, the mean age of presentation is 60. Men account for approximately 60% of cases of PV. Thrombosis is the primary complication associated to PV as a result of increased blood viscosity and altered platelet function. Treatment most often consists of therapeutic phlebotomy, with removal of one unit of blood weekly until a desirable hematocrit (under 45%) is achieved. Treatment with alkylating agents may be needed in some cases, with hydroxyurea being the d rug most frequently used (Damon & Andreadis, 2014).

Acute leukemia is a hematopoietic progenitor cell malignancy causing uncontrolled production of cells that eventually replace normal elements of the bone marrow. Although there is seldom a known cause, ionizing radiation, toxins, such as benzene, and chemotherapeutic agents, especially alkylating agents, have been associated with acute leukemia. Most of the symptoms and physical findings, bleeding, fatigue, infections, and bone pain, stem from the replacement of normal bone marrow with malignant cells. Infiltration of organs with leukemic cells is associated with less common findings. Acute myeloid leukemias are most often found in adults while acute lymphocytic leukemia is most common in children. Laboratory findings in acute leukemia typically demonstrate pancytopenia with evidence of circulating immature or blast cells. Hyperuricemia may also be noted. Flow cytometry is useful to identify leukemia cell phenotypes. Treatment for acute leukemia includes combination chemotherapy and bone marrow transplant (Damon & Andreadis, 2014).

CHRONIC MYELOID LEUKEMIA

Chronic Myeloid Leukemia (CML) is characterized by overproduction of myeloid cells. Specific chromosomal and molecular abnormalities are associated with CML. Early in the course of the disease bone marrow function is preserved, and although demonstrating some abnormalities, WBCs are effective in combating infection. If untreated, an accelerated phase follows, and finally an acute phase resembling acute leukemia often result. CML is most frequently found in middle age. Symptoms that lead patients to seek treatment include fatigue, night sweats, and fever. Splenic enlargement causes abdominal discomfort. Laboratory findings include leukocytosis. In some cases, in the early stage, elevated WBC count is an incidental finding (Damon & Andreadis, 2014).

COAGULATION DISORDERS

Coagulation disorders are typically classified into those that cause bleeding and those that are associated with thrombosis. Bleeding disorders are further broken down into coagulation factor disorders and platelet disorders.

A number of thrombotic disorders cause increased risk for hypercoagulability; for the purposes of this chapter, two disorders with high-prevalence, factor V Leiden mutation and antiphospholipid antibody syndrome (APAS) will be discussed.

When encountering a patient with a report of abnormal bleeding a careful history is required to provide information about the type of bleeding disorder and help in guiding further testing. Questions about life events associated with bleeding, bruising, with and without trauma, procedures, menstruation, and obstetric history provide critical information. The family history, including immediate and extended family members, can offer important information about inherited coagulation disorders. In anticipation of referring an individual with a coagulation disorder to a specialist, screening tests should include platelet count, prothrombin time (PT), activated partial thromboplastin time, thrombin time, and bleeding time to provide essential information regarding platelet function and coagulation factors (Dumas, McKernan, Zacharski, & Ornstein, 2013).

Single coagulation factor disorders are often congenital while there are a number of acquired conditions causing multiple coagulation factor deficiencies. Vitamin K deficiency and warfarin use, heparin, liver disease, and disseminated intravascular coagulation (DIC) are implicated in reducing or inactivating a number of coagulation factors (Van Cott & Laposata, 2014).

von Willebrand disease is the most common congenital bleeding disorder, caused by deficiency of von Willebrand factor (vWF). vWF acts to bind platelets to each other and to areas of injury in blood vessel walls. It also acts as a carrier protein for Factor VIII and has a critical role in thrombus formation. Making the diagnosis of von Willebrand disease may be difficult because the results of PT and aPTT may be normal and certain conditions, including pregnancy, stress, and inflammation may elevate vWF levels. Manifestation of this disorder may include epistaxis, prolonged bleeding from tooth extractions and other minor procedures, and menorrhagia. In addition to CBC, PT and aPTT, when von Willlebrand disease is suspected, additional useful information can be gained by ordering fibrinogen, thrombin time, vWF antigen quantitative assay, vWF activity assay, and Factor VIII activity (Dumas et al., 2013).

Qualitative platelet disorders are associated with abnormal platelet function despite a normal platelet count. Inherited platelet function disorders are rare; however, acquired platelet dysfunction is often associated with commonly used medications, including aspirin and clopidogrel. Uremia induced platelet dysfunction may also be present in patients with kidney disease (Van Cott & Laposata, 2014).

Quantitative platelet disorders may be manifested as thrombocytosis or thrombocytopenia. Thrombocytosis is uncommon but may be associated with myeloproliferative disorders or other malignancies. Thrombocytopenia can occur as result of immune and nonimmune platelet destruction or decreased platelet production. Metastasis from cancer with infiltration into the bone marrow or hematologic malignances may result in thrombocytopenia. Drug-induced thrombocytopenia may be a result of chemotherapy. Sequestration of platelets in the spleen may occur in patients with splenomegaly. Immune disorders may also result in increased platelet destruction (Van Cott & Laposata, 2014).

DIC occurs when uncontrolled localized or systemic activation of coagulation, leading to reduced coagulation factors, fibrinogen, and platelets. Several disorders are associated with development of DIC, including sepsis, cancer, burns, and trauma. Bleeding typically occurs a multiple sites. At the onset, coagulation factors and platelet counts may be within normal range, though reduced from baseline levels. Ultimately, thrombocytopenia, increased aPTT and PT, and decreased fibrinogen levels become apparent. HELLP syndrome (hemolysis, elevated liver enzymes, low platelets), a severe form of DIC that occurs in the peripartum period, includes elevated liver transaminases, and renal dysfunction. Treatment is dependent on the underlying cause as well. Additional treatment with blood products including platelets, cryoprecipitate, and fresh-frozen plasma may be needed to control bleeding (Fogarty & Minichiello, 2014)

There are both acquired and hereditary hypercoagulable states. Hereditary forms stem from either qualitative or quantitative deficiency of anticoagulant proteins, such as protein C (Van Cott & Laposata, 2014).

Factor V Leiden results from a single nucleotide mutation. It is the most common form of inherited coagulopathy and can be found in approximately 30% of people with deep vein thrombosis (DVT). It is primarily noted in those of European descent. When activated, factor V is usually inactivated by protein C. As a result of this mutation, there is a change in the ability of protein c to split factor V, creating increased high levels of factor V and prolonged clot formation. Many individuals with factor V Leiden do not have clinically significant clotting events; there is increased risk for DVT and pulmonary embolism (Rote and McCance, 2010c).

APAS is best described as thrombotic events or obstetric complications occurring in the presence of antiphospholipid antibodies. Antiphospholipid antibodies are acquired autoantibodies directed against phospholipid–protein complexes. Recognized laboratory criteria for APAS include lupus anticoagulant, IgG or IgM anticardiolipin antibodies, and IgG or IgM anti-β2 glycoprotein I antibodies. The cause of thrombosis in patients with APAS is not clear. Individuals with APAS may have one or more episodes of venous arterial or small vessel in any tissue or organ. The most common presentation is venous thromboembolism. Complications of pregnancy can include one or more fetal deaths in an otherwise normal fetus at 10 weeks gestation or more; one or more premature births in a normal neonate before 34 weeks gestation because of placental insufficiency, preeclampsia or eclampsia; or three or more unexplained spontaneous abortions before the tenth week of gestation (Sangle & Smock, 2011).

Diagnostic Studies

COMPLETE BLOOD COUNT

The CBC generally includes the hemoglobin, hematocrit, RBC count, RBC indices, and WBC count. Platelet count, WBC differential, and reticulocyte count are not always included and may need to be ordered separately (Schrier, 2010). An abnormal total WBC count in an individual with anemia should lead the provider to consider referral to a hematologist for further evaluation. Anemia in the presence of a low WBC count may be a result of bone marrow suppression, hypersplenism, or nutritional deficiency. Anemia accompanied by an abnormally high WBC count may be associated with infection, inflammation or hematologic malignancy. Platelet count abnormalities are associated with many conditions accompanied by anemia. Thrombocytopenia may be seen in the presence of hypersplenism, bone marrow malignancy, sepsis, folate, and vitamin B_{12} deficiency, as well as autoimmune platelet destruction. Elevated platelet counts can be indicative of chronic iron deficiency, inflammation or infection, or malignant disorders (Schrier, 2010).

HEMOGLOBIN

Hemoglobin is the oxygen carrying protein found in erythrocytes. Hemoglobin containing cells carry oxygen from the lungs and exchange it for carbon dioxide in the tissues. Hemoglobin is a direct reflection of the oxygen carrying capacity of the blood. The hemoglobin value is frequently used in combination with hematocrit in evaluation of anemia. Normal values in adult males range from 13.2 to 17.3 g/dL. Normal values for adult females range from 11.7 to 16.1 g/dL (Van Leeuwen, Poelhuis-Leth, Bladh, 2011).

HEMATOCRIT

The hematocrit or packed cell volume represents the percentage of RBCs in a volume of whole blood. A low-hematocrit level is associated with anemia. Normal values in adult males range from 38% to 51%; in females, the normal range is 33% to 45% (Van Leeuwen et al., 2011).

RED BLOOD CELL COUNT

The RBC count determines the number of RBCs per cubic millimeter. The RBC multiplied by three approximates the hemoglobin concentration and the hemoglobin multiplied by three should estimate the hematocrit if the RBC cell population is of normal shape and size. A number of drugs and other substances can influence the RBC count (Van Leeuwen et al., 2011).

RED BLOOD CELL INDICES

Four RBC indices are typically measured. MCV, MCH, mean corpuscular hemoglobin concentration (MCHC), and RBC distribution width (RDW) can be measured by most automatic blood cell counters in the laboratory (Schrier, 2010).

The normal range for MCV is 80 to 100 fL. Low MCV is seen in microcytic anemia while higher-than-normal values are seen with macrocytic anemia. Measures over 115 fL are most often associated with vitamin B_{12} or folic acid deficiency (Schrier, 2010).

Usual MCH values range from 27.5 to 33.2 pg of hemoglobin per RBC. Iron deficiency and thalassemia are manifested by lower than normal values while macrocytic anemias of all kinds have higher than normal MCH values (Schrier, 2010).

MCHC reflects the concentration of hemoglobin in each RBC and is noted as the percentage of the cell occupied by hemoglobin Normal MCHC values range from 32 to 36 g/dL in adult males and females (Van Leeuwen et al., 2011).

RDW represents the measurement of cell size distribution throughout the entire cell population measured. RDW is useful in identifying abnormal variations in cell size. The normal values for adult males and females range from 11.6 to 14.8 (Van Leeuwen et al., 2011).

RETICULOCYTE COUNT

The reticulocyte count is another indicator important in identifying the cause of anemia. When elevated it is associated with either hemorrhage or hemolysis. Normal or low reticulocyte counts in the presence of anemia indicate productive disorders including iron or vitamin B_{12} or folate deficiency, ACD, MDS, and aplastic anemia (Damon & Andreadis, 2014; Mais, 2014). Hemolytic anemias are associated with premature destruction of RBCs. Hemolysis can occur within the vascular system (intravascular) or in the reticuloendothelial system (extravascular). The reticulocyte count is an important marker in identifying acute versus chronic anemia. When an increased reticulocyte count is seen with anemia it is most often suggestive of hemorrhage or hemolysis (Mais, 2014). Reticulocytes typically account for less than 1.5% of all red cells. The proportion increases when in the presence of RBC loss in the peripheral circulation as the bone marrow responds to the need for increased RBC production. Anemia with an elevated reticulocyte count reflects the bone marrow's response to continued blood loss or hemolysis. Stable anemia with a low reticulocyte count is most often indicative of impaired RBC production. Hemolysis may be associated with a low reticulocyte count when there is a concurrent problem associated with deficient RBC production (Schrier, 2010). The normal value for reticulocyte count is 1.5% to 2.5% of the RBC count (Van Leeuwen et al., 2011).

Complete Blood Count Reference Values

	Reference Value
Hematocrit	
Male	41–50%
Female	35–45%
Hemoglobin	
Male	13.5–17.5 g/dL
Female	12.0–15.0 g/dL
Mean corpuscular hemoglobin (MCH)	27–33 pg/cell
Mean corpuscular hemoglobin concentration (MCHC)	33–37 gHb/dL
Mean corpuscular volume (MCV)	80–100 μm^3
Red blood cell count	
Male	4.6–6.0 10^6 μL
Female	3.9–5.5 10^6 μL
Platelet count	150–450 10^3 μL
Reticulocyte count	25–75 10^3 μL
White blood cell count	4.5–10 10^3 μL
Neutrophils	56%
Bands	3%
Lymphocytes	34%
Monocytes	4%
Eosinophils	2.7%
Basophils	0.3%

From Laposata, M. (2014). *Laboratory medicine: The diagnosis of disease in the clinical laboratory* (2nd ed.) New York, NY: McGraw-Hill.

SERUM FERRITIN

Ferritin is a protein synthesized in the liver, spleen, and bone marrow that reflects the amount of iron stored in the body. It is the most accurate initial diagnostic test for iron deficiency. A low-ferritin level is the earliest indicator of iron deficiency and continues for the duration of the illness. In the presence of inflammation and hepatic disease, other indicators may be needed to diagnose iron deficiency as ferritin may be falsely elevated (Killip, Bennett, & Chambers, 2007; Mais, 2014).

Levels vary according to age and gender. Levels below 10 are indicative of iron deficiency. Normal values for adult males range from 20 to 250 ng/mL. Values for females 18 to 39 years of age range from 10 to 120 ng/mL and women 40 and over from 12 to 263 ng/mL (Van Leeuwen et al., 2011).

TRANSFERRIN SATURATION

Transferrin is an iron-carrying protein. Transferrin saturation represents the amount of iron being carried. In the presence of iron deficiency, the amount of iron present to bind with transferrin is reduced causing a decrease in transferrin saturation. Transferrin saturation can be calculated using this formula:

$$\frac{\text{Serum iron} \times 100}{\text{TIBC}}$$

Normal values for transferrin saturation range from 15% to 50% (Griffis, 2013).

TOTAL IRON-BINDING CAPACITY

TIBC reflects the amount of iron in the serum in addition to the amount of transferrin available in serum. In the presence of iron deficiency, there is a decrease in transferrin saturation and an increase in iron binding capacity (Killip et al., 2007).

FOLATE LEVEL

Folate, or folic acid, is produced by organisms on the gastrointestinal tract and stored in small quantities by the liver. In addition to its importance in blood cell functions, it is also an important coenzyme in the conversion of homocysteine to methionine. Folate deficiency in pregnancy has been associated with risk for neural tube defects. Folate levels may be increased in the presence of vitamin B_{12} deficiency, pernicious anemia, and excessive dietary intake. Folate deficiency may be present with chronic alcohol abuse, inflammatory bowel disease, and other gastrointestinal disorders marked by malabsorption, hemolytic anemia, liver disease, malnutrition, pregnancy, and malignancies (Van Leeuwen et al., 2011).

VITAMIN B_{12} LEVEL

Vitamin B_{12} comes solely from the diet, with animal products being the most abundant sources. Vitamin B_{12} is essential for hematopoiesis, DNA synthesis, and integrity of nervous system functions. Levels may be increased in the presence of several chronic diseases including diabetes, hepatitis, and chronic obstructive lung disease. Deficiency made be related to decreased dietary intake but is also associated with a variety of gastrointestinal conditions accompanied by malabsorption, including surgery, inflammatory bowel disease, parasites, and bacterial overgrowth (Van Leeuwen et al., 2011).

Nutritional Reference Values

	Reference Value
Ferritin	15–200 ng/mL
Total iron	60–150 µg/dL
Total iron binding capacity	250–400 µg/dL
Folate	5–25 ng/mL
Vitamin B_{12}	160–950 pg/mL

From Laposata, M. (2014). *Laboratory medicine: The diagnosis of disease in the clinical laboratory* (2nd ed.) New York, NY: McGraw-Hill.

HEMOGLOBIN ELECTROPHORESIS

Electrophoresis is the process of separating through the application of electricity. When RBCs are lysed, the primary protein in the lysate is hemoglobin. In the normal adult, the predominant hemoglobin is hemoglobin A_1 with approximately 2% to 3% hemoglobin A_2 (Mais, 2014). Hemoglobin F is the predominant hemoglobin in the fetus; small amounts of hemoglobin F (less than 2%) may be present in adults. Deviations represent hemoglobinopathy or thalassemia (Van Leeuwen et al., 2011).

SICKLE HEMOGLOBIN SCREENING

Two assays are available for rapid screening for sickle hemoglobin without performing electrophoresis. The first can detect insoluble forms of hemoglobin within a lysate of blood. The second detects RBCs with sickling hemoglobin. At least 10% hemoglobin S must be present for the test to yield a positive result so in infants and individuals aggressively transfused the test may be negative. Neither is able to detect genotype information and may be positive in sickle cell disease or with heterozygous (Mais, 2014).

OSMOTIC FRAGILITY TEST

RBCs will expand and lyse in a hypotonic environment; spherocytes do so more quickly than normal biconcave cells. RBCs are placed in progressively more hypotonic solutions along with normal controls. A positive osmotic fragility test results in a more rapid lysis of abnormal cells. The test is most often positive for autoimmune hemolytic anemia, but may be positive in other conditions where spherocytosis is present (Mais, 2014).

DIRECT ANTIGLOBULIN (COOMBS TEST OR DAT)

Direct antiglobulin testing detects antibody sensitization of RBCs. Immunoglobulin G produced in certain disease states, or as a reaction to drugs, attaches to RBCs causing hemolysis. The reagent used in this test is an antibody taken from a mammal that binds to and reacts with human globulins. This reaction may occur in the presence of IgG or complement protein C3 or both. When patient blood is exposed to the reagent, agglutinationor clumping may occur suggesting that the cells are coated with IgG, C3, or both (Mais, 2014; Van Leeuwen et al., 2011).

G6PD DEFICIENCY TESTING

During acute hemolysis, the blood smear will often reveal both bite cells and Heinz bodies with the use of a special stain (Mais, 2014). The diagnosis of G6PD deficiency is made by G6PD assays including quantitative spectrophotometric analysis or more commonly, rapid fluorescent spot test detecting the generation of nicotinamide adenine dinucleotide plus hydrogen (NADPH) from nicotinamide adenine dinucleotide (NAD). The test is positive if bloodspot does not fluoresce under ultraviolet light (Frank, 2005; Minucci et al., 2009).

ENDOSCOPIC EVALUATION

Overt gastrointestinal bleeding is manifested with visible bleeding such as hematochezia or hematemesis and can be further classified as active or inactive. It is often referred to as obscure bleeding, and is recurrent or persistent despite negative findings after initial endoscopic evaluation. Occult refers to bleeding not seen by the patient or provider, which may be manifested as positive FOB or iron deficiency anemia (ASGE Standards of Practice Committee, 2010; Bull-Henry & Al-Kawas, 2013).

Esophagogastroduodenoscopy (EGD) and colonoscopy can identify a source of bleeding in up to 70% of cases (Bull-Henry & Al-Kawas, 2013). EGD is the diagnostic study of choice when an upper gastrointestinal source of bleeding is suspected particularly when there is risk of mucosal disease, such as use of nonsteroidal anti-inflammatory drugs (ASGE, 2010). Colonoscopy is important in identifying lesions in the large intestine; however, small intestine lesions are somewhat more difficult to detect.

Capsule endoscopy is a noninvasive study that may be used to examine the length of the small bowel and able to identify a number of small bowel lesions. It involves swallowing a capsule containing a small, wireless video camera. The device passes through the gastrointestinal tract taking and sending pictures to a recording device (Van Leeuwen et al., 2011).

Deep enteroscopy, also referred to as push endoscopy, uses a longer endoscope, allowing visibility up to the terminal jejunum (ASGE, 2010).

BONE MARROW BIOPSY

The bone marrow biopsy procedure involves the removal of a sample of marrow by aspiration or needle biopsy. The sample is utilized for a more complete hematologic evaluation beyond what can be seen in a CBC. Developing cells in the marrow are evaluated to assess cell morphology, iron stores, stages of cell development, and myeloid to erythroid ratio. Special staining of the sample can be done to identify various types of leukemia. Flow cytometry and cytogenetic studies can also be performed on bone marrow samples to identify leukemias (Van Leeuwen et al., 2011).

COAGULATION STUDIES

A variety of studies can be done to evaluate abnormal bleeding and clotting. Important basic studies are reviewed here.

Activate partial thromboplastin time (aPTT) provides information about the functions of intrinsic and common pathways of the coagulation sequence. aPTT represents the time needed for a firm clot to form when thromboplastin or similar reagents, and calcium are applied to the specimen. Abnormalities are found in most coagulation disorders. It is also important in monitoring the effects of heparin therapy. In combination with prothrombin time (PT), aPTT is used to identify many coagulation disorders (Van Leeuwen et al., 2011).

PT is a measure of the time after Factor III and calcium are applied to a sample of blood. It is used to assess the effects of warfarin therapy. Prothrombin is a protein, dependent on vitamin K produced by the liver. It is useful, as is aPTT to identify individuals who may be at risk for bleeding during invasive procedures. International normalized ratios (INR) are used to standardize PT results using the following formula:

$$INR = (patient\ PT\ result/normal\ patient\ average)^{ISI}$$

The normal patient average is provided by the International Sensitivity Index based on a reference provided by the WHO. This allows for standardization of results from laboratories around the world. Normal INR for patients not receiving anticoagulation therapy is less than two (Van Leeuwen et al., 2011). Conditions for which oral anticoagulation is strongly recommended, in the absence of significant risk for bleeding, include the following:
- Venous thromboembolism
- Antiphospholipid syndrome
- Atrial fibrillation
- Conditions requiring cardioversion
- Valvular heart disease and prosthetic valves
- Peripheral vascular disease
- Myocardial infarction and cardiomyopathy
- Pulmonary embolism
- DVT, including cancer-associated DVT (Keeling et al., 2011)

Fibrinogen is synthesized by the liver. Fibrinogen abnormalities may be congenital of acquired and may involve either decreased production or production of abnormal molecules (Van Cott & Laposata, 2014). It is an acute phase reactant and is often elevated in inflammatory conditions, including cancer, pregnancy, and is associated with increased risk for cardiovascular events. Decreased levels of fibrinogen may be seen in the presence of advanced liver disease and DIC when fibrinogen is rapidly converted to fibrin (Van Leeuwen et al., 2011).

Selected Coagulation Values

	Reference Value
Activated partial thromboplastin time	25–40 sec
Prothrombin time	10–13 sec
Fibrinogen	150–400 mg/dL
von Willebrand factor	70%–140%

From Van Leeuwen, A. M., Poelhuis-Leth, D., & Bladh, M. L. (2011). *Davis's comprehensive handbook of diagnostic tests with nursing implications* (4th ed.). Philadelphia, PA: F. A. Davis.

Recommended Target INR by Condition

Condition	Recommended Target INR
Venous thromboembolism, first episode	2.5
Venous thromboembolism, recurrent	3.5
Antiphospholipid antibody syndrome	2.5
Atrial fibrillation	2.5
Cardioversion	2.5
Mitral stenosis or regurgitation	2.5
Prosthetic heart valves	2.5–3.5

From Keeling, D., Baglin, T., Tait, C., Watson H., Perry, D., Baglin, C., . . . British Committee for
Standards in Haematology (2011). Guideline on oral anticoagulation with warfarin, 4th edition.
British Journal of Haematology, *154*(3), 311–324.

Review Section

Review Questions

1. Which of the following conditions may be noted in older adults with anemia? Select all that apply.

   1. Impaired cognitive function
   2. Alteration in mobility
   3. Falls
   4. Chronic diseases
      a. 1, 2, and 3
      b. 2, 3, and 4
      c. 1, 2, and 4
      d. 1, 2, 3, and 4

2. What is the most important cause of iron deficiency in adults?

   a. Chronic inflammation
   b. Kidney disease
   c. Blood loss
   d. Nutritional deficiency

3. Which of the following are classified as hemolytic anemia? Select all that apply.

   1. Thalassemia
   2. Hereditary spherocytosis
   3. Autoimmune
   4. Iron deficiency
      a. 1 and 2
      b. 2 and 3
      c. 1, 2, and 3
      d. 1, 2, 3, and 4

4. Which medication is most frequently associated with iron deficiency anemia?

   a. Antibiotics
   b. Vitamin B_{12}
   c. Anti-inflammatory drugs
   d. Proton pump inhibitors

5. Which of the following physical findings may be associated with anemia?

   1. Pallor
   2. Paresthesia
   3. Splenic enlargement
   4. Tachycardia
      a. 1 and 2
      b. 1, 2, and 3
      c. 2, 3, and 4
      d. 1, 2, 3, and 4

6. Which of the following treatment approaches is most effective treatment of anemia associated with chronic renal failure or malignancy?

   a. Oral iron supplementation
   b. Vitamin B_{12}
   c. Erythropoietin
   d. Corticosteroids

7. Which of the following is the safest and most cost-effective treatment for individuals with microcytic anemia associated with blood loss after treatment for the source of bleeding?

    a. Transfusion
    b. Parenteral iron supplementation
    c. Oral iron supplementation
    d. Vitamin B_{12} and folate supplementation

8. Which of the following is likely to be associated with hemolysis in an individual with G6PD deficiency?

    1. Trimethoprim–sulfamethoxazole
    2. Fava beans
    3. Penicillin
    4. Avocado
        a. 1 and 2
        b. 1, 2, and 3
        c. 2, 3, and 4
        d. 1, 2, 3, and 4

9. Which of the following blood disorders is known to predispose individuals to development of leukemia?

    a. β-Thalassemia
    b. Myelodysplastic syndrome
    c. Hereditary spherocytosis
    d. Vitamin B_{12} deficiency

10. A 58-year-old male patient is being treated for lung cancer and has chemotherapy-induced anemia, which is treated by his oncologist with darbepoetin. He is seen in the clinic for routine follow-up. Which of the following is an indication for contacting his oncologist because of a possible side effect from the darbepoetin?

    a. New onset of blood pressure elevation
    b. Hemoglobin of 11 g/dL
    c. Hematocrit of 33.2
    d. Complaints of chronic fatigue

Answers with Rationales

1. (d) 1, 2, 3, and 4

    Rationale: Even mild anemia in the elderly can be associated with impaired mobility, deceased cognitive function, depressive symptoms, and risk for falls. Anemia is associated with chronic inflammatory disorders and other chronic diseases, including renal failure.

2. (c) Blood loss

    Rationale: The most important cause of iron deficiency in US adults is chronic blood loss, most often via the gastrointestinal tract. The American Gastroenterology Association suggests that in men and postmenopausal women, iron deficiency should be assumed to be associated with gastrointestinal blood loss until proven otherwise.

3. (c) 1, 2, and 3

    Rationale: Hemolysis can occur in the presence of thalassemia, hereditary spherocytosis, and autoimmune disorders. Iron deficiency is associated with microcytic hypochromic anemia.

4. (c) Anti-inflammatory drugs

    Rationale: Blood loss may be associated chronic use of anti-inflammatory drugs including aspirin, ibuprofen, naproxen, and glucocorticoids.

5. (d) 1, 2, 3, and 4

    Rationale: All of the above findings can be associated with anemia. Pallor and tachycardia may be signs common to all forms of anemia. Splenic enlargement may be found in the presence of hemolytic anemias and myelodysplastic disorders. Paresthesia is often evidence in vitamin B_{12} deficiency.

6. (c) Erythropoietin

    Rationale: Erythropoietin is indicated for treatment of anemia associated with chronic renal failure, anemia associated with treatment for cancer, anemia related to treatment with zidovudine for human immunodeficiency virus infection, and for individuals with anemia, scheduled to have surgery to reduce the need for perioperative transfusions.

7. (c) Oral iron supplementation

    Rationale: Treatment of iron deficiency with oral supplementation is the preferred therapy in most situations. It is cost-effective and generally well tolerated.

8. (a) 1 and 2

    Rationale: Sulfa drugs, antimalarial drugs, nitrofurantoin, dapsone, and legumes, including fava beans, are likely to precipitate hemolysis in individuals with G6PD deficiency.

9. (b) Myelodysplastic syndrome

    Rationale: Myelodysplastic syndromes (MDSs) are one of five major categories of myeloid malignancies. Characterized by dysplastic and ineffective blood cell production, MDS carries the risk of transformation to acute leukemia.

10. (a) New onset of blood pressure elevation

    Rationale: Erythropoiesis-stimulating agents, including erythropoietin and darbepoetin, can precipitate sudden increases in blood pressure, particularly when hypertension is poorly controlled. Both hypertension and seizures have been noted in cases where hematocrit rises quickly.

Suggested Readings

Ackerman, R. (2014). Drugs used in treatment of blood disorders. In W. Tindall, M. Sedrak, & J. M. Boltri (Eds.), *Patient-centered pharmacology* (pp. 135–157). Philadelphia, PA: F. A. Davis.

Agency for Toxic Substances and Disease Registry. (2007). *Toxicology profile for lead*. Atlanta, GA: U.S. Department of Health and Human Services, Public Health Service, Agency for Toxic Substances and Disease Registry.

ASGE Standards of Practice Committee. (2010). The role of endoscopy in obscure GI bleeding. *Gastrointestinal Endoscopy*, 72(3), 471–479.

Banasik, J. L. (2013). Inflammation and Immunity. In L. Copstead & J. Banasik (Eds.), *Pathophysiology* (5th ed., pp. 157–194). St. Louis, MO: Elsevier Saunders.

Bolton-Maggs, P. H., Stevens, R. F., Dodd, N. J., Lamont, G., Tittensor, P., & King, M. J. (2004). Guidelines for the diagnosis and management of hereditary spherocytosis. *British Journal of Haematology, 126*, 445–474.

Brill, J. R., & Baumgardner, D. (2000). Normocytic anemia. *American Family Physician, 62*(10), 2255–2263.

Bross, M. H., Soch, K., & Smith-Knuppel, T. (2010). Anemia in older persons. *American Family Physician, 82*(5), 480–487.

Bull-Henry, K., & Al-Kawas, F. H. (2013). Evaluation of occult gastrointestinal bleeding. *American Family Physician, 87*(6), 430–436.

Carter, D., Levi, G., Tzur, D. Novis, B., & Avidan, B. (2013). Prevalence and predictive value of gastrointestinal pathology in young men evaluated for iron deficiency anemia. *Digestive Diseases and Sciences, 58*, 1299–1305.

Cheerva, A. C., Bleibel, S.A., Jones-Crawford, J. L., Kutlar, A., Leonard, R., & Raj, A. B. (2014). Alpha thalassemia. Retrieved from emedicine.medscape.com

Damon, L. E., & Andreadis, C. (2014). Blood disorders. In M. Papadakis & S. McPhee (Eds.), *Current medical diagnosis and treatment, 2014* (pp. 473–519). New York, NY: McGraw-Hill.

Denny, S. D., Kuchibhatla, M. N., & Cohen, H. J. (2006). Impact of anemia on mortality, cognition, and function in community-dwelling elderly. *American Journal of Medicine, 119*(4), 327–334.

Doll, D. C., & Landaw, S. A. (2010). Clinical manifestations and diagnosis of the myelodysplastic syndromes. Retrieved from http://www.uptodateonline.com.

Dumas, M. M., McKernan, L. Zacharski, L. R., & Ornstein, D.L. (2013). Blood coagulation disorders. In T. M. Buttaro, J. Tryulski, B. P. Bailey, & J. Sandberg-Cook (Eds.), *Primary care: A collaborative practice* (4th ed., pp. 1158–1167). St. Louis, MO: Elsevier Mosby.

Dunbar, L. N., Coleman Brown, L., Rivera, D. R., Hartzema, A. G., & Lottenberg, R. (2012). Transfusion practices in the management of sickle cell disease: A survey of Florida hematologists/oncologists. *ISRN Hematology, 2012*, Article ID 524513, 1–12.

Fogarty, P. F., & Minichiello, T. (2014). Disorders of hemostasis, thrombosis, & antithrombotic therapy. In M. Papadakis & S. McPhee (Eds.), *Current medical diagnosis and treatment, 2014* (pp. 520–546). New York, NY: McGraw-Hill.

Frank, J. E. (2005). Diagnosis and management of G6PD deficiency. *American Family Physician, 72*(7), 1277–1282.

Granick, J. L., Simon, S. I., & Borjesson, D. L. (2012). Hematopoietic stem and progenitor cells as effectors in innate immunity. *Bone Marrow Research*. doi:10.1155/2012/165107.

Griffis, K. P. (2013). Evaluation and management of hematologic disorders. In T. M. Buttaro, J. Tryulski, B. P. Bailey, & J. Sandberg-Cook (Eds.), *Primary care: A collaborative practice*. (4th ed., pp. 1139–1181). St. Louis, MO: Elsevier Mosby.

Guralanik, J. M., Eisenstadt, R. S., Ferrucci, L., Klein, H. G., & Woodman, R. C. (2004). Prevalence of anemia in persons 65 years and older in the United States: Evidence for a high rate of unexplained anemia. *Blood, 104*, 2263–2268.

Hooper, M., Hudson, P., Porter, F., & McCaddon, A. (2004). Patient journeys: Diagnosis and treatment of pernicious anaemia. *British Journal of Nursing, 23*(7), 376–381.

Keeling, D., Baglin, T., Tait, C., Watson H., Perry, D., Baglin, C., . . . British Committee for Standards in Haematology (2011). Guideline on oral anticoagulation with warfarin, 4th edition. *British Journal of Haematology, 154*(3), 311–324.

Killip, S., Bennett, J. M., & Chambers, M. D. (2007). Iron deficiency anemia. *American Family Physician, 75*, 5671–5678.

Kline, N. E. (2010). Alterations of hematologic function in children. In K. L. McCance, S. E. Huether, V. L. Brasher, & N. S. Rote (Eds.), *Pathophysiology: The biologic basis for disease in adults and children* (6th ed., pp. 1062–1090). Maryland Heights, MO: Mosby Elsevier.

Koitke, H., Hama, T., Kawagashira, Y., Hashimoto, R., Tomita, M., Iijima, M., & Soue, G. (2012). The significance of folate deficiency in alcoholic and nutritional neuropathies: Analysis of a case. *Nutrition, 28*, 821–824.

Kotter, M. L., & Trevithick, S. G. (2013). Alterations in oxygen transport. In L. Copstead & J. Banasik (Eds.), *Pathophysiology* (5th ed., pp. 255–293). St. Louis, MO: Elsevier-Saunders.

Lanza, F. L., Chan, F. K., Quigley, E. M.; Practice Parameters Committee. (2009). Guidelines for prevention of NSAID-related ulcer complications. *American Journal of Gastroenterology, 104*, 728–738.

Laposata, M. (2014). *Laboratory medicine: The diagnosis of disease in the clinical laboratory* (2nd ed.) New York, NY: McGraw-Hill.

Mais, D. D. (2014). Diseases of red blood cells. In M. Laposata (Ed.), *Laboratory medicine: The diagnosis of disease in the clinical laboratory* (2nd ed., pp. 221–252). New York, NY: McGraw-Hill.

McEvoy, M. T., & Shander, A. (2013). Anemia, bleeding, and blood transfusion in the intensive care unit: causes, risks, costs, and new strategies. *American Journal of Critical Care, 22*(6) S1–S13.

Minucci, A., Giardina, B., Zuppi, C, & Capoluongo, E. (2009). *IUBMB Life, 61*(1), 27-34.

Muncie, H. L., & Campbell, J. S. (2009). Alpha and beta thalassemia. *American Family Physician*, 80(4), 339–344, 371.

Nau, K. C., & Lewis, W. D. (2008). Multiple myeloma: Diagnosis and treatment. *American Family Physician*, 78(7), 853–859.

National Heart, Lung, and Blood Institute. (2014). Evidence based guidelines for management of sickle cell disease. Retrieved from http://www.nhlbi.nih.gov/sites/www.nhlbi.nih.gov/files/sickle-cell-disease-report.pdf

Orkin, S. H., & Zon, L. I. (2008). Hematopoiesis: An evolving paradigm for stem cell biology. *Cell, 132*, 631–644.

Pharmacology Weekly. (2014). What are common medications that should be avoided in patients with known G6PD deficiency? Retrieved from http://www.pharmacologyweekly.com/articles/G6PD-deficiency-medications-drugs-avoid

Powers, J. M., & Buchanan, G. R. (2014). Iron deficiency in infants and toddlers: How to manage when prevention fails. *Contemporary Pediatrics, 31*(5), 12–17.

Rote, N. S, & McCance, K. L. (2010a). Structure and function of the hematologic system. In K. L. McCance, S. E. Huether, V. L. Brasher, & N. S. Rote (Eds.), *Pathophysiology: The biologic basis for disease in adults and children* (6th ed., pp. 952–988). Maryland Heights, MO: Mosby Elsevier.

Rote, N. S., & McCance, K. L. (2010b). Alterations of erythrocyte function. In K. L. McCance, S. E. Huether, V. L. Brasher, & N. S. Rote (Eds.), *Pathophysiology: The biologic basis for disease in adults and children* (6th ed., pp. 989–1013). Maryland Heights, MO: Mosby Elsevier.

Sabol, V. K., Resnick, B., Galik, E., Gruger-Baldini, A, Gonce Morton, P., & Hicks, P. E. (2010). Anemia and its impact on nursing home residents: What do we know? *Journal of the Academy of Nurse Practitioners, 22*, 3–16.

Sangle, N. A., & Smock, K. J. (2011). Antiphospholipid antibody syndrome. *Archives of Pathology and Laboratory Medicine. 135*(9), 1092–1096.

Renouf, L. S., Sheps, S., Hubley, A., Pick, N., Johansen, D., & Tyndall, M. (2012). The role of diet in predicting iron deficiency in HIV positive women. *Canadian Journal of Diet Practice and Research, 73*(3), 128–133.

Shander, A., Javidroozi, M., Ozawa, S, & Hare, G. M. T. (2011). What is really dangerous: anaemia or transfusion? *British Journal of Anaesthesia, 107*(Suppl 1), i41–i59.

Schauer, P. R., Ikramuddin, S., Gourash, W., Ramanathan, R., & Luketich, J. (2000). Outcomes after laparoscopic Roux-en-Y bypass for morbid obesity. *Annals of Surgery, 323*(4), 515–529.

Schrier, S. L. (2010). *Approach to the adult with anemia.* Retrieved from http://www.uptodateonline.com

Short, M. W., & Domagalski, J. E. (2013). Iron deficiency anemia: Evaluation and management. *American Family Physician, 87*(2), 98–104.

Tefferi, A., & Vardiman, J. W. (2009). Myelodysplastic syndromes. *New England Journal of Medicine, 361*(19), 1872–1885.

Teucher, B., Olivares, M., & Cori, H. (2004). Enhancers of iron absorption: Ascorbic acid and other organic acids. *International Journal of Nutrition Research, 74*(6), 403–419.

Tweet, M. S., & Polga, K. (2010). 44-year-old man with shortness of breath, fatigue, and paresthesia. *Mayo Clinic Proceedings, 85*(12), 1148–1151.

Van Cott, E. M., & Laposata, M. (2014). Bleeding and thrombotic disorders. In M. Laposata (Ed.), *Laboratory medicine: The diagnosis of disease in the clinical laboratory* (2nd ed., pp. 253–290). New York, NY: McGraw-Hill.

Van Leeuwen, A. M., Poelhuis-Leth, D., & Bladh, M. L. (2011). *Davis's comprehensive handbook of diagnostic tests with nursing implications* (4th ed.). Philadelphia, PA: F. A. Davis.

Versteeg, H. H., Heemskerk, J. W. M., Levi, M., & Reitsma, P. H. (2013). New fundamentals in hemostasis. *Physiological Reviews, 93*(1), 327–358. doi:10.1152/physrev.00016.2011

Weinziehr, E. P., & Arber, D. A. (2013). The differential diagnosis and bone marrow evaluation of new-onset pancytopenia. *American Journal of Clinical Pathology, 139*, 9–29.

Wilby, M. L. (2011). Anemia in older adults. *PADONA Journal, 24*(1), 15–19.

World Health Organization. (2001). *Iron deficiency anaemia assessment, prevention, and control: A guide for programme managers.* Geneva, Switzerland: World Health Organization.

World Health Organization. (2011). *Haemoglobin concentrations for the diagnosis of anaemia and assessment of severity.* Geneva, Switzerland: World Health Organization.

Yamazaki, H., & Nakao, S. (2013). Border between aplastic anemia and myelodysplastic syndrome. *International Journal of Hematology, 97*, 558–563.

Young, N. S., Calado, R. T., & Scheinberg, P. (2006). Current concepts in pathophysiology and treatment of aplastic anemia. *Blood, 108*(8), 2509–2519.

Chapter 12

Immune System

Mary L. Wilby

Case Presentation

Directions: Carefully review the case study presented below. At the end of the chapter, answer the review questions. Compare your answers to the correct answers listed in the Review Section.

Chief Complaint: Fever and sore throat

History of Present Illness: A 36-year-old woman presents to the clinic with acute fever, sore throat, and muscle aches for the last several days. She reports that her glands are swollen, and she has a frontal headache. She has fatigue, a decreased appetite, and denies nausea or vomiting. She has intermittent diarrhea. She denies abdominal pain. She also notes a nonpruritic rash on her chest. She denies any other significant health problems. This is her first visit for care in 3 years.

Past Medical History:
Noncontributory, denies any chronic illnesses, no surgeries or hospitalizations. No history of diabetes.

Allergies:
No known medication, food, or environmental allergies

Medications:
Multivitamin daily, acetaminophen as needed

Social History:
She is recently divorced with no children and works as an administrative assistant. She is a lifelong nonsmoker and drinks three to five alcoholic beverages per week. Lives in own home.

Sexual History:
Menarche at age 14 with regular menses every 28 to 30 days, no excessive bleeding. Monogamous with one male partner for 10 years until divorce. Sexual encounter approximately 4 weeks ago with male partner after a party without barrier protection after "way too much to drink." She reports six lifetime partners, all male. Typically uses condoms for contraception. Gravida 0 Para 0.

Health Maintenance:
No recent influenza vaccine, unsure when last tetanus shot given. Last Pap smear 4 years ago.

Review of Systems:
Reports fatigue over the last few days, with acute onset of fever, chills, sore throat as noted earlier. No recent weight changes. Denies visual changes. No dental problems or mouth ulcers. Denies cough, wheezing, chest tightness, or shortness of breath. Notes dysphagia; no nausea, vomiting, or constipation; occasional diarrhea. No blood in stool. No numbness or tingling in extremities, no history of syncope or seizures. Positive frontal headache. Positive muscle aches, but no joint pain, stiffness, or swelling. History of wrist fracture as a teen. Denies history of alcohol or drug abuse, no history of anxiety or depression.

Physical Examination:

Vital Signs: Temperature = 100.8°F   Pulse = 88   Respirations = 14   BP = 116/68   Height = 67 inches
   Weight = 127 lb   BMI = 19.9

General: Well-groomed, thin female, appears stated age, in no acute distress

Head: Normocephalic, atraumatic

Eyes: Sclera white, conjunctiva pink, no discharge

Neck: Supple, trachea midline, no thyromegaly. Enlarged bilateral posterior cervical lymph nodes, 2 to 3 cm in diameter, firm, and mobile

Mouth/Throat: Oral mucosa pink, without lesions. Pharynx erythematous, without exudate

Lungs: Clear to auscultation

Heart: Regular rate and rhythm, no murmurs or gallops

Breasts: No masses or tenderness, no axillary lymphadenopathy

Abdomen: Flat, normal bowel sounds, nontender, liver span 11 cm at mid-clavicular line. No splenomegaly

Extremities: No peripheral edema, no cyanosis or clubbing

Skin: Diffuse erythematous maculopapular rash on chest and back

Genitourinary: Deferred until next visit

Assessment:

- Acute viral syndrome with pharyngitis
- Risk for acute retroviral syndrome
- Need for age-appropriate screening
- Bring immunizations up to date

Differential Diagnoses:

- Acute viral syndrome
- Streptococcal pharyngitis
- Influenza
- Acute HIV infection

Plan:

Screening for HIV, syphilis, chlamydia, gonorrhea. Check complete blood count, chemistry panel, return for review of laboratory results in 2 to 3 days. Return for influenza and tetanus with pertussis vaccines after laboratory tests drawn. Return for Pap smear in next few weeks.

Complete blood count and chemistry panel were within normal limits. HIV RNA viral load and HIV antibody by ELISA were positive. Patient returned in 1 week to discuss results of testing and to receive counseling. Confirmatory testing with Western blot was ordered and was also positive. Patient was referred to HIV specialist services at the local hospital for further evaluation and ongoing follow-up.

Human Immunodeficiency Virus Infection

Human immunodeficiency virus (HIV) infects and depletes a segment of the immune system leaving those infected at significant risk for certain malignancies and infection. Throughout the world HIV infection and Acquired Immune Deficiency Syndrome (AIDS) are major causes of morbidity and mortality. While the number of new cases and deaths in the United States has stabilized in recent years, around the world, particularly in sub-Saharan Africa, the number of cases and deaths continues to grow (Rote & Huether, 2010a).

It has been over 30 years since the first case of AIDS was identified in the United States. Since that time, the care of people infected with the HIV has changed dramatically (Aberg et al., 2013). The CDC AIDS case definition includes opportunistic infections and malignancies that typically do not occur in the absence of severe immune deficiency. Classification of AIDS also includes those with positive HIV serology and certain infections and malignancies that can develop in immunocompetent individuals but are more common in those with HIV infection. Other nonspecific conditions, including wasting and dementia occurring in the presence of positive HIV serology are also included in the definition of AIDS. Additionally, individuals with positive HIV serology who have ever had a CD4 lymphocyte count of 200 cells/μL or less or a CD4 lymphocyte percentage less than 14 are also diagnosed with AIDS (Zolopa & Katz, 2014).

The CDC classifies the following as AIDS defining conditions:
- Multiple or recurrent bacterial infections, in children under 13 years of age
- Candidiasis of esophagus
- Invasive cervical cancer in adolescents and adults 13 years of age or older
- Disseminated or extrapulmonary coccidioidomycosis
- Extrapulmonary cryptococcosis
- Chronic interstitial cryptosporidiosis, greater than 1 month
- Cytomegalovirus (CMV) disease, onset at age greater than 1 month
- CMV retinitis
- HIV-related encephalopathy
- Herpes simplex: Ulcers greater than 1 month's duration or bronchitis, pneumonitis, or esophagitis onset at age greater than 1 month
- Disseminated or extrapulmonary histoplasmosis
- Isosporiasis, greater than 1 month's duration
- Kaposi sarcoma
- Lymphoid interstitial pneumonia or pulmonary lymphoid hyperplasia complex in children under 13 years of age
- Burkitt lymphoma
- Immunoblastic lymphoma
- Primary brain lymphoma
- Disseminated or extrapulmonary *Mycobacterium avium* complex or *M. kansasii*
- *M. tuberculosis* of any site, pulmonary, disseminated, or extrapulmonary
- *Mycobacterium*, other species or unidentified species, disseminated or extrapulmonary
- *Pneumocystis jirovecii* pneumonia
- Recurrent pneumonia, in adolescents and adult 13 years of age or older
- Progressive multifocal leukoencephalopathy (PML)
- Recurrent Salmonella septicemia
- Toxoplasmosis of brain, onset at age greater than 1 month
- Wasting syndrome attributed to HIV (Morbidity and Mortality Weekly Report, 2008)

The availability of highly active antiretroviral therapy (HAART) since the mid-1990s has markedly changed the prognosis for people with HIV/AIDS. Fewer individuals receiving treatment for HIV infection develop a malignancy or infection, or CD4 count low enough to be classified as having AIDS. Many of those who had been diagnosed with AIDS are able to live healthier lives, with higher CD4 counts (Zolopa & Katz, 2014).

Epidemiology

There are over 1 million people in the United States living with HIV infection. Due to advances in care in recent years, the number of newly infected people outweighs the number of deaths. Recent data from the Centers for Disease Control and Prevention (CDC, 2014) reveal that 64% of infections in adolescents and adults are among gay, bisexual, and other men who have sex with men. Approximately 26% of infections occur in heterosexual people, with 67% of those infections among women. An additional 10% of infections are among those who are injection drug users. Less than 1% of living cases of HIV infection are among children. HIV-infected people are disproportionately Black/African American and Hispanic/Latino, living in the Southeast or mid-Atlantic portions of the United States and Puerto Rico, United States Virgin Islands, and some of the country's largest cities (CDC, 2014; Zolopa & Katz, 2014).

There are approximately 33 million people infected with HIV throughout the world. Heterosexual transmission is the most common means of spreading HIV infection among men and women. In some regions of Central and East Africa, nearly 30% of sexually active adults are infected (Zolopa & Katz, 2014).

Transmission of HIV infection can occur through sexual contact, sharing of drug paraphernalia, perinatal routes, needle sticks, and receipt of contaminated blood products. Certain sexual practices, including anal receptive intercourse are significantly riskier than others. Since 1985 universal screening of donated blood using enzyme-linked immunosorbent assay (ELISA) to identify antibodies has been practiced. This coupled with screening of potential donors who have engaged in high-risk behaviors have decreased risk of blood contamination significantly (Zolopa & Katz, 2014).

Between 13% and 40% of children born to HIV-infected mothers contract HIV infection if the mother has not been treated or when the child has not received prophylactic treatment. The availability of antiretroviral drugs for pregnant women since the 1990s has drastically reduced the risk of mother-to-child transmission (Aberg et al., 2013; Zolopa & Katz, 2014).

Progression of HIV-related illness is similar in women and men. Women are also at risk for gynecologic complications including vulvovaginal candidiasis, cervical dysplasia, and pelvic inflammatory disease. Treatment of women is challenging because of issues surrounding pregnancy, drug use, violence against women, and poverty (Zolopa & Katz, 2014).

Etiology

HIV is a blood-borne pathogen found in body fluids, including blood, vaginal fluid, semen, and breast milk. Transmission of the virus can occur through transfusion of contaminated blood and blood products, intravenous drug use with sharing of needles, heterosexual and same sex activity, and from mother to child before or during childbirth (Rote & Huether, 2010a).

HIV is a retrovirus. It carries genetic material in the form of two copies of RNA. Retroviruses are capable of using an enzyme, referred to as reverse transcriptase, to convert RNA into double-stranded DNA. Using an additional enzyme, the newly created DNA is inserted into the infected cell's genetic material, where it may be dormant or become activated. When activated, translation of the viral information occurs, resulting in production of new virons. When viral information is activated, death of the infected cells occurs with subsequent shedding of viral material. HIV-1 is the primary strain of the virus causing infection, but other less virulent strains have been identified (Rote & Huether, 2010a).

Syndromes associated with HIV infection can be explained by one of three alterations in immune activity. Immunodeficiency results from the effects of HIV on immune cells and the influence of generalized inflammation and immune activation associated with chronic viral infection. Autoimmunity results from alterations in cellular immunity and B cell dysfunction. Autoantibody production and lymphocytic infiltration of organs can occur either alone or in combination. Individuals infected with HIV also have higher rates of allergic reactions to unknown allergens in addition to increased rates of hypersensitivity to medications (Zolopa & Katz, 2014)

The primary target of the virus is the CD4 molecule found on the surface of T helper lymphocytes, though other cells may be infected as well. Additional cellular targets include dendritic cells, macrophages, CD 8-positive T lymphocytes, thymic cells which express both CD4 and CD8, natural killer (NK) cells, and neural cells of monocyte origin (Rote & Huether, 2010a).

The virus attaches to the CD4 lymphocyte, creating a cascade of intracellular signals that are believed to facilitate virus replication. Interactions between the virus and chemokine receptors activate changes in the cellular structures. The viral core enters the lymphocyte cytoplasm, and the viral genome is reverse transcribed into the lymphocyte DNA aided by the actions of the virus's reverse transcriptase enzyme. Proliferation of the virus initially takes place in the regional lymph tissue. Infected T lymphocytes or viral particles then migrate through the bloodstream and expand in the gastrointestinal tract, spleen, and bone marrow, resulting in considerable infection of vulnerable cells, resulting in significant increase in viral load in the bloodstream (Simon, Ho, & Abdool Karim, 2006). The virus is also found in T-cells and macrophages found in semen and renal epithelium. Cells in the central nervous system may act as a holding area where HIV-infected cells can be shielded from the effects of antiretroviral drugs (Rote & Huether, 2010a).

There is a significant decrease in CD4 lymphocyte counts during the acute phase of infection along with an increase in HIV viral load once the virus has been transmitted to lymphoid tissue. Acute infection causes a strong inflammatory response characterized by increased amounts of cytokines and chemokines resulting in the symptoms that are associated with acute retroviral syndrome (Cohen, Gay, Busch, & Hecht, 2010). The degree of viremia decreases after the acute infection phase. In addition the number of CD4-positive cells decreases. Gradual destruction of CD4-positive T-lymphocytes is the hallmark of HIV infection, with AIDS being the final disease stage. Although patients may have few symptoms in both early and chronic stages of infection, replication of the virus is ongoing throughout the course of the disease (Simon et al., 2006).

The primary immunologic finding in AIDS is the dramatic effect on the numbers of CD4-positive T lymphocytes. Individuals who are not infected usually have a range of 600 to 1,200 CD4-positive cells per microliter of blood (Rote & Huether, 2010a). HIV causes immunodeficiency through a variety of different mechanisms. As noted above, production of new virons can be directly toxic to the infected cells. Additionally, new surface antigens can serve as targets for other T cells, making them vulnerable to immune mediated lysis. While a number of cells are infected, the majority of CD4-positive T lymphocytes are not infected but still show signs of apoptosis or cell death. It is believed that HIV-infected lymphocytes shed viral proteins that are capable of inducing apoptosis even in uninfected T lymphocytes, neurons, and monocytes (Rote & Huether, 2010a).

Risk Factors

Gay and bisexual men are affected by HIV/AIDS more than any other group in the United States. Gay, bisexual, and other men who have sex with men represent approximately 2% of the United States population yet account for the majority of those infected with HIV. Among all gay and bisexual men, Black/African American men carry a disproportionate burden of HIV infections (CDC, 2014). High-risk sexual risk behaviors account for the majority of HIV infections in gay and bisexual men. Gay and bisexual men acquire HIV through anal sex, which is the riskiest type of sex for becoming infected and transmitting the virus. For sexually active gay and bisexual men, the most effective strategies for prevention of transmission or infection with HIV are to be on antiretroviral medications (to either treat or prevent infection) and to correctly use a condom every time for anal or vaginal sex. Gay men are at increased risk for sexually transmitted infections, including syphilis, gonorrhea, and chlamydia, and the CDC (2014) recommends that all sexually active gay and bisexual be tested at least annually for these infections and obtain treatment, if necessary. Having multiple sex partners increases the risk of infection as there are an increased number of opportunities to have sex with someone who can transmit HIV or another sexually transmitted infection.

Women may be unaware of their male partner's risk factors for HIV infection (including intravenous drug use or having sex with men) and may not use condoms. Women are at higher risk for HIV infection during vaginal sex without a condom than men. Additionally, anal sex without a condom is more risky than vaginal sex without a condom. Women who have been sexually abused are more likely to engage in high-risk sexual behavior than those who have not been abused (CDC, 2014). Infection with sexually transmitted diseases, such as syphilis and gonorrhea can increase the likelihood of becoming infected with HIV. Some women may believe they are unable to talk with their partners about condom use and may even suffer abuse when asking partners to use condoms. Because HIV prevalence is greater in African American and Hispanic/Latino communities and the majority of people tend to have sex with partners of the same race/ethnicity, women from these communities are at greater risk of HIV infection with each new sexual encounter (CDC, 2014).

Others who experience a disproportionate rate of HIV infection in the United States include adolescents and adults, including men and women using drugs, especially those persons who inject drugs, individuals living in areas with high HIV prevalence, young people leaving foster care, and transgender females (CDC, 2014).

Social factors can influence risk for HIV infection. Health-care providers should be aware of that poverty, unemployment, food insecurity, and unstable housing may increase behaviors that increase risk for HIV transmission when these factors prompt decisions to exchange sex for food, housing, and money as well as sharing drug injection materials. Limited education may reduce understanding of information directed at reducing risk for transmission of infection (CDC, 2014).

Mental illness and psychological conditions, including depression, anxiety, and social isolation may coexist with substance use and decrease willingness or ability to seek prevention services or use prevention strategies as well as impairing judgment and increase sexual and drug–injection risk behaviors. Individuals who engage in commercial sex work or are victims of sexual assault may be unable to negotiate condom use or have trauma that may result in blood borne HIV exposure (CDC, 2014).

Signs and Symptoms

Acute HIV infection, or acute retroviral syndrome may present in patients within 2 to 4 weeks of exposure to the virus. Symptoms associated with acute infection including fever, chills, muscle and joint aches, sore throat, lymphadenopathy, and rashes can occur in many, but not all patients. During this early period, viral loads are high and CD4 counts may drop precipitously. Eventually a "viral set point" is reached as a stable level of the virus is achieved. Risk of virus transmission is especially high during this time as the viral load is quite high (Rote & Huether, 2010a).

A clinical latency period follows the acute phase of HIV infection. Especially when individuals are receiving ART, HIV infection may be asymptomatic for many years, even decades. When symptoms do occur they are often variable and nonspecific. It is often a combination of symptoms that is most suggestive of HIV infection. Despite the lack of symptoms, it is possible to transmit the virus during this period (Rote & Huether, 2010; Zolopa & Katz, 2014).

People living with HIV infection may progress through the stages at different rates depending on a variety of factors, including their genetic makeup, their health status prior to infection, how soon after infection they are diagnosed and enter care and treatment, and whether they adhere to their medication regimen and receive follow-up care. Age, HIV subtype, nutritional status, and coinfection with other viruses are other factors that can influence the speed of progression of infection (Rote & Huether, 2010a).

SYSTEMIC COMPLAINTS

Fever, night sweats, and weight loss are common symptoms associated with HIV infection. These may occur with or without opportunistic infection. Nausea with or without vomiting may be present. This may be associated with oral or esophageal candidiasis. Nausea may be present without a clear etiology. Anorexia with associated weight loss can be a very distressing symptoms associated with HIV infection. Concurrent illness, such as hepatitis may be the cause but workup may not identify a specific cause. Diarrhea associated with malabsorption or bacterial, viral, or parasitic enteritis may also be linked to weight loss (Zolopa & Katz, 2014).

PULMONARY COMPLAINTS

Pneumocystis pneumonia is the most common opportunistic infection associated with AIDS. Making the diagnosis can be challenging because symptoms, including fever, cough, and shortness of breath, are nonspecific. Symptoms can also vary widely, from fever with few respiratory symptoms to mild cough or shortness of breath to acute respiratory distress with hypoxemia. Other infectious pulmonary diseases include bacterial, mycobacterial, and viral pneumonias. Community-acquired pneumonia is the most frequent cause of respiratory disease in HIV-infected individuals. Tuberculosis infection has become increasingly more prevalent in urban areas in the United States as a result of HIV infection. Tuberculosis occurs in approximately 4% of persons with AIDS in the United States. In patients with very low CD4 lymphocyte counts, tuberculin skin testing with purified protein derivative (PPD) may yield a false-negative test. When tuberculosis is suspected in an HIV-infected patient and PPD is negative, Quantiferon blood testing is recommended. Noninfectious lung diseases that can be seen in individuals with HIV/AIDS include malignancies such as Kaposi's sarcoma, non-Hodgkin's lymphoma, and interstitial pneumonitis (Zolopa & Katz, 2014).

CENTRAL NERVOUS SYSTEM COMPLAINTS

Central nervous system diseases associated with HIV infection can be manifested as space-occupying lesions, meningitis, and encephalopathy or spinal cord disorders. Cognitive dysfunction especially with advancing age is not uncommon with HIV infection even when patients are receiving adequate antiretroviral therapy (ART) (Zolopa & Katz, 2014). Toxoplasmosis is the most frequent causes of space-occupying lesions in HIV-infected people. A variety of symptoms, including headache, focal deficits, seizures, and changes in mental status, may be seen. Other less common infections include bacterial abscess and cryptococcal, tubercular, or nocardial lesions. Primary non-Hodgkin lymphoma involving the central nervous system is the second most common etiology for space-occupying lesions, with symptoms similar to those of toxoplasmosis. Individuals with HIV-associated dementia may experience problems with memory and attention, emotional and behavioral disturbances, and impaired motor function. PML is associated with a viral infection of the white matter of the brain and may be seen in those with advanced HIV infection and immunosuppression. Signs and symptoms include hemiparesis, aphasia, and vision loss. It is characterized by nonenhancing white matter lesions in imaging studies. With the increased availability of ART, PML is now rare but important to consider in those with acute neurologic symptoms (Zolopa & Katz, 2014).

PERIPHERAL NERVOUS SYSTEM COMPLAINTS

Peripheral mono- and polyneuropathies have identified in individuals with HIV infection. A syndrome marked by demyelinating polyneuropathy, much like Guillain–Barré syndrome can occur in HIV infection before evidence of frank immunosuppression. Improvement with plasmapheresis treatment suggests an autoimmune source for the condition. CMV can cause an ascending polyradiculopathy along with increased neutrophils in cerebrospinal fluid. Transverse myelitis may occur in conjunction with herpes zoster or CMV infection. Peripheral neuropathies are experienced frequently in HIV-infected individuals. Numbness, pain, and tingling in the lower extremities are common symptoms and may be out of proportion to gross motor and sensory examination findings. In addition to HIV infection, neuropathy may be associated with previous treatment with stavudine and didanosine. Alcohol abuse, thyroid disease, vitamin B_{12} deficiency, and syphilis may also contribute to symptoms of neuropathy and should be considered in the differential diagnosis in patients presenting with peripheral neuropathy (Zolopa & Katz, 2014).

MUSCULOSKELETAL AND RHEUMATOLOGIC COMPLAINTS

Arthritis symptoms are a frequent complaint noted by HIV-infected individuals. Involvement of single or multiple joints with or without effusion may be noted. The cause of HIV-related arthritis is not known, but most patients respond well to treatment with nonsteroidal anti-inflammatory drugs. Psoriatic and reactive arthritis have been reported in patients with HIV infection. Thorough evaluation of effusions should be undertaken, with aspiration and culture of fluid for evidence of infection, especially when the joint is erythematous or warm given the increased risk for infection due to immunosuppression (Hellmann & Imboden, 2014; Zolopa & Katz, 2014).

Osteopenia and osteoporosis are also common among HIV-infected patients with chronic infection. Vitamin D deficiency also appears often (Aberg et al., 2014).

OCULAR COMPLAINTS

Changes in visual acuity are cause for concern in HIV-infected individuals. Cotton wool spots are a characteristic lesion associated with microvascular disease and retinal ischemia. CMV retinitis is the most frequently seen retinal infection in persons with AIDS and can progress quickly if diagnosis is delayed (Zolopa & Katz, 2014). Other conditions involving the eye include necrotizing retinitis, caused by varicella zoster, and retinochoroiditis, caused by *Toxoplasma gondii* (Torre, Speranza, & Martegani, 2005).

ORAL COMPLAINTS

The presence of oral lesions, including candidiasis or hairy leukoplakia, often heralds the presence of immunodeficiency. Hairy leukoplakia is associated with Epstein–Barr virus, presenting with white lesions on the lateral aspect of the tongue. Lesions may be flat or elevated and have fine or thick hair-like projections. Oral candidiasis presents with plaque-like lesions, usually white or red. Patients with oral candidiasis often complain of oral discomfort, dry mouth, and an unpleasant metallic taste. Treatment with topical antifungal therapy is often effective in treating candidiasis, but when ineffective oral fluconazole may be used. Angular cheilitis is also often caused by *Candida* and can be treated with ketoconazole cream. Gingival disease is also a common oral complaint for patients with HIV infection. Regular cleaning and chlorhexidine rinses usually prove effective, but more severe cases of gingivitis or periodontitis may require treatment with oral antibiotics effective against oral flora (Zolopa & Katz, 2014).

GASTROINTESTINAL COMPLAINTS

A number of gastrointestinal issues cause an array of troubling symptoms in HIV-infected patients involving the esophagus, stomach, liver, gallbladder, and bowels.

Candida esophagitis is a frequent complication of AIDS. Patients may experience pain and difficulty with swallowing and often have co-occurring oral thrush. Viral infection in the esophagus may be associated with herpes simplex and CMV. Both can also be associated with painful swallowing caused by ulcerative lesions (Zolopa & Katz, 2014).

The liver is a common site of infection and malignancy in HIV-infected individuals. Many infections are not symptomatic. Mild abnormalities in aminotransferases and alkaline phosphatase may be noted. CMV, hepatitis B, hepatitis C, mycobacterial disease, and cancer may cause liver disease resulting in nausea, vomiting, abdominal pain and jaundice. Medications including antibiotics and antirheumatic drugs can be associated with hepatotoxicity (Zolopa & Katz, 2014).

Recommendations for HIV Testing

The HIV Medical Association of the Infectious Diseases Society of America (IDSA) recommends the following diagnostic tests when initiating care for HIV-infected patients (Aberg et al., 2013).

HIV ANTIBODY TESTING

Tests used to detect HIV infection include antibody and antigen studies. Routine HIV antibody testing is done by enzyme-linked immunosorbent assay (ELISA). If the sample is found to be positive, a confirmation test is done using a different test, most often using the Western blot method. ELISA tests may be positive as soon as 3 weeks after transmission of the virus; after 6 weeks, 95% are positive. False-positive tests may be seen in the presence of recent influenza vaccination or other diseases, including connective tissue diseases, some cancers, Epstein–Barr virus infection and improper handling of specimens. The combination of positive antibody test and Western blot yields specificity of greater than 99% (Zolopa & Katz, 2014).

Rapid HIV antibody testing of blood or oral fluids can provide results in as little as 10 minutes. These tests can be done in the outpatient office setting by staff without laboratory training. Positive results should be confirmed with standard HIV testing. Home testing kits using specimens obtained using oral swabs are also available to allow patient privacy (Zolopa & Katz, 2014).

VIRAL LOAD

Quantitative viral RNA or viral load is needed for staging of the disease and for monitoring the efficacy of ART. A number of commercially available tests are available to quantify plasma RNA copies. Viral load is important for determining the rate of immune system deterioration. HIV viral load testing measures the amount of active HIV replication (Simon et al., 2006). Viral load testing should be monitored every 3 to 4 months in untreated patients and those of stable ART, and at 2 to 4 week intervals when starting or adjusting therapy until the viral load becomes undetectable (Aberg et al., 2013)

CD4 LYMPHOCYTE COUNT

The CD4 lymphocyte count is the most widely used marker for identifying prognostic information and influencing therapy decisions. The CD4 count shows the degree of immunodeficiency and is important for determining disease stage. The CD4 count along with clinical manifestations serves as a criteria for HIV disease classification. The CD4 count is a measure of immune function but does not offer an indication of HIV replication in the body. CD4 count is most often measured using flow cytometry. The risk for serious opportunistic infection increases dramatically as the CD4 count decreases. Because there is variability with the CD4 count depending on time of day, concurrent illness, and differences within and between laboratories, ongoing measurements of CD4 counts rather than single measures are usually most important in monitoring patients with HIV infection (Zolopa & Katz, 2014). The frequency of monitoring often depends on the patient's health status and whether they are being treated with antiretroviral drugs. It is recommended that CD4 counts be measured every 3 to 4 months for most patients. For those who have achieved counts well above the threshold for risk of opportunistic infection while on suppressive therapy, monitoring may be decreased to every 6 to 12 months unless a change in their condition warrants earlier assessment (Aberg et al., 2013).

HIV RESISTANCE TESTING

Because drug-resistant virus can be transmitted from one person to another, all patients should be assessed for transmitted drug resistance with an HIV genotype test upon initiation of care.

In the case where ART is deferred, testing should be repeated at the time of ART initiation because of the potential for superinfection. Resistance testing is also indicated for patients who experience drug failure to guide modification of ART (Aberg et al., 2013).

COMPLETE BLOOD COUNT

A complete blood count with differential white blood cell count should be obtained upon initiation of care and periodically during treatment. Anemia, neutropenia, and thrombocytopenia may be evident in cases of advanced disease and as a manifestation of drug toxicity (Zolopa & Katz, 2014). The complete blood count also provides a baseline before starting any medications that may be myelosuppressive (Aberg et al., 2013).

CHEMISTRY PANEL

Baseline electrolyte levels should be noted at diagnosis and initiation of therapy. Alterations in electrolyte balance may be seen in the presence of nutritional disturbances associated with nausea, vomiting, and diarrhea as a result of concomitant illness or treatment toxicity. A baseline chemistry panel also provides information that is necessary before the initiation of any agents that are potentially nephrotoxic or hepatotoxic or those that require adjustment in patients with renal or hepatic dysfunction (Zolopa & Katz, 2014; Aberg et al., 2013).

GLUCOSE-6-PHOSPHATE DEHYDROGENASE SCREENING

Screening for glucose-6-phosphate dehydrogenase (G6PD) deficiency is recommended upon entry into care or before starting therapy with an oxidant drug in patients with a predisposing racial or ethnic background. The drugs frequently used to treat HIV-infected patients that can lead to hemolysis in the presence of G6PD deficiency include dapsone, primaquine, and sulfonamides. Although there are many variants of G6PD deficiency, the most common variants are found in Black men and women, and in men from the Mediterranean, India, and Southeast Asia. The hemolysis associated with some variants of G6PD deficiency can be life-threatening and may preclude the use of oxidant drugs (Aberg et al., 2013).

FASTING LIPID PROFILE

HIV infection itself, many antiretroviral drugs, and other individual factors are associated with increased cholesterol and triglyceride levels. These factors make a fasting lipid profile important when individuals enter HIV-related care. Fasting lipid levels should be obtained prior to and within 1 to 3 months after starting ART. Patients with abnormal lipid levels should be managed according to the National Cholesterol Education Program Guidelines (Aberg et al., 2013).

URINALYSIS AND CALCULATED CREATININE CLEARANCE

A baseline urinalysis and calculated creatinine clearance or estimated glomerular filtration rate (GFR) should be obtained, especially in black HIV-infected patients and anyone with advanced infection or comorbid conditions that are likely to contribute to an increased risk for nephropathy. Urinalysis and calculated creatinine clearance testing should also be performed before initiating drugs that have the potential for renal toxicity (Aberg et al., 2013).

Kidney function is abnormal in up to 30% of HIV-infected patients, and HIV-associated nephropathy is a relatively common cause of end-stage renal disease in black HIV-infected patients. The GFR should be estimated to assist in prescribing antiretroviral agents and other commonly used medications that require dose adjustment based on renal function. Medication doses should be adjusted based on renal function according to their package insert. In addition, a screening urinalysis for proteinuria should be considered at initiation of care and annually thereafter, especially in patients who are at increased risk for developing kidney disease including black patients, those with CD4 cell count less than 200 or viral load greater than 4,000 copies, and those with diabetes mellitus, hypertension, or hepatitis C virus coinfection. Patients with proteinuria of grade or greater by dipstick analysis or reduced kidney function should be referred to a nephrologist for consultation and should have further evaluation, including quantification of proteinuria, renal ultrasound, and possible renal biopsy. Monitoring of renal function and urinary abnormalities is recommended when tenofovir or indinavir are in use (Aberg et al., 2013).

Screening and Treatment of Concomitant Conditions Associated with HIV Infection

TUBERCULOSIS SCREENING

HIV-infected patients without a history of tuberculosis or a prior positive tuberculosis screening test should be tested for *Mycobacterium tuberculosis* infection by either a tuberculin skin test (TST) or by an interferon-γ

release assay. Those with positive test results should be treated for latent *M. tuberculosis* infection after active tuberculosis has been excluded (Aberg et al., 2013).

HEPATITIS SCREENING

HIV-infected patients should be screened for evidence of hepatitis B virus (HBV) infection detection of hepatitis B surface antigen (HBsAg), hepatitis B surface antibody (HBsAb), and antibody to hepatitis B total core antigen (anti-HBc or HBcAb). Patient without evidence of immunity should be vaccinated against HBV. HBsAb should be repeated 1 to 2 months or at the next scheduled visit after the third vaccine was given to assess for immunogenicity. A second series of vaccine is recommended for those whose HBsAb levels are negative or <10 IU/mL after the first vaccine series (Aberg et al., 2013). Vaccination should also be recommended for nonimmune sexual partners of patients who are positive for HBsAg.

Those who are negative for HBsAg and HBsAb but positive for anti-HBc should be screened for chronic HBV infection by testing for of HBV DNA. Vaccination is recommended for those without evidence of chronic infection (Aberg et al., 2013).

HIV-infected patients should be screened for hepatitis C virus (HCV) infection upon initiation of care by a test for HCV antibody and annually thereafter for those at risk.

HCV RNA should be ordered on all those with a positive HCV antibody test to assess for active HCV disease. Infants born to HBV- and/or HCV-infected women should be tested for HBV and HCV transmission. Hepatitis A vaccination is recommended for all susceptible men who have sex with men (MSM), as well as other susceptible individuals with indications for hepatitis A vaccine including injection drug users, those with chronic liver disease, or patients who are infected with hepatitis B and/or C. Hepatitis A total or IgG antibody should be repeated every 1 to 2 months or at the next scheduled visit after the second vaccine to assess for immunogenicity. A repeat vaccine series is recommended in those who remain seronegative. Hepatitis A vaccine should be considered for all other nonimmune patients (Aberg et al., 2013).

SCREENING FOR SEXUALLY TRANSMITTED INFECTIONS

All patients should be screened for syphilis upon initiation of care and periodically thereafter, depending on risk. A lumbar puncture should be performed for patients with a reactive syphilis serology who have neurologic or ocular symptoms or signs, irrespective of past syphilis treatment history (Aberg et al., 2013).

All women should be screened for trichomoniasis, and all women aged 25 years of age and younger should be screened for *Chlamydia trachomatis* infection. Men and women should be screened for gonorrhea and chlamydia infection at initial presentation and then annually if at risk for infection. Retesting in 3 months is indicated in men and women found to be positive for gonorrhea and chlamydial infections and women found to be positive for trichomoniasis on initial screening, because of high-reinfection rates. All of these conditions should be screened for periodically thereafter, depending on the population, reported behaviors, the presence of other STDs in the patient or his/her partner(s), and the prevalence of STDs in the community (Aberg et al., 2013).

CERVICAL CANCER SCREENING AND PREVENTION

HIV-infected women should have a cervical Pap test performed upon initiation of care, and this test should be repeated at 6 months and annually thereafter if results are normal. Women with atypical squamous cells, atypical glandular cells, low-grade or high-grade squamous intraepithelial lesion, or squamous carcinoma noted by Pap testing should have follow up with gynecology and colposcopy and directed biopsy, with additional treatment as indicated by results of evaluation (Aberg et al., 2013).

SCREENING FOR ANAL HUMAN PAPILLOMAVIRUS

HIV-infected men and women with human papillomavirus (HPV) infection are at increased risk for anal dysplasia and cancer. MSM, women with a history of receptive anal intercourse or abnormal cervical Pap test results, and all HIV-infected individuals with genital warts should have an anal Pap test. HPV vaccination is recommended for all females aged 9 to 26 years and all males aged 9 to 21 years. Males aged 22 to 26 years should also be vaccinated if they have not previously been vaccinated at a younger age (Aberg et al., 2014).

SCREENING AND VACCINATION FOR HERPES VIRUSES

Patients at lower risk of CMV infection (those other than MSM or injection drug users, who may be assumed to be seropositive) should be tested for latent CMV infection with an anti-CMV IgG when entering HIV-related care. Patients who are susceptible to varicella zoster virus (VZV), including those who have not been vaccinated, have no history of varicella or herpes zoster, or are seronegative for VZV should receive postexposure prophylaxis with varicella zoster immune globulin (VariZIG) within 10 days after exposure to a person with varicella or shingles. Varicella primary vaccination may be considered in HIV-infected, VZV-seronegative persons over 8 years of age with CD4 cell counts greater than 200 cells/μL and in HIV-infected children aged 1 to 8 years with CD4 cell percentages greater than 15% (Aberg et al., 2013).

OSTEOPOROSIS SCREENING

Baseline bone densitometry (DEXA) screening for osteoporosis in HIV-infected patients should be performed in postmenopausal women and men over fifty years of age. Three primary bone diseases have been identified in HIV-infected individuals. These include osteonecrosis, osteomalacia, and osteoporosis, with osteoporosis being the most common and having the most impact on the long-term health of persons with HIV infection. Low bone mineral density leading to osteoporosis has been recognized in HIV-infected patients. It is believed to be associated with HIV infection itself as well as antiretroviral drug toxicity and comorbid conditions (Powderly, 2012).

Differential Diagnoses

HIV infection may present with symptoms associated with other medical conditions. Since there is a wide spectrum of associated signs and symptoms, a thorough history and physical examination are needed. When individuals present with fever and weight loss, differential diagnoses include cancer, infections such as tuberculosis or endocarditis, and endocrine disorders such as hyperthyroidism. Infectious enteritis, antibiotic associated colitis, malabsorption syndromes, and inflammatory bowel disease should be considered when patients present with diarrhea (Zolopa & Katz, 2014).

Others may present with neurologic conditions including changes in mental status or neuropathy making the diagnosis more challenging. Neurologic conditions also associated with these findings include vitamin deficiency, alcoholism, liver disease, renal disease, and thyroid dysfunction. Peripheral nervous system syndromes associated with HIV infection include inflammatory polyneuropathies, sensory neuropathies, and mononeuropathies. A demyelinating neuropathy similar to Guillain–Barre syndrome can occur prior to evidence of immunodeficiency. CMV can cause polyradiculopathy manifested by lower extremity weakness and the presence of an increased number of neutrophils in cerebrospinal fluid. Transverse myelitis, associated with herpes zoster or CMV infection with symptoms ranging from back pain, to weakness and loss of bowel and bladder function. Peripheral neuropathy is a common occurrence in HIV infection. Patients often note numbness, tingling, and pain in the lower extremities.

Rheumatologic syndromes, including arthritis involving one or more joints can be seen in HIV-infected individuals. The mechanisms of disease are unclear. Inflamed joints with associated effusions should be aspirated to rule out infection. Reactive arthritis, psoriatic arthritis, and systemic lupus erythematosus have been noted on patients with HIV infection (Zolopa & Katz, 2014).

Patient Treatment and Management

ANTIRETROVIRAL THERAPY

HIV-infected individuals will almost inevitably develop immunosuppression without treatment. Progressive immunosuppression, manifested by reduction of CD4 lymphocytes and AIDS-defining illness ultimately will ultimately lead to premature death. The primary goal of treatment is the reduction of morbidity and mortality. Fortunately, advances in treatment since the 1990s have enabled accomplishment of this goal by promoting inhibition of the virus replication. This has promoted improved immune function, lowered risk for AIDS-defining illnesses and other complications of HIV infection, and prolonged life expectancy for those with HIV infection. Treatment regimens have become more effective, more convenient, and more tolerable with these advancements (AIDS Info Panel on Antiretroviral Guidelines for Adults and Adolescents, 2014).

Effective treatment of infection involves use of ART. More than 20 different drugs from six different classes used in various combinations have been most effective. These six FDA-approved classes include:

- Nucleoside reverse transcriptase inhibitors (NRTI)
- Nonnucleoside reverse transcriptase inhibitors (NNRTI)
- Protease inhibitors (PI)
- CCR5 antagonists
- Fusion inhibitors (FI)
- Integrase strand transfer inhibitors (INSTI) (Roche, Tindall, & Sedrak, 2014)

These drugs are active against the virus and are able to suppress viral replication to reduce damage to the immune system and restore immune function, allowing the host to fight opportunistic infections and prolong survival. Individuals with acute primary HIV infection should be treated with a combination of medications capable of suppressing replication of the virus to an undetectable level. Goals of ART treatment include reducing damage and restoring immune system function, reducing HIV- associated morbidity, suppressing HIV viral load and reducing risk for HIV transmission (AIDS Info Panel on Antiretroviral Guidelines for Adults and Adolescents, 2014; Roche et al., 2014).

Federal HIV treatment guidelines recommend ART for all persons with HIV, regardless of CD4 cell count, to improve their health and prolong their lives. Effective treatment also reduces the risk of transmitting HIV to others. Clinical visits that are necessary to prescribe and manage ART provide additional benefits as they offer opportunities to reinforce patient education about risk-reduction and provide other care and prevention services. Providers should offer information to promote understanding of the anticipated risks and benefits of treatment and the expected reduction of transmission of the virus. The need for sustained high adherence to treatment is critical to offering patients the greatest benefit from ART. The importance of making a commitment to uninterrupted therapy must be discussed with patients. The dangers of sharing their ART medications with others, both with and without HIV infection, is an important point of discussion during clinical visits (CDC, 2014).

The most desirable initial ART regimen for a treatment-naive patient consists of two NRTIs in combination with a drug from one of three drug classes: An NNRTI, a PI boosted with ritonavir (RTV), or an INSTI. A number of clinical investigations have shown that this strategy leads to decreases in HIV RNA and CD4 T lymphocyte cell increases in the majority of patients (AIDS Info Panel on Antiretroviral Guidelines for Adults and Adolescents, 2014).

Drug resistance is an issue for all classes of antiretroviral drugs. It has been noted in both patients in whom therapy has failed as well as treatment-naïve patients who are infected with resistant strains, prompting the recommendation for resistance testing at the start of treatment in newly diagnosed patients as well as when changing treatment in the event of drug failure. Many patients, even those who have a history of drug failure can be successfully treated given the number of active antiretroviral agents currently available. It is important to keep in mind that new drugs will continue to be needed given the virus's ability to evolve (Arts & Hazuda, 2012). Medication selection is best when individualized to patient needs based on a number of factors which include:

- Results of HIV genotypic drug resistance testing
- Pretreatment viral load
- The regimen's genetic barrier to resistance
- Potential adverse drug effects
- Potential drug interactions with other medications
- Comorbid conditions including cardiovascular disease, liver or kidney disease, substance abuse, psychiatric illness
- Pregnancy or pregnancy potential
- Patient preferences and adherence potential
- Convenience including pill burden, dosing frequency, availability of fixed dose combination products and food requirements
- Cost (AIDS Info Panel on Antiretroviral Guidelines for Adults and Adolescents, 2014)

The complexity of treatment regimens and need for adherence to medication make patient education and developing strong partnerships with patients essential. Patient education strategies should include instructions for how to take each medication, expected adverse effects, how best to incorporate the treatment regimen into their lifestyle, and managing costs of treatment (Roche et al., 2014).

Knowledge about medications used in treatment of HIV infection is important for primary care providers as well as HIV specialists.

NUCLEOSIDE REVERSE TRANSCRIPTASE INHIBITORS

NRTIs are synthetic substances with the capability of mimicking naturally occurring nucleotides which are essential in producing DNA and RNA. NRTIs compete with naturally occurring nucleotides in the virus that would normally be incorporated into the virus's reverse transcriptase enzyme to form a new viral DNA chain. This process inhibits creation of new viral DNA and limits progression of infection. Each drug in this class has its own side effect profile, but the following are reactions common to all:

- Skin: Rashes
- Gastrointestinal: Abdominal pain, diarrhea, nausea, vomiting, anorexia, dyspepsia, hepatitis
- Hematologic: Thrombocytosis
- Metabolic: Fatigue, lactic acidosis
- Musculoskeletal: Myopathy, back pain
- Neurologic: Headache, tremor, anxiety, confusion, dizziness, depression, restlessness, and syncope

Other drug-specific effects include myelosuppression and hepatotoxicity. Timing of doses around meals also varies between different agents in this class of drugs (Roche et al., 2014)

NONNUCLEOSIDE REVERSE TRANSCRIPTASE INHIBITORS

NNRTIs bind near the site of reverse transcriptase activity and have a combined effect with other antiretroviral drugs to reduce virus replication. Side effects common to NNRTIs include:

- Skin: Rashes, increased perspiration, itching
- Gastrointestinal: Anorexia, nausea, vomiting, diarrhea, increased transaminases
- Neurologic: Headache, fatigue, abnormal dreams, depression, impaired concentration
- Metabolic: Fever

Administration of sedatives, nonsedating antihistamines, calcium channel blockers, ergot alkaloid preparations, and antiarrhythmics carry risk for serious adverse events and are generally contraindicated in combination with NNRTIs (Roche et al., 2014).

PROTEASE INHIBITORS

PIs are active in a different stage of viral replication than the NRTIs. By binding to active sites used by viral protease enzymes, PIs render the virus unable to process precursors needed for development of mature HIV virus. These incomplete viruses are rendered unable to replicate. Resistant mutations of the virus can develop if viral suppression does not occur.

Side effects common to PIs include:

- Gastrointestinal: Diarrhea, vomiting, acid reflux, anorexia, metallic taste, elevated transaminase levels, hyperlipidemia
- Hematologic: Thrombocytopenia with increased risk for bleeding
- Metabolic: Exacerbation of diabetes, lipodystrophy
- Neurologic: Headache, insomnia, dizziness, mood disorders

PIs interact with many drugs metabolized by the liver resulting in increased clearance of non-PI drugs (Roche et al., 2014).

FUSION INHIBITORS

Also referred to as entry inhibitors, FIs block entry of HIV into cells by blocking fusion of the viral envelope to the T lymphocyte cell membrane. Patients who have drug-resistant strains of HIV benefit from the use of such drugs since they have a different mechanism of action from NRTIs, NNRTIs, and PIs. Enfuvirtide is an approved FI in the U.S, and is given by subcutaneous injection (Zolopa & Katz, 2014).

CCR5 ANTAGONISTS

CCR5 antagonists inhibits entry of the virus into uninfected cells by blocking CCR5 coreceptors. Drugs in this class act against what is referred to as CCR5 tropic virus. Testing for the presence of tropism is possible and should be done prior to initiating treatment with a CCR5 antagonist. Maraviroc is an approved CCR5 antagonist in the United States Common side effects include cough, rashes, fever, abdominal discomfort and muscle aches (Zolopa & Katz, 2014).

INTEGRASE STRAND TRANSFER INHIBITORSS

NSTIs affect HIV replication by blocking HIV integrase enzyme needed for the virus to reproduce when used in combination with other drugs, especially in the setting of resistance to at least one drug (Zolopa & Katz, 2014).

PRIMARY PREVENTION IN HIV INFECTION

The CDC (2014) declared that

> the goals of HIV prevention, care, and treatment in the United States are to prevent new HIV infections, increase the proportion n of persons with HIV who are aware of their infection, prevent HIV-related illness and death, and reduce HIV-related health disparities (p.8).

The focus of HIV prevention in the United States has changed because of recent advances in medical, behavioral, and structural prevention strategies, coupled with changes in health care delivery. The availability of ART when used early in the course of illness has been shown to improve health, suppress HIV viral load, and reduce the risk of HIV transmission to others. Offering HIV treatment shortly after diagnosis can also offer opportunities for access to other medical, behavioral and structural interventions that can reduce the risk of transmission of the virus. A wide range of interventions offered by a multidisciplinary team of clinical and nonclinical providers can promote the health of persons with HIV, prevent HIV transmission to their sex and drug-injection partners and offspring, and contribute to the overall health of the community (CDC, 2014).

Education for individuals affected by HIV infection remains an essential intervention in preventing HIV transmission, and while treatment with ART has taken a prominent role in disease prevention in recent years, traditional strategies aimed at prevention remain important.

The use of polyethylene or latex condoms can provide excellent protection from transmission of the HIV virus when used properly. Nonoxynol-9 spermicide use may increase risk. Oil and petroleum-based lubricants should be avoided in combination with latex condoms as they may increase risk of condom breakage (Burgess & Kasten, 2013)

ART is an important element in prevention of HIV transmission. A number of studies have demonstrated that in participants receiving ART, reduced concentrations of HIV RNA in serum and genital secretions have been seen. Studies conducted in communities with relatively high numbers of men engaging in high-risk behaviors have shown that increased use of ART has been associated with reduced rates of new HIV diagnoses. Additionally, data from these studies suggest that the risk of HIV transmission is low when an individual's viral load is below 400 copies per milliliter (AIDS Info Panel on Antiretroviral Guidelines for Adults and Adolescents, 2014).

Postexposure prophylaxis (PEP), entails using a combination of three antiretroviral drugs for 28 days. PEP should commence within 72 hours of exposure. In situations when the individual anticipates ongoing sexual contact with a partner known to be positive for HIV, preexposure prophylaxis (PrEP) can be an option. PrEP may also be considered for individuals who are HIV negative and engage in high-risk behaviors. Primary care providers may wish to consult with an HIV specialist for recommendation about treatment regimens (Burgess & Kasten, 2013).

SECONDARY PREVENTION IN HIV INFECTION

The CDC has recommended HIV screening for all patients ages 13 to 64 in all health care settings after individuals are notified that testing will be done. Patients have the option to decline testing (opt out screening). Recommendations also suggest that people at high risk for infection should be tested at least annually. Screening should be included in routine consent for care. Written consent for testing is not necessary or recommended. Prevention counseling should not be required as part of HIV screening or prevention programs in health-care settings if it is a hindrance to performing testing. However information about HIV infection, testing, and the meaning of test results should be provided. HIV testing should be a routine part of prenatal screening for all pregnant women unless the woman chooses to opt out. In areas with high rates of HIV infection, screening should be repeated in the third trimester of the pregnancy (CDC, 2014).

Prevention and Treatment in Special Populations

MOTHER TO CHILD TRANSMISSION

Infectious Disease Society of America (IDSA) guidelines (Aberg et al., 2013) recommend that for prevention of infection in the fetus, HIV-positive pregnant women should be treated for HIV infection, regardless of their immunologic or virologic status. Additionally, infants exposed to HIV in utero should receive postexposure antiretroviral prophylaxis and undergo HIV virologic testing 14 to 21 days after birth and again at 1 to 2 months of age and 4 to 6 months of age. High-risk exposed infants should have virologic testing at birth.

CHILDREN

Recommendations suggest that HIV-infected infants should undergo HIV resistance testing and because of the rapid progression of disease, should initiate therapy in the first year of life regardless of CD4 cell count, RNA level, or clinical status. After the first year of life, initiation of therapy in HIV-infected children is based on age, CD4 count or percentage, viral load, and symptoms. ART should be initiated in all symptomatic children. CD4 cell counts and viral loads should be monitored at least every 3 to 4 months. Childhood vaccinations should be administered according to the Advisory Committee on Immunization Practices schedules for HIV-infected infants and children. HIV-infected infants and children should be cared for by specialists with knowledge of the unique therapeutic, pharmacologic, behavioral, and developmental issues associated with HIV infection (Aberg et al., 2013).

ADOLESCENTS

Adolescents infected with HIV should receive an individualized and developmental approach to therapy and care given by an HIV specialist with expertise in caring for this age group. HIV-infected adolescents, whether infected perinatally or through behaviors present significant challenges for providers. The mean age of the US cohort of perinatally infected children is the mid-teens, while many others have reached adulthood. Social stigma, difficulty with adherence to treatment, loss of family members, distortion of body image, and negotiation of sexual activity are all challenges faced by HIV-infected adolescents. Incidence of cognitive, psychiatric, and behavioral problems are higher in perinatally infected children. Disclosure of diagnosis can be quite difficult for caregivers but should occur in late childhood. Metabolic changes associated with puberty can affect pharmacodynamics making it important to consider decisions regarding dosing in the context of Tanner staging. Long-term treatment from infancy may result in end-organ toxicity requiring careful monitoring. Special attention should be paid to risk-reduction counseling and secondary prevention in early adolescence. Concomitant psychiatric illness, high rates of substance abuse and sexually transmitted infections are significant issues among behaviorally infected young people (Aberg et al., 2013).

Transition of care to adult providers should be a well-coordinated process involving all members of the health-care team, including the patient. Attention to the unique needs of the adolescent that extend beyond medical care, including employment, independent living, and intimate relationships, is critical in promoting a good quality of life. Emphasis should be placed on helping adolescents to negotiate the health-care system and assume responsibility for their health care. The number of agencies, including the national AIDS Education and Training Centers (AETC) provide resource to assist with these transitions (Aberg et al., 2013).

Early intervention with HIV medical care and antiretroviral treatment (ART) and continued adherence to ART improve health outcomes and survival rates and can prevent HIV transmission. Starting HIV medical care shortly after diagnosis and ongoing care also provide opportunities to offer risk-reduction interventions, services for partners, sexually transmitted disease care, and other services to prevent HIV transmission. Evidence shows that persons who stay in care during their first year of outpatient HIV medical care are more likely to start ART than persons who do not. Those with improved adherence to treatment regimens are more likely to achieve suppression of the virus and practice safer sexual behaviors (CDC, 2014).

Patient Education

All patients with HIV infection should be educated about the benefits of ART for their own health, prolonging lifespan, and reducing the risk of HIV transmission. In addition they should be told about the limitations and risks of ART, including that use of effective ART does not completely eliminate but does substantially reduce the risk of virus transmission. Education should include information about the availability of two different prophylactic regimens of antiretroviral medications, PrEP and nonoccupational postexposure prophylaxis (nPEP) for uninfected partners when clinically indicated to reduce their risk of becoming infected with HIV. When considering PrEP or nPEP, individuals need baseline clinical and laboratory evaluation to test for established or recent HIV infection. Those using PrEP or nPEP need regular follow-up evaluations to monitor for HIV infection status through retesting, identification of possible side effects or other reasons to discontinue prophylaxis, adherence to prescribed medications, as well as adherence to behaviors that may decrease risk of HIV infection, including consistent, correct use of latex or polyurethane condoms. Individuals should be informed about options to obtain ART to minimize the financial burdens associated with treatment. Additionally patients should be informed that use of ART is voluntary and patients can decline ART without risk of being denied medical and social services (CDC, 2014).

Individuals receiving ART should be advised to tell their health care providers about any current or planned use of prescription, nonprescription, or recreational drugs, alcohol, or dietary supplements because these may alter ART effectiveness or cause toxicity (CDC, 2014).

Immune System Review

Immunity against illness is the product of many complex processes. The body's first line of defense against invading pathogens is a layer of epithelium which includes the skin and mucous membranes. When this protective layer is breached, a second defense system of localized and systemic inflammatory response is triggered in an effort to limit the activity of outside organisms. This inflammatory response, sometimes referred to as innate or native immunity, often initiates an adaptive or acquired immunity to the infecting microorganism. Acquired or adaptive immunity is slower to develop but has the ability to target and destroy subsequent infections with particular microorganisms. While these adaptive processes are protective, certain genetic or acquired abnormalities in these processes are associated with disease; a reduced inflammatory response can increase risk for infection while excessive inflammation can be associated with tissue injury. Both can lead to serious illness (Banasik, 2013; Rote & Huether, 2010b).

INNATE IMMUNITY

Inflammation occurs in vascularized tissue when cells are injured. The three primary functions of the inflammatory response include (1) prevention of infiltration by harmful substances, (2) limiting extension of harmful substances into other tissues, and (3) preparing damaged tissue for healing. Inflammation and infection area sometimes confused since they sometimes coexist. Inflammation is frequently associated with infection but inflammation also occurs in the absence of infection, as in arthritis, myocardial infarction, and thrombosis. Characteristic changes in microcirculation include vasodilation, increased vascular permeability with collection of fluid outside of the vessel, followed by movement of white blood cells through the vessel wall to the site of injury. These events result in the onset of the typical signs and symptoms associated with inflammation: redness, heat, swelling, and pain. Aided by biochemical mediators including histamine, bradykinins, and prostaglandins, leukocytes and plasma are able to enter the surrounding tissues. This process allows toxins produced by microorganisms to be diluted, activates plasma proteins to render microorganisms ineffective, and brings neutrophils and macrophages to phagocytize cellular debris. Under normal circumstances, certain plasma proteins limit the inflammatory response and prevent it from extending into unaffected tissue. Inflammatory responses are coordinated with the adaptive immune system to produce a more specific response to the invading organism when macrophages are introduced. Finally, healing is fostered by the removal of cellular debris and other end products of the inflammatory response (Banasik, 2013; Rote & Huether, 2010b).

Three essential plasma protein systems are integral to the inflammatory response. The complement, clotting, and kinin systems each contain inactive plasma proteins that are triggered in the presence of tissue injury. Once activated, each performs essential functions in response to tissue damage. These three systems are closely connected so that activation of one results in activation of the others (Rote & Huether, 2010b).

The complement system contains approximately twenty different plasma proteins that have the ability to kill organisms directly and in collaboration with other elements of the inflammatory response. These proteins are synthesized in the liver and by macrophages and neutrophils. The complement cascade can be activated by antibody–antigen complexes or by substances within the infecting organisms (Rote & Huether, 2010b, Banasik, 2013).

While important in controlling bleeding, the clotting system is also useful in preventing spread of microorganisms to surrounding tissues, confining organisms and foreign objects at the site of inflammation for removal by neutrophils and macrophages. The clotting system may be activated by substances released during cell destruction as well as endotoxins produced by bacteria. Formation of clots is also instrumental in activating fibrinolysis (Banasik, 2013; Rote & Huether, 2010b).

Inflammation is enhanced by the kinin system as well. Kinins are polypeptides capable of causing vasodilation, vascular permeability, and smooth muscle contraction. Bradykinin causes vasodilation and along with prostaglandins stimulates nerve endings to induce pain. Additionally, kinins are linked to the clotting system. Enzymes within the system degrade kinins to control their activity and limit the inflammatory response (Banasik, 2013; Rote & Huether, 2010b).

Another important element of the inflammatory response is the mast cell. Mast cells are found in connective tissue in close proximity to blood vessels and are most abundant in areas with exposure to the external environment, including the skin, respiratory, and gastrointestinal tracts. The inflammatory response can be activated when mast cells are stimulated by physical injury, chemical agents, immune activity, and microbial sensing receptors on the surface of cells, known as toll-like receptors. Once activated, mast cells immediately release histamine, chemotactic factors, and cytokines including tumor necrosis factor and IL-4 (Rote & Huether, 2010b).

Leukocytes including neutrophils, monocytes, and monocyte-derived macrophages phagocytize cellular debris. Neutrophils appear at the site of inflammation within hours of injury, attracted by complement fragments, bacterial proteins, and mast cell chemotactic factors. Macrophages and monocytes arrive at the site later in the process and survive for a longer time period. Macrophages also serve in activation of the adaptive immune system and in producing cytokines that limit inflammation and promote healing. Other leukocytes have important roles in the inflammatory response as well. Eosinophils have some phagocytic function, but act primarily in protecting the body against parasitic infection and controlling vasoactive mediators originating from mast cells (Rote & Huether, 2010b).

Basophils are granulocytes, which are similar in structure to mast cells found in the vascular system which have receptors that enable them to bind to IgE antibodies and release proinflammatory substances. Release of granules from mast cells and basophils is an initiating factor in the response seen in allergic responses (Banasik, 2013).

The relationship between these many types of cells is critical in both inflammatory and acquired immune responses. Cellular products are secreted by cells contributing to the acquired immune system. These include chemokines and cytokines with either proinflammatory or anti-inflammatory activity. When bound to their target cells, reactions may occur that lead to production of other mediators. Some cellular products may have different actions when bound to different types of target cells (Rote & Huether, 2010b). For the purpose of this chapter, discussion of cytokines will be limited to interleukins (ILs).

ILs are chemical messengers derived primarily from lymphocytes and macrophages as they respond to the presence of invading organisms or other products of the inflammatory response. Their role is important in augmenting the acquired immune response to pathogens and other foreign substances. For example, IL-1 is a proinflammatory agent secreted by macrophages that have identified substances associated with infection. It has the ability to activate lymphocytes and phagocytes as well as promote increased production of neutrophils. It also is able to act on receptors in the hypothalamus to increase body temperature. IL-10 is an anti-inflammatory agent that acts to down regulate the activities of both the inflammatory and acquired immune responses by suppressing the production of lymphocytes and proinflammatory cytokines (Rote & Huether, 2010b).

ACQUIRED (ADAPTIVE) IMMUNITY

Acquired immune functions work in concert with inflammatory responses. Many components of the inflammatory response assist in mounting an acquired immune response, making the interaction of the two systems to provide adequate protection against many diseases essential.

The body is continuously bombarded with substances that are recognized as foreign. These substances, referred to as antigens are frequently linked to pathogens including bacteria, viruses, parasites, and fungi. An antigen is a molecule that can react with antibodies or T- and B-cell receptors. Most antigens are immunogenic, or capable of stimulating an immune response that results in production of functional T cells or antibodies. Antigens function as such because a portion of the molecule is recognized and bound to an antibody or lymphocyte receptor. Some antigens may be noninfectious and can include environmental allergens, while others are related to medications, vaccines, transfusion products, and transplanted tissue. What sets acquired immunity apart from inflammation is that it has the ability to provide long-term protection against particular agents. This ability stems from the presence of immunoglobulins and lymphocytes. This specificity and long-term "memory" characterize acquired immune response (Rote & Huether, 2010c; Banasik, 2013).

The acquired immunity response system has two components: (1) antibody, or humoral immunity, and (2) cell-mediated immunity. Acquired immunity can be achieved by way of active or passive processes. Active immunity occurs as a result of exposure to an antigen either by natural means or after immunization. Passive immunity occurs when antibodies or T lymphocytes are transferred from a donor to a recipient. Examples of transfer of antibodies include transfer of maternal antibodies to a fetus through the placenta or treatment with immunotherapy as in the case of an individual exposed to hepatitis A who receives immunoglobulin to provide temporary immunity (Rote & Huether, 2010c).

An effective immune response depends on the ability of specific antibodies or receptors on T cells or B cells to recognize an antigen. This is followed by additional intercellular responses among antigen presenting cells and lymphocytes. A number of variables determine the degree to which antigens are immunogenic. These include (1) foreignness to the host; (2) size of the antigen; (3) having significant chemical complexity; and (4) present in an adequate amount, with foreignness being the most significant. Molecular size, particularly those large in size, more often affects immunogenicity. Antigens that are composed of a variety of chemical components are more likely to be immunogenic than those composed of only one. Lastly, when antigens are present in very small or very large concentrations they may be unable to trigger an immune response since they may generate a state of tolerance instead of immunity (Rote & Huether, 2010c).

Antigens are recognized by three types of molecules. These include (1) circulating antibodies and (2) antigen receptors on the surfaces of B lymphocytes and (3) T-lymphocyte antigen receptors.

Antibodies and Antibody Function

Antibodies or immunoglobulins are glycoproteins produced by plasma cells in response to the presence of an immunogen. Immunoglobulin is a term used to describe all molecules known to have specificity for antigen, while antibody is a term used to describe a specific group of immunoglobulins that act on a particular antigen. There are five classes of immunoglobulins including, IgA, IgM, IgE, IgG, and IgD, each with structural and functional differences (Rote & Huether, 2010c; Banasik, 2013).

The most plentiful immunoglobulin in the body is IgG, accounting for approximately 80% to 85% of circulating immunoglobulin. It is the most active immunoglobulin in protection against infection. Maternal IgG is the primary class of antibody found in fetal and infant blood as it crosses the placenta (Rote & Huether, 2010c).

IgA is most often found under the skin and attached to mucosal epithelial cells and is found in tears, saliva, tracheobronchial secretions, colostrum and breast milk, as well as gastrointestinal and genitourinary secretions (Rote & Huether, 2010c; Banasik, 2013).

IgM is the largest immunoglobulin in size and is the first immunoglobulin produced in response to an antigen. It is primarily found in intravascular fluid. It is the primary antibody found on B cell surfaces and is important in activating complement (Banasik, 2013)

IgD is found in low concentrations in the blood, primarily on the surface of immature B cells in addition to IgM. It acts as a cellular antigen receptor, stimulating B-cell proliferation, differentiation, and secretion of additional immunoglobulins (Banasik, 2013).

IgE is the least concentrated immunoglobulin in the circulation. It functions as a mediator in allergic responses and in fighting against parasitic infections. It is found on receptors on the surface of basophils and mast cells, causing cell degranulation when antigens are detected (Rote & Huether, 2010c; Banasik, 2013).

Antibodies function in several different ways to contain and eliminate antigens from the body. Successful immune response against antigen requires that antigens be processed and be expressed on cell surfaces in a particular manner. Some types of antigen are processed by specialized cells referred to as antigen presenting cells while others are processed and presented by a variety of different cells. Some sets of cell-surface molecules are responsible for presenting antigens for immune activity. Clusters of differentiation (CD) are a group over 200 proteins which are found on the surface of cells that influence the immune response. Major histocompatibility complexes (MHC) are molecules consisting of glycoproteins that are found on most human cells which are active in presenting antigens to be identified. MHC in humans is also known as human leukocyte antigen (HLA) (Rote & Huether, 2010c; Banasik, 2013). MHC and CD1 play significant roles in mounting an immune response against antigens (Rote & Huether, 2010c).

The immune system typically responds to two types of antigens, those that are exogenous and those that are endogenous. Exogenous antigens come from outside the cell and are trapped and phagocytized. Endogenous antigens are formed inside a cell. This can occur with viral infection when the viruses infect cells and use cellular material, such as protein synthesizing mechanisms, to translate viral genes into viral proteins. This process is also seen in malignancy, when cells undergo malignant change and begin producing proteins specific to cancer cells that are presented as foreign antigens on cell surfaces. Exogenous and endogenous antigens are presented by different types of MHCs (Rote & Huether, 2010c).

T CELLS

The thymus is the primary lymphoid organ involved with T-cell development. Precursor cells are generated early in embryonic life from the yolk sac and fetal liver and then later in the bone marrow. These cells then travel to the thymus. Influenced by thymic cells and hormones, they mature and develop the characteristics of T cells. These changes include developing the T-cell receptor sites and surface molecules. T cells recognize foreign antigens offered by antigen presenting cells by using specialized T-cell receptors specific for single antigens. T cells are eventually released into the blood and stored in secondary lymphoid tissue until needed to process antigens (Banasik, 2013; Rote & Huether, 2010c).

A subpopulation of T lymphocytes is helper T cells, which function in both cellular and humoral immunity. These specialized T lymphocytes are helpful in antigen-driven maturation of both T and B cells by assisting in the interactions between antigen-presenting cells and immunocompetent lymphocytes. Cells that become helper T cells have particular features, including the expression of CD4 molecules on their surfaces. CD4 protein allows T-helper cells to bind with MHC type 2 proteins while T-cell receptors allow identification of antigens. The role of helper T cells in this process includes interaction with antigen-presenting cells through various receptors, undergoing differentiation which allows activation a number of cytokines and working with either immunocompetent T cells or B cells to augment their response to antigens. Helper T cells are a critical component of many immune responses. Subsets of helper T cells carry out different functions in relationship to development or cellular humoral immunity and inflammation. The mechanism by which helper T cells differentiate into the various subtypes is not well understood (Rote & Huether, 2010c).

Cytotoxic T cells recognize antigens that are associated with MHC type 1 proteins. CD8 protein is required for the cells to bind with MHC while T-cell receptors are bound to the corresponding antigen. The cytotoxic process is augmented by the presence of IL-2 cytokines secreted by activated T-helper cells (Banasik, 2013).

Peripheral or secondary lymphoid tissue includes the spleen, lymph nodes, tonsils, and Peyer patches in the gastrointestinal tract. Lymphocytes move into secondary lymphoid tissue through the blood and are bound to the endothelium by way of adhesion molecules. Once in the lymphoid tissue, T and B cells that come in contact with antigen differentiate further and proliferate, creating specialized centers (Banasik, 2013; Rote & Huether, 2010c).

HUMORAL IMMUNE RESPONSES

B cells are responsible for antibody-mediated immunity. The two major subtypes of cells are memory cells and plasma cells. Memory cells contain antigen receptors and function in a way similar to that of T memory cells. Plasma cells are short-lived antibody producing cells. These antibodies circulate and bond to the specific antigens that triggered their production (Banasik, 2013).

The primary site of B-cell development in humans is in segments of the bone marrow. The process of differentiation and maturation is similar to that of T cells. Lymphoid stem cells in the bone marrow are influenced by substances in the marrow and develop and differentiate into mature cells acquiring the necessary surface molecules, with B-cell receptors on their cell surfaces. The proliferation of cells that recognize antigens are regulated by T-helper lymphocytes. Some of the cells involved in the inflammatory response influence immature T and B cells to initiate processes needed for specific, long-acting immunity through direct contact in peripheral lymphoid tissues (Banasik, 2013; Rote & Huether, 2010c).

When the mature B cell comes in contact with a particular antigen, it is stimulated to multiply and differentiate, developing many copies of that B cell. This cell then becomes a plasma cell that can be found in blood, secondary lymphoid tissue, and some sites of inflammation. Each plasma cell, in turn becomes a site of antibody production specific to one antigen (Rote & Huether, 2010c).

A primary immune response occurs in which IgM against the antigen is produced within 5 to 7 days after antigen exposure followed by IgG. If there is no further exposure to the antigen, the circulating antibody is eventually broken down and measureable quantities are not detectable in blood samples, but the immune system has been prepared for future contact with the antigen. A second encounter with the same antigen results in a secondary immune response typified by quicker production of a larger amount of antibody than in the primary response. This quick secondary response is made possible by memory cells. IgM is produced during the secondary response, but IgG is the primary antibody, produced in large quantities. When the antigen challenge is produced by infection or immunizations, the levels of antigen specific (IgG) antibody can be elevated for many years (Rote & Huether, 2010c).

CELL-MEDIATED IMMUNE RESPONSES

The binding of antigens to specific T-cell receptors initiates the cell-mediated immune responses. The primary functions of these activated T cells are direct killing of foreign and abnormal cells and activation of other cells. Cytotoxic T lymphocytes are responsible for destroying certain target cells including tumor cells and cells infected by viruses. Apoptosis, or death of the target cells, is provoked by receptors on the cell surface and enzymes that penetrate the cell membranes (Rote & Huether, 2010c).

Other cells capable of causing target cell death include NK cells. NK cells supplement the actions of cytotoxic T lymphocytes with the ability to recognize abnormal proteins on the surfaces of infected or otherwise abnormal cells. Once attached, the NK cell acts in a manner similar to that of cytotoxic cells with the additional ability to attach to MHC-bearing cells that may be otherwise resistant to the effects of cytotoxic T lymphocytes. NK cells and macrophages also have the ability to destroy specific target cells with the aid of antibodies (Rote & Huether, 2010c).

Other Immune System Alterations

AUTOIMMUNE DISEASES

A number of autoimmune diseases exist and description of each of them is beyond the scope of this chapter. Rheumatoid arthritis (RA) is discussed as an example of the systemic effects that are often associated with autoimmune disorders.

RA is a systemic, chronic inflammatory disease characterized by synovitis affecting multiple joints. RA is more common in women than men with a ratio of three to one. The peak age of onset for women is between 40 and 50 in women and 60 and 80 in men, but it can occur at any age. While the specific cause in not known, there are a number of genetic factors associated with RA. Joint effusions are often seen in acute exacerbations. Proliferation of synovial cells and infiltration with T and B cells, macrophages and plasma cells occurs. The synovial membrane eventually becomes hypertrophied, forming a pannus which invades the surrounding tissues. Chronic synovial membrane inflammation can ultimately lead to damage to cartilage, bone, tendons and ligaments, leading to decreased function and disability (Hellmann & Imboden, 2014; Johnson & Quismorio, 2013).

Autoimmune activity includes activation of the complement system, triggering kinins, prostaglandins, cytokines, and other substances to increase permeability of vessels and draw white blood cells to the joint. As neutrophils phagocytize immune complexes, enzymes released by the cells damage joint structures. Rheumatoid factor (RF) and autoantibodies are produced in the joint triggering further damage. A number of autoantigens are attacked by the immune system including some that are T-cell targets. Activated T cells multiply and stimulate additional secretion of cytokines and production of immunoglobulins including RF (Johnson & Quismorio, 2013).

Symptoms involving the joints are the primary complaint in most patients with RA. Additionally, multiple systemic symptoms also occur. Morning joint stiffness, often lasting for hours, swelling of multiple joints, associated with tenderness are often predominant symptoms of synovial inflammation. The proximal interphalangeal joints in the fingers and metacarpophalangeal joints are most often involved.

Metatarsophalangeal joints in the feet may also be affected. Nerve entrapment syndromes including carpal tunnel syndrome are also common (Hellmann & Imboden, 2014).

The differential diagnosis for RA should include other conditions known to cause inflammatory arthritis including systemic lupus erythematosus, psoriatic arthritis, ankylosing spondylitis, and reactive arthritis. Extra-articular symptoms are often helpful in differentiating RA from other diseases. Tendinitis, bursitis, and other soft tissue conditions, and polymyalgia rheumatic in older adults may present a similar picture to early stages of RA. Viral infections including HIV and hepatitis may cause symmetric polyarthralgia and should also be included in the differential diagnosis (Johnson & Quismorio, 2013).

Multiple other extra-articular signs and symptoms highlight the systemic nature of RA. The physical examination often reveals warm, tender, and swollen joints that feel boggy due to swollen synovial membranes. Skin over the affected joint is typically reddened. Subcutaneous rheumatoid nodules are seen in a significant number of patients. While most common over bony prominences, nodules may also be found in extra-articular tissue including the lungs and sclerae. Dryness of the eyes, mouth, and other mucous membranes are often noted in more advanced disease. Inflammation involving the eye is also associated with scleritis and episcleritis. Cough and progressive shortness of breath may be associated with interstitial lung disease which affects a significant number of patients. Pericarditis, pleural effusion and vasculitis are also sometimes evidenced in RA (Hellmann & Imboden, 2014).

Preliminary diagnosis is often made based on the history and physical examination findings. Diagnostic tests including radiologic examination are important in confirming the diagnosis, predicting prognosis, and establishing a treatment plan. Baseline information including CBC, ESR, and C-reactive protein, as well as electrolytes, renal functions, liver functions, and urinalysis are important. Normocytic anemia is often associated with RA. Impaired renal or hepatic function may pose limits on which antirheumatic drugs may be used in treatment. Additionally, more specific immunologic testing to the presence of RF, anticyclic citrullinated peptide antibodies is useful in establishing the diagnosis. Not all patients with RA are RF positive at the onset of the disease, but may become positive as the disease progresses. High RF titers at the onset of the disease often have more severe symptoms and a poorer prognosis. Radiologic tests at the time of diagnosis are helpful in establishing a baseline for determining disease progression and response to treatment (Johnson & Quismorio, 2013).

Treatment objectives in RA include reducing inflammation and discomfort, preserving function, and preventing joint deformities that may result in permanent disability. Disease-modifying antirheumatic drugs (DMARDs) are synthetic or biologic agents that are able to reduce disease activity and induce remission in some cases. Referral to a rheumatologist and treatment with DMARD should begin as soon as possible to reduce disease activity. Frequent monitoring of disease status and for treatment toxicity is necessary. A number of drugs in different classes are utilized in treatment (Hellmann & Imboden, 2014; Johnson & Quismorio, 2013).

Glucocorticoids are often used at the onset of treatment to control inflammation until DMARDs, which are typically more slow acting, take effect. Long-term use of glucocorticoids is associated with many adverse consequences and should be avoided whenever possible. Synthetic DMARDs including methotrexate, sulfasalazine, and antimalarials are often used in initial therapy. Other synthetic drugs including leflunomide, and minocycline are useful in selected cases (Hellmann & Imboden, 2014).

Biologic DMARDS including tumor necrosis factor inhibitors, rituximab, abatacept, and tocilizumab may be used alone or more often in combination with other DMARDs. Combination therapies typically show greater efficacy than single agents (Hellmann & Imboden, 2014).

NSAIDS and COX-2 inhibitors have a limited role in RA but are beneficial in reducing pain and promoting mobility. They carry the increased risk of cardiovascular events. This coupled with known risk for cardiovascular disease associated with RA makes their use on a long-term basis less desirable (Johnson & Quismorio, 2013).

Nonpharmacologic therapy for individuals with RA should include education about joint protection, strength training, range of motion exercise and conserving energy. Consultation with physical and occupational therapists for their expertise in promoting function and independence can help to promote physical as well as psychological well-being. Patient and family education about the disease process, managing symptoms, and medications are critical in treatment of RA (Johnson & Quismorio, 2013).

HYPERSENSITIVITY

Hypersensitivity reactions are altered immunologic responses that result in tissue damage or disease. Such reactions are typically categorized by the type of antigen the immune system is responding to (either allergy, autoimmune or alloimmune) and by the mechanisms that trigger the response. Allergy refers to the effects of hypersensitivity to antigens from the environment while autoimmunity is an abnormal response to self-antigens or autoantibodies. Alloimmunity refers to the response against tissues of another person including blood, transplanted tissues, or fetus in pregnancy (Rote, 2010).

When hypersensitivity reactions are classified by the immune mechanism that triggers the response, four types of reactions are recognized. Type I reactions are mediated by IgE. Type II reactions are tissue specific, while Type III are immune complex mediated, and Type IV reactions are cell mediated. The four types of reactions are related and most reactions are associated with more than one mechanism. Hypersensitivity requires sensitization against an antigen to produce immune responses. Sensitization occurs when a sufficient number antibodies or T cells mount a response when reexposed to the antigen. Hypersensitivity reactions can occur immediately after reexposure, occurring in minutes to hours, or delayed, occurring hours or day later. Anaphylaxis is the most rapid and severe immediate hypersensitivity reaction, having generalized or localized manifestations. Generalized anaphylaxis symptoms include itching, erythema, headache, vomiting, cramps, diarrhea, and dyspnea. Bronchospasm, laryngeal edema, and vascular collapse may be life threatening (Rote, 2010).

Type I reactions are mediated by antigen-specific IgE and substances released from tissue mast cells. Many common environmental allergies are type I reactions, but type I reactions also contribute to some autoimmune and alloimmune diseases. Not all common allergies are IgE mediated (Rote, 2010). Degranulation of mast cells releases inflammatory response mediators and the most potent is histamine. By acting on H1 receptors, histamine causes vascular permeability, vasodilation and edema and bronchoconstriction. Actions affecting H2 receptors cause increased gastric secretions and decreases release of more histamine from basophils and mast cells. Histamine also has an effect on other chemotactic factors such as eosinophils, attracting them into sites of allergic inflammation (Rote, 2010).

Tissue-specific, type II reactions are typically characterized by particular cells or tissues targeted in the immune response. Symptoms associated with type II reactions depend on which tissues or organs express a particular antigen. Autoimmune thrombocytopenia, Grave disease, and autoimmune hemolytic anemia are examples of type II reactions (Rote, 2010).

Type III reactions are caused by antigen–antibody complexes that are formed in the circulation and then deposited in blood vessel walls and in extravascular tissues. Unlike type II reactions in which the antibody binds to cell surface antigens, in type III reactions the antibody binds to soluble antigen that has been released into blood or body fluids and the immune complex is then delivered to the tissues. These reactions are not organ specific. Harmful effects of the immune response stem from complement activation, especially by stimulating neutrophilic chemotactic factors. Neutrophils bind to the complexes where they attempt to destroy them but are unable to do so because they are bound to large amounts of tissue. Serum sickness-type reactions are systemic syndromes caused by repeated administration of drugs and other antigens causing development of immune complexes that are then deposited in tissues including blood vessels, joints, and kidney. Symptoms of this type of reaction include fever, lymphadenopathy, and rashes. Arthus reaction is an example of a localized type III reaction resulting from repeated localized exposure an antigen that reacts with immune complexes in local blood vessel walls. Reactions are characterized by pain, edema, and hemorrhage, with accumulation of neutrophils in the damaged tissue. Arthus reaction may last for 1 to 2 days; this type of reaction is sometimes associated with administration of vaccines such as tetanus toxoid. Tissue damage associated with systemic lupus erythematosus with glomerulonephritis, vasculitis, and arthritis exemplifies a disease caused by a type III response (Rote, 2010).

Type IV reactions are mediated by T lymphocytes, without the involvement of antibodies. Cytotoxic T lymphocytes or lymphokine-producing T lymphocytes promote cell destruction directly. Examples of type IV reactions include graft versus host disease and allergic reactions resulting from direct contact with substances including metals and poison ivy. The TST is also an example of a delayed hypersensitivity reaction. Infiltration of the injection site with macrophages and T lymphocytes results in the indurated erythematous lesion typical of a positive skin test (Rote, 2010).

PRIMARY IMMUNODEFICIENCY

Primary immunodeficiency (PI) refers to a group of disorders associated with inadequate or absent functions of one or more elements of the immune system. Most are the result of genetic mutations that are not inherited. PIs are quite different from acquired immunodeficiencies that are the result viral infection or treatment with immunosuppressive drugs. With the exception of IgA deficiency, PIs are quite rare. PIs are categorized based on the components of the immune system that are affected. Five categories identified by the National Institutes of Health include T-lymphocyte deficiencies, B-lymphocyte deficiencies, combined T- and B-lymphocyte deficiencies, complement deficiencies, and phagocyte deficiencies (McCusker and Warrington, 2011; Rote, 2010).

Symptoms often appear in the first few years of life. Clinical presentations vary greatly depending on the condition but risk for infection is common to most PI disorders. Ear, sinus, and skin infections are common. (Rote, 2010; McCusker & Warrington, 2011).

T-cell disorders typically increase risk for infection with viruses, fungi, parasites, and some bacteria. Mutation of T cells can affect maturation or activation of cells as well as communication among cells through defects on receptors or production of cytokines. B-cell deficiencies are more likely to be associated with altered humoral immunity and increased rates of infection with bacteria such as *Streptococcus*, *Staphylococcus*, and *Haemophilus* organisms. Combined deficiencies are linked to more severe infections at an early age. Multiple immune pathways are affected and if unrecognized, such deficiencies are associated with drastically shortened lifespans (Bowdish, 2013).

Evaluation should include complete blood count looking for lymphopenia and other hematologic abnormalities as well as lymphocyte proliferation assays and flow cytometry to identify the number of B cells, T cells, and NK cells, and the evaluation of lymphocyte markers, T-cell variability, and adhesion receptors that may be associated with specific immune defects. When B-cell deficiency is suspected the evaluation should include the measurement of serum IgG, IgA, IgM, and IgE levels, which is important (McCusker & Warrington, 2011).

Selective IgA deficiency is the most common of the PIs. It is defined as decrease or absence of serum levels of IgA with preservation of other types of immunoglobulins. Many individuals with the condition are healthy with the condition being found incidentally while others have recurrent respiratory and gastrointestinal infections, allergies, and autoimmune symptoms. Secretory IgA is the most abundant form in the body and is found primarily in the mucosal secretions of the respiratory, gastrointestinal, and genitourinary tracts. Although the functions of IgA are not completely understood, it is clear that it performs important protective functions in preventing of invasive bacteria from penetrating the mucosa. Individuals with IgA deficiency manifest increased incidence of sinus infection and pneumonia, and other conditions affecting the gastrointestinal tract, including giardiasis, malabsorption syndromes, ulcerative colitis, and celiac disease, as well as allergic disorders including asthma and atopic dermatitis (Yel, 2010).

SECONDARY IMMUNODEFICIENCIES

Secondary immunodeficiencies are acquired or associated with other diseases. In addition to HIV infection, malnutrition is a common cause of secondary immunodeficiency. Aging can lead to decline in immune function. Systemic inflammatory diseases such as systemic lupus erythematosus, cancer, and immunosuppressive drugs are causes of secondary immunodeficiency. Whenever patients present with recurrent infection, secondary immunodeficiency should be considered (Bowdish, 2013).

Treatment of immunodeficiency includes minimizing risk of infection and enhancing immune system function. Appropriate use of antibiotics after obtaining cultures is essential with prolonged therapy often necessary. Overgrowth of *Clostridium difficile* and fungal infections and other adverse effects of antibiotics should be monitored. Education regarding avoidance of infection and recognizing signs and symptoms of infection is an essential part of patient care. Enhancing immune function may be accomplished in a variety of ways depending on the components that are deficient. Treatment with cytokines, immunoglobulins, plasma infusion, growth factors, or gene therapy may be required (Bowdish, 2013).

Diagnostic Studies

Evaluation of a suspected immunodeficiency disorder should include a complete blood count to identify neutropenia and lymphopenia. Cultures of sputum, urine, blood, and wounds are necessary to identify infecting organisms. Erythrocyte sedimentation rate (ESR) and C-reactive protein are important markers of inflammation. Quantitative serum immunoglobulins can also be useful in screening for antibody disorders. Based on findings of initial testing, referral to an immunologist is warranted in the presence of immunodeficiency. Additional testing might include antibody responses to antigens, T-cell functional assay, evaluation of T-cell subtypes, phagocyte function, flow cytometry for abnormal cell markers, and complement levels. Delayed-type hypersensitivity skin testing is useful in ruling out T-cell disorders (Bowdish, 2013).

ERYTHROCYTE SEDIMENTATION RATE

ESR is a measure of the rate of sedimentation of RBCs in an anticoagulated whole blood sample over a designated time period. The foundation of the test is that proteins in blood are altered in the presence of inflammation, causing the RBCs to aggregate and become heavier and settle more rapidly at the bottom of a calibrated tube. The test is a nonspecific marker of inflammation and is often the first test ordered to identify the presence of an inflammatory condition (Van Leeuwen, Poelhuis-Leth, & Bladh, 2011).

C-REACTIVE PROTEIN

C-reactive protein is a glycoprotein produced in the liver in response to inflammation. It is frequently used along with the ESR to determine the existence of inflammation. Though not specific, it is more sensitive and appears more quickly than the ESR. It is used in assessment and monitoring the course of inflammatory conditions (Van Leeuwen et al., 2011).

RHEUMATOID FACTOR

RF is an antibody associated with RA; however, patients with other inflammatory diseases such as systemic lupus erythematosus, hepatitis, infectious mononucleosis, and endocarditis may also test positive for RF. A number of factors can influence the results of the test. Older adults often have increased RF levels. Multiple vaccines and recent transfusion may influence results. In some cases false-positive results have been found in individuals with high serum lipid levels. A level of less than 14 international units per milliliter is a normal result (Van Leeuwen et al., 2011).

ANTICYCLIC CITRULLINATED PEPTIDE

Anticyclic citrullinated peptide is an enzyme-linked immunoassay important in the diagnosis and monitoring of RA. This assay is more sensitive and more specific than RF and is helpful in the diagnosis of patients with RA who may be RF negative at the early stage and moderately positive results range between stages of disease. It is also more sensitive in identifying individuals with erosive joint disease. A result of less than 20 units is a negative test. Levels between 20 and 39 are considered weakly positive, while results ranging between 40 and 59 are moderately positive. Greater than 60 units is a strongly positive result (Van Leeuwen et al., 2011).

IMMUNOGLOBULIN E

The primary response of IgE is associated with allergic reactions and parasite infections. Most available IgE is stored in the tissues and not circulating in the blood. Serum IgE levels are useful in evaluating allergies. Levels may be elevated in allergy, asthma, dermatitis, eczema, sinusitis, and rhinitis as well as parasitic infections. Reduced levels may be seen in the presence of advanced cancer when there may be a generalized decrease in immune responses and immunodeficiency syndromes. Normal serum IgE levels vary with age.

IMMUNOGLOBULINS A, D, G, AND M

Quantitative serum immunoglobulins are useful in the evaluation of humoral immunity. Assessment of immunoglobulins is useful in diagnosis and monitoring the status of some cancers including multiple myeloma and macroglobulinemias during treatment. Reference ranges vary with age and other factors.

Review Section

Review Questions

1. A 25-year-old male presents to the clinic complaining of fever to 101°F, chills and body aches associated with nausea, and a maculopapular rash. He denies recent sick contacts and denies use of intravenous drugs. He does report multiple sex partners and inconsistent use of condoms. He has otherwise been well, has no significant medical history, and takes no medications. He has bilateral, painless, enlarged cervical lymph nodes. His physical examination is otherwise unremarkable. His laboratory results are within normal limits with the exception of a platelet count of 86,000. Which of the following is the best diagnostic test to order?

   a. HIV antibodies
   b. CD4 count
   c. HIV viral load
   d. Erythrocyte sedimentation rate

2. A 34-year-old male with HIV infection asks your opinion about starting antiretroviral therapy (ART) suggested by a specialist. He feels well and is working full-time. His most recent most recent CD4 counts on two separate occasions are 586 and 547. Viral loads are 5,000 and 3,965. Which of the following statements guides your conversation with the patient?

   a. There is no need to start therapy given his current laboratory results.
   b. The patient should be followed closely and start treatment when his CD4 count falls below 500.
   c. The side effects of therapy will preclude the patient from being able to function at the level he is accustomed to.
   d. Current recommendations suggest that all persons infected with HIV infection should be offered ART.

3. A 28-year-old African American male diagnosed with AIDS will require prophylactic treatment against pneumocystis pneumonia. The medication usually prescribed in this situation is trimethoprim/sulfamethoxazole. Before prescribing the drug, the Nurse Practitioner orders laboratory testing to avert an adverse drug reaction. Which of the following is the most appropriate test?

   a. G6PD-deficiency screening
   b. Complete blood count
   c. Viral load
   d. CD4 count

4. A 46-year-old patient with AIDS presents with cough, fatigue, and shortness of breath. His oxygen saturation is 95% on room air. A chest X-ray demonstrates infiltrates and a tuberculin skin test is negative. Which action by the Nurse Practitioner is most appropriate?

   a. Initiate treatment for pneumocystis pneumonia.
   b. Initiate treatment for bacterial pneumonia.
   c. Order Quantiferon blood testing to rule out tuberculosis.
   d. Order supplemental oxygen while further workup continues.

5. A 26-year-old woman is diagnosed with acute HIV infection. To complete her evaluation, several screening tests are required. Which of the following are appropriate for this patient?

   a. Testing for syphilis, gonorrhea, and chlamydia
   b. Testing for hepatitis B and C
   c. Cervical cancer screening with Pap smear
   d. a and b
   e. a, b, and c

6. Which of the following describes a process involved in a typical acute inflammatory response?

   a. Arteriolar constriction
   b. Influx of mast cells
   c. Influx of macrophages
   d. Influx of neutrophils

7. Type 1 hypersensitivity reactions are most often mediated by which type of antibody?

   a. IgA
   b. IgE
   c. IgG
   d. Ig M

8. Which of the following best exemplifies passive immunity?

   a. Injection of immune globulin
   b. Passage of IgG antibodies from mother to fetus
   c. Infusion of a weak antigen
   d. a and b
   e. a, b, and c

9. After exposure to infection, the primary antibody produced providing long-term protection when reexposed to the same antigen is which of the following?

   a. IgA
   b. IgE
   c. IgG
   d. IgM

10. The Nurse Practitioner is caring for a 78-year-old patient who has had recurrent lung infections despite standard treatment. His pulmonary function tests are normal. A chest CT scan is negative for evidence of malignancy. Which of the following should the Nurse Practitioner consider in the differential diagnosis?

   a. Primary immunodeficiency
   b. Secondary immunodeficiency
   c. Drug resistant organisms causing infection
   d. None of the above

Answers with Rationales

1. (c) HIV viral load

   Rationale: The patient's signs and symptoms are consistent with acute HIV infection. The appropriate test to order in this situation is the HIV viral load. HIV antibodies may not be evident in acute infection.

2. (d) Current recommendations suggest that all persons infected with HIV infection should be offered ART.

   Rationale: The most recent recommendations for initiating treatment suggest that treatment with ART should be offered to all persons with HIV, regardless of CD4 cell count, to improve their health and prolong their lives. Effective treatment also reduces the risk of transmitting HIV to others.

3. (a) G6PD-deficiency screening

   Rationale: G6PD deficiency is more likely to occur in African American males. The risk of hemolytic anemia associated with G6PD deficiency is increased with sulfa drugs, so the Nurse Practitioner should assess for the presence of the disorder prior to prescribing the medication.

4. (c) Order Quantiferon blood testing to rule out tuberculosis.

   Rationale: In the setting of immunodeficiency, tuberculin skin tests are often falsely negative. Additional testing to rule out tuberculosis is needed. The results of sputum samples for acid–fast bacillus smear and culture will also yield useful information.

5. (e) a, b, and c

   Rationale: Risk factors for coinfection with other sexually transmitted infection and hepatitis B and C are the same as those for HIV infection making screening important. Women with HIV infection are also at greater risk for cervical cancer, making screening warranted.

6. (d) Influx of neutrophils

   Rationale: Neutrophils are attracted to a site of inflammation by factors released from mast cells.

7. (b) IgE

   Rationale: Type 1 sensitivity reactions are mediated by IgE.

8. (d) a and b

   Rationale: Passive immunity refers to receiving antibodies from an external source rather than producing them through their own immune system.

9. (c) IgG

   Rationale: IgM is produced during the secondary response, but IgG is the primary antibody, produced in large quantities. When the antigen challenge is produced by infection or immunizations, the levels of antigen specific (IgG) antibody can be elevated for many years.

10. (b) Secondary immunodeficiency

    Rationale: Secondary immunodeficiencies are acquired or associated with other diseases. In addition to HIV infection, malnutrition is a common cause of secondary immunodeficiency. Aging can lead to decline in immune function. Systemic inflammatory diseases such as systemic lupus erythematosus, cancer, and immunosuppressive drugs are causes of secondary immunodeficiency. Whenever patients present with recurrent infection, secondary immunodeficiency should be considered.

Suggested Readings

Aberg, J. A., Gallant, J. E., Ghanem, K. G., Emmanuel, P., Zingman, B. S., & Horberg, M. A. (2013). Primary care guidelines for the management of persons infected with HIV: 2013 update by the HIV Medical Association of the Infectious Diseases Society of America. *Clinical Infectious Disease, 58,* e1–e35. Retrieved from http://cid.oxfordjournals.org

AIDS Info Panel on Antiretroviral Guidelines for Adults and Adolescents. (2014). *Guidelines for the use of antiretroviral agents in HIV-1 infected adults and adolescents.* Retrieved from http://aidsinfo.nih.gov/guidelines

Arts, E. J., & Hazuda, D. J. (2012). HIV-1 Antiretroviral drug therapy. *Cold Spring Harbor Perspectives in Medicine, 2*(4):a007161, 1–24.

Banasik, J. L. (2013). Inflammation and immunity. In L. Copstead & J. Banasik (Eds.), *Pathophysiology* (5th ed., pp. 157–194). St Louis, MO: Elsevier Saunders.

Bowdish, M. S. (2013), Immunodeficiency. In T. M. Buttaro, J. Trybulski, B. P. Bailey, & J. Sandberg-Cook (Eds.), *Primary care: A collaborative practice* (4th ed., pp. 1224–1230). St. Louis, MO: Elsevier Mosby.

Burgess, M. J., & Kasten, M. J. (2013). Human immunodeficiency virus: What primary care clinicians need to know. *Mayo Clinic Proceedings, 88*(12), 1468–1474.

Centers for Disease Control and Prevention. (2014). Recommendations for HIV Prevention with Adults and Adolescents in the United States, 2014. Retrieved from http://stacks.cdc.gov/view/cdc/26062

Chu, C., & Selwyn, P. A. (2010). Diagnosis and initial management of acute HIV infection. *American Family Physician, 15*(81), 1239–1244.

Cohen, M. S., Gay, C. L., Busch, M. P., & Hecht, F. M. (2010). The detection of acute HIV infection. *Journal of Infectious Diseases, 202*(S2), S270–S277.

Hellmann, D. B., & Imboden, J. B. (2014). Rhematologic & immunologic disorders. In M. A. Papadakis & S. J. McPhee (Eds.), *Current medical diagnosis and treatment 2014* (pp. 786–836). New York, NY: McGraw Hill.

Johnson, D. K., & Quismorio, F. P. (2013). Rheumatoid arthritis. In T. M. Buttaro, J. Trybulski, B. P. Bailey, & J. Sandberg-Cook (Eds.), *Primary care: A collaborative practice* (4th ed., pp. 1196–1200). St. Louis, MO: Elsevier Mosby.

Maartens, G., Celum, C., & Lewin, S. R. (2014). HIV infection: epidemiology, pathogenesis, treatment, and prevention. *Lancet, 384,* 258–271.

McCusker, C., & Warrington, R. (2011). Primary immunodeficiency. *Allergy, Asthma & Clinical Immunology, 7*(Suppl 1), S11.

Morbidity and Mortality Weekly Report. (2008). AIDS defining conditions: Appendix A. *MMWR Recommendations and Reports, 57*(RR10), 9.

Powderly, W. G. (2012). Osteoporosis and bone health in HIV. *Current HIV/AIDS Reports, 9*(3), 218–222. doi: 10.1007/s11904-12-0119-7.

Roche, W. P., Tindall, W. N., & Sedrak, M. M. (2014). Drugs used in the treatment of nonbacterial infections. In W.N. Tindall, M.M. Sedrak, & J. M. Boltri (Eds.), *Patient Centered Pharmacology: Learning System for the Conscientious Prescriber* (pp. 338–361). Philadelphia, PA: F.A. Davis.

Rote, N. S. (2010). Alteration in immunity and inflammation. In K. L. McCance, S. Huether, V. L. Brashers, & N. S. Rote (Eds.), *Pathophysiology: The biologic basis for disease in adults and children* (6th ed., pp. 256–292). Maryland Heights, MO: Mosby Elsevier.

Rote, N. S., & Huether, S. E. (2010a). Infection. In K. L. McCance, S. Huether, V. L. Brashers, & N. S. Rote (Eds.), *Pathophysiology: The biologic basis for disease in adults and children* (6th ed., pp. 293–335). Maryland Heights, MO: Mosby Elsevier.

Rote, N. S., & Huether, S. E. (2010b). Innate immunity: inflammation. In K. L. McCance, S. Huether, V. L. Brashers, & N. S. Rote (Eds.), *Pathophysiology: The biologic basis for disease in adults and children* (6th ed., pp. 183–216). Maryland Heights, MO: Mosby Elsevier.

Rote, N. S., & Huether, S. E. (2010c). Adaptive immunity. In K. L. McCance, S. Huether, V. L. Brashers, & N. S. Rote (Eds.), *Pathophysiology: The biologic basis for disease in adults and children* (6th ed., pp. 217–255). Maryland Heights, MO: Mosby Elsevier.

Simon, V., Ho, D. D., & Abdool Karim, Q. (2006). HIV/AIDS epidemiology, pathogenesis, prevention and treatment. *Lancet, 368,* 489–504.

Torre, D., Speranza, F., & Martegani, R. (2005). Impact of highly active antiretroviral therapy on organ-specific manifestations of HIV-1 infection. *HIV Medicine, 6,* 66–78.

Van Leeuwen, A. M., Poelhuis-Leth, D., & Bladh, M. L. (2011). *Davis's comprehensive handbook of diagnostic tests with nursing implications* (4th ed.). Philadelphia, PA: F. A. Davis.

Yel, L. (2010). Selective IgA deficiency. *Journal of Clinical Immunology, 30,* 10–16.

Zolopa, A. R., & Katz, M. H. (2014). HIV infection and AIDS. In M. A. Papadakis & S. J. McPhee (Eds.), *Current medical diagnosis and treatment 2014* (pp. 1273–1304), New York, NY: McGraw Hill.

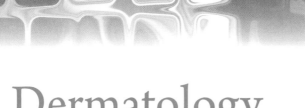

Chapter 13

Dermatology

Joanne Schwartz

Case Presentation

Directions: Carefully review the case study presented below. At the end of the chapter, answer the review questions. Compare your answers to the correct answers listed in the Review Section.

Chief Complaint and History of Present Illness:
A 68-year-old, obese, African-American female comes to the health clinic complaining of irritation and itching of the skin under her breasts and in her groin. The patient reports that the problem has started approximately 2 weeks ago, has gotten worse with the recent hot weather, and simply "won't go away." She reports that she has applied petroleum jelly to the affected area with no relief. Her health history includes hypothyroidism, hypercholesterolemia, and hypertension. She visited her primary care provider approximately 6 months ago. She comes to the clinic today because she no longer has health insurance.

Medication:
Levothyroxine (Synthroid) 50 mcg daily, furosemide (Lasix) 40 mg daily, simvastatin (Zocor) 20 mg daily

Medical History:
Patient reports generally good health. Patient denies polyuria, polydipsia, polyuria, or blurred vision. Patient denies slow healing/nonhealing breaks in skin integrity. Patient denies numbness or decreased sensation in lower extremities.

Physical Examination:
A 5-feet-2-inch, 170-lb woman. Her physical examination is remarkable for moist, glistening patches of bright red erythema with satellite macules bilaterally on the submammary area and intertriginous areas in groin. Both areas have numerous excoriations, but are without any exudate. Lungs are CTA. +S1, S2. −S3, −S4. No murmurs. +BS. No tenderness, no organomegaly of abdomen. LE without edema and warm to touch. Skin intact. +3 pedal pulses. +sensation to pin pricks.

Laboratory Studies/Serum Chemistry:
Glucose: 250 mg/dL
Total cholesterol: 142 mg/dL
TSH: 2.4 mIU/L
Total (serum) T3: 112 ng/dL
Total (serum) T4: 8.1 µg/dL

Vital Signs:
Blood pressure = 128/84 mm Hg   Temperature = 98.8°F   Respirations = 16/minute   Pulse = 82 beats/minute

Diagnostic Studies:
None necessary

Diagnoses:
Cutaneous/intertrigo candidiasis
Type 2 diabetes mellitus
Healing excoriations in submammary and intertriginous areas

Treatment:
Ketoconazal (Nizoral) cream
Apply a thin coat to affected area b.i.d. for 5 days.
Metformin (Glucophage) 500 mg daily
Patient should be seen in 1 week for follow-up to assess the state of the candidiasis infection and to make sure the excoriations have not become infected. Patient should be assessed for compliance with metformin and to assess progress with weight reduction.

Patient Teaching Regarding Prevention of Cutaneous Candidiasis:
Patient should be instructed to do the following:
- Air dry after bathing and use a blow-dryer on a cool setting to thoroughly dry the affected areas.
- Wear nonrestricting cotton clothes and no underwear when sleeping.
- Utilize air-conditioning during warm weather or stay in air-conditioned environments such as shopping centers or libraries.
- Avoid conditions that cause candidiasis to flourish: high serum glucose, moisture, heat, and darkness.

Patient Teaching Regarding Diabetes Mellitus Type 2 Management:
Patient needs:
- A referral to a dietician for education regarding weight reduction
- Guidelines for exercise
- Teaching regarding the connection between weight and diabetes mellitus type 2

Acne Vulgaris

Description of the Disease: A relatively common skin condition characterized by increased sebaceous gland activity and bacteria presence in hair follicles, resulting in closed (whiteheads) and open (blackheads) comedones, papules, pustules, nodules, cysts, and in severe cases, scarring.

Epidemiology:
- The most common skin disease in the United States. Approximately 80% of individuals will have acne during their lifetime.
- Most commonly found in white males aged 14 to 18, but a substantial number of male and female aged 20 to 40 may also be affected.
- Adolescent acne is more common in males and adult acne more common in females.

Etiology:
- The etiology of acne vulgaris is not entirely clear. However, the disease is correlated with an increase in androgen production during adolescence, androgen-sensitive lipid synthesis in the pilosebaceous follicle, follicular shedding of epithelial cells resulting in obstruction and proliferation of the bacteria *Propionibacterium acnes*, which thrives on sebum, and chemical inflammatory mediators.
- These factors work together to contribute to the follicular inflammatory process, resulting in skin lesions that may be painful and can cause scarring.

Risk Factors:
- Male gender, increased androgen activity, increased sebaceous production, stress, genetics, medications, diet, smoking, and environmental factors such as clothing and touching or rubbing of affected areas.

Signs and Symptoms:
- Presence of noninflamatory lesions (comedones) and inflammatory lesions (papules, pustules, nodules, and cysts) on areas with increased sebaceous gland activity such as the face, neck, back, and chest most often during adolescence or adulthood

- Patients with acne may experience depression and suicidal ideation related to self-esteem; these individuals should always be assessed for depression and suicidal risk.

Differential Diagnoses:
- Acne rosacea, acneiform, seborrheic dermatitis, contact dermatitis, millia, and periorbital dermatitis

Diagnostic Studies:
- Generally none. However, hormonal testing may be indicated to rule out increased androgen production (testosterone) particularly in adult women with severe acne, dysmenorrhea, or hirsutism.

Treatment:

Mild Acne
- Mild noninflammatory comedonal acne is usually treated with topical agents such as benzoyl peroxide which decreases *P. acnes*, salicylic acid which decreases desquamation of cells, or azelaic acid which decreases *P. acnes*. Improvement should be seen in 4 to 8 weeks.
- Additionally, the topical retinoid and retinoid analogues (Retin-A, Tazorac, Differin) which decrease hyperkeratinization and inflammation can be applied nightly to affected areas.
- For mild inflammatory acne (papules and pustules) topical antibiotics which decrease bacteria and inflammation: erythromycin (Erygel), clindamycin (Clindagel), or metronidazole (Metrogel) may be used by themselves or added to the treatment plan for mild acne

Moderate Acne
- Moderate acne (papules and pustules) is usually treated with topical agents and an oral antibiotic such as a tretracyline (Acnecycline) or erythromycin (E-mycin) which help to decrease *P. acnes*.
- Women using an oral contraceptive may benefit from a combination pill (estrogen and progestin).
- The FDA has approved three combination pills for treatment of acne for women who need contraceptive: estrogen/norgestimate (Ortho Tri-Cyclen), estrogen/norethindrone (Estrostep), and estrogen/drospirenone (YAZ).
- Some research has indicated an increased risk of blood clots with drospirenone compared to other progestins.

Severe Acne
- For severe (nodules and cysts) acne or mild or moderate acne that has been treated long-term without success, the oral retinoids may be indicated as they have numerous mechanisms of action: decrease the size of sebaceous glands and decrease sebum production, decrease follicular *P. acnes*, decrease desquamation of skin, and have anti-inflammatory properties.
- Absolute contraindications are pregnancy, lactation, renal, or liver disorders. Oral retinoids are a pregnancy category X. A strict protocol must be followed for the female patient of childbearing age who is using an oral retinoid. Hepatic, renal, and triglyceride levels must be assessed regularly.
- If the female patient does not have the maturity to reliably follow the protocol, a retinoid should not be used. The use of isotretinoin (Accutane) has been associated with increased rates of suicide. Patients on isotretinoin should be regularly monitored for suicidal thoughts.
- Acne scarring may affect up to 20% of individuals. Patients with acne scarring, but without acute lesions, who have expressed interest in scar revision should be referred to a dermatologist or plastic surgeon for further treatment.
- Patients should be aware that hyperpigmentation may occur after an inflammatory acne lesion has resolved. These areas are caused by thinning of the dermis and the increased vascularity of the area. These hyperpigmented areas will fade usually within 3 to 6 months of the lesion's resolution.

Patient Teaching for Patients with Acne
- Patients should be taught that topical agents such as benzoyl peroxide, salicylic acid, and azelaic acid, and the retinoids may cause erythema of the skin. The patient may need to decrease frequency of application, amount of time skin is exposed to medication, or strength of medication until it is better tolerated.
- As each classification of topical drug works via a different mechanism, the patient may be on one or more of these drugs concurrently. Daily use of a water-based broad spectrum sunscreen of at least SPF 30 is strongly recommended.
- Some patients will notice an exacerbation about 2 weeks after starting a topical medication. This exacerbation indicates the topical agent is working and the patient should continue to use the medication as instructed.

- A patient with acne should be instructed on proper face washing. A patient with acne has sensitive skin—not dirty skin. The patient should be instructed to wash face two to three times a day with soap for sensitive skin and warm water and pat skin dry.
- The patient should be instructed not to pick at skin as this can aggravate acne and increase likelihood of scarring. The patient should also be instructed to replace oil-based cleansers, moisturizers, and makeup with oil-free or water-based products.
- The patient should also be instructed regarding food choices. Recent research has indicated that there may be some relationship between certain foods and beverages and acne. Patients should be advised to look for patterns between oral intake and an acne exacerbation. Simple sugars, dairy products, and carbonated beverages may be found to worsen acne.

Acrochordon (Skin Tag)

Description of the Disease: A benign, small, soft, pedunculated, flesh-colored skin tumor commonly found in intertriginous areas of the body

Epidemiology:
- An estimated prevalence rate of 25% to 46% in the general population

Etiology:
- Usually appear in areas of friction—where skin or clothes rub skin

Risk Factors:
- Female gender, middle age or older, obesity, elevated insulin levels/prediabetes, type 2 diabetes mellitus, genetics, pregnancy, possibly human papillomavirus (HPV) 6 or 11.

Signs and Symptoms:
- Regular or irregular painless, skin growth generally 2 to 5 mm usually with a peduncular base commonly found in the intertriginous areas of the neck, axillae, under breasts, groin, and eyelids. A patient may have a few to a hundred in number.

Differential Diagnoses:
- Some common skin conditions that can mimic skin tags include seborrheic keratoses, moles, warts, cysts, milia, neurofibromas, and nevus lipomatosus. Rarely, skin cancers like basal cell carcinoma, squamous cell carcinoma, and malignant melanoma may mimic skin tags.

Diagnostic Studies:
- None generally required. However, a biopsy may be indicated when diagnosis is in question.

Treatment:
- No treatment is generally necessary. Referral for removal if patient expresses cosmetic concerns or if tags become irritated from clothing, jewelry, shaving, seatbelts, etc. Tags may be removed via cauterization, cryosurgery, excision, or ligation. While they may commonly reoccur, removal itself does not cause an increase in number.

Actinic Keratosis (Solar Keratosis)

Description of the Disease: Thick, scaly, rough, precancerous lesions, approximately 2 to 10 mm in size and may range from flesh-colored and tan to red and occurs in sun-exposed areas of the skin such as the scalp, face, lips (actinic keratosis), posterior hands, chest, and back. Itching, burning, and bleeding may also be present. Lesions may go away without treatment. Between 0% and 0.5% of actinic keratoses develop into squamous cell carcinoma.

Epidemiology:
- Approximately 58 million individuals in the United States and approximately half of the world's population have actinic keratoses.

Etiology:
- Actinic keratosis is characterized by dysplasia and disorder of the epidermis.

Risk Factors:

- Age, HPV infection, history of skin cancer, fair skin, immunosuppressive drugs

Signs and Symptoms:

- Actinic keratosis may begin as rough spots with a sandpaper texture that are easier felt than see on sun-exposed areas of the skin. Lesions may coalesce to areas larger than several centimeters. The patient may report that lesions are tender or itchy.

Differential Diagnoses:

- Seborrheic keratosis, squamous cell carcinoma, basal cell carcinoma, melanoma, warts

Diagnostic Studies:

- Biopsy if diagnosis is uncertain; if lesions reoccur after treatment; or are unresponsive to treatment. Increasing thickness, pain, and ulceration are possible signs that an actinic keratosis may be transforming to squamous cell carcinoma. Actinic keratoses will emit a pink fluorescence under wood lighting.

Treatment:

Patient Teaching

Patient should be instructed to:

- use a broad-spectrum sunblock of at least SPF 30 or sunscreens containing titanium dioxide or zinc oxide (preferred over chemical sunblocks due to broader protection).
- wear hats, long-sleeve tops, and pants.
- avoid the sun between the hours of 12 and 3 PM.
- maintain regular follow-up appointments to evaluate for changes in existing lesions and appearance of new ones as 10% of actinic keratoses progress to squamous cell carcinoma.

Laser, cryosurgery, electrocautery, curettage, shave excision, chemical peels, and excision are all methods for removal.

Cutaneous Candidiasis

Description of the Disease: A proliferation of the normal skin fungi, *Candida albicans*, often causing erythema, pruritus, irritation and/or soreness

Epidemiology:

- In one Japanese study, cutaneous candidiasis was found in 755 (1%) of 72,660 outpatients.

Etiology:

- *Candida* is often present on the skin in low levels, but its growth is normally limited by a healthy immune system and competing microorganisms. When the normal balance is disturbed, Candida flourishes, causing an infection of the skin (cutaneous candidiasis), intertrigionous areas (intertrigo candidiasis), and the paronychia (paronychiasis). *Candida albicans* accounts for 80% to 90% of candidiasis infections in humans.

Risk Factors:

- Obesity, diabetes, immunosuppression, pregnancy, antibiotics, hot and humid weather, tight clothing, poor hygiene, perspiration, wearing wet clothing such as bathing suits and workout clothes

Signs and Symptom:

- Erythematous, glistening, pruritic areas particularly in warm, intertriginous areas not exposed to air or light such as the abdominal folds, groin, axillae, rectal area, and under pendulous breasts. Satellite lesions are often present and may coalesce with larger lesions.

Differential Diagnoses:

- Cutaneous tinea infections, seborrheic dermatosis, psoriasis

Diagnostic Studies:

- Clinical assessment is usually enough to make the diagnosis. KOH testing and histologic examination will confirm diagnosis.

Treatment:

Candidiasis is treated with topical antifungals such as clotrimazole (Lotrimin AF), nystatin (Mycostatin), and ketoconazole (Nizoral) applied to affected areas.

Patient Teaching
- The patient should be instructed to keep the skin dry when possible, taking particular care with drying after washing. A blow-dryer set on a cool setting may help in thoroughly drying skin. The use of antifungal powders may assist in preventing infections.
- Patients should use caution when applying powders as inhalation may lead to pneumonia. The patient should be instructed that maintaining a healthy weight and a normal blood sugar will also help decrease the likelihood of infections.

Cherry Angioma

Description of the Disease: A cluster of capillaries at the skin.

Epidemiology:
- Present in up to 50% of adults; present in both genders and all races

Etiology:
- Unknown; possibly hormonal; possibly exposure to chemicals such as mustard gas, 2-butoxyethanol, bromides, and cyclosporine

Risk Factors:
- First appear in early adulthood and increase with age

Signs and Symptoms:
- Initially a red to dark red, nonblanching pinpoint macula that may grow to a papule approximately 1 to 2 mm in diameter; usually found on the trunk and extremities

Diagnostic Studies:
- None necessary; visual inspection is generally enough to make the diagnosis.

Treatment:
May be removed by laser or electrocautery if bleeding or a cosmetic concern

Patient Teaching
- A cherry angioma, because it is a cluster of capillaries, may bleed profusely if it is injured

Atopic Dermatitis/Eczema

Description of the Disease: Inflammation of the skin characterized by pruritic, erythematous, vesicular, exudative, fissures, lichenification, and crusting. Chronic dermatitis is often referred to as atopic dermatitis or atopic eczema.

Epidemiology:
- Affects 3.5% of the world population. It is most prevalent in infants, females of reproductive age, individuals with higher levels of education, and health-care and social service workers. The rates of eczema have risen significantly since the latter half of the 20th century particularly in developing countries.

Etiology:
- Exact cause unknown. Theories suggest that a faulty epidermal barrier due to structural and functional abnormalities or an immune function disorder in which an inflammatory response is mounted in response to environmental factors.

Risk Factors:
- History of hay fever or asthma; limited exposure to allergens during childhood, having celiac disease, or having a relative with celiac disease

Signs and Symptoms:
- Extremely pruritic, erythematous, dry, scaly, excoriated, lichenified patches of skin. The areas of the body most commonly affected are the flexor and extensor areas of the body, arms, wrists, knees, face, hands, and genitalia.

Differential Diagnoses:
- Seborrheic dermatitis, contact (allergic) dermatitis, eczema herpeticum, scabies

Diagnostic Studies:
- Generally none indicated.

Treatment:
- Drying soaps and detergents should not be used on affected skin because they can remove skin oils further exacerbating the itch. Perfumes should be avoided on the affected area. Moisturizing products should be used frequently. Thicker, heavier moisturizing creams (oil-based), are preferred over thinner, lighter (water-based) moisturizing lotions. Moisturizers should be used even during lesion-free periods as a preventive measure.
- Patients experiencing intense itching are at risk for skin infections due to breaks in skin integrity from scratching. If concerns about infection arise, consider the use of topical antibiotics such as fusidic acid (Fuscidan) and mupirocin (Bactroban) or oral antiobiotics such as penicillin, erythromycin (E-mycin), and flucloxacillin (Floxapen). Antibiotics should be prescribed no longer than 2 weeks.
- Severe scratching will injure skin cells, causing histamine to be released. First-generation oral antihistamines such as diphenhydramine (Benadryl) may help to control the pruritus as well as aid in sleeping.
- Environmental and behavioral changes and the use of moisturizers are the first line of defense. Topical corticosteroids may only be needed during periods of exacerbation. The severity of the eczema should determine the potency of the steroid, with oral steroids being reserved for severe cases with numerous or widespread lesions.
- The topical calcineurin inhibitors and immunosuppressants, pimecrolimus (Elidel) and tacrolimus (Protopic), may be used as an alternative if the patient has not responded satisfactorily to gluccocorticoids. Tacrolimus has proven more effective than picrolimus, but it has been associated with an increased risk of skin cancer and lymphoma.
- When eczema is severe and does not respond to steroids or topical immunosuppressants, oral immunosuppressants may need to be considered. Light therapy using ultraviolet light has been used but has minimal evidence supporting its effectiveness. Additionally, ultraviolet light increases risk for skin cancer. A daily dosage of vitamin D 2,000 IU also may minimize the symptoms of eczema.

Patient Teaching
- Wet dressings are helpful to decrease inflammation, pruritus and burning. Wet dressings may be made using: cool tap water, Burrow solution (Domeboro astringent solution powder packets), or acetic acid (mix half cup of white vinegar with 1 pint of water).
- Instruct patient to apply emollient to area. Immerse a clean cloth and wring excess solution. Apply to affected area for 30 to 60 minutes for three to four times a day. As wet compresses may dry skin, limit their use if skin becomes too dry. A low to medium potency topical steroid may be applied in place of emollient; however, this should be limited to one time per day and last no longer than 1 week as the wet compress may increase systemic steroidal absorption.

Cellulitis/Erysipelas

Description of the Disease: Cellulitis and erysipelas (St. Anthony fire) are skin infections that occur when bacteria enter to deeper skin tissues. Erysipelas affects the upper dermis and superficial lymphatics; cellulitis involves the deeper dermis and subcutaneous fat.

Epidemiology:
- Erysipelas most commonly affects children and older adults, with peak incidence at 60 to 80 years of age. Cellulitis most commonly affects adults older than 45.

Etiology:
- Bacteria gain entrance to deeper skin tissues via a break in skin integrity. The most common bacteria is group A *Streptococcus*. The blood flow to the deeper tissues, rich in oxygen and nutrients, allows the bacteria to grow rapidly. The source of the bacteria may be the patient's nasal passages.

Signs and Symptoms:
- Bright red, shiny erythema, warmth, edema, tenderness, and pain in the affected area, as well as fever, fatigue, and general ill feeling. The lower legs are most commonly affected, though in erysipelas the face can often be affected. Because it affects the more superficial layers of the dermis, erysipelas usually has a clear line of demarcation with raised borders (Peau de Orange).

- Erysipelas usually presents with an acute onset of symptoms with fever, chills, anorexia, and vomiting within 48 hours of initial infection; cellulitis has a slower onset of symptoms that tend to be more localized in nature.
- Erysipelas may present with a butterfly rash over cheeks or affect the ear (Milian ear sign) due to the ears' more superficial dermis. Lymphadenopathy with streaking from lymph nodes, vesicles, and bullae may be noted in both. While cellulitis may produce pus, erysipelas will generally only produce serous exudate.
- Desquamation of the skin may occur with both on resolution of the infection. If left untreated, erysipelas and cellulitis may rapidly spread to deeper tissues and enter the lymphatic system leading to septicemia and a high risk of death.

Differential Diagnoses:
- Systemic lupus erythematosus, herpes zoster, angioedema, drug allergy, necrotizing fasciitis, and contact dermatitis

Diagnostic Studies:
- None generally required. Elevation of the antistreptolysin O (ASO) titer occurs approximately 10 days after start of infection.

Risk Factors:
- Diabetes, immunosuppression, surgery, bug bites, shaving, tattoo or piercing, any condition that causes a disruption in the skin integrity such as eczema, psoriasis, obesity, edema, tinea, IV drug use, impaired lymphatic drainage, radiation therapy, chemotherapy, pregnancy, recent streptococcal pharyngitis. Up to 50% of patients with erysipelas/cellulitis will experience repeat episodes often at the same site of infection.

Treatment:
Patient Teaching
Patient should be instructed to do the following:
- Elevate the affected limb and use cold compresses several times daily for the first 48 hours.
- Notify primary care provider if they are experiencing an increase in erythema, discomfort, vomiting, chills, or fever.

Treatment involves either oral or intravenous antibiotics with IV antibiotics and hospitalization being used for more severe cases. While the drug of choice is penicillin (Pen VK) first line in uncomplicated infection, erythromycin (E-Mycin) if allergic to penicillin, and clindamycin (Cleocin) if intolerant to erythromycin may also be used. Consider adding ciprofloxacin or doxycycline if there has been exposure to freshwater at the site of infection. Symptoms resolve within a day or two after initiation of antibiotic therapy, the skin may take weeks to return to normal. Appropriate treatment of streptococcal throat and wound infections will aid in preventing further episodes. Patients should be instructed to do the following:
- Wear protective clothing during activities which may disrupt the skin integrity such as those encountered during work or sports.
- Moisturize dry skin to prevent cracking.
- Keep wounds clean and protected.
- Observe for signs of infection.
- Wear shoes that fit well.
- Trim nails properly to prevent injury to skin.

When a break in skin integrity occurs, patients should be instructed to do the following:
- Clean the break carefully with soap and water.
- Apply antibiotic ointment daily.
- Cover with bandage and change daily until a scab forms.
- Observe for signs of infection and report to health provider.

Contact Dermatitis: Allergic and Irritant

Description of the Disease: Contact dermatitis is an inflammatory response of the skin caused by contact with a substance either through skin or systemic exposure. If there has been previous contact that resulted in an immune response with sensitization to an allergen, it is known as allergic contact dermatitis (ACD). If it is an immediate response to a single exposure without an immune response, it is known as irritant contact dermatitis (ICD).

Epidemiology:
- Data from the National Health Interview Survey showed a 12-month prevalence for occupational contact dermatitis of 1,700/100,000 workers.
- Allergic dermatitis: More common in women than in men due to allergy to nickel, which is more common in women

Etiology:
- Allergic dermatitis: A delayed hypersensitivity reaction in which a substance comes into contact with the skin and forms an antigen complex that leads to sensitization. Upon subsequent exposures of the epidermis to the antigen, the sensitized T cells initiate an inflammatory cascade.
- Irritant dermatitis: Exposure of the epidermis to an irritant affects the barrier properties of the epidermis through several different mechanisms: removal of fat emulsion, cellular damage, transepidermal water loss, and DNA damage. Damage to the epidermis results in inflammation.

Triggers/Risk Factors:
- Common triggers for ACD include nickel (the most common of all allergens), gold, perfumes, neomycin, formaldehyde, thimerosal, bacitracin, poison ivy, poison oak, aromatherapy, sunscreens, rubber or latex gloves, and dyes.
- Common triggers for ICD include solvents, rubbing alcohol, bleach, soaps, deodorants, cosmetics, sawdust, rubber gloves, pesticides.
- Some occupations are at greater risk for contact with an allergen or irritant that causes dermatitis. These include hairdresser, cosmetologist, chef, construction worker, gardener, cleaners, health-care workers.
- Individuals with a history of eczema are more likely to experience ICD.

Signs and Symptoms:
- The first sign of ACD is the presence of a pruritic rash at the site of exposure. The rash may present as erythema, papules, vesicles, bullae with exudate and usually occurs where the contact with the allergen occurred. Usually, the lesion appears a day or two after exposure and may last for up to a month after exposure.
- ICD: Presents as dry, red, and rough skin. Lesions may appear as a burn. Fissures may form on the affected areas. The affected area is usually more irritated than pruritic.

Differential Diagnoses:
- Allergic dermatitis: Seborrheic dermatitis, contact dermatitis, tinea corporus, drug-induced photosensitivity, urticaria
- Irritant dermatitis: Atopic dermatitis, scabies, erysipelas, drug eruptions, seborrheic dermatitis

Diagnostic Studies:
- Clinical assessment may be enough for diagnosis. A patch test may be used to identify specific allergens. Histologic examination and culture of the lesions may assist with diagnosis.

Treatment:
- Assist the patient in attempting to identify the allergen/irritant. It is essential that the allergen/irritant be avoided to avoid a reoccurrence.
- In mild to moderate cases, topical glucocorticoids will be able to decrease the inflammation and relieve the pruritus. Topical glucocorticoids may be used for 1 to several weeks.
- Cool compresses may assist in relieving the itch.
- Oral diphenhydramine (Benadryl) is helpful for nighttime itching.
- Severe cases are generally treated with systemic corticosteroids (prednisone) which may be tapered gradually up to 2 to 3 weeks. A topical steroid may be used as well.
- Tacrolimus (Protopic) ointment or pimecrolimus (Elidel) cream can also be used in addition to the corticosteroid creams or in place of them.

Ecthyma/Impetigo

Description of the Disease: Bullous and nonbullous impetigo are common infections in the epidermis that usually occur in childhood and occasionally in adults primarily caused by *Staphylococcus aureus*, but sometimes by *Streptococcus pyogenes*.

Ecthyma is an ulcerative pyoderma of the skin commonly caused by either *Pseudomonas, Streptococcus S. pyogenes,* or *Staphylococcus aureus.* While impetigo affects the epidermis, ecthyma involves the dermis.

Epidemiology:
- There is no gender or racial preference in ecthyma or impetigo. Young and old are more frequently affected. Impetigo affected approximately 140 million people (2% of the population) in 2010. The incidence of ecthyma is not known.

Etiology:
- Infection is spread by direct contact with lesions or items such as towels, toys, clothes that harbor the bacteria. Scratching may cause the infection to spread.

Risk Factors:
- Break in skin integrity, diabetes, immunosuppression, crowding, poor hygiene, high temperature, and humidity

Signs and Symptoms:
- *Impetigo contagiosa,* also called *nonbullous impetigo,* is the most common form of the skin infection. Nonbullous impetigo most often begins as an erythematous lesion ranging from the size of a pimple to the size of a coin that often appears near the nose or mouth, but may appear on the neck, hands, and diaper region. The lesions are generally not painful, but may be pruritic. The lesion fills with fluid and then breaks, leaving a honey-colored scab. Usually there is no scarring. Lymphadenopathy may be present.
- Bullous impetigo is characterized painless, fluid-filled blisters, mostly on the arms, legs and trunk, surrounded by red and itchy (but not sore) skin. The blisters may be large or small. After they break, they form yellow scabs.
- Ecthyma is characterized by painful fluid- or pus-filled sores with redness of skin, usually on the arms and legs, which become ulcers that penetrate deeper into the dermis. After they break open, they form hard, thick, gray–yellow scabs, which may cause scarring. Ecthyma may be accompanied by swollen lymph nodes in the affected area.

Differential Diagnosis:
- Nonbullous impetigo: Perioral dermatitis, seborrheic dermatitis, herpes simplex, ACD, and scabies
- Bullous impetigo: ACD, herpes simplex or zoster, folliculitis, bullous pemphigoid, and porphyria cutanea tarda
- Ecthyma: Insect bites, leishmaniasis, *Mycobacterium marinum* infection, papulonecrotic tuberculid

Diagnostic Studies:
- Clinical presentation is usually enough to make diagnosis. If diagnosis is in question, culture is indicated. Histologic examination may also confirm diagnosis.

Treatment:
- Treatment may involve washing the lesions with soap and air-drying. Mild cases may be treated with bactericidal ointment, such as mupirocin (Bactroban). More severe cases require oral antibiotics, such as dicloxacillin, flucloxacillin, or erythromycin.
- Individuals with recurrent impetigo should have a nasal culture, and those who are found to be carriers of staphylococci should be started on mupirocin (Bactroban) applied three times a day to the nares, umbilicus, and anal region for approximately 1 week.
- Opinions on the duration and frequency of therapy vary from 5 to 10 days in a one-time treatment to 1 week/month for 6 months. Persistent infections or recurrent cases should be cultured to rule out MRSA.

Folliculitis

Description of the Disease: Folliculitis is the infection and inflammation of one or more hair follicles by bacteria, fungi, or parasites.

Epidemiology:
- Folliculitis usually affects those in their teens and may persist till the early 30s. Japanese and males are at greater risk for eosinophilic folliculitis. Women are possibly at greater risk for *Pityrosporum* folliculitis.

Etiology:

- Folliculitis starts when hair follicles are damaged by friction from clothing, an insect bite, blockage of the follicle, shaving, or tight hair braids. In most cases of folliculitis, the damaged follicles are then infected with the bacterium *Staphylococcus*, though the etiological cause may also be fungi or parasites. "Hot tub folliculitis" may occur approximately 72 hours after use of a poorly maintained hot tub and often presents with infection of follicles over the stomach, arms, or legs and possibly fever. Hot tub folliculitis is usually caused by the bacteria *Pseudomonas aeruginosa*.

Risk Factors:

- Warm weather, shaving, clothing friction, makeup, machine oils, hot tubs, immunosuppression, and iron deficiency anemia (chronic cases)

Signs and Symptoms:

- Erythema, pruritis, or burning papules or pustules near a hair follicle occurring in a variety of places: chest, back, arms, legs, head, neck, axillae, groin, or genitals. They may appear as red dots with hairs in the center that come to white tips. The lesions may drain pus or blood.
- Folliculitis should not be confused with irritated bumps known as pseudofolliculitis barbae caused by hairs curling back into the skin often after shaving. Razor bumps are common in people with tightly coiled hair such as African Americans. Treatment is avoidance of shaving, use of lasers, removal of ingrown hair, and medications such as allantoin, axulene, tretinoin salicylic acids, and antibotic gels.

Differential Diagnoses:

- Acne vulgaris, cutaneous candidiasis, ICD, impetigo, rosacea

Diagnostic Studies:

- Clinical assessment is usually enough to determine the diagnosis. A culture of the pus will identify the bacterial etiology. If a fungal infection is suspected, potassium hydroxide slide will assist in identification. Histologic examination can also determine pathology.

Treatment:

- Folliculitis may resolve with no intervention. Topical antiseptic treatment such as mupirocin 2% (Bactroban) or neomycin (*Neo-Fradin*) is adequate for most cases. Oral antibiotics are indicated when the folliculitis is more resistant. The infecting organism may be resistant to a number of commonly used antibiotics. A culture of the bacteria may be indicated to select the most appropriate antibiotic.
- Topical antifungal agents such as econazole nitrate (Spectazole) are indicated if the pathogen is a fungus.
- Postinflammatory hyperpigmentation may be treated with skin lightening creams.

Furuncle (Boil)

Description of the Disease: A furuncle (boil) is an infection of the hair follicle most commonly caused by *S. aureus* extending from the dermis to the subcutaneous tissues and involving the pilosebaceous unit. A cluster of furuncles is a carbuncle.

Epidemiology:

- More common in males than females; peak incidence 14 to 18 years

Etiology:

- Most furuncles and carbuncles are caused by *S. aureus.* This bacterium gains entrance through a break in skin integrity to the pilosebaceous unit where large numbers of leukocytes travel to the site to fight the infection.

Risk Factors:

- Obesity, malnutrition, immunosuppression, family history, diabetes, HIV/AIDS, alcoholism, antibiotic therapy, hospitalization, anemia, and other skin conditions

Signs and Symptoms:

- Erythematous, extremely tender, warm, pus-filled nodule commonly found on the face, neck, thighs, and buttocks

Differential Diagnoses:

- Allergic dermatitis, folliculitis, tinea infection, herpes simplex virus, hidradenitits suppurativa

Diagnostic Studies:
- Diagnosis usually made through clinical assessment. Pathogen can be confirmed with cultures.

Treatment:
- Smaller furuncles may resolve with no treatment. Antibiotics such as *sulfamethoxazole 800 mg and trimethoprim* 160 mg (Bactrim DS) or *clindamycin* (Cleocin) are advisable for larger or recurrent boils on the face or near lymph nodes.
- More severe boils should be treated with intralesional steroid injections. If antibiotics and steroid injections do not resolve the lesion, incision and drainage are usually necessary.
- Signs of sepsis such as fever and chills should be treated immediately. A furuncle that is on the lip, ear, scalp or near the spine are considered serious as the infection can spread to the brain or other organs.

Herpes Zoster (Shingles)

Description of the Disease: Herpes zoster is the reactivation of latent varicella zoster virus (HZV) in the dorsal root ganglia. The reactivation causes painful blisters in a dermatome on the body.

Epidemiology:
- In the United States, approximately one of every three individuals will get shingles, with a strong correlation with risk and advancing age. Half of those affected are older than 50. The increased risk associated with aging populations is theorized to be related to the decrease in cellular immunity.

Etiology:
- The varicella zoster virus lies dormant in the nerve cell bodies after initial infection. After the initial infection, the virus may travel to nerve axons to cause viral infection of the skin in the region (dermatome) of the spinal nerve.
- The virus may spread from one or more ganglia along nerves of an affected segment and infect the corresponding dermatome causing its characteristic rash upon reactivation.
- Postherpetic neuralgia occurs in about 20% of shingle cases. It should be noted that herpes zoster only occurs in a person who has had chickenpox (varicella zoster).
- An individual who has never been infected with the varicella zoster virus and is exposed to someone with herpes zoster is at risk to get chicken pox, not shingles.

Risk Factors:
- Age, immunosuppression, psychological stress, physical trauma, and immunotoxins

Signs and Symptoms:
- The initial symptoms of herpes zoster are flu-like symptoms without fever, diarrhea, stomach discomfort, and lymphadenopathy. These symptoms are commonly followed by sensations of pain, burning, itching, tingling, or numbness, which may present days to weeks before the appearance of the rash.
- The pain may be described as mild to severe. A band of rash appears on one side of the body only. The rash may appear on the forehead, cheek, nose, or around one eye (herpes zoster ophthalmicus).
- Herpes zoster ophthalmicus is an emergency requiring immediate attention. Blisters with clear fluid will form; the fluid may become cloudy in several days. The rash may be severe, mild, or nonexistent. Blisters will break, ooze, and crust over in about 5 days. The rash often causes piercing or stinging pain and will resolve in about 2 to 4 weeks. Scars may develop.

Differential Diagnoses:
- Herpes simplex virus, contact dermatitis, renal calculi, conjunctivitis

Diagnostic Studies:
- Visual inspection is often enough as the rash has a distinctive appearance with its dermatomal distribution. The Tzanck smear can diagnose a herpes virus, but does not distinguish between HSV, which can sometimes present with a rash similar to VZV.
- Blood tests can test for chickenpox or herpes zoster during active infection. Exudate from blisters can be tested by polymerase chain reaction for VZV DNA or examined with an electron microscope for virus particles.

Treatment:
- The zoster vaccine (Zostavax) is considered the first line of defense in reducing incidence of herpes zoster. The vaccine reduces the rate of shingles by 50% and reduces the incidence of herpatic neuralgia by 66%. Duration of vaccine protection is unknown.

- Antiviral drug treatment may reduce the severity and duration. Antiviral agents must be given for 7 to 10 days and be given no later than 72 hours after appearance of lesions.
- Wet dressings soaked in Burrow solution applied for 30 to 60 minutes four to six times daily may decrease discomfort. People with mild to moderate pain can usually be treated with over-the-counter pain medications. Calamine lotion, can be used on the lesions. Corticosteroids appear to alleviate acute, but not long-term, pain.
- Postherpetic neuralgia is a complication more likely to occur in older patients. The majority of patients are pain free within 1 year after shingles.

Herpetic Whitlow

Description of the Disease: A painful infection of one or more fingers caused by the herpes simplex virus 1 (HSV-1) or herpes simplex virus 2 (HSV-2)

Etiology:
- Exposure to infected body fluids via a break in the skin, most commonly a torn cuticle. In adults, exposure to HSV-2 via the genitalia is the most common causative viral agent.

Epidemiology:
- In the United States, annual incidence is estimated at 2.4 to 5.0 cases per 100,000 population. Males and females are equally affected.

Etiology:
- In the general adult population, herpetic whitlow is most often due to autoinoculation from genital herpes.

Risk Factors:
- Individuals with HSV-1 or HSV-2; health-care workers with occupational exposure to oral or genital secretions; contact sports; immunosuppression

Signs and Symptoms:
- Symptoms include swelling, reddening, and tenderness of the skin of the infected finger usually at the distal phalanx. This may be accompanied by fever and swollen lymph nodes.
- Small, clear vesicles initially form individually, then merge and become cloudy. Associated pain often seems large relative to the physical symptoms. The herpes whitlow lesion usually heals in 2 to 3 weeks.
- Lymphangitic streaking and possibly adenopathy of the epitrochlear and axillary nodes may be present. After 10 to 14 days, symptoms usually improve significantly and lesions crust over and heal. Preexisting herpetic lesions may be noted in mouth or on genitals.

Differential Diagnoses:
- Cellulitis, felon, paronychia

Diagnostic Studies:
- Diagnosis of herpetic whitlow usually is through clinical assessment.
- Definitive diagnostic testing may include Tzanck testing, viral cultures, serum antibody titers, fluorescent antibody testing, or DNA hybridization.

Treatment:
- Oral antiviral agents are typically used.
- Lancing or surgically debriding the lesion may make it worse by causing a secondary bacterial infection or spread of the herpes infection to other areas of the body.
- Antibiotics are indicated when secondary infections are present.
- Analgesics should be used for pain control.

Hidradenitis Suppurativa

Description of the Disease: Hidradenitis suppurativa is a chronic skin disease that is associated with blocked apocrine and pilosebaceous gland.

Epidemiology:

- Affects at least 1% of the population. Condition begins after puberty, with the most common ages affected being 20 to 40 years of age.

Etiology:

- Unknown etiology. Theories suggest that the condition results as a blockage of the apocrine (sweat) gland or the hair follicle. The gland or follicle expands, ruptures, and infection ensues.

Risk Factors:

- Age, female gender, African ancestry, hormones, alcohol intake, family history, cigarette smoking, obesity, and hot and humid climates

Signs and Symptoms:

- Multiple open comedones are often the first sign. The development of one lesion and then multiple lesions as sweat and bacteria are forced into the surrounding area. Lesions usually are erythematous, firm, tender, pus-filled and vary in size from 1 cm to 3 cm.
- They may be interconnected with sinus tracts. The lesions often rupture and drain a malodorous pus. Dermal contractures and cord-like scarring that causes limitation of movement of the affected area may occur.
- The lesions usually appear in areas where skin rubs together such as the submammary area, axillae, thighs, buttocks, and groin. While the disease is often distressing, it is rarely life-threatening. Arthropathy, while uncommon, may be present.

Differential Diagnoses:

- Furuncle, carbuncle, acne, pseudofolliculitis, erysipelas

Diagnostic Studies:

- Clinical assessment is usually enough to make diagnosis. Histologic examination may be done when diagnosis uncertain.

Treatment:

- Oral antibiotics such as erythromycin (E-Mycin), tetracycline (Sumycin), minocycline (Minocin) can help improve the symptoms and possibly reduce the risk of future outbreaks. Generally, topical antibiotics are not helpful.
- Isotretinoin (Accutane) may be helpful in less severe cases.
- Intralesional or oral steroids should also be considered, particularly if lesions are painful.
- Surgery may be indicated for severe or chronic cases. Due to the condition's chronic nature, wide local excision is recommended.

Patient Teaching:

Patients should be instructed to do the following:

- Practice proper hygiene of affected area.
- Wear loose-fitting clothing, which should be encouraged.

Patients who smoke or are obese should be made aware of their increased risk for the disease.

Keratosis Pilaris

Description of the Disease: Is a common follicular condition that is characterized by the appearance of rough, light or slightly red in color, hard bumps on the skin that are sometimes pruritic, but not painful. It most often appears on the back and outer sides of the upper arms, buttocks, thighs, and, occasionally, face.

Epidemiology:

- It is more common in women than in men and is often present in otherwise-healthy individuals. The skin condition is equally prevalent in persons of all races. It usually appears within the first decade of life and is more common in young children.

Etiology:

- Keratosis pilaris occurs when there is an excess production of the protein keratin. The excess keratin encapsulates the hair follicles. This causes the formation of hard plugs. If the keratinized hair follicle blocks the hair before it exits the hair follicle, an ingrown hair may result.

Risk Factors:
- Childhood, cold temperatures, pregnancy, childbirth, dry skin, eczema

Signs and Symptoms:
- Keratosis pilaris results in small bumps on the skin that feel like rough sandpaper. They are skin-colored bumps the size of a grain of sand, many of which are surrounded by a slight pink color. Generally keratosis pilaris is sometimes itchy, but not painful.

Differential Diagnoses:
- Acne vulgaris, atopic dermatitis, folliculitis, milia

Diagnostic Studies:
- None generally are indicated.

Treatment:
- Keratosis pilaris is harmless and generally only a cosmetic concern. Topical exfoliants may help to remove dead skin cells from the affected area, though they may cause redness and burning. These include α-hydroxy acid, glycolic acid, salicylic acid, or urea.
- Steroid creams can also be used to reduce redness. Topical retinoids tretinoin and tazarotene may help to unplug the hair follicles. These agents also may cause redness, burning, or peeling. Exfoliating the affected area with a wash cloth after a bath may help to unplug the hair follicles.
- Laser therapy may help some cases of severe keratosis pilaris.

Lentigo Senilis

Description of the Disease: Age spots (also known as liver spots) are lesions on the skin associated with aging and exposure to sun.

Epidemiology:
- More commonly found in midlife and older, fair-skinned individuals

Etiology:
- Histologic findings may include hyperplasia of the epidermis and increased pigmentation of the basal layer. A lentigo senilis resembles a freckle (ephelides). While both lesions are associated with sun exposure, a lentigo senilis has more melanocytes and a freckle has an increase in melanin, though no change in the number of melanocytes.

Risk Factors:
- Sun exposure including a history of sunburns or chronic sun exposure; fair skin; advancing age

Signs and Symptoms:
- Benign, nonpuritic macular round or oval lesions usually less than 5 mm in diameter that may be homogenous or variegated in color ranging from tan, light brown to black and are located in areas most often exposed to the sun, particularly the hands, face, shoulders, arms and forehead, and the scalp in midlife to older adults. Lesions may increase in size and number over time.

Differential Diagnoses:
- Seborrheic keratosis, actinic keratosis, ephelides

Diagnostic Studies:
- Biopsy should be considered if there is a concern regarding skin cancer.

Treatment:
- Generally considered harmless and more of a cosmetic concern. However, the lesions may make detection of skin cancer more difficult. Electrosurgery, laser treatment and cryotherapy may be used for removal. Bleaching creams are usually not substantively effective.

Patient Teaching:
Patient should be instructed to do the following:
- Use a broad-spectrum sunblock of at least SPF 30.
- Wear hats, long-sleeve tops, and pants.
- Avoid the sun between the hours of 12 and 3 PM.

Lichen Planus

Description of the Disease: A skin condition that resembles lichen and affects the skin and mucous membranes. The term lichenoid reaction is used when the triggering event is identified.

Epidemiology:
- The disease usually arises between ages 30 to 60. It is more common in women than men at a ratio of 3:2. US prevalence is approximately 1% to 4%.

Etiology:
- Unknown; evidence suggests that inflammation and autoimmunity are key factors.

Risk Factors:
- Middle age, nonsteroidal anti-inflammatory drugs, influenza vaccine, hepatitis B vaccine, hepatitis C infection, graft-versus-host disease

Signs and Symptoms:
- Presentation varies depending on affected site. Lesions are found in cutaneous or mucosal areas.
- Cutaneous lesions may appear on the scalp, nails, anterior forearm, dorsum of hand, wrist, ankle, or the external genitals. They present as shiny, red–purple, firm lesions often found on the wrists, lower back, and ankles.
- The lesions may manifest as: annular, linear, hypertrophic, atrophic, bullous, ulcerative, and pigmented. A common presentation is known as the "6Ps" of lichen planus: *p*lanar (flat-topped), *p*urple, *p*olygonal, *p*ruritic, *p*apules, and *p*laques. The lesions may have white lines throughout (Wickham striae).
- Lesions may be few or many. In areas were lesions reoccur, thick, scaly, pruritic skin may develop. Rarely, blisters may appear. Postinflammatory hyperpigmentation is often present and resolves slowly. Scalp lesions may appear as tender, erythematous lesions with hair loss and possible scarring.
- Nail lesions may cause grooving, ridging, thinning, subungal hyperpigmentation and keratosis, and possibly loss of the nail plate. External genital lesions may present as painful sores.
- Mucosal lesions are commonly white, lacey, and painful and occur on the GI mucosa, larynx, bladder, peritoneum, eyes, ears, nose, and genitals. Oral lesions, while they can appear on the tongue and gums, usually appear on the buccal mucosa and often are painful. Erythema, edema, and sloughing of the gums are often present.

Differential Diagnoses:
- Cutaneous lichen planus: Psoriasis, tinea corporis, syphilis, pityriasis rosea
- Oral lichen planus: Candidiasis, leukoplakia, stomatitis, lupus erythematosus

Diagnostic Studies:
- Clinical assessment is usually enough to make a diagnosis. A histology examination may be indicated if diagnosis is uncertain. Testing for hepatitis may be indicated due to the disease's strong association with Hepatitis C. Oral lichen planus may increase risk for mouth cancers.

Treatment:
- There is no cure for lichen planus. Treatment is for comfort or cosmetic reasons. Cutaneous lesions will generally resolve in 6 to 9 months without any treatment. Mucosal lesions tend to be more resistant and prone to reoccur.
- Commonly used medications include corticosteroids, retinoids, topical calcineurin inhibitors such as tacrolimus (Protopic) and pimecrolimus (Elidel), or antihistamines or phototherapy.

Patient Teaching:
- *Patients* with cutaneous lichen planus should be instructed to do the following:
  - Decrease stress.
  - Avoid scratching or injuring lesions.
  - Take oatmeal bath.
- *Patients* with oral lichen planus should be instructed to do the following:
  - See a dentist twice a year.
  - Maintain oral hygiene.
  - Avoid foods that are citrusy, spicy, salty, or crispy and those that contain caffeine as these may aggravate lichen planus.

Lipoma

Description of the Disease: Composed of adipose tissue, lipomas are usually slow-growing, smooth, solitary tumors with a firm, rubbery consistency occurring on the trunk, shoulders, posterior neck, and axillae approximately 1 to 3 cm, but may grow to 10 to 20 cm and weigh several kilograms.

Epidemiology:
- Approximately 1% of the population has a lipoma. They are most often found from ages 40 to 60. Single lipomas occur equally in males and females. Multiple lipomas may occur and are more common in males.

Etiology:
- Not completely understood; genetics appear to play a role; trauma may be a trigger.

Risk Factors:
- Middle age; defects in chromosome 12; genetics; possibly trauma

Signs and Symptoms:
- Often a lipoma is easy to identify because it moves readily with slight finger pressure. It has a rubbery feel. Lipomas are usually painless, unless they press on nerves.

Differential Diagnoses:
- Liposarcoma

Diagnostic Studies:
- Generally none necessary. If liposarcoma, X-rays, CT scan, and MRI may be indicated.

Treatment:
- Generally none needed. Characteristics consistent with a malignant liposarcoma include size larger than 5 cm in diameter, deep, rapid growth, or location on the thigh. Lipomas may be removed via standard excision, squeezing the lipoma through a small incision, and liposuction. Because lipomas generally do not infiltrate into surrounding tissue, they can be easily removed. Lipomas may reoccur.

Melasma

Description of the Disease: Melasma (chloasma or mask of pregnancy) is an irregular patch of tan, brown, or gray–blue hyperpigmentation commonly found on the face—particularly the forehead, cheeks, or jaw.

Epidemiology:
- In the United States, over 5 million people have the condition, with the majority of cases being diagnosed during pregnancy.

Etiology:
- Not completely understood. Possibly the stimulation of melanocytes by estrogen and progesterone when the skin is exposed to sun.

Risk Factors:
- Female gender (over 90% of individuals with melasma), pregnancy, oral or patch contraceptive, hormone replacement therapy (HRT), genetics, Native American, Hispanic, Arab, German Russian, and Jewish descent, sun exposure, thyroid disease, perimenopause, medication (tetracycline, quinine derivatives).

Signs and Symptoms:
- Appearance of macular or patches of darkened skin often on the face, but also may appear on the trunk and limbs.

Differential Diagnoses:
- Postinflammatory hyperpigmentation, actinic lichen planus, contact dermatitis, drug-induced photosensitivity, lupus erythematosus

Diagnostic Studies:
- Usually diagnosed via clinical assessment. A Wood lamp may assist in determining if excess melanin is present in the epidermis or dermis.

Treatment:

- The area of hyperpigmentation usually gradually fades over several months once the increased/fluctuating hormones stop (end of pregnancy, cessation of oral or patch contraceptive or HRT). Treatments to lighten the area of hyperpigmentation include skin lightening agents, dermabrasion, chemical peels, or laser skin rejuvenation.

Patient Teaching:

Patient should be instructed to do the following:

- Use a broad-spectrum sunblock of at least SPF 30 or sunscreens containing titanium dioxide or zinc oxide (preferred over chemical sunblocks due to broader protection).
- Wear hats, long-sleeve tops, and pants.
- Avoid the sun between the hours of 12 and 3 PM.

Molluscum Contagiosum

Description of the Disease: A benign viral infection of the epidermis or the mucous membranes. The virus is spread via person to person contact or contact with objects that harbor the virus.

Epidemiology:

- Approximately 122 million people were affected worldwide by molluscum contagiosum as of 2010 (1.8% of the population).

Etiology:

- There are four types of MCV, MCV-1 to MCV-4; MCV-2 is seen usually in adults.

Risk Factors:

- Children aged 1 to 10, sexually active adults, immunosuppression, crowded living conditions, warm or humid climates, possibly swimming pools

Signs and Symptoms:

- Flesh-colored solitary or clustered, soft lesions that are about 1 to 5 mm in diameter, with a pit in the center and commonly found on the face, neck, trunk, arms, groin, and legs. They may be tender, but usually do not itch.
- The lesions usually spontaneously resolve within 1 year, but can last for several years and may leave a crater-like scar. There is no life-long immunity to the virus nor is there a dormant state. An individual is only infectious when the lesions are present.

Differential Diagnoses:

- Acrochordons, umbilicated lesions, wart

Diagnostic Studies:

- Clinical assessment is usually enough for a diagnosis. A histology examination may be done when the diagnosis is uncertain.

Treatment:

- Treatments that rupture the lesions may facilitate spread of the infection.
- Topical medications to destroy the lesions include salicylic acid, potassium hydrochloride, and cantharidin. Imiquimod, an immunotherapeutic, has had varying success.
- Surgical treatments include cryosurgery, curette scraping, and laser surgery.

Patient Teaching:

- Patients should be instructed to avoid scratching lesions as this may cause rupture and spread of infection.

Onychomycosis

Description of the Disease: An infection of the toenails that may be caused any one of several different pathogens.

Epidemiology:

- Most common nail disease; affects 10% of the population; more common in males than females

Etiology:

- A number of pathogens may be the causative infecting agent including dermatophytes, *Candida*, and nondermatophytic molds. Dermatophytes are fungi most commonly responsible for onychomycosis in the temperate western countries. If the infection is due to a dermatophyte, the term tinea unguium may be used.

Risk Factors:

- Age, decreased blood circulation, diabetes mellitus, extended periods of immersion in water, heat, family history, immunosuppression, tinea pedis, break in skin integrity

Signs and Symptoms:

- Nails thicken and change in color to white, yellow, or green. The nails may be brittle and are often difficult to cut.

Differential Diagnoses:

- Nail deformity (half of all suspected cases of onychomycosis), nail psoriasis, lichen planus, contact dermatitis, melanoma

Diagnostic Studies:

- Clinical assessment is usually enough for diagnosis. KOH testing with direct microscopy, histopathologic examination, or culture to confirm diagnosis

Treatment:

- Oral antifungals are generally the first line of treatment. Fungi are imbedded deeply in the nail; topical agents lack ability to penetrate the nail. The use of topical agents should be limited to cases involving less than half of the distal nail plate or for patients unable to tolerate systemic treatment.
- Removal of the affected portion of the nail may improve outcomes. Laser surgery, which destroys fungi through increased temperatures, shows promise but has limited evidence to date.

Paronychia

Description of the Disease: Is an infection affecting the skin tissue around the finger or toe nail.

Epidemiology:

- Accounts for 35% of hand infections making it the most common hand disease in the United States; affects women more than men at a ratio of 3:1

Etiology:

- The infection is caused by bacteria (acute paronychia) or fungi (chronic), such as candidiasis. The pathogen gains access to the tissue through a break in skin integrity in acute infection or as the result of immersion in water or irritant chemicals in chronic infections.

Risk Factors:

- Acute paronychia: manicuring, thumb-sucking, nail-biting, application of artificial nails
- Chronic paronychia: occupations such as dishwasher, hairdresser, nurse, bartenders, florists, bakers, swimmers, or housekeepers; immunosuppression; and steroid therapy

Signs and Symptoms:

- Erythema, warmth, tenderness, and possible exudate in the tissues surrounding the nail. Bacterial infection will present more rapidly and usually only involves one finger or toe, fungal infection will have a slower presentation and will often affect more than one finger or toe. Rarely the infection may spread to tendons, bones, and bloodstream and cause systemic symptoms such as chills, fever, joint and muscle pain.

Differential Diagnoses:

- Herpetic whitlow, psoriasis, malignant melanoma, squamous cell carcinoma, foreign object, chancres

Diagnostic Studies:

- None generally indicated; culture of exudate may be done to identify pathogen. Tzanck smear may be necessary to differentiate a paronychia from a herpetic whitlow.

Treatment:

- Acute paronychia:
  - A paronychia without an accumulation of pus may be treated simply with warm water soaks of affected area two to four times per day for 15 minutes until resolution. Elevation of affected digit will facilitate healing.

- Moderate to severe acute paronychia will require oral antibiotics such as antistaphylococcal penicillin (cloxacillin/Cloxapen) or a first-generation cephalosporin (cefalexin/Keflex). If an abscess has formed, it will require incision and drainage.
- Chronic paronychia:
  - The probable pathogen in chronic paronychia is candidiasis and therefore should be treated with a topical antifungal medication, such as clotrimazole (Lotrimin) or ketoconazole (Nizoral). Topical antifungal ointments are usually effective; however, oral antifungal medications may be necessary.

Patient Teaching:
The patient should be instructed:
- Not to bite or pick the nails.
- To wear rubber or plastic gloves when hands are immersed in water.
- To avoid cutting of cuticles.

Head, Body, and Pubic Lice

Description of the Disease: An infestation of the blood-feeding insect, the louse. The infestation may occur on the scalp (*pediculus humanus capitis*), body (*pediculus humanus humanus* or *pediculus humanus corporis*), and pubic area (*phthiriasis pubis*).

Etiology:
- Head lice are generally spread through direct head-to-head contact with an infested person. While transmission can occur through contact with an infested person's combs, hats, helmets, wigs, or other personal items, it is much less common than head-to-head transmission.
- Head lice feed on human blood by piercing the skin with their mouths and excreting saliva. The saliva causes an inflammation process in the host resulting in intense itching. Lice that infest humans cannot live without a human host beyond approximately 2 days.
- The nits from head lice can live for approximately 1 week. Infestation is not related to cleanliness. Some head lice in Africa have been known to be vectors of disease.
- Body lice are spread through direct contact with the body, clothing, bed or other personal items of a infested person. Adult body lice can live no longer than approximately 3 days without a host.
- Nits from body lice need body heat in order to hatch. If infested clothes are not worn, the nits won't hatch and may die. Body lice move from clothing to the skin surface to feed. They are a disease of the unclean. Body lice may be vectors of disease such as typhus, trench fever, and relapsing fever.
- Pubic lice occur most commonly on the hair near the groin or in other areas of the body with coarse hair such as eyebrows, eyelashes, beard, chest, and axillae. They are most often spread by intimate contact, though sharing of personal items such as towels, bedding, and clothing may be enough for transmission. They can live up to 1 day without a human host. They do not transmit disease.

Epidemiology:
- Head lice: About 14 million people, mainly children, are treated annually for head lice in the United States alone. Infestation is most frequent on children aged 3 to 10 and their families. Females are more frequently infested than males by a ratio of two to four times due to their longer hair. Lice infestations do not generally occur in African hair due to hair texture.
- Body lice: Severe outbreaks of body lice, and associated louse-borne diseases, have historically occurred during wars, in prisons, on crowded ships, and under similar crowded and unsanitary situations but are less common today.
- Pubic lice: Current worldwide prevalence has been estimated at 2% of the human population, mostly adults, though infestation may be underreported.

Risk Factors:
- Head lice: Close contact activities, childhood, female gender, number of children in family, long hair; non-African ethnicity
- Body lice: Poor hygiene, close and crowded living quarters, homeless, war refugees/those experiencing social upheaval
- Pubic lice: Adulthood, intimate contact, and sharing of clothes, bedding, and towels

Signs and Symptoms:
- Head lice: Itching is the most prominent sign of infestation. However, itching may not occur during a first infestation or until after several weeks in a repeat infestation. Infection may occur secondary to disruption in skin integrity from intense scratching. A mature louse is about 2 to 4 mm in size and grey to brown in color. Lice are attracted to warm areas of the scalp such as around the ears or at the nape of the neck. Lice do not jump, fly, or swim. Nits are about the size of a thread knot, creamy to white in color, and often found on the hair shaft about a quarter of an inch from the scalp. Nits may be mistaken for dandruff or hair product residue. Nits are difficult to remove, even if the nymph has hatched. Pets have no role in the human infestation of head lice.
- Body lice: Resemble those of head lice. Lice and nits are generally easy to see in the seams of an infested person's clothing, particularly around the waistline and arm holes.
- Pubic lice: Like head lice, itching is the most prominent sign of infestation. However, itching may not occur during a first infestation or until after several weeks in a repeat infestation. Pubic lice can be distinguished from head and body lice as pubic lice are slightly smaller (1 to 2 mm), round, and have six legs. They are often called "crabs" due to their resemblance to the crustacean.

Differential Diagnoses:
- Head lice: Dandruff, hair product residue, dermatophyte infection
- Body lice: Folliculitis, insect bites, scabies, impetigo, postinflammatory hyperpigmentation
- Pubic lice: Dermatophyte infection, folliculitis, contact dermatitis

Diagnostic Studies:
- Live lice are necessary to make the diagnosis of infestation; nits alone are not enough to make a diagnosis. A comb specifically for removing lice and a magnifying glass are helpful in making a diagnosis. Combing the hair over white paper makes it easier to identify any lice.

Treatment:
- Chemical treatment of head lice: A pediculicide should only be used if a living louse is found. However, some prophylactic treatment using a pediculicide for persons who share the same bed with an infested individual may need to be considered. There are a number of medications that can kill lice: malathion (Ovide), invermectin (Stromectol), and dimeticone. Dimeticone (Hedrin Lotion) works via a mechanical means—possibly suffocation or dehydration of the lice rather than neurotoxicity—and is often preferred due to the low risk of side effects. Pyrethroids, such as permethrin (Elimite), have been commonly used; however, resistance is increasing. Some evidence indicates creams work better than shampoos. Swimming or washing the hair within 1 to 2 days after treatment may render some treatments less effective. Swimming and washing of hair has no effect on lice or nits.
- Nonchemical treatment of head lice: Shaving the head will eliminate lice. Also, combing with a nit comb hair that has been soaked with conditioner will remove lice. The hair should be combed through in sections and wiped after each stroke. This should be repeated every 3 to 4 days for about 3 to 4 weeks until no more live lice are found. Alternative methods of lice removal including tea tree oil, vinegar, butter, mayonnaise, isopropyl alcohol, and olive oil have not been shown to be effective.
- Body lice: Can be eliminated with washing of clothes in hot water and detergent. There is generally no need for insecticides, if hygiene is maintained.
- Public lice: Treat pubic lice in the same manner as head lice with medicated lice shampoo and nit combing. The sexual partners of an infested person should be treated as well.

Patient Teaching:
- Adult lice cannot live without a human blood source. Special chemical treatments are not essential. Wash all bedding, linens and clothing for 30 minutes in 140°F. Items that cannot be washed should be put in isolation for 2 weeks or dry cleaned. Combs and brushes may be deloused by putting in boiling water for 5 to 10 minutes. Vacuum any furniture which may have come into contact with the lice.

Pityriasis Rosea

Description of the Disease: A common, benign, often pruritic rash that affects the back, chest, and abdomen and usually lasts approximately 6 to 8 weeks but may last as long as several months.

Epidemiology:
- Occurs equally in men and women and all races. Most prevalent in individuals aged 10 to 40.

Etiology:
- Unknown cause; possible viral etiology

Risk Factors:
- Respiratory tract infection; human herpes virus 6 and 7; pregnancy

Signs and Symptoms:
- The rash often begins with a herald or "mother" patch. This single lesion is a round or oval, pink-to-gray scaly patch with a raised, well-defined border often found on the abdomen. The size of the patch ranges from 2 to 10 cm.
- Days to weeks later, pink- or salmon-colored, 1 to 2 cm oval "daughter" patches appear on the neck, abdomen, chest, back, arms, legs, and infrequently the face. Lesions generally do not appear on the palmar or plantar surfaces. Patches on the back are often vertical and angled to form a "Christmas tree" or "fir tree" appearance. The rash may be papular or vesicular in presentation. Approximately 50% of patients experience pruritus.
- The rash may be accompanied by flu-like symptoms of lethargy, low-grade fever, headache, nausea, sore throat, and loss of appetite. As many as 69% of patients may have an upper respiratory infection prior to any other symptoms. Postinflammatory hyperpigmentation may occur on dark skin after rash has resolved.

Differential Diagnoses:
- Eczema, psoriasis, tinea corporis, tinea versicolor, secondary syphilis rash

Diagnostic Studies:
- Diagnosis is usually made on visual inspection. If diagnosis is in question, a KOH wet mount can be performed. Histopathology examination or culture can also be performed to confirm diagnosis. A rapid plasma reagent (RPR) may be indicated to rule out syphilis.

Treatment:
- Usually resolves without treatment. Skin lotions, oral anithistamines and topical corticosteroids may be used to decrease itching. Antiviral medicines like acyclovir (Valtrex) may shorten the duration of rash, especially if taken at first sign of rash. Sunlight may shorten duration of rash, but caution must be used regarding increased risk of skin cancer and sunburn.

Patient Teaching:
Instruct patient to do the following:
- Avoid becoming overheated as this may worsen rash and increase the itch.
- Take an oatmeal bath in lukewarm water and apply calamine lotion to the rash when skin is still moist to decrease skin irritation and itch.
- Use small amounts of mild soap when bathing/showering.

Psoriasis

Description of the Disease: Immune-mediated, chronic skin condition characterized by erythema with silvery-white scaly papules, patches, and plaques that are often pruritic and may be painful.

Epidemiology:
- The disease affects 2% to 4% of the general population. The condition commonly first appears between the ages of 15 and 25, but all ages may be affected. It affects European whites much more commonly than other races; it affects both genders equally.

Etiology:
- Not completely known, but believed to be immune mediated. Normally, skin cells take several weeks to turnover. In psoriasis, the skin cells overturn every few days and accumulate on the skin's surface.

Risk Factors:
- Crohn disease, ulcerative colitis, cessation of systemic or topical corticosteroids, genetics, alcohol, smoking, obesity, stress, infections (such as strep throat), skin dryness, skin injury, sunburn, cold and dry climate, and numerous drugs including nonsteroidal anti-inflammatory agents, lithium, β-blockers.
- Psoriasis has been associated with a significant increase in numerous cancers including basal cell, squamous cell, lung, bronchus, upper GI tract, urinary tract, pancreatic, and liver. Psoriasis has also been associated with an increased risk of Crohn disease and ulcerative colitis.

Signs and Symptoms:
- Psoriasis vulgaris is the most common form of psoriasis and presents as plaques commonly found on the elbows, knees, scalp, and back.
- Psoriatic erythroderma (erythrodermic psoriasis) is characterized by psoriatic plaques over most of the body. It is usually an exacerbation of psoriasis vulgaris. This form of psoriasis can be life-threatening as the disruption of the skin integrity may cause inability to regulate body temperature.
- Pustular psoriasis appears as raised bumps filled with noninfectious pus.
- Generalized pustular psoriasis is a rare and acute form of psoriasis that is characterized by many pustules on top of tender red skin often accompanied by a fever, muscle aches, nausea, and an elevated white blood cell count. This type of psoriasis may require hospitalization.
- Psoriatic arthritis involves painful inflammation of the joints. Often the fingers and toes are affected, but the hips, knees, and spine may also be affected. Approximately 30% of individuals with psoriasis will develop psoriatic arthritis.
- Psoriasis can affect the nails and produces a variety of changes including pitting, discoloration, thickening, loosening, crumbling, and separation of the in the appearance of finger and toe nails.

Differential Diagnoses:
- Seborrheic dermatitis, eczema, pityriasis rosea, cutaneous T-cell lymphoma (50% of individuals with this cancer are incorrectly diagnosed with psoriasis), secondary syphilis, and onychomycosis (nail psoriasis).

Diagnostic Studies:
- A visual assessment of the skin is often enough to make the diagnosis. Auspitz sign where pinpoint bleeding occurs when a scale is removed is a physical exam technique that may help with diagnosis. Additionally, a patient history of Koebner phenomenon—where psoriatic lesions arise along lines of skin trauma—is also helpful in making the diagnosis.

Treatment:
There are numerous treatment options available for psoriasis.
- Moisturizers containing aloe vera, jojoba, zinc pyrithione, or capsaicin help control scaling and dryness and may relieve itching.
- Bath solutions containing oil, oatmeal, or Dead Sea salts can help remove scales.
- Scale lifters containing salicylic acid, lactic acid, or urea also remove scales.
- Calamine, hydrocortisone, camphor, or menthol creams may help relieve itching.
- For mild cases, topical corticosteroids are the cornerstone of treatment as they decrease the skin cell turnover and decrease inflammation. Very potent steroids have greater efficacy than lower potency corticosteroids. HPA insufficiency may occur with higher potency steroids used over larger surface areas.
- For moderate cases, light therapy, both natural and artificial light, are used. Ultraviolet light B (UVB) slows the rate of skin cell turnover and is the primary source of the benefits of light therapy. A commonly used treatment for management of psoriasis is PUVA (*p*soralen and *u*ltra *v*iolet *A* light). Ultraviolet light A is relatively ineffective in the treatment of psoriasis unless used with topical or oral psoralen. Psoralen renders the skin more sensitive to UVA light, which slows the rate of skin cell turnover. Psoralens should not be used with tanning beds as it may result in severe sunburn resulting in worsening of psoriasis on the sun-damaged skin (Koebner Phenomenon).
- Coal tar, a keralytic agent, is one of the oldest treatments for psoriasis. There is mixed evidence regarding its efficacy. Coal tar products soften the skin and decrease the rate of skin cell turnover. Coal tars are available in a variety of formulations: shampoos, soaps, gels, lotions, creams, and oils. Coal tar may cause skin irritation and photosensitivity to UVA light waves. Coal tar has an unpleasant odor and may cause black staining to skin, nails, clothes and give a yellow cast to white hair.
- Calciprotriene (Dovenix), a topical preparation of vitamin D, appears to improve psoriasis by inhibiting skin cell reproduction.
- Salicylic acid moisturizers, creams, and shampoos help remove some of the scales seen in psoriasis. Caution must be taken to avoid toxicity if used over large areas or at high doses. Salicylic acid is often combined with topical corticosteroids and coal tar.
- Anthralin is used to treat psoriasis as it slows down the growth of the skin cells and has anti-inflammatory actions. It is available as a cream, ointment and scalp lotion. Anthralin can cause brown staining to skin, nails, and clothes.
- For severe psoriasis, oral glucocorticoids are indicated.
- A combination approach often yields the most effective results and allows the use of lower doses.

Rosacea

Description of the Disease: A chronic condition characterized by facial erythema and sometimes pimples.

Epidemiology:
- It primarily affects people of northwestern European descent. Women are affected nearly three times more than men, but men generally have more severe symptoms possibly due to delay in seeking treatment. The peak age of incidence is the fourth to seventh decade.

Etiology:
- Precise etiology is unknown. *Helicobacter pylori* and *Demodex folliculorum* mites mites may play a role in pathology.

Risk Factors:
- Family history, changing temperatures and temperature extremes, exercise, sunburn, stress, anxiety, alcohol, caffeine, spicy foods, and foods high in histamine (red wine, aged cheeses, yogurt, beer, cured pork products such as bacon, etc.), microdermabrasion, chemical peels, and medications such as isotretinoin (Accutane), tretinoin (Retin-A), and topical and oral steroids.

Signs and Symptoms:
- Rosacea typically begins as redness in the forehead, cheeks, nose, or chin and less frequently the ears, scalp, neck, and chest. It is also characterized by telangiectasia, papules, pustules, reddened, irritated eyes, rhinophyma (thickening of the skin of the nose). Unlike acne, comedones are not present in rosacea.

Differential Diagnoses:
- Acne vulgaris, lupus erythematosus, seborrheic dermatitis, psoriasis, eczema

Diagnostic Studies:
- The diagnosis is made based on clinical findings.

Treatment:
- Rosacea is not curable; lifelong treatment is often necessary.
- Mild cases are often not treated. In moderate and severe cases, the cornerstone of treatment is antibiotic therapy such as oral tetracycline (Sumycin) and topical metronidazole (Flagyl).
- Topical *azelaic acid* (Finacea) may help reduce inflammation.
- Using α-*hydroxy acid* peels may help relieve redness caused by irritation, and reduce papules and pustules.
- Isotretinoin (Accutane) in low doses may be helpful in treating papules and pustules.
- Lasers are commonly used to destroy capillaries to decrease erythema and to vaporize excess tissue in rhinophyma.
- Oral antibiotics may help to relieve symptoms of ocular rosacea.
- Antihistamines may be helpful for those patients who identify foods rich in histamine as a trigger.

Patient Teaching:
- Explain to patients the importance of identifying triggers and then avoiding them.

Seborrheic Dermatitis

Description of the disease: A common, chronic inflammatory condition of the skin characterized by scales on sebum-rich skin. Seborrheic dermatitis of the scalp is commonly referred to as dandruff.

Etiology:
- Involves an inflammatory reaction, possibly to the yeast *Malassezia*.

Epidemiology:
- It affects 1% to 3% of healthy adults. It occurs more often in men than women. Caucasian race and Celtic ethnicity are more often affected.

Risk Factors:
- Genetics, hormones, and immunodeficiency, stress, fatigue, poor sleep, poor hygiene, alcohol, high-fat diet, Parkinson's Disease, CVA, CHF, epilepsy, and depression have been associated with the development of seborrheic dermatitis.

Signs and Symptoms:

- Presents with yellow or white flakes on the scalp, eyebrows, ears, nasolabial folds, chest, back, or groin in areas where sebaceous glands are numerous. Scales may attach to the hair shaft. Patches of erythema are often present. Occasionally, pruritus may be present. Periods of remission and exacerbation are common.

Differential Diagnoses:

- Eczema, cutaneous candidiasis, ACD, impetigo, rosacea

Diagnostic Studies:

- Clinical assessment is usually enough for diagnosis.

Treatment:

- A topical agent containing selenium sulfide, zinc pyrithione, coal tar, antifungals, or corticosteroids may be utilized in the form of a shampoo for seborrheic dermatitis affecting the scalp.
- Antifungal and corticosteroid topical agents may be applied to the affected areas on the face and body. In severe cases not responding to conventional therapy, the retinoid, isotretinoin (Accutane) or the immunosuppressive medications, pimecrolimus (Elidel) or tacrolimus (Protopic), may be used.
- Phototherapy can be utilized as a treatment method, as both natural and artificial UV light impede the growth of Malassezia.

Seborrheic Keratosis

Description of the Disease: A common benign scaly lesion of the epidermis

Epidemiology:

- Associated with advancing age. Men and women are affected equally affected. Lesions are more common in whites than blacks.

Etiology:

- Not established

Risk Factors:

- Possibly sunlight, genetics, pregnancy, and estrogen therapy

Signs and Symptoms:

- Scaly, benign lesions of the epidermis, approximately 2 mm to 3 cm in diameter, ranging in color from light tan to black with a well-circumscribed border, round to oval in shape, which often appear to be "stuck on" the surface of the skin, most commonly on the trunk, but also found on the scalp, face, and extremities.
- Lesions may be flat or raised; usually rough. Sometimes called the "barnacles of old age." The sudden appearance of many or an increased size of exiting seborrheic keratoses (Leser–Trélat sign) may be indicative of an internal malignancy. Dermatosis papulosa nigra is a varient of seborrheic keratosis consisting of numerous small, brown or black papules often found on the face of dark-skinned persons.

Differential Diagnoses:

- Malignant melanoma, actinic keratosis, basal cell carcinoma, lentigo, acrochordon

Diagnostic Studies:

- Clinical assessment is usually enough for diagnosis. Biopsy should be done to confirm diagnosis, particularly if a concern of malignant melanoma exists.

Treatment:

- No treatment is necessary. If the lesion becomes excessively itchy or is irritated by clothing or jewelry, it can be removed. Lesions may be removed with electrocautery, curettage, or cryosurgery.

Scabies

Description of the Disease: An intensely pruritic, highly contagious skin condition caused by the mite *Sarcoptes scabiei*.

Epidemiology:
- A health problem with 300 million new cases globally each year

Etiology:
- Transmission of the mites involves close and prolonged person-to-person contact of the skin-to-skin variety (the mites are unable to fly or jump); brief contact such as shaking hands or contact with clothing or personal items that an infected person has used are unlikely to result in infection.

Risk Factors:
- Homelessness; institutional environment often of immunocompromised where symptoms of infection are not initially readily apparent: nursing homes, hospitals, long-term care facility; sexual contact. Animals are not a vector for scabies that infect humans.

Signs and Symptoms:
- A skin rash characterized by severe itching and small red bumps and blisters and commonly affects such areas of the body as the wrists and back of the elbows, the knees, waist, umbilicus, axillary folds, the area around the nipples, the sides and backs of the feet, the genital area, and the buttocks. The itch may be mild for weeks and then become unbearable, particularly at night, when sleep is impossible. Gray, brown, or red 2 mm to 15 mm burrows may be present, but are usually very difficult to see. Linear excoriation marks are often mistaken for burrows. Frequent scratching of the lesions may lead to secondary infections.
- Norwegian scabies (also called crusted scabies) is a severe form of scabies in which thousands of mites can be found in crusts. This type of scabies usually affects people with a compromised immune system (advanced age, AIDS, lymphoma, etc.). The infestation may cover the entire body, but usually does not affect the face. Itch is usually minimal or absent.

Differential Diagnoses:
- Eczema, psoriasis, drug eruption, lichen planus, urticaria, syphilis

Diagnostic Studies:
- The diagnosis is usually made on diagnostic exam and history of intense, unrelenting itch. The definitive diagnosis is made by scraping the skin with a scalpel blade over an area of a burrow and examining the scrapings (covered with a drop of mineral oil) microscopically to identify mites, eggs, or pellets.

Treatment:
- Topical scabicidal agents are the cornerstone of treatment. Permethrin (Elimite) cream is one of the safest and most effective treatment for scabies. Lindane (Kwell) cream may cause seizures, it is not considered a first line of treatment. Treatment failure is increasing. *Ivermectin* (Stromectol) is an antiparasitic and scabicide. Ivermectin, while comparable to permethrin in efficacy, poses a greater risk of toxic side effects. It is not considered a first line of treatment, but used when other agents are ineffective or not tolerated. Crotamiton (Eurax, Crotan) is another scabicide, but may not be as effective as permethrin.
- Within a couple of weeks after treatment, the itch should decrease. If the itch does not improve after treatment, another diagnosis must be considered. Antihistamines and oral or topical steroids can help with itching.
- Mites may live only up to 72 hours without a human host. Clothing, bedding, and towels can be decontaminated by laundering in hot water and drying in the hot cycle or dry-cleaning. Alternately, items can be placed in isolation for 72 hours. Vacuuming of furniture and carpets is recommended in cases of Norwegian scabies.
- Treat sexual contacts or relevant family members (who either have either symptoms or have the kind of relationship that makes transmission likely).

Skin Cancer

Description of the Disease: The proliferation of abnormal cells in the skin that have the ability to invade or spread to other parts of the body. The three most common types of skin cancer are basal cell carcinoma, squamous cell carcinoma, and malignant melanoma.

Epidemiology:
- Basal cell carcinoma is the most common cancer in the United States. An estimated 2.8 million are diagnosed annually in the United States. An estimated 700,000 cases of SCC are diagnosed each year in the United States. An estimated 76,100 new cases of invasive melanoma will be diagnosed in the United States in 2014.

- The mortality rate of basal cell and squamous cell carcinoma are around 0.3% causing 2,000 deaths/year in the United States. In comparison the mortality rate of melanoma is 15% to 20%, and it causes 6,500 deaths/year.

Etiology:

- Alterations in DNA are implicated in all three types of skin cancer. UV light is strongly associated with this alteration of DNA. Compared to other malignant melanoma and squamous cell cancers, they have a lesser chance of metastasis. While they may cause significant destruction of tissue, they rarely are fatal.

Risk Factors:

- Basal cell skin cancer: UV light exposure, exposure to radiation, family history, age greater than 50, male gender, immunosuppressing drugs, xeroderma pigmentosum, psoriasis
- Squamous cell carcinoma: Natural or artificial (tanning beds) UV light exposure, immunocompromised status, fair skin and eye color, history of sunburns, weakened immune system, arsenic, history of blistering sunburn, history of precancerous lesions, personal history of skin cancer, xeroderma pigmentosum, psoriasis
- Malignant melanoma: Natural or artificial (tanning beds) UV light exposure, fair skin and eye color, genetics, history of blistering sunburn, weakened immune system, many (50 or more) or unusual moles, living close to the equator or at higher elevations, family history of melanoma

Signs and Symptoms:

- Basal cell skin cancers are often slow-growing and may appear as a pink, friable, eczema-like lesion; a shiny, pearly nodule with telangiectasia; or as a skin or scar thickening. In 80% of all cases, basal cell cancers are found on the head and neck. The lesions do not heal; they do not spread to other parts of the body until they invade into deeper tissue layers.
- Squamous cell skin cancers appear as rough, pink patches that can appear suddenly or grow from actinic or solar keratoses. They also may appear as ulcerated lesions. They may bleed or be described by the patient as lesions that "won't heal." Squamous cell skin cancer lesions have a significant risk of metastasis if untreated.
- Melanoma skin cancer lesions often are changing in appearance—color, shape, size, or thickness. Approximately 20% to 30% arise from moles. The lesions may itch or bleed. Most commonly found on the legs in woman and the backs in men. A method for remembering the signs and symptoms of melanoma is the mnemonic "ABCDE":
    - Asymmetry
    - Border irregularity
    - Color variegation
    - Diameter greater than 6 mm (size of pencil eraser)
    - Enlarging or evolving

Differential Diagnoses:

- Seborrheic dermatoses, senile lentigines, actinic keratoses

Diagnostic Studies:

- Biopsy will confirm diagnosis.

Treatment:

- Referral to a specialist is warranted. Treatment options generally include surgery, chemotherapy, electrodesiccation and curettage, immunotherapy, cryosurgery, photodynamic therapy.

Tinea Corporis (Ringworm)

Description of the Disease: A superficial dermatophyte infection characterized by lesions on the glabrous skin

Epidemiology:

- Tinea corporis can occur in all populations. It is common in childbearing women probably due to interaction with infected children. It is also common in preadolescents.

Etiology:

- A superficial fungal infection of the skin caused by a dermatophyte. The dermatophyte is a natural inhabitant of the skin. Certain conditions (heat, moisture) can cause an overgrowth. The infection can be acquired via person-to-person contact, animal-to-person contact, and object-to-person contact (clothing, towels, bedding, combs). Dermatophytes may also reside in soil.

Risk Factors:
- Perspiration, humid and crowded living conditions, heat, contact sports, constrictive clothing, immunosuppression

Signs and Symptoms:
- Usually presents with scaly, raised, red rings with a central clearing and loss of hair in infected areas. Pruritus may be present. Papules, vesicles, and bullae may appear especially at the border. Often occurs in the armpits, groin, and intertriginous areas
- Infection may occur on the scalp (tinea capitis), beard area (tinea barbae), or groin (tinea cruris). Unlike cutaneous candidiasis, tinea cruris generally does not involve the scrotum or penis or have satellite lesions.

Differential Diagnoses:
- Atopic dermatitis, cutaneous candidiasis, impetigo, psoriasis, tinea versicolor

Diagnostic Studies:
- Usually clinical assessment is enough to make diagnosis. KOH tests with direct microscopy, histology examination, PCR assay, and culture can confirm diagnosis.

Treatment:
- Topical antifungal agents are usually first line of treatment, with oral antifungals being reserved for more severe or extensive cases. Any pet that has been identified as a possible source of infection should be treated.

Patient Teaching:
Patient should be instructed to do the following:
- Wash hands thoroughly after petting or grooming pets and touching soil or plants.
- Avoid close contact with infected individuals.
- Wash workout clothes, swimsuits, and undergarments after one wearing.
- Wear loose-fitting clothes made of cotton or synthetic material that wicks moisture away from skin.
- Do not share towels, clothes, or combs/brushes with others.

Tinea Pedis (Athlete's Foot)

Description of the Disease: A superficial dermatophyte infection of the interdigital areas or soles of the feet.

Epidemiology:
- Tinea pedis is the most common dermatophytosis globally. Age increases prevalence. Males are two to four times more affected than females. Races are equally affected.

Etiology:
- Dermatophytes invade the superficial keratin of the skin. Dermatophytes can inhibit the body's immune response and may reduce keratinocyte proliferation, resulting in decreased sloughing and a chronic state of infection.

Risk Factors:
- Diabetes, heavy foot perspiration, occlusive footwear, recent break in skin integrity of the foot, immersion of feet in water for long periods of time, poor circulation

Signs and Symptoms:
- Most common presentation is a toe-web maceration, most commonly the space between the fourth and fifth digit, that may be pruritic and painful. Vesicles and bullae may be present usually on the soles. Moccasin-type tinea pedis presents with erythema and hyperkeratotic lesions on the soles and sides of feet.
- Patients may report the scaly lesions as "dry skin." Many people with tinea pedis have tinea cruris, perhaps due to autoinoculation. It is theorized that after showering/bathing, a towel is used to dry the infected feet first, and then the genitals, permitting spread of the infection.

Differential Diagnoses:
- ACD, friction blisters, psoriasis, cutaneous candidiasis

Diagnostic Studies:
- Usually clinical assessment is enough to make diagnosis. KOH testing with direct microscopy or a culture can confirm diagnosis. Culture and histology examination can also confirm diagnosis. A Wood light is generally not helpful in diagnosing tinea infections of the skin as the dermatophytes do not fluoresce under ultra violet light.

Treatment:
- Topical antifungal agents are usually first line of treatment with oral antifungals being reserved for more severe, moccasin-type infection, or in cases not responsive to topical antifungals.
- Clotrimazole–betamethasone (Lotrisone) combines an antifungal agent with a potent steroid that may be indicated in patients with clinical features of inflammation such as erythema, pruritus, and burning. Caution must be used given the complications of long-term steroid use. The cream should be only used for 2 weeks; tinea pedis typically needs to be treated with an antifungal agent for 4 weeks.
- Tinea pedis provides breaks in the integrity of the epidermis through which bacteria can cause a secondary infection; scratching of infected feet may also contribute to a secondary infection. Secondary bacterial infections are usually caused by *S. pyogenes* or *S. aureus*. The clinician should monitor for signs and symptoms of a secondary bacterial infection.

Patient Teaching:
Instruct patient to do the following:
- Use shower shoes on wet floors or showers to prevent becoming infected or spreading infection to others.
- Clean bathroom surfaces with bleach to prevent spread of the disease and reinfection.
- Wash feet thoroughly each day with soap and water and dry completely paying special attention to area inbetween toes.
- Wear shoes that are well-ventilated and made of natural material.
- Wear clean cotton socks or socks made with synthetic materials that wick away perspiration, and change socks and shoes as often as needed to keep feet dry.
- Frequently use antifungal powders.
- Nails should be kept short. Scratching of the feet may permit transfer of dermatophytes from feet to nails. Loosened scales may spread infection to others.

Tinea Versicolor

Description of the Disease: Overgrowth of a fungus that normally grows on the skin.

Epidemiology:
- Adolescents and young adults are most commonly affected.

Etiology:
- The causative infection is usually caused by *Malassezia globosa* fungus; *Malassezia furfur* is the causative fungus in a lesser number of cases. Acidic bleach from the growing yeast causes changes in skin color.

Risk Factors:
- Hot, humid climates, heavy perspiration, oily skin, immunosuppression

Signs and Symptoms:
- Macules or patches that may appear anywhere or the body but most often appear on the neck, chest, back, and arms. The affected areas are white, pink, red, or brown and can be lighter or darker than the skin around them. Scaling may be present. The affected lesions may improve during cool weather and worsen during warm weather. While not common, pruritis and pain may be present.

Differential Diagnoses:
- Psoriasis, seborrheic dermatitis, vitiligo, tinea corporis

Diagnostic Studies:
- Clinical assessment is usually enough to make diagnosis. Wood lamp will cause the fungus to fluoresce yellow–green. KOH testing with direct microscopy, histology examination, or culture will confirm diagnosis.

Treatment:
- Topical antifungal agents are usually first line of treatment with oral antifungals being reserved for more severe cases or those not responsive to topical antifungals.

Patient Teaching:
Patient should be instructed to do the following:
- Avoid using oil-based products on the skin.
- Avoid the sun as this may exacerbate the condition, and tanning of the unaffected skin will contrast more sharply with the skin that is affected by the fungus and cannot tan.

- When possible, avoid activities that increase perspiration.
- Wear loose, cotton clothing or clothing made of synthetic materials that wicks moisture away from the skin.

Urticaria

Description of the Disease: Wheals in the epidermis and dermis resulting from the release of histamine or other vasoactive substances into capillaries.

Epidemiology:
Acute urticaria affect 15% to 20% of the general population at some time during their lifetime. Chronic urticaria occur slightly more frequently in women and in the fourth and fifth decade.

Etiology:
Caused by an allergic or nonallergic trigger.

Risk Factors:
- Common triggers for acute urticaria include foods such as nuts, eggs, fish, tomatoes, berries, soy, wheat, milk, and food preservatives; insect stings, perfumes/fragrances, nickel, rubber, latex, detergents; or viruses (hepatitis).
- Medication that may cause urticaria include aspirin, NSAIDs, ACE inhibitors, penicillin, and codeine. Less common causes of acute urticaria include exercise, perspiration, friction, pressure, water, emotional distress, cold, and sunlight.
- Risk factors for chronic urticaria may include autoimmunity (lupus and rheumatoid arthritis), chronic infections, hormonal disorders, and malignancy.

Signs and Symptoms:
- White to erythematous, raised, pruritic, blanching, edematous lesions that may be pinpoint to several inches in diameter and may coalesce into larger lesions. They can appear anywhere on the body, including the face, lips, tongue, throat, or ears and may be linear, annular, or serpiginous. There are two major subsets: acute (less than 6 weeks duration) and chronic (more than 6 weeks duration, sometimes lasting for months and years). There is no difference in the appearance of acute and chronic urticaria.
- Acute urticaria are often caused by an allergic trigger or an infection, and chronic urticaria are often associated with autoimmunity. Urticaria are often confused with other dermatologic lesions that are pruritic such as drug eruptions and eczema. A distinguishing diagnostic feature of urticaria is that the lesions blanch.
- Similar to urticaria, but at a deeper tissue layers is angioedema. Angioedema is characterized by nonerythematous edema and stinging or burning around the eyes, lips, tongue, and pharynx and may cause difficulty breathing. It is a medical emergency.

Differential Diagnoses:
- Atopic dermatitis, allergic dermatitis, drug eruptions, scabies, pityriasis rosea

Diagnostic Studies:
- Generally, diagnosis can be made on history and physical examination.

Treatment:
- Acute urticaria should be closely monitored as angioedema or anaphylaxis may occur.
- Identification and avoidance of urticarial triggers is essential.
- Begin first-generation H1 blocker such as diphenhydramine (Benadryl) or hydroxyzine (Atarax) for acute urticaria and second-generation H1 blockers such as fexofenadine (Allegra), loratadine (Claritin), desloratadine (Clarinex), cetirizine (Zyrtec) for chronic urticaria.
- If no improvement, increase the dose of the H1 blocker, add another H1 blocker, or add a leukotriene receptor antagonist such as montelukast (Singulair).
- If no or minimal improvement, consider adding doxepin which blocks both H1 and H2 receptors. If the patient's symptoms do not improve, they should be referred to a dermatologist.
- Oral glucocorticoids may be used short-termly to manage acute urticaria.

Verruca

Description of the Disease: A rough growth in the epidermis caused by the HPV, usually of the skin or genitals. The virus is transmitted by contact.

Epidemiology:
- Nine out of every 10 individuals will experience a wart in their lifetime. Verruca are more common in children and are related to their immature immune systems.

Etiology:
- There are about 130 known types of HPVs. Each HPV is typically only able to infect a few specific areas on the body. HPV is contagious and usually enter the body through a break in skin integrity.

Risk Factors:
- Conditions that are associated with immunodeficiency such as AIDS, cancer, diabetes, chemotherapy and break in skin integrity related to injury, atopic dermatitis, and use of public showers and pools

Signs and Symptoms:
Appearance of wart varies by anatomic location:
- Common wart (verruca vulgaris): A raised wart with a roughened surface
- Flat wart (verruca plana): A small, smooth, flesh-colored, flattened wart which can occur in large numbers and that occur most commonly on the face, neck, hands, wrists, and knees
- Filiform or digitate wart, a thread- or finger-like wart, most common on the face, especially near the eyelids and lips
- Genital wart (venereal wart, condyloma acuminatum, verruca acuminata): Raised, rough warts on or near the genitals or anus. They may occur singly or in clumps and are often described as being cauliflower-like.
- Mosaic wart, a group of tightly clustered plantar-type wart, commonly on the hands or soles of the feet
- Periungual wart: A cluster of rough warts that occurs around the nails
- Plantar wart (verruca, verruca plantaris): A hard, smooth, sometimes painful lesion, often with multiple black specks in the center (capillaries) that are usually found on pressure points on the soles of the feet

Differential Diagnoses:
- Verucca vulgaris: molluscum contagiosum, actinic keratosis, seborrheic keratosis, squamous cell carcinoma

Diagnostic Studies:
- Physical inspection is usually enough to make diagnosis. Biopsy may be indicated if diagnosis uncertain.

Treatment:
- There are many methods for wart removal with varying degrees of success, pain, and scarring. Salicylic acid can be prescribed or found over the counter. Salicylic acid softens the outer layers of a wart so that the wart can be rubbed off with a pumice stone or file. It is also thought that the irritation of the acid triggers an immune response which fights the virus.
- Imiquimod is a topical cream that helps the body's immune system fight the wart virus by encouraging interferon production. Dinitrochlorobenzene (DNCB) induces an allergic immune response resulting in inflammation that wards off the wart-causing virus. Silver nitrate applied topically acts as a chemical cauterization. Staining of clothes and skin is a problem.
- Duct tape occlusion therapy involves placing a piece of duct tape over the wart. While effectiveness is inconclusive, it is a simple technique with limited side effects and is still utilized. The irritation of the duct tape is thought to stimulate the body's immune system and fight the virus.
- Other methods for wart removal include electordesiccation, cryosurgery, curettage, laser, and infrared coagulator.

Patient Teaching:
- Gym locker rooms, swimming pools, showers, and other public areas where people convene with bare feet are common sites for infection to occur. Wearing foot attire in such places will help to avoid infection with HPV.

Vitiligo

Description of the Disease: A condition in which melanocytes lose their ability to produce melanin resulting in depigmentation of the skin.

Etiology:
- Unknown, but possibly an autoimmune disorder, genetics, or a trigger event such as exposure to sun, a virus, chemicals, or stress.

Epidemiology:

- The incidence worldwide is less than 1%, with some populations averaging between 2% and 3% and as high as 16%. Vitiligo most often appears before age 20. Vitiligo affects all racial groups; however, it is more noticeable in people with darker skin.

Risk Factors:

- Autoimmune disorders, family history

Signs and Symptoms:

- Patches of skin discoloration that may occur anywhere on the body. The discoloration first shows on sun-exposed areas, such as the hands, feet, arms, face and lips. It may also present with graying of the hair, eyelashes, eyebrows, or beard, inside the mouth and nose, loss of color in the retina, and axillae, navel, genitals, and rectum.

Differential Diagnoses:

- Pityriasis alba, tuberculoid leprosy, postinflammatory hypopigmentation, tinea versicolor, albinism

Diagnostic Studies:

- Visual assessment is usually enough for diagnosis. Skin with vitiligo will glow blue under a Wood lamp. Individuals with vitiligo may have an increased risk of hearing loss; hearing tests should be considered.

Treatment:

- While the appearance of the skin can be improved with treatment, vitiligo is not curable. There are numerous medical and surgical treatment options.
- Repigmenting the affected skin using UVB light is a common treatment for vitiligo.
- Psoralen with light therapy (photochemotherapy) will help to repigment the affected areas.
- A topical corticosteroid may help with repigmentation of the skin.
- Calcineurin inhibitors, tacrolimus (Protopic) or pimecrolimus (Elidel), may be effective particularly with small areas of depigmentation.
- A medication with monobenzone lightens the unaffected skin so that it blends with the discolored areas. Depigmentation is permanent and increases the patient's risk for sunburns and melanoma.
- Skin grafts, autologous melanocyte transplants, and micropigmentation (tattooing) may also be possible treatments.

Review Section

Review Questions

1. Which of the following treatments is typically utilized for severe, cystic acne not responding to other treatments?

   a. Benzoyl peroxide gel
   b. Topical antibiotic solution
   c. Oral antibiotic
   d. Oral retinoid

2. A commonly used over-the-counter treatment for verruca is:

   a. imiquimod.
   b. tretinoin.
   c. dinitrochlorobenzene.
   d. salicylic acid.

3. Common causes of allergic dermatitis include all of the following except:

   a. gold.
   b. wood.
   c. perfumes.
   d. poison oak.

4. To distinguish urticaria from contact dermatitis, the clinician knows that urticaria:

   a. are erythematous.
   b. are pruritic.
   c. blanch upon pressure.
   d. have raised lesions.

5. Treatment for rosacea may include all of the following medications except:

   a. antibiotics.
   b. glucocorticoids.
   c. tretinoins.
   d. benzoyl peroxide.

6. A patient diagnosed with head lice should be instructed to:

   a. place all nonwashable items in a bag and place in isolation for 2 weeks.
   b. apply butter to head to "suffocate" lice.
   c. apply isoethyl alcohol to the lice bites.
   d. shave head.

7. All of the following markers of a lesion are associated with melanoma skin cancer except:

   a. enlarging.
   b. increase in size.
   c. uniform color.
   d. asymmetry.

8. Vitiligo may be associated with:

   a. hearing loss.
   b. arthritis.
   c. mood elevation.
   d. cystic lesions.

9. The infective causative agent in seborrheic dermatitis is believed to be:

   a. fungus.
   b. yeast.
   c. virus.
   d. bacterium.

10. A risk factor for molluscum contagiosum is:

    a. crowded living conditions.
    b. cool, dry climates.
    c. middle age.
    d. poor hygiene.

Answers with Rationales

1. (d) Oral retinoid

   Rationale: Oral antibiotics are used for moderate to severe acne, and oral retinoid is reserved for severe cases of recalcitrant, nodular/cystic acne. Topical benzoyl peroxide gel is usually a first-line treatment for mild, noninflammatory acne. Topical antibiotics are usually reserved for mild to moderate inflammatory acne.

2. (d) Salicylic acid.

   Rationale: Salicylic acid is found over the counter and is commonly used as a first-line treatment. Imiquimod, tretinoin, and dinitrochlorobenzene are not found over the counter. Furthermore, tretinoin is not used in the treatment of warts.

3. (b) Wood.

   Rationale: Gold, perfumes, and poison oak are all common causes of allergic dermatitis. Wood is not.

4. (c) Blanch upon pressure.

   Rationale: The lesions associated with contact dermatitis are erythematous, pruritic, and raised. The lesions do not blanch with pressure.

5. (d) Benzoyl peroxide.

   Rationale: Commonly used agents in the treatment of rosacea include antibiotics, glucocorticoids, and tretinoins. Benzoyl peroxide is used in the treatment of acne vulgaris as it assists in decreasing the comedones associated with acne. Comedones are not present in the pathology of rosacea. Benzoyl peroxide plays no role in the treatment of rosacea.

6. (a) Place all nonwashable items in a bag and place in isolation for 2 weeks.

   Rationale: Lice and nits need human blood for survival. Nonwashable items should be placed in isolation for 2 weeks to ensure the death of all viable nits and lice. Butter has not been shown to be effective in the treatment of lice. While secondary infection related to scratching is a concern with head lice, isoethyl alcohol may cause stinging or burning sensations of the inflamed lesions. Topical or oral antibiotics would be an appropriate treatment choice. While shaving of head will remove the head lice, there are less drastic treatment modalities that can resolve the problem.

7. (c) Uniform color.

   Rationale: The markers for malignant melanoma are *A*symmetry, *B*order Irregularity, *C*olor Variegation, *D*iameter greater than 6 mm, *E*nlarging or *E*volving.

8. (a) Hearing loss.

   Rationale: Vitiligo may be associated with hearing loss. Psoriasis is a skin condition that may be associated with arthritis. Patients with vitiligo are at increased risk for depression due to social stigma. Cystic lesions are often present with rosacea or acne vulgaris.

9. (b) Yeast

   Rationale: It is believed that the yeast *Malassezia* is responsible for seborrheic dermatitis.

10. (a) Crowded living conditions.

   Rationale: Crowded living conditions which promote spreading of bacteria are a risk factor for molluscum contagiosum. Warm, wet climates, rather than cool, dry climates are a known risk factor. Childhood, aged 1 to 10, not middle age, is another risk factor. Poor hygiene is not correlated with molluscum contagiosum.

Suggested Readings

Acne Vulgaris:

Boyce, N. (2012). Shakespeare under water. *Lancet, 379*(9813), 361–372.

Collier, C. N., Harper, J. C., Cafardi, J. A., Cantrell, W. C., Wang, W., Foster, K. W., & Elewski, B. E. (2008). The prevalence of acne in adults 20 years and older. *Journal of the American Academy of Dermatology, 58*(1):56–59.

Hay, R. J., Johns, N. E., Williams, H. C., Bolliger, I. W., Dellavalle, R. P., Margolis, D. J., … Naghavi, M. (2014). The global burden of skin disease in 2010: An analysis of the prevalence and impact of skin conditions. *The Journal of Investigative Dermatology, 134*(6), 1527–1534. doi:10.1038/jid.2013.446

http://www.medscape.org

http://www.acne.org

http://www.webmd.com

http://www.best-treatment-for-acne.com

Marshall, S. J. (1998). On being a ginseng connoisseur. *Lancet, 351*(9119), 1871–1876.

Acrochordon (Skin Tag):

Gupta, S., Aggarwal, R., Gupta, S., & Arora, S. K. (2008). Human papillomavirus and skin tags: Is there any association? *Indian Journal of Dermatology, Venereology and Leprology, 74,* 222–225.

Habif, T. P. (2009). Benign skin tumors. In: T. P. Habif (Ed.), *Clinical dermatology* (5th ed.). Philadelphia, PA: Mosby Elsevier.

Higgins, J. C., Maher, M. H., Douglas, M. S. (2015). Diagnosing Common Benign Skin Tumors. *American Family Physician, 92*(7), 601-607.

Actinic Keratosis (Solar Keratosis):

Berhane, T., Halliday, G. M., Cooke, B., & Barnetson, R. S. (2002). Inflammation is associated with progression of actinic keratoses to squamous cell carcinomas in humans. *The British Journal of Dermatology, 146*(5), 810–815.

http://misc.medscape.com

The Lewen Group. (2005). *The burden of skin diseases 2005.* Cleveland, OH and Washington, DC: The Society for Investigative Dermatology and the American Academy of Dermatology Association.

Roewert-Huber, J., Stockfleth, E., & Kerl, H. (2007). Pathology and pathobiology of actinic (solar) keratosis: An update. *The British Journal of Dermatology, 157*(Suppl 2), 18–20.

Cutaneous Candidiasis:

Edwards, J. E., Jr. (2009). Candida species. In G. L. Mandell, J. E. Bennett, & R. Dolin (Eds.), *Principles and practice of infectious diseases* (7th ed.). Philadelphia, PA: Elsevier Churchill Livingstone.

http://www.merckmanuals.com/professional/dermatologic_disorders/fungal_skin_infections/candidiasis_mucocutaneous.html

Kauffman, C. A. (2011). Candidiasis. In L. Goldman, & A. I. Schafer (Eds.), *Cecil medicine* (24th ed.). Philadelphia, PA: Saunders Elsevier.

Nishimoto, K. (2006). An epidemiological survey of dermatomycoses in Japan, 2002. *Nihon Ishinkin Gakkai Zasshi, 47*(2), 103–111.

Cherry Angioma:

Cohen, A. D., Cagnano, E., & Vardy, D. A. (2001). Cherry angiomas associated with exposure to bromides. *Dermatology, 202*(1), 52–53.

De Felipe, I., & Redondo, P. (1998). Eruptive angiomas after treatment with cyclosporine in a patient with psoriasis. *Archives of Dermatology, 134*(11), 1487–1488.

http://www.aafp.org/afp/2003/0215/p729.html

Atopic Dermatitis/Eczema:

Berke, R., Singh, A., Guralnick, M. (2012). Atopic dermatitis: An overview. *American Family Physician, 86*(1), 35–42.

Bufford, J. D., & Gern. J. E. (2005). The hygiene hypothesis revisited. *Immunology and Allergy Clinics of North America, 25*(2), 247–262. doi:10.1016/j.iac.2005.03.005

Goodyear, H. M., Spowart, K., & Harper, J. I. (1991). "Wet-wrap" dressings for the treatment of atopic eczema in children. *British Journal of Dermatology, 125,* 604.

http://pediatrics.about.com/od/ezema/a/0408_wet_drsngs.htm

http://www.ncbi.nlm.nih.gov

Kim, B. S. (2014). In P. Fritsch, R. P. Vinson, V. Perry, C. M. Quirk, W. D. James (Eds.), *Atopic dermatitis.* http://emedicine.medscape.com/article/1049085-overview

Mallon, E., Powell, S., & Bridgman, A. (1994). "Wet-wrap" dressings for the treatment of atopic eczema in the community. *Journal of Dermatological Treatment, 5,* 97–98.

Niwa, Y., Terashima, T., & Sumi, H. (2003). Topical application of the immunosuppressant tacrolimus accelerates carcinogenesis in mouse skin. *The British Journal of Dermatology, 149*(5), 960–967.

Pfeiffer, N. (2004). Tacrolimus vs. pimecrolimus: Which is better for eczema? *Drug Topics, 148,* 36.

Samochocki, Z., Bogaczewicz, J., Jeziorkowska, R., Sysa-Jędrzejowska, A., Glińska, O., Karczmarewicz, E., … Woźniacka, A. (2013). Vitamin D effects in atopic dermatitis. Journal of the American Academy of Dermatology, 69(2), 238–244.

Cellulitis/Erysipelas:

Bisno, A. L., & Stevens, D. L. (1996). Streptococcal infections of skin and soft tissues. *The New England Journal of Medicine,* 334(4), 240–245. doi:10.1056/NEJM199601253340407

Morris, A. D. (2008). Cellulitis and erysipelas. *BMJ Clinical Evidence, 2008,* 1708.

Huerter, C., Sherman, R. N., Willis, W., & Talarico, L. D. (1997). Helpful clues to common rashes. Patient Care, 31(8).

Contact Dermatitis: Allergic (ACD) and Irritant (ICD):

Behrens, V., Seligman, P., Cameron, L., Mathias, C. G., & Fine, L. (1994). The prevalence of back pain, hand discomfort, and dermatitis in the US working population. *American Journal of Public Health, 84*(11), 1780–1785.

Belsito, D. V. (2000). The diagnostic evaluation, treatment, and prevention of allergic contact dermatitis in the new millennium. *The Journal of Allergy and Clinical Immunology, 105,* 409–420.

Belsito, D. V. (2005). Occupational contact dermatitis: Etiology, prevalence, and resultant impairment/disability. *Journal of the American Academy of Dermatology, 53,* 303–313.

English, J. S. (2004). Current concepts of irritant contact dermatitis. *Occupational and Environmental Medicine, 61,* 722–726.

http://www.mayoclinic.org

Usatine, R. P. (2009). Contact dermatitis. In R. P. Usatine, M. Smith, E. J. Mayeaux, & H. Chumley. (Eds.), *Color atlas of family medicine.* New York, NY: McGraw-Hill.

Ecthyma/Impetigo:

http://emedicine.medscape.com

Vos, T. (2012). Years lived with disability (YLDs) for 1160 sequelae of 289 diseases and injuries 1990–2010: A systematic analysis for the Global Burden of Disease Study 2010. *Lancet, 380*(9859), 2163–2196. doi:10.1016/S0140-6736(12)61729-2

Folliculitis:

http://www.webmd.com

http://emedicine.medscape.com/article/1070456-overview#a0199

Nervi, S. J., Schwartz, R. A., & Dmochowski, M. (2006). Eosinophilic pustular folliculitis: A 40 year retrospect. Journal of the American Academy of Dermatology, 55(2), 285–289.

Furuncle (Boil):

Bernard, P. (2008). Management of common bacterial infections of the skin. *Current Opinion in Infectious Diseases,* 21(2), 122–128. doi:10.1097/QCO.0b013e3282f44c63

Demos, M., McLeod, M. P., & Nouri, K. (2012). Recurrent furunculosis: A review of the literature. *The British Journal of Dermatology, 167*(4), 725–732. doi:10.1111/j.1365-2133.2012.11151.x

El-Gilany, A. H., & Fathy, H. (2009). Risk factors of recurrent furunculosis. *Dermatology Online Journal, 15*(1), 16.

http://www.nlm.nih.gov/medlineplus

Head, Body, and Pubic lice:

http://www.cdc.gov/parasites/lice/
http://www.emedicinehealth.com/lice/article_em.htm
http://www.webmd.com/children/tc/lice-topic-overview

Herpes Zoster (Shingles)

Dworkin, R. H., Johnson, R. W., Breuer, J., Gnann, J. W., Levin, M. J., Backonja, M., … Whitley, R. J. (2007). Recommendations for the management of herpes zoster. *Clinical Infectious Diseases,* 44(Suppl 1), S1–S26.

http://emedicine.medscape.com

Herpetic Whitlow:

http://emedicine.medscape.com

Hidradenitis Suppurativa:

http://www.mayoclinic.org
http://emedicine.medscape.com
http://www.webmd.com
http://dermatology.about.com

Keratosis Pilaris:

Cysts, lumps, bumps, and your skin. http://www.webmd.com/skin-problems-and-treatments/guide/cysts-lumps-bumps#1. Retrieved July 29, 2016.

http://www.nhs.uk/conditions/keratosis-pilaris/Pages/Introduction.aspx

Mayo Clinic Staff. Tests and diagnosis. *Mayo Clinic.* Retrieved October 31, 2013.

Park, J., Kim, B. J., Kim, M. N., & Lee, C. K. (2011). A pilot study of Q-switched 1064-nm Nd:YAG laser treatment in the keratosis pilaris. *Annals of Dermatology, 23*(3), 293–298. doi:10.5021/ad.2011.23.3.293

Lentigo Senilis:

Bolognia, J. L. (Ed.). (2003). *Dermatology* (pp. 983, 1760–1761). New York, NY: Mosby.

Freedberg, I. M. (Ed.). (2003). *Fitzpatrick's dermatology in general medicine* (6th ed., pp. 721, 823, 863–865, 888–889). New York, NY: McGraw-Hill.

Lichen Planus:

Asch, S., & Goldenberg, G. (2011). Systemic treatment of cutaneous lichen planus: An update. *Cutis,* 87(3), 129–134.

Boyd, A. S., & Neldner, K. N. (1991). Lichen planus. *Journal of the American Academy of Dermatology, 25,* 593–619.

Cheng, S., Kirtschig, G., Cooper, S., Thornhill, M., Leonardi-Bee, J., & Murphy, R. (2012). Interventions for erosive lichen planus affecting mucosal sites. *The Cochrane Database of Systematic Reviews, 2*: CD008092. doi:10.1002/14651858.CD008092.pub2

http://www.skindermatologists.com

https://www.aad.org

Sharma, A., Białynicki-Birula, R., Schwartz, R. A., & Janniger, C. K. (2012). Lichen planus: An update and review. *Cutis, 90*(1), 17–23.

Usatine, R. P., & Tinitigan, M. (2011). Diagnosis and treatment of lichen planus. *American Family Physician, 84*(1), 53–60.

Lipoma:

Hakim, E., Kolander, Y., Meller, Y., Moses, M., & Sagi, A. (1994). Gigantic lipomas. *Plastic and Reconstructive Surgery, 94*(2), 369–371. doi:10.1097/00006534-199408000-00025

http://emedicine.medscape.com

http://www.mayoclinic.org/diseases-conditions/lipoma

Salam, G. A. (2002). Lipoma excision. *American Family Physician,* 65(5), 901–904.

Melasma:

Grimes, P. E. (1995). Melasma. Etiologic and therapeutic considerations. *Archives of Dermatology, 131*(12), 1453–1457.

http://emedicine.medscape.com

Molluscum Contagiosum:

Hanson, D., & Diven, D. G. (2003). Molluscum contagiosum. *Dermatology Online Journal, 9*(2), 2.

Vos, T. (2012). Years lived with disability (YLDs) for 1160 sequelae of 289 diseases and injuries 1990-2010: A systematic analysis for the Global Burden of Disease Study 2010. *Lancet, 380*(9859), 2163–2196. doi:10.1016/S0140-6736(12)61729-2. Retrieved from http://www.cdc.gov/ncidod/dvrd/molluscum/faq/everyone.htm#whogets

Onychomycosis:

Gupta, A., Lynde, C., Jain, H., Sibbald, R., Elewski, B., Daniel, C. R., III, … Summerbell, R. (1997). A higher prevalence of onychomycosis in psoriatics compared with non-psoriatics: A multicentre study. *The British Journal of Dermatology, 136*(5), 786–789. doi:10.1046/j.1365-2133.1997.6771624.x

http://emedicine.medscape.com/article/1105828-treatment

Roberts, D. T., Taylor, W. D., Boyle, J., & British Association of Dermatologists. (2003). Guidelines for treatment of onychomycosis. *The British Journal of Dermatology, 148*(3), 402–410. doi:10.1046/j.1365-2133.2003.05242.x

Szepietowski, J. C., & Salomon, J. (2007). Do fungi play a role in psoriatic nails? *Mycoses, 50*(6), 437–442. doi:10.1111/j.1439-0507.2007.01405.x.

Westerberg, D. P., & Voyack, M. J. (2013). Onychomycosis: Current trends in diagnosis and treatment. *American Family Physician, 88*(11), 762–770.

Paronychia:

Fung, V., Sainsbury, D. C., Seukeran, D. C., & Allison, K. P. Squamous cell carcinoma of the finger masquerading as paronychia. *Journal of Plastic, Reconstructive and Aesthetic Surgery, 63*(2), e191–e192.

http://emedicine.medscape.com

Rockwell, P. G. (2001). Acute and chronic paronychia. *American Family Physician, 63*(6), 1113–1116.

Pityriasis Rosea:

http://www.webmd.com/skin-problems-and-treatments/tc/pityriasis-rosea-topic-overview?page=2

https://www.aad.org/dermatology-a-to-z/diseases-and-treatments/m---p/pityriasis-rosea

Sharma, P., Yadav, T., Gautam, R., Taneja, N., & Satyanarayana, L. (2000). Erythromycin in pityriasis rosea: A double-blind, placebo-controlled clinical trial. *Journal of the American Academy of Dermatology, 42*(2), 241–244. doi:10.1016/S0190-9622(00)90132-4

Psoriasis:

Kupetsky, E. A., & Keller, M. (2013). Psoriasis vulgaris: An evidence-based guide for primary care. *Journal of American*

Board of Family Medicine, 26(6), 787–801. doi:10.3122/jabfm.2013.06.130055

Menter, A., Gottlieb, A., Feldman, S. R., Van Voorhees, A. S., Leonardi, C. L., Gordon, K. B., … Bhushan, R. (2008). Guidelines of care for the management of psoriasis and psoriatic arthritis: Section 1. Overview of psoriasis and guidelines of care for the treatment of psoriasis with biologics. *Journal of the American Academy of Dermatology, 58*(5), 826–850. doi:10.1016/j.jaad.2008.02.039

Parisi, R., Symmons, D. P., Griffiths, C. E., Ashcroft, D. M., & Identification and Management of Psoriasis and Associated ComorbidiTy (IMPACT) Project Team (2013). Global epidemiology of psoriasis: A systematic review of incidence and prevalence. *Journal of Investigative Dermatology, 133*(2), 377–385. doi:10.1038/jid.2012.339

Richard, M. A., Barnetche, T., Horreau, C., Brenaut, E., Pouplard, C., Aractingi, S., … Paul C. (2013). Psoriasis, cardiovascular events, cancer risk and alcohol use: Evidence-based recommendations based on systematic review and expert opinion. *Journal of the European Academy of Dermatology and Venereology, 27*(Suppl 3), 2–11. doi:10.1111/jdv.12162

Richard, W., Hunter, J. A. A., Savin, J., & Dahl, M. (2008). *Clinical dermatology* (4th ed., pp. 54–70). Malden, MA: Blackwell.

Stanway, A. Erythrodermic psoriasis. http://dermnetnz.org/scaly/erythrodermic-psoriasis.html. Retrieved March 16, 2014.

Rosacea:

Barankin, B., & Guenther, L. (2002). Rosacea and atopic dermatitis. Two common oculocutaneous disorders. *Canadian Family Physician, 48*, 721–724.

Cuevas, T. (2001). Identifying and treating rosacea. *Nurse Practitioner, 26*, 13–15, 19–23.

http://rosacea.org

http://www.mayoclinic.org

McDonnell, J. K., & Tomecki, K. J. (2000). Rosacea: An update. *Cleveland Clinic Journal of Medicine, 67*, 587–590.

Pray, W. S., & Pray, J. J. (2004). Differentiating between Rosacea and Acne. *US Pharmacist, 29*(4).

Wollina, U., & Verma, S. B. (2009). Rosacea and rhinophyma: Not curse of the Celts but Indo Eurasians. *Journal of Cosmetic Dermatology, 8*(3), 234–235. doi:10.1111/j.1473-2165.2009.00456.x

Seborrheic Dermatitis:

Calzavara-Pinton, P. G., Venturini, M., & Sala, R. (2005). A comprehensive overview of photodynamic therapy in the treatment of superficial fungal infections of the skin. *Photochemistry and Photobiology* 78(1), 1–6.

Dessinioti, C., & Katsambas, A. (2013). Seborrheic dermatitis: Etiology, risk factors, and treatments: Facts and controversies. *Clinics in Dermatology, 31*(4), 343–351. doi:10.1016/j.clindermatol.2013.01.001

Gupta, A. K., Bluhm, R., Cooper, E. A., Summerbell, R. C. & Batra, R. (2003). Seborrheic dermatitis. *Dermatologic Clinics, 21*, 401–412.

McMichael, A. J. (2003). Hair and scalp disorders in ethnic populations. *Dermatologic Clinics, 21*, 629–644.

Seborrheic Keratosis:

http://emedicine.medscape.com

http://health.usnews.com/health-news/family-health/allergy-and-asthma/articles/2009/05/19/got-a-skin-rash-how-to-tell-eczema-from-seborrheic-dermatitis

Schwartz, R. A. (1996). Sign of Leser-Trélat. *Journal of the American Academy of Dermatology, 35*(1), 88–95. doi:10.1016/S0190-9622(96)90502-2

Scabies:

Chosidow, O. (2006). Clinical Practices. Scabies. *New England Journal of Medicine, 354*(16), 1718–1727.

Hay, R. J. (2009). Scabies and pyodermas—diagnosis and treatment. *Dermatology and Therapy, 22*(6), 466–474. doi:10.1111/j.1529-8019.2009.01270.x.

Hicks, M. I., & Elston, D. M. (2009). Scabies. *Dermatology and Therapy, 22*(4), 279–292. doi:10.1111/j.1529-8019.2009.01243.x.

http://www.cdc.gov/parasites/scabies

Vos, T. (2012). Years lived with disability (YLDs) for 1160 sequelae of 289 diseases and injuries 1990–2010: A systematic analysis for the Global Burden of Disease Study 2010.*Lancet, 380*(9859), 2163–2196. doi:10.1016/S0140-6736(12)61729-2

Skin Cancer:

American Cancer Society. (2014). *Cancer facts & figures 2014.* Atlanta, GA: American Cancer Society. Retrieved June 2, 2014 from http://www.cancer.org/acs/groups/content/@research/documents/webcontent/acspc-042151.pdf

Jerant, A. F., Johnson, J. T., Sheridan, C. D., & Caffrey, T. J. (2000). Early detection and treatment of skin cancer. *American Family Physician, 62*(2), 357–368, 375–376, 381–382.

http://www.mayoclinic.org

National Institute of Cancer. http://www.cancer.gov/types/skin/hp/skin-treatment-pdq

Rogers, H. (2010, March 31). Your new study of nonmelanoma skin cancers. *Email to the Skin Cancer Foundation.*

Wong, C. S., Strange, R. C., & Lear, J. T. (2003). Basal cell carcinoma. *British Medical Journal, 327*(7418), 794–798. doi:10.1136/bmj.327.7418.794

World Health Organization. (2014). *World cancer report 2014* (Chapter 5.14). Geneva, Switzerland: World Health Organization.

Tinea Corporis (Ringworm):

http://emedicine.medscape.com

Likness, L. P. (2011). Common dermatologic infections in athletes and return-to-play guidelines. *Journal of the American Osteopathic Association, 111*(6), 373–379.

Tinea Pedis (Athlete's Foot):

Al Hasan, M., Fitzgerald, S. M., Saoudian, M., & Krishnaswamy, G. (2004). Dermatology for the practicing allergist: Tinea pedis and its complications. *Clinical and Molecular Allergy, 2*(1), 5. doi:10.1186/1476-7961-2-5

Bell-Syer, S. E., Khan, S. M., & Torgerson, D. J. (2012). Oral treatments for fungal infections of the skin of the foot. *Cochrane Database of Systematic Reviews, 10*, CD003584. doi:10.1002/14651858.CD003584.pub2.

Habif, T. P. (1996). Superficial fungal infections. In T. P. Habif (Ed.), *Clinical dermatology: A color guide to diagnosis and therapy* (3rd ed., pp. 362–408). St. Louis: Mosby.

http://emedicine.medscape.com

http://www.aafp.org

http://www.ncbi.nlm.nih.gov

McAleer, R. (1980). Fungal infection as a cause of skin disease in Western Australia. *Australasian Journal of Dermatology, 21*, 25–46.

TIougan, B. E., Mancini, A. J., Mandell, J. A., Cohen, D. E., & Sanchez, M. R. (2011). Skin conditions in figure skaters, ice-hockey players and speed skaters: Part II—cold-induced, infectious and inflammatory dermatoses. Sports Medicine, 41(11), 967–984.

Tinea Versicolor:

http://emedicine.medscape.com

http://www.dermnetnz.org/fungal/pityriasis-versicolor.html

http://www.webmd.com/skin-problems-and-treatments/tinea-versicolor-cause-symptoms-treatments?page=2

Morishita, N., & Sei, Y. (2006). Microreview of pityriasis versicolor and *Malassezia* species. *Mycopathologia, 162*(6), 373–376. doi:10.1007/s11046-006-0081-2.

Prohic, A., & Ozegovic, L. (2007). *Malassezia* species isolated from lesional and non-lesional skin in patients with pityriasis versicolor. *Mycoses, 50*(1), 58–63. doi:10.1111/j.1439-0507.2006.01310.x.

Rapini, R. P., Bolognia, J. L., & Jorizzo, J. L. (2007). *Dermatology* (2-volume set; Chapter 76). St Louis: Mosby.

Urticaria:

Bernstein, J. A., Lang, D. M., Khan, D. A., Craig, T., Dreyfus, D., Hsieh, F., ... Blessing-Moore, J. (2014). The diagnosis and management of acute and chronic urticaria: 2014 update. *Journal of Allergy and Clinical Immunology, 133*(5), 1270–1277.

Frigas, E., & Park, M. A. (2009). Acute urticaria and angioedema: Diagnostic and treatment considerations. *American Journal of Clinical Dermatology, 10*(4), 239–250.

http://emedicine.medscape.com

Verruca:

de Villiers, E. M., Fauquet, C., Broker, T. R., Bernard, H. U., & zur Hausen, H. (2004). Classification of papillomaviruses. *Virology, 324*(1), 17–27. doi:10.1016/j.virol.2004.03.033.

Gibbs S., Harvey I., Sterling J., Stark R. (2002). Local treatments for cutaneous warts: systematic review. *British Medical Journal, 325*(7362), 461.

Kwok, C. S., Gibbs, S., Bennett, C., Holland, R., & Abbott, R. (2012). Topical treatments for cutaneous warts. *Cochrane Database Systematic Reviews, 9*, CD001781. doi:10.1002/14651858.CD001781.pub3.

Vitiligo:

Berti, S., Buggiani, G., & Lotti, T. (2009) Use of tacrolimus ointment in vitiligo alone or in combination therapy. *Skin Therapy Letter, 19*(4), 5–7.

http://www.mayoclinic.org/diseases-conditions/vitiligo

http://www.medicinenet.com/vitiligo

Krüger, C., & Schallreuter, K. U. (2012). A review of the worldwide prevalence of vitiligo in children/adolescents and adults. *International Journal of Dermatology, 51*(10), 1206–1212. doi:10.1111/j.1365-4632.2011.05377.x.

National Institute of Arthritis and Musculoskeletal and Skin Diseases. (2007, March). *What is vitiligo? Fast facts: An easy-to-read series of publications for the public additional.* Bethesda, MD: Author

Scherschun, L., Kim, J. J., Lim, H. W. (2001). Narrow-band ultraviolet B is a useful and well-tolerated treatment for vitiligo. *Journal of the American Academy of Dermatology, 44*(6), 999–1003. doi:10.1067/mjd.2001.114752

Chapter 14

Gerontology

Julie Kinzel • Catherine Nowak • Ryan J. Clancy • and Claire E. Pisoni

Case Presentation

Directions: Carefully review the case study presented below. At the end of the chapter, answer the review questions. Compare your answers to the correct answers listed in the Review Section.

History of Present Illness: Mrs. Jones is an 86-year-old widow who lives alone in a two-bedroom apartment. She has been doing well since her husband died 6 years ago and is able to care for herself and her home without assistance. Her daughter lives nearby and calls her mother every other day to check in. The daughter takes her mother food shopping once a week. Mrs. Jones has a history of hypertension, which has been well controlled with medication for 25 years. In addition, she has DM type 2, also well controlled with diet and medication. She also has glaucoma for which she takes eyedrops. Mrs. Jones sees her primary care practitioner every 2 months. Today, the daughter became alarmed when her mother did not answer the phone over the course of an hour's time, so she went to her mother's home to check that everything was alright. She found her mother sitting in her nightclothes at the kitchen table with her medications strewn across the table. Her mother was muttering incoherently to herself and seemed very distressed. Mrs. Jones did not seem to recognize her daughter and actually appeared frightened when she realized her daughter was standing in the kitchen. When the daughter tried to calm her mother, Mrs. Jones yelled, "Get out of my house or I will call the police!" Mrs. Jones then attempted to get up from the table but appeared weak and unable to do so. The daughter noticed that Mrs. Jones had been incontinent of very foul-smelling urine.

Within a few minutes, the daughter was able to calm her mother and help her to the bathroom where she assisted her mother in bathing and dressing. Mrs. Jones seemed to improve, but still did not seem quite right. The daughter called Mrs. Jones' primary care physician (PCP) and scheduled an appointment for later in the day.

The Following Findings Were Made at the PCP Office:
Vital Signs: Temperature = 97.6 PO   HR = 104   RR = 16   BP = 136/82
    Pulse Ox = 97% on RA   BMI = 21 (decreased from last visit 6 weeks ago)
General Survey: Alert woman appearing her stated age. Seems fearful and suspicious of staff and does not
    recognize the PCP; she does not appear in acute distress. She is dressed neatly and appropriately for weather.
Skin: Warm and dry, turgor slow
Head, Eyes, Ears, Nose, Throat (HEENT): Within normal limits with the exception of dry, cracked lips
Pulmonary: Clear in all fields; no adventitious breath sounds
Cardiovascular: No lifts, heaves, or visible pulsations. S1 > S2, RRR without murmurs. Lower extremity distal
    pulses intact
Abdomen: Nondistended, normoactive bowel sounds; soft; nontender
Extremities: Ecchymosis and mild edema to right lateral elbow and anterior right knee
Neurologic: Gait is steady. Mini mental status examination: 21/30

Workup:
CXR: No infiltrates or effusions
Urine dip: Leukocytes 3+; nitrates +; protein −

Assessment:

Urinary tract infection (Midthun, 2004)

Throughout this chapter, we will be discussing some theories of the aging process, the physiology of aging, a few of the most common medical conditions of the elderly patient, and recommendations for screening tests in older adults.

Theories of Aging

The main theories of aging can be separated into two paths of thinking: programmed theory and error theory. Both modern theories attempt to provide a rationale behind the aging process. The rationale of the programmed theory hypothesizes that there is a finite timetable of physiologic events that control the aging process. Error or damage theories point to an external environmental exposure that impacts the individual cumulatively (Jin, 2010).

Program theory can be subdivided into the following three categories:

- Programmed Longevity: We age due to certain genes turning off and no longer functioning after a set time point (Davidovic et al., 2010).
- Endocrine Theory: Insulin/IGF-1 are the hormones that control the aging process by up- and downregulating the timing of the aging process (van Heemst, 2010).
- Immunologic Theory: Over time, the immune system no longer functions optimally due to deterioration, which decreases protection against diseases and infection (Cornelius, 1972).

Damage and error theory can also be subdivided:

- Wear and Tear Theory: The body and its components break down and no longer function (Rozemuller, van Gool, & Eikelenboom, 2005).
- Rate of Living Theory: The faster the metabolic rate, the sooner expiration of cells occurs (Brys, Vanfleteren, & Braeckman, 2007).
- Cross-link: First proposed in 1942 by Johan Bjorksten; an increase in the number of cross-linked proteins causes increased cell damage (Bjorksen, 1990; Gerschman, Gilbert, Nye, Dwyer, & Fenn, 1954).
- Free Radicals Theory: This theory pioneered by Dr. Denham Gerschman in the early 1950s states that an accumulation of free radicals in a person's cells causes progressive damage to the cells affected, leading to organ death (Harman, 1956; Hayflick & Moorhead, 1961).
- DNA Damage Theory: Genetic mutations in DNA occur throughout the life of an individual to the point where defects are unable to be corrected by the normal repair mechanisms, leading to cell deterioration and malfunction. Included in this theory is the shortening telomere theory pioneered by Dr. Hayflick in 1961. His limit theory (Hayflick & Moorhead, 1961) stated each telomere has a finite ability to divide before it ceases the replication process and ultimately continued survival.

Physiologic Changes with Aging

Everyone experiences changes which are considered part of normal aging. The rate at which a person undergoes the change consistent with the physiologic aging process will vary among individuals. This is most likely due to genetic makeup. Some of the changes expected in body systems with normal aging are listed below.

Dermatologic Changes:

- Epidermis becomes thinner (Hurd, 2014).
- The stratus corneum loses the ability to retain water; the skin becomes dry and feels rough; cell replacement, barrier functions, and wound healing decline.
- The dermis becomes thinner, loses elasticity.
- Eccrine sweat glands shrink and secrete less.
- Collagen and elastic tissue in dermis lose integrity and sag or droop.
- Senile purpura (also known as solar or traumatic purpura) is a common benign condition of blood in the dermis.
- Seborrheic keratosis—very common brown hyperkeratotic "stuck on" lesions
- Angiomas—red-appearing macules which are benign vascular growths

Body Temperature:
- Core body temperature tends to be lower in older men and women (Blatteis, 2012).
- Less ability to tolerate extremes in temperature and greater risk of developing hypo- or hyperthermia
- There are fewer sweat glands, resulting in less total body sweat produced.
- Overall ability of the cardiorespiratory system to adjust blood flow in response to changes in body temperature is reduced.
- Loss of muscle mass and increase in fat mass reduces capacity to generate heat when needed.

Hematologic:
- There is an increased prevalence of anemia in older adults; much of this goes unexplained. This is not a normal physiologic finding; however, it tends to be more common. It may be a result of decreased hematopoietic cell proliferation and ability for hematopoiesis (Pawlec, 2008).
- Reduced lymphocyte function, less numbers of immune cells such as antigen-presenting cells, dendritic cells, and a lower production of natural killer cells (Pawlec, 2008)
- Poor response to vaccinations
- Age-associated thymic involution contributes to reduction in naive T-cell production (Pawlec, 2008).
- General decline in cellular protein synthesis which can affect immune function
- Arterial wall thickening, increased stiffness, increased systolic pressures (Navaratnarajah & Jackson, 2013)
- Increased systemic resistance and increased cardiac afterload (Navaratnarajah & Jackson, 2013)

Cognitive Function and Brain:
- In general, there is a decline in brain volume and reduced synapse density (Navaratnarajah & Jackson, 2013).
- Conceptual reasoning, memory, processing speed decline gradually (Harada, Natelson Love, & Triebel, 2013)
- Reduced ability to focus on a specific task while ignoring irrelevant distractions, such as concentrating on a conversation in a noisy room or driving. Also, divided attention such as doing two things at once, preparing a meal while talking on the phone (Harada, Natelson Love, & Triebel, 2013)
- Overall language ability remains intact.

Renal System:
- There is a wide variation in kidney function with age. Typically, kidney size decreases; the number of nephrons is lower.
- Atherosclerotic blood vessels result in changes to renal blood flow, which seems to be more profound in the renal cortex. Increased resistance in afferent and efferent arterioles
- The functional reserve of the kidneys is less, and therefore, when elderly people are sick, the patient may be at higher risk of kidney failure. Less ability to respond to changes in water/salt intake
- Bladder volume decreases with less bladder elasticity.
- The female urethra shortens and becomes thinner.
- Male prostate enlarges (Jaipaul, n.d.).
- Decrease in glomerular filtration rate (GFR) and glomerular capillary flow rate and ultrafiltration coefficient. This decline may be the result of many factors including systemic hypertension, inflammation, and atherosclerosis (Weinstein & Anderson, 2010).
- Decline in creatinine clearance (Weinstein & Anderson, 2010)
- Increase in glomerular basement membrane permeability, which can result in proteinuria (Weinstein & Anderson, 2010)

Respiratory System:
- Chest wall and thoracic changes lead to an increased effort of breathing, reduced chest wall and lung compliance, kyphosis, decline in respiratory muscle strength and endurance (Lalley, 2013; Sharma & Goodwin, 2006)
- Reduced ability to clear airways with cough
- Alveolar dead space increases, increased residual volume, lower diffusing capacity
- Decline in lung function reduces FEV (Blatteis, 2012).
- Decline in gas exchange and diffusing capacity of carbon dioxide
- No change in total lung volume with age, and minute ventilation is maintained with increased respiratory rates.
- β-receptor affinity is reduced.
- Decline in maximal oxygen consumption or Vo_{2max}
- Respiratory system reserve is limited and decreases in response to hypercapnia; hypoxia cause increase stress with illnesses such as pneumonia

Cardiovascular System:
- Increased stiffness of aorta and all vessels (Nicolle, 2009)

- Increases in systolic blood pressure; diastolic may increase slightly, and then with older age will likely decrease, resulting in a widened pulse pressure
- Increases in left ventricular mass and wall thickness
- Fibrosis and collagen accumulation occurs in the myocardium, calcification of valvular leaflets, and coronary artery calcifications.
- Loss of pacemaker cells, fibrosis of the A-V node
- Declines in cardiac output

Gastrointestinal:

- Oropharynx: Tendency for more difficulty transfer of food bolus to the pharynx, normal swallowing function declines (Nicolle, 2009)
- Taste buds diminish in sensitivity, more quickly with sweet and salty tastes
- The mucosa tends to be more dry as less saliva is produced.
- Increased gastric-emptying time
- Decrease in gastric mucosal blood flow
- Liver size declines as well as blood flow. Metabolism of many medications through the liver is slowed.
- There tends to be an increase in cholelithiasis.
- Small bowel changes are minimal. Some studies suggest people have less tolerance for lactose with aging, resulting in difficulty digesting dairy products (DiStefano, Veneto, Malservisi, Strocchi, & Corazza, 2001).
- Changes occurring with the colon may be related to medications or diet in an elderly person, but typically, gastrointestinal transit time is slowed, which results in constipation with aging.

Age-Related Hearing Loss

Hearing loss is very common in the elderly. Age-related hearing loss is most commonly sensorineural, resulting in a gradual decline of hearing bilaterally. Sudden or unilateral hearing loss in a patient should be evaluated thoroughly. Age-related hearing loss typically occurs first with high pitches and is worse in loud areas. There are both genetic and environmental factors associated with presbycusis. Risk factors include frequent exposure to loud noises, smoking, certain medications, and other chronic medical conditions such as diabetes mellitus. The American Academy of Family Physicians recommends periodic screening for individuals over the age of 60 during routine examinations (Cacchione, 2005; DeStefano, Gates, Heard-Costa, Myers, & Baldwin, 2003; Garringer, Pankratz, Nichols, & Reed, 2006; Walling & Dickson, 2012).

Age-Related Vision Changes

With age, the lens gradually yellows, resulting in some difficulty with color discrimination, a reduced capacity to adapt to glare and light or see at night. The lens also becomes increasingly rigid, resulting in a significant loss of accommodation and the ability to judge contrasts when changing terrain such as walking off curbs or steps. The older person has difficulty shifting focus from distance to near. People commonly develop cataracts, which further impair vision. Certainly, chronic diseases contribute to vision loss, such as diabetic retinopathy, atherosclerotic disease, hyperlipidemia, and hypertension. Other eye-related diseases are more common as people age, such as macular degeneration and glaucoma.

Osteoporosis and aging

With aging, men and women are both at risk for fractures due to osteoporosis or a decline in bone mass. Osteoporosis affects more women than men. Risk factors that lead to increased bone fragility are age, female gender, family history of hip fracture, Caucasian or Asian ethnicity, poor nutrition and low calcium intake, physical inactivity, tobacco use, and excessive alcohol intake. Certain disease states resulting in malabsorption, estrogen deficiency, or medications such as chronic corticosteroid use contribute to the onset of osteoporosis. The goal for practitioners is to identify patients at risk and counsel on preventative measures or initiate medications that may decrease fracture risk (Ferri, 2015).

Pressure Ulcers

Elderly people have a combination of factors that increase their risk of developing pressure sores. The fact that the skin is thinner and more susceptible to tearing or shear stress along with immobility and the resultant pressure of bony prominences result in an increased development of pressure ulcers.

The National Pressure Ulcer Advisory Panel lists four stages of pressure ulcers:

- **Category/Stage I: Nonblanchable erythema**—Intact skin with nonblanchable redness of a localized area usually over a bony prominence. Darkly pigmented skin may not have visible blanching; its color may differ from the surrounding area. The area may be painful, firm, soft, warmer, or cooler as compared to adjacent tissue. Category I may be difficult to detect in individuals with dark skin tones.
- **Category/Stage II: Partial thickness**—Partial thickness loss of dermis presenting as a shallow open ulcer with a red–pink wound bed, without slough. May also present as an intact or open/ruptured serum-filled or serosanginous-filled blister. Presents as a shiny or dry shallow ulcer without slough or bruising.[1] This category should not be used to describe skin tears, tape burns, incontinence-associated dermatitis, maceration, or excoriation.
- **Category/Stage III: Full-thickness skin loss**—Full-thickness tissue loss. Subcutaneous fat may be visible but bone, tendon, or muscle are *not* exposed. Slough may be present but does not obscure the depth of tissue loss. *May* include undermining and tunneling. The depth of a category/stage III pressure ulcer varies by anatomical location. The bridge of the nose, ear, occiput, and malleolus do not have (adipose) subcutaneous tissue, and category/stage III ulcers can be shallow. In contrast, areas of significant adiposity can develop extremely deep category/stage III pressure ulcers. Bone/tendon is not visible or directly palpable.
- **Category/Stage IV: Full-thickness tissue loss**—Full-thickness tissue loss with exposed bone, tendon, or muscle. Slough or eschar may be present. Often includes undermining and tunneling. The depth of a category/stage IV pressure ulcer varies by anatomical location. The bridge of the nose, ear, occiput, and malleolus do not have (adipose) subcutaneous tissue, and these ulcers can be shallow. Category/stage IV ulcers can extend into muscle and/or supporting structures (e.g., fascia, tendon, or joint capsule), making osteomyelitis or osteitis likely to occur. Exposed bone/muscle is visible or directly palpable.

Source: National Pressure Ulcer Advisory Panel (2013).

"Pressure sores are the second commonest cause of bacteremia, which is usually polymicrobial in elderly people and can be regarded as the source of the sepsis in the absence of any other proved source and especially in the presence of foul smelling discharge and necrotic tissue" (Htwe 2007 Infections in the Elderly).

Frailty

The aging process has been subdivided into components that align with a person's functional capacity, physiologic reserve and ability to maintain homeostasis. The functional capacity of a group of people all at age 80 or 85 is vastly different. Many aging theories have attempted to explain these differences. The term "frailty" has come about to include basically five measures in a validated screening tool (Fedarko, 2011). To be considered frail, a person must have three or more of these.

- Self-reported exhaustion
- Slowed performance by walking speed
- Weakness by grip strength
- Unintentional weight loss (4.5 kg in the last year)
- Low physical activity

The frail older adult is generally in high need for health care and support services from the community. The expectation is that the number of frail adults will greatly increase as the majority of the baby boomers age.

Alterations in Disease Presentations in Elderly Patients

Urinary Tract Infection:
- Urinary Tract Infection (UTI) is the most common bacterial infection in the geriatric patient. The majority of UTIs in the elderly are asymptomatic.
- Epidemiology: As women get older the prevalence of asymptomatic UTI increases. The prevalence of bacteriuria increases threefold in women over 65 and then doubles after 80. Men develop higher

---

[1]Bruising indicates deep tissue injury.

incidences of bacterimia when they develop benign prostatic hypertrophy. When looking at the epidemiology of UTIs in the elderly, there are significantly more UTI cases in institutionalized persons than independent adults in the community. There are several factors in an older adult that predispose them to UTIs. Loss of estrogen affects the genitourinary mucosa. Prostatic hypertrophy, bacterial prostatitis, prostatic calculi, urethral strictures, and external urine-collecting devices can contribute to UTIs in men. Patients requiring urinary catheters (intermittent, indwelling), those with genitourinary structural abnormalities, bladder diverticulae, neurogenic bladder, or chronic disease such as diabetes mellitus will have an increased risk for UTI.

- The most common bacterial organism causing UTI in the elderly is the same as in the young. *Escherichia coli* accounts for 68% to 72% and 19% to 50% in women and men, respectively, in the community and 47% to 77% and 11% to 27% in women and men, respectively, in patients in institutions.

Mortality and Morbidity Associated with UTI in the Elderly

Asymptomatic UTI	No Decreased Survival
Symptomatic UTI (noninstitutionalized)	Mental status changes, tachycardia, and hypotension Morbidity is significantly higher and includes complications of pyelonephritis and sepsis. Mortality is 2.6%.
Symptomatic UTI (institutionalized)	Deterioration in functional status may contribute to morbidity, although it is an infrequent cause of mortality.

Myocardial Infarction:
- Coronary artery disease and myocardial infarction are common in the geriatric patient. The presentation can be atypical. Usually a younger patient predominately presents with crushing chest pain, which can radiate to their left arm along with diaphoresis.

Pneumonia

Incidence:
- Pneumonia in older adults can be classified as community acquired, hospital acquired, or skilled nursing facility acquired. The incidence of pneumonia is nearly 20% in adults 65 to 69 years of age but increases to over 50% in those older than 85 years of age. Some recent data suggest that respiratory infections have surpassed UTI as the most common infection among skilled nursing home residents.
- CURB65: Risk index to predict mortality from community-acquired pneumonia (Lim et al., 2003)

Etiology:
- Aspiration is a common cause of pneumonia in elderly patients. This may be a result of swallowing dysfunction, regurgitation of gastric contents, and poor dentition.

Risk Factors for Pneumonia:
- Older age
- Male gender
- History of aspiration
- Functional disability
- History of smoking, COPD
- Heart disease
- Cancer
- History of CVA
- Recent surgery or intensive care unit stay
- Presence of a feeding tube

Clinical Signs:
- About 25% of older patients with pneumonia present without a fever. Atypical symptoms may also include fatigue, loss of appetite, decrease functional capacity, and mental status changes.

Symptom	Points
Confusion	1
Urea >7 mmol/L	1
Respiratory rate >30 breaths/min	1
Systolic BP <90 mm Hg, diastolic pressure <60 mm Hg	1
Age >65	1
Total 30-day mortality	0 (0.6%), 1 (3.2%), 2(13%), 3(17%), 4(41.5%), 5(57.5%)

Surgery: (Surgical Considerations)
- Physiologic age, not chronologic age, should be considered prior to accessing risk for various surgical procedures. The presence of diminished functional status and comorbidities are the predictors of morbidity and mortality.
- In acute settings requiring surgical intervention, it is vital to be aware that an older patient may exhibit atypical symptoms. For example, when an elderly patient presents with cholecystitis, one-third lack fever, elevated white blood cell count, and physical findings of peritonitis.

Depression:
- In older adults, a diagnosis of major depression has been increasing, and by 2020 depression will rank second to cardiovascular disease as the leading cause of disability in the elderly. Women are twice as likely to suffer from depression as men.

Depression Screen

Two-Question Case-Finding Instrument	
During the last month, have you often been bothered by feeling down, depressed, or hopeless?	Yes/No
During the last month, have you often been bothered by having little interest or pleasure in doing things?	Yes/No
Directions: Yes to either question is a positive screen for depression.	

Risk Factors for Depression
- Prior history of depression
- Family history of depression
- Lack of social support
- Use of alcohol or other substances
- Recent loss of a loved one

Geriatric patients usually have more somatic complaints and fewer mood complaints, making it difficult to differentiate from underlying chronic disease processes.

Delirium and Dementia

Clinical Features	Delirium	Dementia
Onset	Acute	Insidious
Course	Fluctuating, with lucid intervals; worse at night	Slowly progressive
Duration	Hours to weeks	Months to years
Sleep/wake cycle	Always disrupted	Sleep fragmented
General medical illness or drug toxicity	Either or both present	Often absent, especially in Alzheimer disease

Examples of Causes:
- Delirium
  - Delirium tremens (due to withdrawal of alcohol)
  - Uremia
  - Acute hepatic failure
  - Acute cerebral vasculitis
  - Atropine poisoning
- Dementia
  - Reversible: Vitamin B_{12} deficiency, thyroid disorders
  - Irreversible: Alzheimer disease, vascular dementia (from multiple infarcts), dementia due to head trauma

Urinary Incontinence in the Geriatric Patient:
- Older adults are more likely to experience urinary incontinence (UI). UI is defined as simply the involuntary loss of urine. It is a syndrome, not a disease. UI happens more in women than in men. Patients typically underreport symptoms of UI because of embarrassment. It also has been shown to be undertreated by practitioners.

Characteristic of the Elderly Patient	Incidence of Incontinence (%)
Healthy older adults	15–30
Frail elderly community dwellers	Nearly 50
Institutionalized elderly adults	50–75

Table 14-1 provides recommendations for screening tests in older adults..

Table 14-1: Screening Test Recommendations in Aging Patients

Screening	Men	Women	Rationale
Hepatitis C testing	Always	Always	Everyone born between 1945 and 1965 needs to be screened for the hepatitis C virus (USPSTF).
Pneumonia vaccination	Always	Always	Anyone over 65 yr old or with significant risk factors (ACIP)
Influenza vaccination yearly	Always	Always	For yearly flu protection
Shingles vaccination	Always	Always	To protect against herpes zoster complications starting at age 60
Td vaccination	Always	Always	Vaccinate once every 10 yr to protect against tetanus, diphtheria infection.
Tdap vaccination	Always	Always	Vaccinate once if have not had the vaccine to protect against tetanus, diphtheria, and pertussis (ACIP).
Colorectal cancer screening	Always	Always	Get checked regularly for colorectal cancer, starting at age 50 (USPSTF).
Blood pressure screening	Always	Always	Get your blood pressure checked at least once every 2 yr starting at age 18 (USPSTF).
Cholesterol screening	Always	Always	Get your cholesterol checked once every 5 yr, starting at age 35 (USPSTF).
Daily aspirin administration	Always	Always	To help lower your risk of heart attack, men 45–79 yr and women 55–79 yr old (USPSTF)
HIV testing	Always	Always	Get tested at least one time and more often depending on your risk (USPSTF).

(continued)

Table 14-1: Screening Test Recommendations in Aging Patients (*continued*)

Screening	Men	Women	Rationale
Breast cancer screening		Always	A mammogram every 2 yr from 50 to 74 yr old (USPSTF)
Cervical cancer screening		Always	Pap test every 3 yr. If you get a Pap test and an HPV test, then may be screened every 5 yr until age 65 (USPSTF).
Lung cancer	Sometimes	Sometimes	Screen from ages 55 to 80 if you have a 30 pack-year smoking history, smoke now, or have quit within the past 15 yr (USPSTF).
Alcohol use screening	Sometimes	Sometimes	
Dietary screening	Sometimes	Sometimes	If your provider has told you that you are at risk for heart disease or diabetes, ask about dietary counseling (USPSTF).
Fall screening/prevention	Sometimes	Sometimes	If you are worried about falls, ask how exercise, physical therapy, and vitamin D supplements might help you prevent falls (USPSTF).
Hepatitis B screening	Sometimes	Sometimes	Risk factors for hepatitis B (like any injection drug use or if you were born in a country where hepatitis B is common) then test (USPSTF)
Tobacco abuse screening	Sometimes	Sometimes	Ask about smoking cessation at every visit and provide counseling (USPSTF).
Diabetes screening	Sometimes	Sometimes	If there is chronic elevated blood pressure, then screen for type 2 diabetes (USPSTF).
Abdominal aortic aneurysm screening	Sometimes		Men aged 65–75 who have ever smoked tobacco (USPSTF)
Depression screening	Sometimes	Sometimes	Yearly screening for sad, down, or hopeless feelings only if depression counseling services are in place in office (USPSTF)
Healthy diet and physical activity screening	Sometimes	Sometimes	If you are overweight, ask your medical provider about screening and counseling for obesity (USPSTF).
Sexually transmitted infections screening	Sometimes	Sometimes	Testing and prevention counseling for chlamydia, gonorrhea, and syphilis (USPSTF)

From Guide to Clinical Preventive Services (2014). *Recommendations of the U.S. Preventive Services Task Force, June 2014.* Rockville, MD: Agency for Healthcare Research and Quality. Retrieved from http://www.ahrq.gov/professionals/clinicians-providers/guidelines-recommendations/guide/index.html; myhealthfinder (web-based tool) Copyright 2015 National Health Information Center, Washington, DC. Retrieved from http://www.healthfinder.gov/myhealthfinder/

Review Section

Case Summary

The care of the elderly patient must be considered unique and not that of simply old adults. Evaluating the ill elderly patient can sometimes be a challenge in a variety of ways. Often, new symptoms are vague and difficult to correlate to a specific problem. A family member may report that the patient "just doesn't seem right" when a bacterial infection may be brewing.

Because the elderly patient's immune system is no longer robust enough to launch an appropriate response to infection, clinicians cannot rely on the usual signs of elevated temperature or white blood cell count to aid in diagnosis. Practitioners must realize that the elderly may not present the same symptoms of illness as those of younger adults.

Review Questions

1. Which of the following age groups require one-time hepatitis C testing?

   a. Born before 1935
   b. 1935to 1944
   c. 1945 to 1965
   d. 1965 to 1985
   e. 1985 to present

2. At what age is it recommended to stop screening for colorectal cancer in a female without any risk factors?

   a. 65
   b. 69
   c. 70
   d. 75
   e. 79

3. Which of the following screenings is recommended by the USPSTF for a nonsexually active, nonsmoking 68-year-old female?

   a. Cervical cancer
   b. HIV
   c. Syphilis
   d. Lung cancer
   e. Chlamydia and gonorrhea

4. An 85-year-old patient presents for 3-month checkup. Which of the following positive findings on examination would be considered pathologic?

   a. Increased skin turgor, and oral mucosa dryness
   b. Lower extremity bilateral edema
   c. Decreased visual and auditory acuity
   d. Elevated systolic blood pressure
   e. Oral temperature of 97.4

5. Which of the following is a measure of frailty in an elderly patient?

   a. Recent fall
   b. Memory loss
   c. Inability to perform ADLs
   d. Unintentional weight loss
   e. Cognitive decline

6. A stage II pressure ulcer has which of the following identifying features?

   a. Blanchable area of erythema
   b. Slow-healing wound
   c. Visible muscle or connective tissue
   d. Significant area of sloughing
   e. Shallow dry ulcer without exudate

7. Skin tears in elderly patients are related to which physiologic change?

   a. Seborrheic dermatitis
   b. Several actinic keratosis
   c. Fewer sweat glands
   d. Epidermal thinning
   e. Increase in benign angiomas

8. Which of the following is not considered one of the criteria to define frailty?

   a. Grip weakness
   b. Slowed walking speed
   c. Need for daytime naps
   d. Weight loss

9. A 66-year-old female presents to the emergency department and is diagnosed with pneumonia. Using the CURB65 mortality risk, what is her mortality risk if she is confused and has a respiratory rate of >30 breaths per minute?

   a. >5%
   b. >10%
   c. >15%
   d. >20%
   e. >30%

10. What are considered normal physiologic changes in the patient in the above case presentation?

    a. Urinary incontinence
    b. Glaucoma
    c. Mini mental status 21/30
    d. Temp 97.6°F
    e. Delirium

Answers with Rationales

1. (c) 1945 to 1965

   Rationale: The US Preventive Services Task gives a Grade B recommendation to offer first-time hepatitis C screening to anyone born between 1945 and 1965. The recommendation is due to the fact that this age cohort is at risk of potential exposure to hepatitis C virus prior to universal blood screening (Guide to Clinical Preventive Services, 2014).

2. (d) 75

   Rationale: The US Preventive Services Task Force gives a Grade A recommendation to screen for colorectal cancer in any patient starting at age 50 and continuing to age 75. Screening may be done by fecal occult blood testing, colonoscopy, or sigmoidoscopy. Evidence has found that screening in this age group has decreased colorectal cancer mortality. There is a Grade C recommendation to not routinely screen those individuals 76 to 85 years of age (Guide to Clinical Preventive Services, 2014).

3. (b) HIV

   Rationale: The US Preventive Services Task Force provides a Grade A recommendation to screen all adolescents and adults 15 to 65 years of age for HIV infection. Any further screening after this age range would be determined by patient risk assessment such as having a new sexual partner (Guide to Clinical Preventive Services, 2014).

4. (b) Lower extremity bilateral edema

   Rationale: With aging, there is a reduced ability of the cardiovascular efficiency due to increased vessel stiffness and lack of compliance. Venous return decreases and is less capable of handling changes in intravascular volume. Further evaluation of the cause of the bilateral edema is warranted. All of the other choices above are considered a part of normal physiologic changes with aging.

5. (d) Unintentional weight loss

   Rationale: According to Fedarko in the article "The Biology of Aging and Frailty" (2011), "The validated and widely used 5-item frailty criteria for screening—self-reported exhaustion, slowed performance (by walking speed), weakness (by grip strength), unintentional weight loss (4.5 kg in the past year), and low physical activity—are composite outcomes of multiple organ systems."

6. (e) Shallow dry ulcer without exudate

   Rationale: A stage II pressure ulcer is characterized by partial thickness loss of the dermis, is open and shallow with a pink wound bed, and may or may not have slough. A stage I ulcer is characterized by intact skin with nonblanchable redness, a stage III ulcer by full-thickness tissue loss and possible appearance of subcutaneous fat, and a stage IV ulcer by full-thickness loss with exposed bone, tendon, or muscle (Dementia, 2008).

7. (d) Epidermal thinning

   Rationale: Physiologic changes of the skin with aging include reduced epidermal cell turnover, reduced vascularization, and skin atrophy, making the skin more susceptible to injury and skin tears (Navaratnarajah & Jackson, 2013).

8. (c) Need for daytime naps

   Rationale: The American Geriatrics Society defines frailty as a clinical syndrome including the evaluation of self-reported exhaustion, slowed walking speed, weakness, unintentional weight loss, and low physical activity. They recommend using an assessment tool to identify patients at high risk of loss of independence and frailty.

9. (c) >15%

   Rationale: The CURB-65 risk stratification identifies patients at low risk for community-acquired pneumonia mortality. It takes into account mental status, BUN >20 mg/dL, respiratory rate >30, systolic blood pressure < 90 mm Hg or diastolic <60 mm Hg and age ≥65. A single point is given to each value based on the numbers of each. A score of 0 to 1 indicates low mortality risk, and the patient may be managed as an outpatient. A score of 2 is moderate to high, and the patient may require short inpatient stay or be supervised outpatient, a score of 3, 4, or 5, generally requires inpatient stay and possibly ICU admission. Each of these scores is assigned a mortality risk from 0.6% to the highest at 27.8%. This patient is over 65, confused, and her respiratory rate is >30 or a score of 3, which indicates a mortality risk of close to 15%.

10. (d) Temp 97.6°F

    Rationale: Core body temperature tends to be lower as people age. This is thought to be a result of decreased vasomotor responses in skin as well as the ability of skin to detect changes in temperature. In addition, as we age, the ability to increase heat production by shivering is diminished as is hepatic thermogenesis. Older people are at risk of suffering from extremes in temperature (Navaratnarajah & Jackson, 2013; Blatteis, 2012). The other symptoms listed above are not a part of normal aging and should be further evaluated.

Suggested Readings

Theories of Aging:

Bjorksten, J. (1968). The crosslinkage theory of aging. *Journal of the American Geriatrics Society, 16*, 408–427.

Bjorksten, J., & Tenhu, H. (1990). The crosslinking theory of aging—Added evidence. *Experimental Gerontology, 25*, 91–95.

Brys, K., Vanfleteren, J. R., & Braeckman, B. P. (2007). Testing the rate-of-living/oxidative damage theory of aging in the nematode model Caenorhabditis elegans. *Experimental Gerontology, 42*, 845–851.

Cornelius, E. (1972). Increased incidence of lymphomas in thymectomized mice—evidence for an immunological theory of aging. *Experientia, 28*, 459.

Davidovic, M., Sevo, G., Svorcan, P., Milosevic, D. P., Despotovic, N., & Erceg, P. (2010). Old age as a privilege of the "selfish ones". *Aging and Disease, 1*, 139–146.

Gerschman, R., Gilbert, D. L., Nye, S. W., Dwyer, P., & Fenn, W. O. (1954). Oxygen poisoning and x-irradiation: A mechanism in common. *Science, 119*, 623–626.

Harman, D. (1956). Aging: A theory based on free radical and radiation chemistry. *Journal of Gerontology, 11*, 298–300.

Hayflick, L., & Moorhead, P. S. (1961). The serial cultivation of human diploid cell strains. *Experimental Cell Research, 25*, 585–621.

Jin, K. (2010). Modern biological theories of aging. *Aging and Disease, 1*, 72–74.

Rozemuller, A. J., van Gool, W. A., & Eikelenboom, P. (2005). The neuroinflammatory response in plaques and amyloid angiopathy in Alzheimer's disease: Therapeutic implications. *Current Drug Targets CNS Neurological Disorders, 4*, 223–233.

van Heemst, D. (2010). Insulin, IGF-1 and longevity. *Aging and Disease, 1*, 147–157.

Altered Disease Presentations:

Bickley, L. S. (2008). *Bates' guide to physical examination and history taking* (10th ed., p. 931). Philadelphia, PA: Lippincott-Raven.

Gammack, J. K. (2014). Urinary incontinence. In B. A. Williams, A. Chang, C. Ahalt, H. Chen, R. Conant, C. S. Landfeld, . . . M. Yukawa. (Eds.), *Current diagnosis and treatment: Geriatrics* (2nd ed., pp. 375–383). New York, NY: Mcgraw Hill Medical.

Hardin, R. E., & Zenilman, M. E. (2014). Surgical considerations in the elderly. In F. C. Brunicardi, D. K. Andersen, T. R. Billiar, D. L. Dunn, J. G. Hunter, J. B. Matthews, & R. E. Pollock (Eds.), *Schwart's principles of surgery* (10th ed.). New York, NY: McGraw-Hill Education.

Lim, W. S., van der Eerden, M. M., Laing, R., Boersma, W. G., Karalus, N., Town, G., . . . Macfarlane, J. (2003). Defining community acquired pneumonia severity on presentation to hospital: An international derivation and validation study. *Thorax, 58*(5), 377–382. doi:10.1136/thorax.58.5.377.

Liu, D., Norman, M. A., Singh, B., & Lee, K. (2014). Depression & other mental health issues. In B. A. Williams, A. Chang, C. Ahalt, H. Chen, R. Conant, C. S. Landfeld, . . . M. Yukawa. (Eds.), *Current diagnosis and treatment: Geriatrics* (2nd ed., pp. 328–331). New York, NY: Mcgraw Hill Medical.

Midthun, S. J. (2004). Criteria for urinary tract infection in the elderly: Variables that challenge nursing assessment. *Urologic Nursing, 24*(3), 157–162.

Mody, L., Riddell, J., Kaye, K., & Chopra, T. (2014). Common infections. In B. A. Williams, A. Chang, C. Ahalt, H. Chen, R. Conant, C. S. Landfeld, . . . M. Yukawa. (Eds.), *Current diagnosis and treatment: Geriatrics* (2nd ed., pp. 352–353). New York, NY: Mcgraw Hill Medical.

Nicolle, L. E. (2009). Urinary tract infections. In J. B. Halter, J. G. Ouslander, M. E. Tinetti, S. Studentski, K. P. High, & S. Asthana (Eds.), *Hazzard's geriatric medicine and gerontology* (6th ed., pp. 1547–1560). New York, NY: McGraw Hill Medical.

Sinclair, D. (1994). Myocardial infarction. Considerations for geriatric patients. *Canadian Family Physician, 40*, 1172–1177.

The Physiologic Changes with Aging and the Hearing Loss, Pressure Ulcers and Frail Elderly:

Besdine, R. W. (n.d.). *Changes in the body with aging.* Retrieved from http://www.merckmanuals.com/home/older_peoples_health_issues/the_aging_body/changes_in_the_body_with_aging.html?qt=aging%20and%20the%20colon&alt=sh

Blatteis, C. M. (2012). Age dependent changes in temperature regulation—A mini review. *Gerontology, 58*, 289–295. doi:10.1159/000333148.

Cacchione, P. (2005). Want to know more: Sensory changes. Retrieved from http://consultgerirn.org/topics/sensory_changes/want_to_know_more retrieved 1/18/2015

DeStefano, A. L., Gates, G. A., Heard-Costa, N., Myers, R. H., & Baldwin, C. T. (2003). Genomewide linkage analysis to presbycusis in the Framingham Heart Study. *Archives of Otolaryngology—Head and Neck Surgery, 129*(3), 285–289. doi:10.1001/archotol.129.3.285.

DiStefano, M., Veneto, G., Malservisi, S., Strocchi, A., & Corazza, G. (2001). Lactose malabsorption and intolerance in the elderly. *Scandinavian Journal of Gastroenterology, 36*(12), 1274–1278.

Fedarko, N. S. (2011). The biology of aging and frailty. *Clinics in Geriatric Medicine, 27*, 27–37. doi:10.1016/j.cger.2010.08.006.

Ferri, F. (2015). Osteoporosis. In F. Ferri (Ed.), *Ferri's clinical advisor 2015* (pp. 860–862). Philadelphia, PA: Mosby/Elsevier Inc.

Ferrucci L., & Studenski, S. (2012). Clinical problems of aging. In D. L. Longo, A. S. Fauci, D. L. Kasper, S. L. Hauser, J. Jameson, & J. Loscalzo (Eds.), *Harrison's principles of internal medicine* (18th ed.). Retrieved December 30, 2014 from http://accessmedicine.mhmedical.com.ezproxy2.library.drexel.edu/content.aspx?bookid=331&Sectionid=40726805

Fillit, H. M., Rockwood, K., & Woodhouse, K. (2010). *Brocklehurst's textbook of geriatric medicine and gerontology* (7th ed., pp. 30–37). Philadelphia, PA: Saunders/Elsevier, Inc.

Fletcher, K. (2008). Dementia. In E. Capezuti, D. Zwicker, M. Mezey, & T. Fulmer (Eds.). *Evidence-based geriatric nursing protocols for best practice* (3rd ed., pp. 83–109). New York, NY: Springer Publishing Company.

Garringer, H. J., Pankratz, N. D., Nichols, W. C., & Reed, T. (2006). Hearing impairment susceptibility in elderly men and the

DFNA18 locus. *Archives of Otolaryngology—Head and Neck Surgery, 132*(5), 506–510. doi:10.1001/archotol.132.5.506.

Guide to Clinical Preventive Services. (2014). *Recommendations of the U.S. Preventive Services Task Force, June 2014.* Rockville, MD: Agency for Healthcare Research and Quality. Retrieved from http://www.ahrq.gov/professionals/clinicians-providers/ guidelines-recommendations/guide/index.html

Ham, R. J., Sloane, P. D., Warshaw, G. A., Potter, J. F., & Flaherty, E. (2014). *Ham's primary care geriatrics: A case-based approach* (6th ed.). Philadelphia, PA: Saunders/Elsevier Inc.

Harada, C. N., Natelson Love, M. C., & Triebel, K. L. (2013). Normal cognitive aging. *Clinics in Geriatric Medicine, 29*(4), 737–752. doi:10.1016/j.cger.2013.07.002.

Hoffman, R., Benz, E. J., Silberstein, L. E., Heslop, H. E., Weitz, J. I., & Anastasi, J. (2013). *Hematology: Basic principles and practice* (6th ed.). Philadelphia, PA: Elsevier.

Hurd, R. (2014). *Aging changes in skin.* Retrieved from http://www. nlm.nih.gov/medlineplus/ency/article/004014.htm

Jaipaul, N. (n.d.). *Effects of aging on the urinary tract.* Retrieved from http://www.merckmanuals.com/home/kidney_and_urinary_ tract_disorders/biology_of_the_kidneys_and_urinary_tract/ effects_of_aging_on_the_urinary_tract.html

Lalley, P. M. (2013). The aging respiratory system pulmonary structure function and neural control. *Respiratory Physiology and Neurobiology, 187*, 199–210.

Melmed, S., Polonsky, K. S., Larsen, P. R., & Kronenberg, H. M. (2011). *Williams textbook of endocrinology* (12th ed.). Philadelphia: Saunders/Elsevier.

National Pressure Ulcer Advisory Panel. (2013). Retrieved January 19, 2015 from http://www.npuap. org/resources/educational-and-clinical-resources/ npuap-pressure-ulcer-stagescategories/

Navaratnarajah, A., & Jackson, S. (2013). The physiology of ageing. *Medicine, 41*(1), 5–8.

Nicolle, L. E. (2009). Urinary tract infections. In J. B. Halter, J. G. Ouslander, M. E. Tinetti, S. Studentski, K. P. High, & S. Asthana (Eds.), *Hazzard's geriatric medicine and gerontology* (6th ed., pp. 1547–1560). New York, NY: McGraw Hill Medical.

Pawlec, L. (2008). Immunity and aging in man: Annual review 2006/2007. *Experimental Gerontology, 43*, 34–38.

Sharma, G., & Goodwin, J. (2006). Effect of aging on respiratory system physiology and immunology. *Clinical Interventions in Aging, 1*(3), 253–260.

Walling, A. D., & Dickson, G. M. (2012). Hearing loss in older adults. *American Family Physician, 85*(12), 1150–1156. Retrieved January 15, 2015 from http://www.aafp.org/ afp/2012/0615/p1150.html

Weinstein, J. R., & Anderson, S. (2010). The aging kidney: Physiological changes. *Advances in Chronic Kidney Disease, 17*(4), 302–307. doi:10.1053/j.ackd.2010.05.002.

Chapter 15

Pediatric and Adolescent Review

Kristen A. Altdoerffer and MaryKay Maley

Growth and Development

Age	Milestones
2 mo	Lifts head, follows to midline, vocalizes, responsive smile
4 mo	Sits with head steady, starts to roll over, grasps rattle, laughs
6 mo	Starts to sits without support, rolls over, reaches, turns to rattling sound, starts to feed self
9 mo	Pulls to stand and stands holding on, transfers cube, says nonspecific Dada/Mama, waves bye-bye, feeds self
1 yr	Stands alone, bangs two cubes, imitates sounds and vocalizations, babbles, starts to wave bye-bye, plays pat-a-cake, imitates
15 mo	Walks well, stoops and recovers, 1–3 words
18 mo	Walks backward, scribbles, tower of 2 cubes, 3–6 words, helps in house, starts removing garments
2–2.5 yr	Kicks ball, walks upstairs, jumps up, starts to throw ball, points to 6 body parts, combines words, speech more understandable, puts on clothes, knows 2 actions
3 yr	Broad jump, overhand ball throw, imitates vertical line, tower of 6–8 cubes, understandable speech, names 1 color, names 4 pictures, names a friend, brushes teeth with help
4 yr	Hops, balances for 2 sec on one foot, draws a person with 3 parts, tower of 8 cubes, names 4 colors, understandable speech, copies a circle/cross
Early adolescence (11–14 yr)	Onset of puberty, menarche (females), growth spurt (females) Concrete thought Preoccupied with friends, rapid body changes, sexual identity, increasing independence, but parents still have strong control
Middle adolescence (15–17 yr)	Ovulation (females), growth spurt (males) Abstract, future thinking, sense of invincibility Preoccupied with sexual identity, narcissism, increased peer relationships over parental control, health-risk behaviors
Late adolescence (18–21 yr)	Growth complete Future oriented; independence; prepares for career, marriage, parenting Individual agenda over peers, transition to own home Transition in relationships with parents

American Academy of Pediatrics. (2016). *Bright futures*. Retrieved from www.brightfutures.aap.org

Figure 15-1 shows current recommended immunization schedule.

Recommended immunization schedule for persons aged 0 through 18 years – **United States, 2015.**

(FOR THOSE WHO FALL BEHIND OR START LATE, SEE THE CATCH-UP SCHEDULE [FIGURE 2]).

These recommendations must be read with the footnotes that follow. For those who fall behind or start late, provide catch-up vaccination at the earliest opportunity as indicated by the green bars in Figure 1. To determine minimum intervals between doses, see the catch-up schedule (Figure 2). School entry and adolescent vaccine age groups are shaded.

Vaccine	Birth	1 mo	2 mos	4 mos	6 mos	9 mos	12 mos	15 mos	18 mos	19–23 mos	2-3 yrs	4-6 yrs	7-10 yrs	11-12 yrs	13-15 yrs	16-18 yrs
Hepatitis B[1] (HepB)	1st dose	←2nd dose→			←3rd dose→											
Rotavirus[2] (RV) RV1 (2-dose series); RV5 (3-dose series)			1st dose	2nd dose	See footnote 2											
Diphtheria, tetanus, & acellular pertussis[3] (DTaP: <7 yrs)			1st dose	2nd dose	3rd dose			←4th dose→				5th dose				
Tetanus, diphtheria, & acellular pertussis[4] (Tdap: ≥7 yrs)														(Tdap)		
Haemophilus influenzae type b[5] (Hib)			1st dose	2nd dose	See footnote 5		←3rd or 4th dose, See footnote 5→									
Pneumococcal conjugate[6] (PCV13)			1st dose	2nd dose	3rd dose		←4th dose→									
Pneumococcal polysaccharide[6] (PPSV23)																
Inactivated poliovirus[7] (IPV: <18 yrs)			1st dose	2nd dose	←3rd dose→							4th dose				
Influenza[8] (IIV; LAIV) 2 doses for some: See footnote 8					Annual vaccination (IIV only) 1 or 2 doses						Annual vaccination (LAIV or IIV) 1 or 2 doses		Annual vaccination (LAIV or IIV) 1 dose only			
Measles, mumps, rubella[9] (MMR)					See footnote 9		←1st dose→					2nd dose				
Varicella[10] (VAR)							←1st dose→					2nd dose				
Hepatitis A[11] (HepA)							←2-dose series, See footnote 11→									
Human papillomavirus[12] (HPV2: females only; HPV4: males and females)														(3-dose series)		
Meningococcal[13] (Hib-MenCY ≥ 6 weeks; MenACWY-D ≥9 mos; MenACWY-CRM ≥ 2 mos)			See footnote 13											1st dose		Booster

- Range of recommended ages for all children
- Range of recommended ages for catch-up immunization
- Range of recommended ages for certain high-risk groups
- Range of recommended ages during which catch-up is encouraged and for certain high-risk groups
- Not routinely recommended

This schedule includes recommendations in effect as of January 1, 2015. Any dose not administered at the recommended age should be administered at a subsequent visit, when indicated and feasible. The use of a combination vaccine generally is preferred over separate injections of its equivalent component vaccines. Vaccination providers should consult the relevant Advisory Committee on Immunization Practices (ACIP) statement for detailed recommendations, available online at http://www.cdc.gov/vaccines/hcp/acip-recs/index.html. Clinically significant adverse events that follow vaccination should be reported to the Vaccine Adverse Event Reporting System (VAERS) online (http://www.vaers.hhs.gov) or by telephone (800-822-7967). Suspected cases of vaccine-preventable diseases should be reported to the state or local health department. Additional information, including precautions and contraindications for vaccination, is available from CDC online (http://www.cdc.gov/vaccines/recs/vac-admin/contraindications.htm) or by telephone (800-CDC-INFO [800-232-4636]).

This schedule is approved by the Advisory Committee on Immunization Practices (http//www.cdc.gov/vaccines/acip), the American Academy of Pediatrics (http://www.aap.org), the American Academy of Family Physicians (http://www.aafp.org), and the American College of Obstetricians and Gynecologists (http://www.acog.org).

NOTE: The above recommendations must be read along with the footnotes of this schedule.

Figure 15-1: Recommended immunization schedule for persons aged 0 through 18 years—United States, 2015.
Source: Centers for Disease Control and Prevention. (2015). *Recommended immunization schedule for persons aged 0 through 18 years.* Retrieved from http://www.cdc.gov/vaccines/schedules/hcp/child-adolescent.html

Case Presentation

Directions: Review the case studies presented throughout this chapter carefully. At the end of each case study, answer the questions. Proceed then to the Review Section. Compare your answers to what you find in the Review Section along with the rationales.

Infant Case Presentation

You are caring for a 2-week-old female patient at a well-child physical. Her current weight is 6 lb 15 oz. Her mother feels that she has a strong latch during breast-feeding, her milk supply is in, and she nurses on both sides until the breasts are emptied. She has about eight wet diapers a day with yellow, seedy stools with every diaper change. She is sleeping for about 18 to 20 hours a day, but easily arousable.

Past Medical History: 38 weeks' gestation, a vaginal delivery, without complications. No oxygen required at birth. Birth weight was 7 lb 2 oz

Medications: None

Allergy: None

Social: Home: Lives with parents, no siblings

Immunizations: HBV first dose at 1 day of age

Family History: Unremarkable

Review of Systems/Health Promotion:
Constitutional: Denies fevers, fatigue
Head, Eyes, Ears, Nose, Throat (HEENT): **Head:** Denies head injury. **Eyes:** Denies eye problems. **Ears:** Appears responsive to sound. **Nose:** Denies nasal congestion
Neck: Denies neck problems
Respiratory: Denies difficulty breathing
Cardiovascular: Denies pale or blue skin discoloration
Gastrointestinal: Denies v/d; strong latch during breast-feeding, mother's milk supply is in, nurses on both sides until the breasts are emptied, seedy stools with every diaper change
Musculoskeletal: Denies injuries
Neurology: Denies seizures
Genitourinary: Eight wet diapers/day
Integumentary: Denies rashes, open sores, nail problems. + newborn acne on face, +yellow skin tone

Physical Examination:
Vital Signs: Temperature = 98.2°F BP = Not obtained HR = 135 bpm RR = 52 Height = 21 inches Weight = 6 lb 15 oz
General/Psych: Awake and alert; crying with examination. Accompanied to visit by mom.
Skin: Dry, cool to touch, closed comedones on nasal bridge, jaundice down to the umbilicus, acyanotic
HEENT: **Head:** Normocephalic, anterior and posterior fontanels are open and flat. **Eyes:** PERRL. **Ears:** No drainage, TMs pearly gray bilaterally. **Nose:** Patent, turbinates pink, no discharge, septum intact and midline. **Mouth/Throat:** Mucous membranes are moist, pharynx pink, tonsils +1, uvula midline
Thoracic/Lungs: CTA bilaterally, no wheezing noted. No signs of increased work of breathing, +belly breathing
Cardiovascular: Soft systolic murmur left sternal border, femoral and brachial pulses +2 bilaterally
Abdomen: Soft, nontender, +BS, no masses, palpable liver edge, no splenomegaly.
Musculoskeletal: Full range of motion in all joints of the upper and lower extremities, negative Ortolani/Barlow, normal tone; spine: straight
Neurologic: Newborn reflexes intact, +suck
Genitalia: Tanner I, no lesions, discharge, or rashes noted

Case Study Review Questions

1. The mother is concerned with her daughter's weight and asking what her percentage is on the growth chart. What is your response?

   At 2 weeks she should be up to her birth weight, but it is reassuring that she is nursing well and has wet diapers. Her weights should be plotted on the World Health Organization Growth Curve Standards. She is at the 10th percentile for weight (Fig. 15-2).

2. What additional education would you include for breast-feeding?

   1. Vitamin D supplementation of 400 IU/day
   2. Exclusive breast-feeding should occur for about 6 months, and once foods are introduced, it is encouraged to continue breast-feeding until age 1 or longer.
   3. Review with the mother the health benefits of nursing, the economic benefits, adapting nursing to the workplace, and ensuring proper techniques.
   4. Implement routine weight checks to verify adequate calorie intake and ensure proper weight gain.
   5. Refer to lactation and possibly observe breast-feeding for an adequate latch.

3. What are your concerns after completing the physical examination?

   Jaundice: It is normal for about 30% to 40% of predominately breastfed infants to present with jaundice for the first 4 weeks (Maisels et al., 2014), as exclusive breast-feeding and prematurity are the most predictive factors of jaundice. Although they should be considered as differentials, acute bilirubin encephalopathy and kernicterus are fortunately rare.

   Murmur: Up to 90% of children have a cardiac murmur, but only 8 to 10 per 1,000 have a structural heart disease. Therefore, the primary care provider must determine which patients with murmurs need further evaluation (Turiy, 2012).

4. What is your treatment plan?

> Jaundice: A risk score, transcutaneous bilirubin, or total serum bilirubin should be ordered. If the level is elevated in comparison to the risks on a total serum bilirubin nomogram, phototherapy could be initiated. Breast-feeding should continue to be encouraged with hyperbilirubinemia.

> Murmur: It is imperative to investigate the perinatal history and family history. This includes prenatal ultrasounds, medications, use of drugs and alcohol, maternal pregnancy comorbidities, a family history of congenital abnormalities, inheritable cardiac diseases, childhood deaths, or first-degree relatives with structural heart disease. The patient's vital signs, disposition and color, feeding habits, and a thorough cardiac physical examination should be evaluated. Four extremity blood pressures should be measured. In a patient with a difference of 20 mm Hg in the arms than the legs, further evaluation for coarctation of the aorta or interrupted aortic arch should be conducted. Preductal and postductal pulse oximetry (right upper extremity and either right or left lower extremity) should be evaluated for discrepancies. The use of EKGs and chest radiography is controversial. An echocardiogram remains the gold standard.

5. What anticipatory guidance would be appropriate to include?

> Anticipatory guidance would include screening for postpartum depression, coping strategies for older siblings, breast-feeding guidance and hunger cues, do not prop a bottle, signs of an infection and illness prevention, reduce sun exposure, parental bonding, education on SIDS prevention, and bathing, feeding, car seat, and sleep safety.

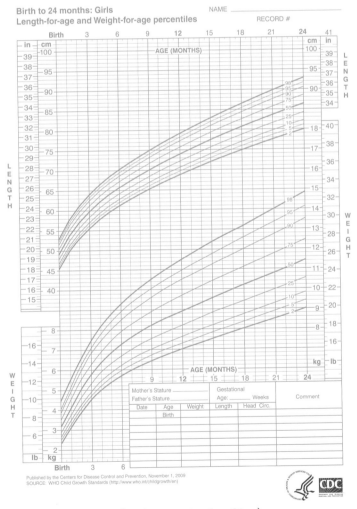

Figure 15-2: Pediatric Girls Growth Chart (Birth to 24 Months of Age).

Common Infant Diagnoses

Congenital Heart Disease

Description of the Disease: While congenital heart disease (CHD) is the most common congenital disease in newborns, about 25% require invasive interventions. Newborns with critical CHD are symptomatic and require interventions quickly after birth. A prolonged lack of treatment increases the risk of morbidity and mortality.

Epidemiology/Etiology:
- The prevalence of CHD ranges from 6 to 13 per 1,000 live births (Altman, 2015)
- The prevalence is two to three times more likely in premature infants (born <37 weeks' gestation)
- Maternal risk factors include maternal multifetal pregnancy, diabetes mellitus, hypertension, maternal CHD, thyroid disorders, epilepsy, and mood disorders (Altman, 2015)
- One of the leading congenital malformation causes of perinatal and infant death

Signs and Symptoms:
- Asymptomatic
- Critical CHD: Shock, cyanosis, or pulmonary edema
- Abnormal heart rate (sinus tachycardia, supraventricular tachycardia, ventricular tachycardia, bradycardia, atrial and ventricular arrhythmias)
- Precordial activity
- Abnormal heart sounds
- Pathologic murmurs (grade 3 or higher, harsh quality, pansystolic duration, loudest at upper left or right sternal border, or apex, abnormal S2)
- Diminished or absent peripheral pulses
- Respiratory abnormalities
- Tachypnea
- Coughing and wheezing
- Extracardiac abnormalities
- Pulse oximetry less than 95%
- Difficulty with feeding
- Central cyanosis or persistent pallor
- Excessive, unexplained irritability
- Excessive sweating, increased with feeds
- Poor weight gain
- Decreased activity/excessive sleeping
- Delayed motor milestones

Differential Diagnoses:
- Hypoplastic left heart syndrome (HLHS)
- Pulmonary atresia (PA)
- Tetralogy of Fallot (TOF)
- Total anomalous pulmonary venous return (TAPVR)
- Transposition of the great arteries (TGA)
- Tricuspid atresia (TA)
- Truncus arteriosus (TAC)
- Pulmonary etiology
- Genetic disorders
- Metabolic myopathies

Diagnostic Studies:
- Pulse oximetry screening on the right hand (preductal) and either foot (postductal) after 24 hours of life
- Refer to cardiology
- Echocardiographic evaluation

Treatment (Both Pharmacologic and Nonpharmacologic):
- Management specific on diagnosis

Croup

Description of the Disease: Croup is usually a self-limiting disease, but could present with respiratory distress and upper airway occlusion. The typical presentation of croup is inspiratory stridor, cough, and hoarseness, resulting from inflammation of the larynx and subglottic airway. The typical pathogenesis of croup is the viral infection of the nasal and pharyngeal mucosal epithelia spreading along the respiratory epithelium to the larynx and trachea. Laryngotracheitis (croup) is inflammation of the larynx and trachea. Spasmodic croup usually coincides with a mild upper respiratory infection with the sudden onset of inspiratory stridor occurring at night, lasting for a short duration, and suddenly resolves, without fever or inflammation. Spasmodic croup can also be referred to as "frequently recurrent croup" and "allergic croup" because of its recurrent nature and its overlap with atopic diseases.

Epidemiology/Etiology:
- Peaks between ages 6 and 36 months, but can affect children between 3 months and 6 years of age
- Peaks in the fall and early winter with a major peak in October, coinciding with the parainfluenza type 1 virus (the most common cause)
- More common in boys than girls, with boys to girls ratio of 1.4:1

Risk Factors:
- Family history; anatomic narrowing of the airway, hyperactive airways, and acquired airway narrowing; parental smoking is not a risk factor

Signs and Symptoms:
- Narrowing of the trachea in the subglottic region (Table 15-1).

Differential Diagnoses:
- Acute epiglottitis
- Peritonsillar and retropharyngeal abscesses
- Foreign body aspiration or ingestion
- Laryngeal diphtheria
- Allergic reaction
- Acute angioneurotic edema
- Upper airway injury
- Congenital anomalies of the upper airway (Woods, 2015)

Diagnostic Studies:
- Based on clinical evaluation
- Radiographic confirmation or laboratory tests are not necessary.

Table 15-1: Comparison between Laryngotracheitis and Spasmodic Croup

Laryngotracheitis Gradual onset of symptoms	Spasmodic Croup Abrupt onset and cessation of symptoms
• Nasal irritation, congestion, and coryza ↓ *12–48 hr* • Fever, hoarseness (older children), barking cough (younger children), stridor ↙ ↘	• Occurs at night, short duration (often subsides by time of medical attention) • Afebrile • Mild upper respiratory symptoms • Recurrent episodes during same night or subsequent nights
If progresses • Upper airway obstruction:	*Symptoms resolve* • Cough: 3 d, other symptoms: 7 d	
• Respiratory distress • Restless/anxious • Retractions • Diminished breath sounds • Hypoxia • Cyanosis	

Treatment (Both Pharmacologic and Nonpharmacologic):
- Identify patients at risk for significant upper airway obstruction
- Mild:
  - No therapy or improve with humidified air
  - Consider single dose of dexamethasone (0.6 mg/kg) to prevent worsening systems
  - Manage at home, but educate on indications of when to seek medical treatment
- Moderate/severe:
  - Refer to the emergency department

Bronchiolitis

Description of the Disease: Bronchiolitis is a lower airway disease commonly occurring in infants and children less than 2 years of age. The epithelial cells lining the small airway become inflamed, edematous, and necrotic, in combination with increased mucus and bronchospasm.

Epidemiology/Etiology:
- Occurs in children less than 2 years of age, with a peak between 3 and 6 months
- Peaks during the fall and winter, with increased hospitalizations during the winter and early spring
- Respiratory syncytial virus (RSV) is the most common cause. Other causes include adenovirus, influenza, and parainfluenza.
- Transmitted by direct contact or immediate inhalation of a cough or sneeze

Risk Factors:
- Being younger than 6 months, a history of prematurity ($<$37 weeks' gestation), a cardiopulmonary disease, cigarette smoke exposure, not being breastfed, and immunodeficiency

Signs and Symptoms:
- Begins with mild upper respiratory symptoms
- Within 2 to 3 days wheezing and coughing
- Improves after the third day with symptoms resolving in a week
- Copious secretions
- Increased work of breathing
- Respiratory distress: Cyanosis, intercostal retractions, nasal flaring, tachypnea

Differential Diagnoses:
- Reactive airway disease
- Pneumonia
- Croup
- Foreign body
- Allergic reaction

Diagnostic Studies:
- Based on history and clinical evaluation

Treatment (Both Pharmacologic and Nonpharmacologic):
- The initial treatment for bronchiolitis is prevention of RSV by administering the palivizumab prophylaxis vaccine, if appropriate.
- Mild: Symptomatic treatment
  - Hydration
  - Monitoring respiratory effort
  - Humidified air
  - Rest
- Moderate/severe:
  - Oxygen supplementation if needed
  - Rehydration therapy
  - Bronchodilators, corticosteroids, or ribavirin should not be used as routine treatment.
  - α-Adrenergics or β-adrenergics can be used as an option with close monitoring.
  - Antibiotics should only be used for comorbidities.

Pyloric Stenosis

Description of the Disease: Pyloric stenosis is forceful vomiting in young infants related to a near-complete gastric obstruction resulting from hypertrophy of the pylorus.

Epidemiology/Etiology:
- Occurrence rate of approximately 2 to 3.5/1,000 live births, but varies between regions
- More common in males than in females (4:1 to 6:1), premature infants, and the first-born child
- Etiology is probably multifactorial:
  - Environmental: Maternal smoking during pregnancy, bottle-feeding
  - Genetic
  - Use of macrolide antibiotics by the infant and maternal use during pregnancy and breast-feeding

Signs and Symptoms:
- Symptoms present between 3 and 5 weeks and rarely after 12 weeks of age.
- Postprandial nonbilious projectile vomiting
- Demands to be refed
- Emaciated and dehydrated
- Palpable "olive-like" mass RUQ abdomen
- Hyperbilirubinemia

Differential Diagnoses:
- Gastroesophageal reflux
- Cow's milk protein intolerance
- Adrenal crisis
- Intestinal obstruction
- Liver disease

Diagnostic Studies:
- Detailed history of appetite, urine output, stools, medications
- Palpable "olive" is pathognomonic
- Electrolytes
  - Low serum chloride and potassium, elevated bicarbonate, hyper- or hyponatremia
  - BUN and creatinine to evaluate hydration and renal insufficiency
- CBC: Normal
- If jaundice: Total and conjugated bilirubin, AST, ALT, alkaline phosphatase or GGTP
  - Unconjugated hyperbilirubinemia is consistent
  - Other elevations, evaluate for liver disease
- Abdominal ultrasound as confirmation or upper gastrointestinal contrast study as alternative
  - Barium studies if nondiagnostic
  - Upper endoscopy if results inconclusive

Treatment (Both Pharmacologic and Nonpharmacologic):
- Pyloromyotomy

Colic

Description of the Disease: Crying with no evident cause for more than 3 hours a day and more than 3 days a week, persisting for more than 3 weeks in a healthy infant less than 3 months of age, without failure to thrive.

Epidemiology/Etiology:
- Prevalence ranges from 8% to 40% depending on the diagnostic criteria, population, and parental perception.
- No differences between gender, breast- or bottle-fed, or full-term or preterm infants
- Increased association between siblings
- Etiology is unknown. Gastrointestinal, biologic, and psychosocial are proposed etiologies.
  - Gastrointestinal: Faulty feeding techniques, cow's milk protein intolerance, lactose intolerance, gastrointestinal immaturity, intestinal hypermotility, alternations in fecal microflora
  - Biologic: Immature motor regulation, increased serotonin, tobacco smoke and nicotine exposure, early form of migraine
  - Psychosocial: Temperament, hypersensitivity, parental variables

Signs and Symptoms:
- Cry/fuss paroxysmal behavior
- Colic cry qualitatively different from normal cry (urgent, piercing, distressing)
- Hypertonia
- Difficult to console

Differential Diagnoses:
- Heart failure
- Infection
- Trauma
- Neuromuscular disease
- Central nervous system (CNS) disorder
- Metabolic disease
- Bacterial meningitis
- Failure to thrive
- Gastrointestinal obstruction
- Cow's milk or soy-induced colitis
- Anal fissure
- Intussusception

Diagnostic Studies:
- Suspected based on history, confirmed retrospectively after the course
- History and examination to rule out (r/o) other causes
- Laboratory or imaging studies are not standard.

Treatment (Both Pharmacologic and Nonpharmacologic):
- Parental support
  - Reassurance that colic is common and will spontaneously resolve by 3 to 4 months of age.
  - Reassurance child is not sick
  - Reassure the parents it is not their fault.
  - Encourage the parent to take breaks when needed.
- Decrease environmental stimuli
- Modify feeding technique
- Soothing techniques
  - Using a pacifier
  - Car rides or stroller walks
  - Holding the infant or using a front carrier
  - Rocking
  - Changing the scenery
  - Infant swing
  - Warm bath
  - Rubbing the abdomen
  - Hip-healthy swaddling
  - Providing "white noise"
  - Playing an audiotape of heartbeats
- Alternative interventions that are not supported by literature:
  - Probiotics, soy protein formula, fiber-enriched formula, lactase, sucrose, infant massage, simethicone, herbal remedies, homeopathic remedies, manipulative therapies

Cryptorchidism

Description of the Disease: Cryptorchidism, the failure of one or more testicles to descend into the scrotum by birth, is one of the most common genital disorders identified at birth. The majority of testicles descend prior to 9 months of age. Some males have retractile testes from a strong cremasteric reflex, and are able to be manipulated from the inguinal canal into the scrotum. This is normal and descends at puberty.

Epidemiology/Etiology:
- Risk factors: Prematurity (at 36 weeks of fetal life the testicles descend from the abdomen to scrotum), genetic and environmental contributing factors
- When testes are nonpalpable, 50% are in the inguinal canal or abdomen and 50% are absent secondary to a testicular torsion and infarct.
- 35% to 43% of congenital cryptorchid testes spontaneously descend (Kolon et al., 2014)
- Increased risk for testicular malignancy (4- to 10-fold), even status postsurgical correction, fertility potential, testicular torsion, and inguinal hernia

Signs and Symptoms:
- Asymptomatic
- Empty scrotum

Differential Diagnoses:
- Retractile testes
- Disorder of sex development
- Congenital adrenal hyperplasia

Diagnostic Studies:
- Clinical evaluation. Testes should be palpated at each well-child visit.
- If cryptorchidism is detected at birth, if no spontaneous descent by 6 months, refer to urology.
- Imaging testing by ultrasound or CT scan (risk of radiation and needs sedation) should not be performed prior to referral.
- If nonpalpable, surgical exploration, followed by orchidopexy if indicated.

Treatment (Both Pharmacologic and Nonpharmacologic):
- Usually will spontaneously descend prior to age 1.
- If it does not:
  - Refer to urology
  - Orchidopexy is the main treatment.
  - Human chorionic gonadotropin or luteinizing hormone-releasing hormone injections as an alternative

Developmental Dysplasia of the Hip

Description of the Disease: Developmental dysplasia of the hip (DDH) is an orthopedic condition when the femoral head is not aligned properly within the acetabulum.

Epidemiology/Etiology:
- Prevalence of 5 of every 1,000 infants
- Six to eight times more common in girls
- Three times more common in the left than right, and 20% bilateral
- Unknown etiology; suspected developmental etiology
  - Genetic: 12 times more likely with a family history
  - Birth position: Breech positions cause more pressure on the hips
  - Prolonged swaddling

Risk Factors:
- More common in breech and cesarean deliveries, family history of DDH

Signs and Symptoms:
- Asymmetry of the thigh or gluteal folds
- Hip click or pop
- Leg length discrepancies
- Limited hip abduction
- Limp when cruising or walking
- Pain
- Limited range of motion
- Swayback

Differential Diagnoses:
- Teratogenic anomalies
- Femoral neck fracture
- Traumatic hip subluxation (child abuse)
- Avascular necrosis
- Septic hip
- Contusions
- Slipped capital femoral epiphysis
- Snapping hip syndrome

Diagnostic Studies:
- Hip ultrasound for breech baby girls at 6 weeks of age
- The hips should be evaluated at every well-child examination through 1 year of age.

- Hip stability is evaluated by the Ortolani and Barlow tests. Each hip should be evaluated separately. If a palpable clunk or dislocation of the femoral head posteriorly out of the acetabulum occurs, an orthopedist referral should be made.
- In younger infants ultrasonography could evaluate the hips, but after 4 to 6 months, radiographs are more accurate.

Treatment (Both Pharmacologic and Nonpharmacologic):
- Referral to orthopedics for harness or casting
- Pavlik harness: Infants less than 6 months old, worn for up to 5 months
- Casting: Infants older than 6 months
- Surgery if harness and casting are not successful

Diaper Dermatitis

Description of the Disease: Diaper dermatitis or diaper rash is not a specific disorder, but is an umbrella term for a reaction of the skin from numerous factors, both systemic and local.

Epidemiology/Etiology:
- Prevalence: One in four infants and toddlers
- Associated factors:
  - Skin wetness decreases the ability to tolerate friction
  - Elevated pH level of the skin
  - Fecal enzymes lead to skin maceration and increased permeability
  - Microorganisms, especially *Candida*

Etiology:
- *Candida albicans*: Causes a primary infection and can spread as a secondary invader of other systematic conditions
- *Staphylococcus aureus*
- Risk Factors:
- Diarrhea, frequency of diaper change, use of rubber or plastic pants, recent illness, antibiotic use, exposure to contagious disease

Signs and Symptoms:
- Irritant dermatitis
  - Erythematous desquamative rash
  - Involves convex surfaces touching the skin, spares the inguinal folds
  - Mild erythema without papules
  - Shiny glazed skin appearance
  - Meatitis
- Atopic dermatitis
  - Eczematoid appearance with lichenification
  - Pruritus
  - Atopic dermatitis elsewhere
  - Involves skin folds, spares convex surfaces
- Secondary *Candida* dermatitis
  - Moist, macerated skinfolds
  - Satellite lesions, bright red and confluent, raised borders
  - Satellite lesions on the trunk and legs
  - Painful and tender
- Seborrheic dermatitis
  - Erythematous, salmon-colored patches
  - Greasy scales
  - Involves convex surfaces and creases
- Tidemark dermatitis
  - Elastic band presentation from too tight diapers

Differential Diagnoses:
- Seborrhea dermatitis
- Atopic dermatitis

- Hand-foot-and-mouth disease
- Herpes simplex infection
- Psoriasis
- Varicella
- Miliaria
- Scabies
- Congenital syphilis
- Kawasaki disease

Diagnostic Studies:
- Based on clinical diagnosis
- Laboratory tests are not necessary, but potassium hydroxide preparation and fungal culture of skin scrapings could be diagnostic for *Candida,* or a bacterial culture for *Staphylococcus.*

Treatment (Both Pharmacologic and Nonpharmacologic):
- Minimize contact with wet diapers
- Children changed eight or more times a day have less diaper rash.
- Breathable diapers with water absorbance keep the skin drier.
- Wipe stool off skin immediately and allow skin to dry.
- Use wipes containing water, an emollient, and surfactants.
- Barrier pastes and ointments to create friction barriers
- Apply topical nystatin for 5 to 10 days if *Candida* is suspected.
- 1% hydrocortisone could be used to decrease inflammation (nothing stronger).

Toddler Case Presentation

An 18-month-old male presents to your clinic for a well-child visit. His mother thinks he might be behind in some vaccines, but is not sure if he can get them caught up today because he has a runny nose currently.

Past Medical History: 36 weeks' gestation, a vaginal delivery, without complications. No oxygen required at birth. Birth weight was 6 lb 4 oz.

Medications: None

Allergy: None

Social: Home: Lives with parents, 1 younger brother

Immunizations: 3 Hep B, 2 rotavirus, 3 DTAP, 2 Hib, 3 PCV 13, 3 IPV, 2 LAIV, 1 MMR, and 1 VAR

Family History: Unremarkable

Review of Systems/Health Promotion:
Constitutional: Denies fevers, fatigue,
HEENT: **Head:** Denies head injury. **Eyes:** Denies eye problems. **Ears:** No ear pulling. **Nose:** Denies nasal congestion.
Neck: Denies neck problems
Respiratory: Denies difficulty breathing
Cardiovascular: Denies pale or blue skin discoloration
Gastrointestinal: Denies v/d; eats three meals a day with snacks in between, has a bottle of milk when he goes to sleep at night
Musculoskeletal: Denies injuries
Neurology: Denies seizures
Genitourinary: Six wet diapers/day
Integumentary: Denies rashes, open sores, nail problems
His current weight is 9.9 kg and height is 31 inches.

Physical Examination:
Vital Signs: Temperature = 98.4°F   BP = Not obtained   HR = 110 bpm   RR = 41   Height = 31 inches   Weight = 9.9 kg
General/Psych: Awake and alert; playful with examination. Accompanied to visit by mom.
Skin: Dry, cool to touch, acyanotic, race appropriate

HEENT: **Head:** Normocephalic, anterior and posterior fontanels closed. **Eyes:** PERRL, sclera clear, conjunctiva pink. **Ears:** No drainage, TMs pearly gray bilaterally. **Nose:** Patent, turbinates pink, + clear nasal discharge, septum intact and midline. **Mouth/Throat:** Mucous membranes are moist, pharynx pink, tonsils +1, uvula midline

Cardiovascular: S1, S2, no murmur, regular rate, radial pulses +2 bilaterally, warm and well perfused

Abdomen: Soft, nontender, nondistended +BS, no masses, no hepatomegaly, no splenomegaly

Musculoskeletal: Full range of motion in all joints of the upper and lower extremities, normal tone; Spine: Straight

Neurologic: CN II-X grossly intact

Genitalia: Tanner I, no lesions, discharge, or rashes noted.

Case Study Review Questions

1. His mother is worried if he is eating enough since his 16-month-old cousin is much heavier. How would you respond?

   He is doing fine. Every child is different. He is at the 25th percentile for weight and the 20th percentile for height. I would recommend continuing to offer three meals a day with healthy snacks in between.

   Since he was 36 weeks' gestation, up to the age of 2 years old, his growth chart will be adjusted back 4 weeks. Therefore, his corrected weight is at the 25th percentile and his corrected height is at around the 20th percentile (Fig. 15-3).

2. What developmental milestones should this child have achieved at 18 months?

   Pointing to direct others' attention to an interest

   Saying six words

   Pointing to a body part

   Walking up steps and starting to run

   Stacking two small blocks

   Using spoon and cup without spilling the majority of the time

   Laughing appropriately in response to others

3. What other screenings should be completed?

   A structured developmental screen

   An autism-specific screen

   A dental risk assessment

   A lead, anemia, and tuberculosis risk assessment

4. What vaccines should this child receive during the visit to make his immunizations up to date? How would you address the concern with the runny nose?

   According to the CDC's 2015 immunization schedule, he should receive the DTAP, Hib, PCV 13, HAV. (CDC, 2015)

   A runny nose is not a contraindication, and all vaccines should be administered. True contraindications include being immunocompromised (MMR, VAR) and a history of a severe allergic reaction. A precaution would be to administer the vaccine to a patient with a moderate or severe illness with or without a fever.

5. What anticipatory guidance should be offered to the parents during this examination?

   Read and sing often. Describe pictures found in books. Talk in simple words and use simple commands.

   Encourage family time. He could cling to his parents, which is normal.

   Continue to offer new foods and allow him to mouth and touch them to learn new consistencies and tastes.

   Continue to use a rear-facing car seat until the age of 2 years or until he outgrows the growth recommendations stated by the car seat's manufacturer.

   Safety-proof the house: lock up medications, poisons, cleaning supplies; place gates on stairs; and guard windows

   Call Poison Help (1-800-222-1222) if concerned with any ingestions.

   Keep guns out of the home. If there is a gun in the home, make sure it is stored unloaded and locked up, with the ammunition locked away from the gun.

   A working smoke detector is needed on every floor.

   He is ready to toilet train when he notifies adults when he is wet or dry, he is dry for 2 hours, he pulls his pants up and down, and shows an interest in using the toilet. Have a parent or sibling of the same sex take him to the bathroom. Praise him for sitting on the toilet, even if he is clothed.

   Set limits and be consistent. Praise him for good behavior. Make time-outs brief with simple explanations of the poor behavior. When he gets upset, redirect his focus to another activity.

   Stop using a bottle, especially to go to bed.

   Recommend teeth brushing twice daily. If the dental risk assessment demonstrates he is at risk for caries, he should be referred to a dentist.

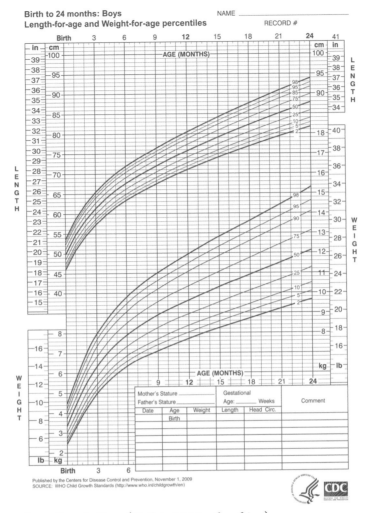

Figure 15-3: Pediatric Boys Growth Chart (Birth to 24 Months of Age).

Common Toddler Diagnoses

Febrile Seizures

Description of the Disease: A simple febrile seizure is the most common seizure in children. A child has a fever without a CNS infection and no history of febrile seizures and has a brief, generalized, tonic–clonic or clonic seizure, which is either simple or complex.

Epidemiology/Etiology:
- Occurs in children ranging from 1 month to 5 years of age, but 93% occur between 6 months and 3 years
- 2% to 4% of children have febrile seizures
- Unknown etiology
  - Excludes seizures from intracranial illness or underlying CNS causes

Risk Factors:
- Family history, NICU stay more than 30 days, developmental delay, day care attendance

Signs and Symptoms:
- Concurrent illness
- Generalized seizure lasting less than 15 minutes
- Rapid rising fever higher than 102.2°F
- Most seizures occur 1 to 24 hours after fever onset
- Minimal postictal confusion

Differential Diagnoses:
- Sepsis
- Meningitis
- Metabolic or toxic encephalopathies
- Hypoglycemia
- Anoxia
- Trauma
- Tumor
- Hemorrhage
- Febrile delirium
- Febrile shivering
- Breath-holding spells

Diagnostic Studies:
- Clinical diagnosis
- Children younger than 12 months of age should receive a lumbar puncture. It is not recommended in children above 18 months of age.
- An EEG or neuroimaging, serum electrolytes, calcium, phosphorus, magnesium, CBC, or blood glucose is not recommended on healthy children.

Treatment (Both Pharmacologic and Nonpharmacologic):
- Protect the airway, breathing, and circulation if seizure persists.
- Administer a fever reducer, acetaminophen or ibuprofen, after the seizure resolves.
- Emergency room evaluation if seizure lasted more than 10 minutes
- Anticonvulsant therapy is not recommended.
- Antipyretics have not proven to decrease the chance of recurrent febrile seizures.

Conjunctivitis

Description of the Disease: Inflammation of the conjunctiva often presents with hyperemia and exudate, but can range in severity. Conjunctivitis occurs when there is a disruption of the eyes' natural defenses.

Epidemiology/Etiology:
- Etiology:
  - Viral: Adenovirus
  - Bacterial: *S. aureus, S. epidermidis, Streptococcus pneumonia, Moraxella catarrhalis, Pseudomonas, and Haemophilus influenza type b* (less frequent since Hib vaccine)
  - Irritants
  - Allergens

Signs and Symptoms:
- Hyperemia (injection of the conjunctivae)
- Epiphora (tearing)
- Subconjunctival hemorrhage
- Chemosis (conjunctival edema)
- Copious purulent discharge
- Eyelid edema
- Foreign body sensation
- Itching
- Burning
- Photophobia
- Preauricular and submandibular lymphadenopathy

Differential Diagnoses:
- Infectious conjunctivitis (bacterial, viral, parasitic)
- Allergic (seasonal) conjunctivitis
- Drug or toxin exposure
- Trichiasis (eyelash irritation)
- Nasolacrimal duct obstruction
- Congenital glaucoma

- Orbital cellulitis
- Blepharitis (eyelid inflammation)
- Uveitis
- Foreign body
- Trauma (corneal abrasion, subconjunctival hemorrhage)

Diagnostic Studies:
- Based on clinical examination
- A bacterial Gram stain and culture are not required, unless gonococcal conjunctivitis is suspected or conjunctivitis is severe, recurrent, or refractory.

Treatment (Both Pharmacologic and Nonpharmacologic):
- Bacterial
  - Acute bacterial: Fluoroquinolone or polymyxin B/trimethoprim
  - Ophthalmology referral if no improvement after 7 days
  - *Neisseria gonorrhoeae or N. meningitidis*: Hospital admission with parenteral antibiotics
- Viral
  - Cool compresses
  - Preservative-free artificial tears four times a day for comfort
  - Antibiotic drops are not recommended.
  - Corticosteroid drops are contraindicated.
  - Education:
    ○ Worsens for the first 4 to 7 days and may take 2 weeks to heal
    ○ Transmission prevention
- Parasitic
  - Refer to ophthalmologist for management
- Allergic
  - Cold compresses
  - Preservative-free artificial tears four times a day for comfort
  - Topical antihistamines
  - Mast cell stabilizers
  - Topical nonsteroidal anti-inflammatory agents
  - Selective use of topical corticosteroids (ophthalmologist)

Strabismus

Description of the Disease: Strabismus is ocular misalignment. It includes esotropia (eye turned inward), exotropia (eye turned outward), or vertical strabismus (eye turned up or down). Infantile esotropia is congenital. Accommodative esotropia is when farsighted children increase focus (accommodate) to see better causing convergence, thus leading to esotropia. Intermittent exotropia, when the eyes drift apart, is the most common between the ages of 2 and 8 years.

Epidemiology/Etiology:
- Infantile esotropia:
  - Onset prior to 6 months
  - Multifocal etiology: Variability in inheritance patterns
- Accommodative esotropia:
  - Children 12 months to 5 years of age
  - Acquired
- Intermittent exotropia:
  - Common in children between ages 2 and 8 years
  - Etiology unknown, but occurs when child is tired, daydreaming, or ill

Signs and Symptoms:
- Poor eye alignment
- Diplopia (children over age 5 years)
- Blurred vision
- Amblyopia (poor vision)
- Asthenopia (vague vision discomfort)

- Visual fatigue
- Photophobia
- Squints one eye
- Limited abduction
- Motor anomalies (nystagmus)

Differential Diagnoses:
- Duane syndrome
- Congenital fibrosis or extraocular muscles
- Sixth nerve palsy
- Myasthenia gravis
- Intracranial tumor
- Hydrocephalus
- Mastoiditis
- Viral
- Arnold–Chiari malformation

Diagnostic Studies:
- Infantile esotropia: If persistent after 2 months, refer to an ophthalmologist
- Accommodative esotropia: Refer to ophthalmologist
- Intermittent exotropia: Cover test detects better than corneal light reflex test, refer to ophthalmologist

Treatment (Both Pharmacologic and Nonpharmacologic):
- Infantile esotropia
  - Surgical repair between 6 months and 2 years of age
- Accommodative esotropia
  - Prescription of full hypermetropic corrective lenses
  - If spectacles do not correct, then surgical repair
- Intermittent exotropia
  - Elective eye muscle surgery
  - Part-time occlusion of the dominant eye
  - Correction for myopia
  - Eye exercises

Intussusception

Description of the Disease: Telescoping of a section of the intestine with the proximal bowel trapped in the distal segment. Intussusception is the most common cause of intestinal obstruction in children and, if not treated, can lead to bowel perforation.

Epidemiology/Etiology:
- Idiopathic etiology
- Medical predisposing factors: Polyps, Meckel diverticulum, Henoch–Schonlein purpura, constipation, lymphomas, lipomas, parasites, rotavirus, adenovirus, and foreign bodies (Burns, Dunn, Brady, Starr, & Blosser, 2013).
- Peaks between 5 and 10 months of age, but common among children between 5 months and 3 years

Signs and Symptoms:
- Classic triad: Paroxysmal colicky abdominal pain, vomiting, and currant jelly stools
- Screaming, legs drawn up for relief
- Periods of calm between episodes
- Glassy eyed and groggy between episodes
- History of UTI
- Lethargy
- Fever
- Sausage-like mass in RUQ of abdomen
- Emptiness in RLQ
- Abdominal distention
- Abdominal tenderness
- Guaiac-positive stools

Differential Diagnoses:
- Incarcerated hernia
- Testicular torsion
- Acute gastroenteritis
- Appendicitis
- Colic
- Intestinal obstruction

Diagnostic Studies:
- Abdominal ultrasound is very accurate. Abdominal flat-plate radiograph can appear normal.
- Air contrast enema is diagnostic and treatment of choice.

Treatment (Both Pharmacologic and Nonpharmacologic):
- Refer to pediatric surgeon
- Radiologic reduction via air contrast enema under fluoroscopy
- Prophylactic IV antibiotics
- If peritonitis, perforation, or hypovolemic shock, then surgery
- Monitored 12 to18 hours postreduction, followed by discharge instructions to return; contact surgery if symptoms reoccur.

Wilms Tumor

Description of the Disease: Most common malignancy of the genitourinary track that manifests as a solitary growth on one or both kidneys

Epidemiology/Etiology:
- 5% of all pediatric malignancies
- Approximately 500 new cases a year in the United States
- Equal occurrence among boys and girls
- More common in black children, less common in Asian children
- Average age for presentation: 3 years
- Associated disorders: WAGR syndrome (Wilms tumor, aniridia, genitourinary anomalies, developmental retardation), hypospadias, cryptorchidism, gonadal dysgenesis
- 5% have bilateral kidney involvement

Signs and Symptoms:
- Asymptomatic abdominal masses
- Hematuria
- Abdominal pain
- Fever
- Dyspnea
- Diarrhea
- Vomiting
- Weight loss
- Malaise
- Firm smooth abdominal mass, not crossing midline

Differential Diagnoses:
- Multicystic kidney
- Hydronephrosis
- Renal cyst
- Mesoblastic nephroma
- Neuroblastoma
- Hepatoblastoma
- Sarcoma
- Lymphoma
- Germ cell tumors
- Benign masses

Diagnostic Studies:
- Ultrasound to evaluate abdominal mass: Reveals intrinsic renal mass
- Refer to pediatric oncologist

- CT: Solid, intrinsic renal mass with the "claw sign"
- Further evaluation for metastatic involvement: CT of chest, abdomen, pelvis, lymph nodes, lungs, and liver
- Ultrasonography with Doppler flow: Evaluate vasculature of tumor
- Urinalysis: Evaluate for hematuria, proteinuria

Treatment (Both Pharmacologic and Nonpharmacologic):
- Individualized treatment based on staging and metastasis
- General approach: Surgical resection and chemotherapy and/or radiotherapy
- Initial therapy cure rates
  - Stage I and II: 90%
  - Stage III: 85%
  - Stage IV: 66%

Preschool Case Presentation

A 4-year-old female patient presents to the urgent care clinic with complaints of upper airway congestion and coughing for the past 4 days. She has had a decreased appetite and her mother reports her daughter wakes up coughing a few times a night over the past 2 days. She recently has been diagnosed with asthma, and her primary care provider prescribed her an albuterol and Flovent 44 mcg inhaler. Currently she is using samples and has not gotten her prescriptions filled. Mom states she has been using the "albuterol one puff twice a day, once in the morning and once at night and the Flovent one puff as needed with her 'coughing fits.'" She admits to using the Flovent only twice in the past 4 days.

Past Medical History: Newly diagnosed asthmatic approximately 3 weeks back, history of otitis media (approximately 15 months ago)

Medications:
Albuterol inhaler, according to mom "taking one puff twice a day"
Flovent inhaler 44 mcg, according to mom "taking one puff as needed for coughing fits"

Allergy:
No medication allergies + environmental allergies: Dust, mold, pollen, pet dander

Immunizations: All immunizations are up to date.

Family History: Unremarkable

Social History:
Goes to early preschool, three mornings a week
Denies recent travel
Has pet fish and a rescued cat

Review of Systems: (History provided by mom)
Constitutional: Diminished appetite, is drinking fine, playful, not sleeping well due to nighttime cough
HEENT: **Head:** Denies complaints of headache. **Eyes:** Denies eye pain or discharge. **Ears:** Denies ear pain or discharge. **Nose:** Has slight runny nose with mild nasal stuffiness. **Throat:** Denies sore throat
Neck: Denies neck pain
Respiratory: Mom states + wet cough more during night, does not hear wheezing unless she puts her ear to chest
Cardiovascular: Denies chest pain
Gastrointestinal: Not eating as well as she did a few days ago, drinking normally; no complaints of belly pain, diarrhea, vomiting
Integumentary: Denies any rashes

Physical Examination:
Vital Signs: Temperature = 98.2°F   Pulse = 98   Respirations = 22   BP = 104/60   Weight = 35 lb
General/Psych: Happy, pleasant, talkative cooperative with examination

HEENT: **Head:** Normocephalic. **Eyes:** PERRLA, Sclera white, conjunctivae without redness. **Ears:** TMs intact, pink, landmarks visible bilaterally. **Nose:** Turbinates slightly swollen with pallor, minor clear mucoid discharge noted, no nasal flaring. **Throat:** Buccal mucosa moist, Pharynx without redness, Tonsils +1, + post nasal drip.

Neck: No lymphadenopathy

Thoracic/Lungs: No retractions noted; mild end expiratory wheeze throughout. Respirations = 22, Pulse O_2 = 99%

Cardiovascular: RRR, + S1, S2, no murmur, apical rate 98, pulses +2 bilaterally

Abdomen: + BS all four quadrants, soft, nontender, nondistended

Skin: Warm to touch, no rashes noted

Case Study Review Questions

1. Her mother is insisting you start her on an antibiotic. What treatment would you offer this patient?

> At this point she should be treated as having a viral illness. She has not had a fever or otalgia, and her lungs reflect an upper airway infection triggering her asthma. Educate the mother on the risk of antibiotic resistance and educate her on supportive treatment.
>
> History and symptomatology points to the fact that the child's asthma may be still uncontrolled, mainly due to lack of understanding of medication management by the mother. Also, exacerbation of symptoms may be due to onset of a mild upper respiratory infection.

2. What education would you provide to this parent with regard to her child's diagnosis and the use of antibiotics?

> The mother needs to understand the underlying pathophysiology of asthma and that it is a hyperresponsiveness to a trigger and not an infection. Common triggers are exposure to pets, dusts, smoke, mold, air pollution, to name a few. Onset of a viral illness such as an upper respiratory infection often can cause an asthma flare-up in children. Asthma is not caused by bacteria and therefore will not respond to antibiotics.

3. What education would you provide to this parent regarding her medication management?

> It seems that the mother has been administering her daughter's medication incorrectly. Albuterol is a short-acting β2 agonist and should be used as a rescue inhaler on an as-needed basis. Flovent is an inhaled corticosteroid and should be utilized twice daily. Proper dosage for a 4-year-old is Flovent 88 mcg twice daily. Not only has the parent mixed up how to use the two medications, but she was also underdosing, which might be the reason for exacerbation of her symptoms.

4. How would you treat this young patient at this point in time?

> The child is playful and speaking well, has mild wheeze, and is not in any apparent distress. Recommended treatment for this mild exacerbation according to current guidelines for the management of asthma (National Institute of Health, 2007) would be to initiate albuterol nebulizer therapy via mask in clinic. If improvement is noted, then continue at home every 4 to 6 hours for the next 24 hours. Inhaled corticosteroids will be increased to Flovent 44 mcg two puff via areochamber twice a day. Patient to follow up with primary care health provider in 24 hours.

5. A week later the patient and her mother return to the urgent care clinic with left ear pain and a temperature of 101.5 for 2 days. On physical examination you notice the left tympanic membrane is red and bulging. Her mother is concerned since she has never had any problems with her ears before. What is your diagnosis and treatment plan?

> Acute otitis media. She has acute onset and symptoms with evidence of a middle ear effusion (TM bulging) and symptoms of inflammation (erythema and otalgia).
>
> Treatment for a child older than 2 years of age with certain diagnosis of otitis media is antibacterial therapy. Amoxicillin 90 mg/kg/day twice daily is the antibiotic of choice for otitis media. Younger children and children who have severe illnesses should be treated for 10 days. If she does not improve within 3 days of treatment, high-dose amoxicillin–clavulanate would be the next therapy.
>
> 14.5 kg × 90 mg/kg/day = 1,305 mg/day/two doses = 652.5 mg/dose (round to 650 mg)
>
> Follow up if no relief in 2 days. A 2-week follow-up is not needed if patient is asymptomatic.

Common Preschool Diagnoses

Pediatric Asthma

Description of the Disease: Asthma is a chronic, reversible inflammatory disease of the airway passages. This disorder is characterized by cough and wheezing. It is typically classified according to level of severity: mild intermittent, mild persistent, moderate persistent and severe persistent.

Epidemiology:
- 9.6% of children under the age of 18
- Males affected more
- Seen in 11% to 16% of African, American Indian, Hispanic children
- Prevalence in the Northeastern and Midwestern states

Etiology:
- Airway inflammation from trigger
  - Allergy: Number one cause in up to 70% of cases
  - Viral infections: Number one cause in children under 5
  - Exercise induced
  - Exposure to cold air
- Leads to bronchoconstriction, airway hyperresponsiveness, airway mucosal wall swelling and mucus production → narrowing of airways (airway obstruction)
- Process is reversible

Risk Factors:
- Allergy
- History of atopic dermatitis
- Exposure to secondhand smoke
- Exposure to strong odors, dust, and cockroaches
- Family history of asthma or atopy
- Early onset of viral respiratory illness
- Gastroesophageal reflux

Signs and Symptoms:
- Cough (worsens at night)
- Wheezing
- Shortness of breath
- Chest tightness

Classification of Asthma according to the National Institute of Health (NIH; National Heart, Lung, and Blood Institute [NHLB], 2007):

Mild intermittent	Symptoms: ≤2 days/wk Nighttime awakenings: ≤2 days/mo No interference with daily activities Peak Expiratory Flow Rate (PEFR): >80% of normal
Mild persistent	Symptoms: >2 days/wk but not every day Nighttime awakenings: • 0–4 yr: 1–2 times/mo • 5–11 yr: 3–4 times/mo Minor limitations in activities PEFR: >80% of normal
Moderate persistent	Symptoms: daily Nighttime awakenings: • 0–4 yr: 3–4 times/mo • 5–11 yr: ≥1 night/wk but not nightly Some limitations in activities PEFR: 60%–80% of normal
Severe persistent	Symptoms: throughout the day Nighttime awakenings: • 0–4 yr: >1/wk • 5–11 yr: occurs nightly Extremely limited in activities PEFR: <60%

Differential Diagnoses:
- Upper airway diseases (sinusitis and URI)
- Respiratory illnesses
  - Bronchiolitis/bronchitis
  - RSV
  - Pneumonia
- Cystic fibrosis
- Gastroesophageal reflux
- Foreign body obstruction
- Vocal cord dysfunction

Diagnostic Studies:
- Detailed history and physical examination
  - Since those under the age of 5 can be difficult to diagnose by spirometry, consider possibility of asthma diagnosis after four confirmed cases of cough and/or wheezing.
- Spirometry: Essential for diagnosis: usually cannot be successfully performed under age 5.
  - >5 years perform pre- and post- short-acting beta agonist
  - Peak flow meters are not diagnostic.
- Peak expiratory flow rate: Used for monitoring only
- Referral to specialist for bronchial provocation test with methacholine or histamine if spirometry is not diagnostic
- Chest X-ray: R/o other diagnoses.
- CBC to r/o other diagnoses; may also show increased eosinophil count if allergic
- Allergy testing to determine possible allergen etiology for those with persistent asthma classification

Treatment:
- NHLB recommends a stepwise approach to asthma management.
- Recommends consultation with asthma specialist at step 3 and 4 for all children younger than 4
- NHLB requires for asthma management by an asthma specialist for children 5 to 11 years old
- If symptoms are controlled for at least 3 months, may implement a step-by-step down approach

Pharmacologic:
- **Pharmacologic Routine Management** (NIH, 2007)
  - *Mild intermittent* (Step 1)
    - Ages: ≤11 years of age
    - *Preferred:*
    - Short-acting β_2-agonist (SABA) for exacerbations (AKA "rescue inhaler" due to its fast-acting onset)
      - Example: Albuterol (nebulizer or inhaler)
    - No need for preventative or long-term medication

If using rescue inhaler more than twice a week for more than 1 month *or* 1 exacerbation requiring oral corticosteroid in a year, need to step up to Step 2
  - *Mild persistent* (Step 2)
    - Geared to prevention of attacks. SABA continues as rescue inhaler.
    - Age: ≤4 years
    - *Preferred:*
      - Low dose of inhaled corticosteroids (ICS) up to twice daily
        - Example: ICS budesonide nebulizer solution (approved for 4 years and younger)
    - *Alternative:*
      - Leukotriene modifier daily
        - Recommended: Montelukast (use in children 6 months and above)
      - Cromolyn nebulizer (may be used as second alternative)
    - Age: 5 to 11 years
    - *Preferred:*
      - Low dose of ICS daily
      - Examples:
        - Budesonide DPI (>4 years)
        - ICS fluticasone HFA (≥4 years)

Alternative:
  ○ Leukotriene modifier daily
  ○ Examples:
    ○ Montelukast
    ○ Zafirlukast (not recommended for children under 7)
  ○ Cromolyn or sustained-release theophylline may be substituted for leukotriene modifier.

If having more than two exacerbations requiring oral corticosteroids in 6 months or less; OR >4 wheezing episodes in year, need to step up therapy to Step 3
  ● *Moderate persistent* (Steps 3 and 4)
    ○ Step 3: Age: ≤4 years (guidelines require consultation with specialist for all children ≤ 4 starting at step 3)
    Preferred:
      ○ Medium dose of ICS
    Alternative:
      ○ None
    ○ Step 3: Age: 5 to 11 years
    Preferred:
      ○ Low dose ICS *plus* either long acting β_2-agonist (LABA), leukotriene modifier or sustained-release theophylline
      ○ Examples of LABA:
        ○ Salmeterol (>4 years of age)
        ○ Formoterol (>5 years of age)
    Or
      ○ Medium dosing ICS

If symptoms persist, step up therapy to step 4.
      ○ Step 4: Age: ≤4 years (managed by asthma specialist)
      Preferred:
        ○ Medium dose of ICS *plus* LABA or montelukast
      Alternative:
        ○ None
      ○ Step 4: Age: 5 to 11 years (consultation with an asthma specialist is required at this stage for all children.)
      Preferred:
        ○ Medium dosing ICS *plus* LABA
      Alternative:
        ○ Medium dose of ICS *plus* leukotriene modifier or sustained-release theophylline
  ● *Severe Persistent*: (Steps 5 and 6)
    ○ Should be managed by asthma specialist
    ○ Treatment centers on high-dose ICS, long-term β_2-agonists, and use of oral corticosteroids.
● **Pharmacologic Acute Office Management** (NIH, 2007)
  ● Assess lung function (if over 5 years) by PEFR or spirometry.
  ● SABA via nebulizer (albuterol: 0.10 to 0.15 mg/kg; up to 2.5 mg); may give nebulizer every 20 minutes up to three doses
  ● Administer supplemental oxygen if needed.
  ● If lung functions improve to >70%, may discharge patient.
    ○ Nebulizer treatments every 4 hours for the next 24 hours,
    ○ Systemic corticosteroids (Prednisone 1 to 2 mg/kg/day divided into three dosages for 3 days; maximum dose 60 mg/day) depending on severity (the use of systemic corticosteroids should be reserved to those <5 years experiencing moderate to severe acute asthma exacerbation in consultation with a physician.)
    ○ Recheck in 48 hours.
    ○ Consider initiation of ICS at follow-up visit.
  ● If lung function worsens or is without improvement, transport to ER.
● **Pharmacologic Treatment for Exercise-Induced Asthma** (NIH, 2007)
  ● Pretreat prior to exercise with any of the following:
    ○ Inhaled SABA: Two inhalations prior to exercise, then repeat in 2 hours if needed (first-line treatment)
    ○ Leukotrienes: Take 2 hours prior to exercise.
    ○ Inhaled cromolyn: Two inhalations prior to exercise

Nonpharmacologic:
- Use of peak flow monitoring for persistent asthma (readings below 80% indicate airway inflammation and need for revision in current treatment)
- Avoid allergens.
  - Instruct families way to decrease environmental factors that can worse asthma (i.e., rugs, pets sleeping with child, avoiding playing outside when air quality is poor)
- Spirometry should be ordered every 1 to 2 years to monitor lung function.
- Medication education:
  - Proper use and cleaning of metered dose inhalers
  - Use of spacers or aerochambers
  - Proper use of nebulizer
  - Review side effects of specific medications:
    - Since ICS are the mainstay of treatment, emphasize rinsing of mouth after use to prevent thrush.
  - Review proper daily medication, proper adjustment of medication for increasing symptom, and when to call health care provider.
- Use written asthma action plan for parents and for school as well.
- Routine follow-up visits every 3 to 6 months as needed
- For exercise-induced asthma:
  - Warm-up exercises before exercise have been shown to decrease exercise-induced asthma symptoms.
  - Wearing a mask or scarf during cooler and cold weather days has also shown to diminish symptoms.

Epiglottitis

Description of the Disease: Inflammation of the epiglottis is a rare disorder, but a pediatric otolaryngologic medical emergency.

Epidemiology/Etiology:
- Caused by *H. influenza* type B (HIB), drastically reduced since HIB vaccine
- Occurs in children between age 1 and 5 years
- 4 to 10 times higher in Navajo Native Americans and Alaskan Eskimos

Signs and Symptoms:
- Abrupt fever
- Severe sore throat
- Dyspnea
- Inspiratory and sometimes expiratory stridor
- Drooling
- Toxic appearance
- Aphonia
- Rapid respiratory obstruction
- Nasal flaring and retractions
- Hyperextension of neck positioning (tripod position)
- Dysphagia
- Irritability, restlessness
- Brassy cough
- Cherry-red epiglottis
- Hoarse cough

Differential Diagnoses:
- Strep pharyngitis
- Acute laryngotracheitis
- Laryngotracheobronchitis
- Diphtheria
- Foreign body

Diagnostic Studies:
- If suspected, do not examine the posterior pharynx. It could cause the epiglottis to spasm and obstruct the airway, leading to respiratory distress.
- Blood cultures

- Lateral neck radiograph with respiratory professionals presence (evaluating for the "thumb sign")
- Otolaryngologist evaluation of cherry-red epiglottis

Treatment (Both Pharmacologic and Nonpharmacologic):
- Prevention: Vaccination of the HIB series
- Transfer to emergency department, notify otolaryngologist of arrival
- Evaluate in the OR with trained otolaryngologist
- Establish an airway via nasotracheal or tracheostomy
- Broad-spectrum IV antimicrobials

Hand–Foot–Mouth Disease

Description of the Disease: Hand–foot–mouth disease is an infectious disease seen in pre- and school-age children caused by the Coxsackievirus A (enterovirus). Characteristic symptoms include vesicular-type lesions on the hand, foot and in the mouth, hence the name.

Epidemiology:
- Commonly seen in preschoolers
- Seen more in late spring through early fall

Etiology:
- Coxsackievirus A or enterovirus 71
- Spread by fecal–oral route or respiratory route
- Incubation is 3 to 6 days post exposure

Risk Factors:
- Age (under 5)
- Crowded conditions (day care, school)
- Seasonal (tepid climates)
- Contact with infected person or object

Signs and Symptoms:
- Fever and general feeling of malaise
- Poor appetite
- Occasional abdominal pain
- Sore throat: vesicular lesions found within the mouth structures (tongue, gums, buccal membranes, palate, etc.). Lesions ulcerate with erythemic circumference.
- Erythemic rash: Macular → vesicular lesions (approx. 2 to 3 mm) mainly appear on palms and soles of feet and occasionally on buttocks
- May only have 5 to 10 lesions

Differential Diagnoses:
- Herpangina (similar in signs/symptoms but no lesions on palms and soles of feet)
- Herpes simplex
- Fifth disease
- Scarlet fever
- Aphthous ulcers

Diagnostic Studies:
- None indicated; diagnosed by clinical presentation

Treatment
Pharmacologic:
- Symptomatic treatment: Acetaminophen for fever and pain relief

Nonpharmacologic:
- Popsicles, ice water, and sherbet for pain relief
- Warm saline gargles
- Encourage fluids

Impetigo (Nonbullous Type)

Description of the Disease: Impetigo is a contagious skin infection seen mainly in children but can occur in adults. The nonbullous type is mainly seen in primary care.

Epidemiology:
- Most commonly seen in the 2 to 6 year age group, but can occur at any age
- Occurs equally in girls and boys
- Higher incidence in summer months or in warm, humid climates
- 10% of all primary pediatric care visits

Etiology:
- *S. aureus* (major cause in up to 70%)
- Group A β-hemolytic Streptococcus (GABHS)
- Two main classifications: Nonbullous and bullous (Koning et al., 2012)
  - Nonbullous:
    - More commonly seen and more contagious
    - Affects any age group but still prevalent in the preschool and early-school-age child
    - Most cases caused by *S. aureus*, although can see GABHS
    - Occurs mainly on the face and extremities
    - Mainly vesicular lesions and pustules
  - Bullous:
    - Mostly seen in neonates and infants
    - Seen mainly on the trunk and in moist areas (groin, axillae, neck folds)
    - Much larger lesions than those seen in the nonbullous (bullae) type
    - All cases caused by *S. aureus* that releases a toxin that formulates bullae

Risk Factors:
- Warm climates
- Breakage in the skin, scratch, minor cut, insect bite
- Poor hygiene
- Contact with infected lesions
- Household members
- Co-skin conditions such as eczema

Signs and Symptoms:
- Nonbullous:
  - Classic presentation: Initially appears as a maculopapular lesion → 1 to 2 mm vesicle → pustule → ruptures quickly (forming shallow weeping erythemic ulcers and spreads → produces classic honey colored crusts)
  - Common areas on the face are around mouth, nose.
  - May have regional lymphadenopathy
- Bullous:
  - Initially begins as a vesicular lesion → rapidly increases in size forming a bullae → lesion changes from clear to cloudy and stays intact longer; base is not erythemic → ruptures centrally forming honey color crusts while outer area becomes scaly
  - Favors moist areas, axillae, diaper area, groin

Differential Diagnoses:
- Herpes simplex
- Varicella
- Insect bites
- Contact and atopic dermatitis
- Bullous impetigo:
  - Second-degree burns
  - Bullous pemphigoid reactions
  - Steven–Johnson Syndrome
  - Bullous erythema multiforme

Diagnostic Studies
- None indicated; diagnosed by clinical presentation
- Wound culture only if unusual presentation, severe presentation, or treatment failure

Treatment:
Pharmacologic:
- Topical antibiotics are preferred over systemic for mild cases.
- Recommend removal of crusts with gentle washing two to three times a day to promote absorption of topical antibiotics.

- Nonbullous: (topical)
  - Mupirocin 2% ointment:
    - Apply to affected area three times daily for 7 to 14 days.
    - Approved use in children 3 months or older
  - Retapamulin 1% ointment:
    - Apply to affected skin twice daily for 5 days.
    - Total treatment area should not exceed 2% of total body surface area in children.
    - Approved use in children 9 months or older
- Systemic antibiotics recommended for moderate/severe cases of nonbullous impetigo, those cases not responding to topical treatment, and all bullous impetigo. Recommended length of treatment is 7 days.
  - Dicloxacillin:
    - Children: 12.5 to 25 mg/kg/day p.o. given in divided doses every 6 hours
  - Cephalexin:
    - Children: 25 to 50 mg/kg/day orally given in divided doses every 6 hours
  - If penicillin allergy:
    - Macrolides: (increasing incidence of resistance)
      - Children: 40 mg/kg/day orally given in divided doses every 6 hours
  - If MRSA is suspected or confirmed, Infectious Diseases Society of America recommends doxycycline, clindamycin, or sulfamethoxazole–trimethoprim (SMX-TMP) to be prescribed (Stevens et al., 2014)
    - Adjunct therapy: Intranasal topical antibiotics
      - If repeated occurrences, treat, or if MRSA is suspected in addition to above:
        - Mupirocin topical 2%, apply to nares three times daily for 7 days.

Nonpharmacologic:
- Good hygiene; thorough hand washing
- Removal of crusts by gentle washing two to three times a day, preferably before application of topical treatments
- Contagious until treated with antibiotics for 48 hours
- Keep fingernails short so as to not to scratch lesions
- Avoid sharing of towels and washcloths

Rubeola (Measles)

Description of the Disease: Measles is a highly contagious viral illness preventable by vaccination. However, due to parental opposition to vaccinating their children, resurgence of this almost eradicated disease is making a comeback.

Epidemiology: (Chen, 2015)
- Measles is still a global concern with approximately 400 deaths/day occurring in young children in foreign countries (WHO, 2015).
- 30 million cases a year
- Measles as an epidemic no longer exists; however in 2014 there were 644 reported cases in the United States.
  - 97% of these cases were from foreign travelers into the country.
- Most outbreaks occur in unimmunized individuals.
- Incubation 7 to 10 days from exposure; child is contagious from 3 to 5 days before the rash appears to 4 days after the onset of rash.

Etiology
- Exposure to the paramyxovirus (an RNA virus) of genus *Morbillivirus*
- Transmission is airborne and by droplet contact.

Risk Factors:
- Unimmunized or partially immunized child (vaccination is initially given between 12 and 15 months with a second dose between 4 and 6 years)
- Immunocompromised

Signs and Symptoms:
- Prodromal phase
  - High fever
  - Classic 3 "Cs" presentation:
    - Conjunctivitis (may have photosensitivity)

○ Coryza
○ Cough
- Koplick spots (diagnostic): whitish–bluish miniscule spots with reddened ring found on the buccal mucosa
- Rash
  - Erythemic maculopapular and confluent in nature
  - Occurs 3 to 5 days after prodromal phase
  - Begins on face, progresses downward to trunk, then upper extremities, buttocks, and finally lower extremities involves hands and feet
  - Rash lasts approximately 5 days

Differential Diagnoses:
- Rubella
- Scarlet fever
- Drug rash
- Erythema infectiosum
- Roseola (if seen in under 2)
- Kawasaki disease
- Dengue fever
- Rocky Mountain spotted fever

Diagnostic Studies:
- Diagnosed by clinical presentation
- Measles serology: IgM titer after day 3 of rash (preferred)
- IgG titer can be ordered 7 days after rash showing a fourfold increase from acute to convalescence levels.

Treatment:
Prevention is the best treatment. Immunization is usually given at 12 to 15 months of age and then between 4 and 6 years of age. Second dose can also be given 28 days after first dose if trying to catch up on vaccinations.

Pharmacologic: (WHO, 2009)
- Antivirals are not effective with measles.
- WHO recommends the administration of vitamin A in all acute cases of measles to decrease mortality, given in two dosages 24 hours apart:
  - 50,000 IU for infants younger than 6 months of age
  - 100,000 IU for infants 6 to 11 months of age
  - 200,000 IU for children 12 months of age and older
- Recommended treatment for exposure: (McLean et al., 2013)
  - For children older than 12 months of age and exposed or individuals not adequately immunized, give MMR vaccine within 72 hours of exposure.
  - Any nonimmune individual exposed to measles, administer immunoglobulin (IG) within 6 days of exposure.
  - Recommended dosage is 0.5 mL/kg of body weight (maximum dose = 15 mL).
  - High-risk individuals for IG include infants <12 months, unvaccinated pregnant women, and those who are immunocompromised.
  - If an outbreak affects preschool-aged children or adults with community-wide transmission, a second dose should be considered for children aged 1 through 4 years or adults who have received 1 dose.

Nonpharmacologic:
- Symptomatic treatment
  - Acetaminophen for fever
  - Oral fluids
  - Air humidification to help with respiratory signs/symptoms
  - Saline drops and sunglasses for photosensitivity

Constipation

Description of the Disease: Constipation occurs often in childhood and is regarded as a normal occurrence, which will resolve with age. Anticipatory guidance including a healthy diet, toilet training, and toileting behaviors can often prevent constipation. Often painful bowel movements can lead to stool withholding, which worsens the constipation, leading to fecal impaction. Ninety-five percent of children with constipation have functional constipation.

Epidemiology/Etiology:
- Functional constipation occurs often with the introduction of solid foods and cow's milk, toilet training, and entry into school.
- Trigger: Painful defecation, toilet training too vigorous, diet with high-processed foods, rice cereal, cow's milk
- Less than 5% of pediatric constipation has an organic cause.

Signs and Symptoms:
- Two or less defecations per week
- Incontinence
- Dyschezia (straining)
- Encopresis
- Abdominal pain
- Abdominal distention
- Vomiting
- Hard stools
- Painful stools
- Small- or large-diameter stools
- Anal fissures
- Palpable stool in abdomen
- Presence of large fecal mass in rectum
- Perianal irritation
- Hemorrhoids
- Absent anal wink

Differential Diagnoses:
- Functional constipation
- Low dietary fiber
- Inadequate fluid intake
- Anorexia nervosa
- Starvation
- Cerebral palsy
- Spinal cord injury
- Myelomeningocele
- Neurofibromatosis
- Hypokalemia
- Juvenile systemic sclerosis
- Drugs
- Hirschsprung disease
- Cow's milk intolerance
- Cystic fibrosis
- Anorectal anomalies
- Celiac disease
- Infantile botulism
- Lead poisoning
- Hypothyroidism
- Neurologic disorder

Diagnostic Studies:
- Thorough clinical history and physical examination
- Digital rectal examination, abdominal ultrasound, and abdominal radiography is not routinely necessary.

Treatment (Both Pharmacologic and Nonpharmacologic):
- Encourage adequate amounts of fiber (5 g/day for children under 2 years; 11 to 16 g/day for a 6-year-old) and fluid
- Decrease milk intake, limit to less than 24 oz/day
- Delay toilet training if withholding stool, "child-oriented" approach
- Parents should ask routinely about bowel movements, especially if the child goes by himself/herself.
- Routine toilet time after meals
- Sorbitol-containing juices (apple, prune, or pear)

- Substitute barley or whole-grain cereal for rice cereal
- Medications:
  - Infants: Glycerin suppositories, polyethylene, lactulose, or sorbitol
  - Toddlers and children: Sodium phosphate enema for impaction, polyethylene glycol 0.4 to 0.8 g/kg/day, lactulose, mineral oil, magnesium hydroxide, or stimulant laxative
  - Fecal impaction: Sodium phosphate enema for impaction, polyethylene glycol 1 to 1.5 g/kg/day for 6 days, or lactulose

Acute Gastroenteritis

Description of the Disease: Diarrhea in children can have numerous etiologies. Diarrhea is three or more loose stools per day. Its severity ranges from acute diarrhea, lasting less than a few days; acute bloody diarrhea; and persistent diarrhea, lasting 14 days or more.

Epidemiology/Etiology:
- Pediatric diarrhea: 1.5 million outpatient visits, 200,000 hospitalizations, and 300 deaths annually in the United States
- Acute gastroenteritis: On average, children less than 5 years have about two episodes of gastroenteritis annually.
- Rotavirus: One-third of all hospitalizations for children less than 5 years with diarrhea
- Common causes:
  - Viral: Rotavirus, norovirus, enteric adenoviruses, astrovirus, enterovirus
  - Bacteria: *Campylobacter jejuni, Salmonella, Escherichia coli, Shigella*
  - Protozoa: *Cryptosporidium, Giardia lamblia, Entamoeba histolytica*

Signs and Symptoms:
- Dehydration: Sunken eyes, dry mucous membranes, poor skin turgor, decreased alertness
- Diarrhea
- Vomiting
- Fever
- Anorexia
- Abdominal cramps
- Blood in stool
- Decreased food intake

Differential Diagnoses:
- Diabetes
- Metabolic disorders
- Urinary tract infections
- Meningitis
- Gastrointestinal obstruction
- Ingestion

Diagnostic Studies:
- Clinical history and examination:
  - Viral: Low-grade fever, watery diarrhea without blood
  - Bacterial: High fever, diarrhea with blood
- Laboratories are not routinely indicated.
  - Electrolytes are beneficial in patients who are severely dehydrated and need intravenous fluid therapy.
  - Stool studies are beneficial during outbreaks or recent foreign travel.

Treatment (Both Pharmacologic and Nonpharmacologic):
- Drug therapy is not recommended for most cases of gastroenteritis, except zinc supplementation and probiotics could be considered.
  - Exceptions: Antibiotic for acute enteritis with sepsis, cholera, shigellosis, amebiasis, giardiasis
  - Ondansetron, a selective serotonergic 5-HT3 receptor antagonist, as a single-dose antiemetic
- Oral rehydration therapy as soon as diarrhea starts
  - Rehydration phase: Fluids replaced over a 3- to 4-hour period.
  - Maintenance phase: Fluids and calories are continued at baseline rate.
  - Breast-feeding should be continued.

- Fruit juice, sports drinks, soft drinks, and tea should be avoided.
- Admit for inpatient hydration therapy if intractable emesis, severe dehydration (loss of more than 9% of body weight), less than 1 year old with lethargy/irritability, complicated disease course, or concern of reliable caregivers.

Enterobiasis (Pinworms)

Description of the Disease: In the United States, enterobiasis is the most common worm infection. Humans are the only vector to transfer the parasite. The eggs can survive indoors for 2 to 3 weeks.

Epidemiology/Etiology:
- Highest occurrence in school-aged children and institutionalized children
- Transmitted via ingestion of pinworm eggs
  - Deposit around the anus and transmitted to mouth by hands, toilet seats, or personal belongings
  - Directly ingest eggs when breathing
- Incubation period of 1 to 2 months to mature in the small intestines, spreads to the colon, and lays eggs around the anus at night
- Reinfection is common in children.

Signs and Symptoms:
- Asymptomatic
- Perirectal and/or vaginal pruritus
- Secondary bacterial infection
- Teeth grinding
- Insomnia
- Abdominal pain
- Urethritis
- Vaginitis
- Salpingitis
- Pelvic peritonitis
- Irritability
- Hyperactivity

Differential Diagnoses:
- Urethritis
- Vaginitis
- Salpingitis
- Pelvic peritonitis
- Alternative intestinal parasite
- Atopic dermatitis
- Diaper dermatitis
- Candidiasis
- Allergic dermatitis

Diagnostic Studies:
- Transparent adhesive on perianal skin during the night for three consecutive nights; microscopic evaluation for eggs present on tape
- Serologic or stool studies are not recommended.

Treatment (Both Pharmacologic and Nonpharmacologic):
- Transmission prevention: Shower every morning, good hand washing, cut fingernails regularly, frequent changing of linens and underclothing
- Mebendazole, pyrantel pamoate, or albendazole
  - One dose initially followed by second dose in 2 weeks
- If more than one household member is infected, the whole household should be treated.

Nocturnal Enuresis

Description of the Disease: Urinary incontinence or "bedwetting" occurs in approximately 15% of children at 5 years of age, with spontaneous resolution often occurring.

Epidemiology/Etiology:

- Decreases in occurrence as children get closer to adolescence
- 10% to 15% of children still have nocturnal enuresis by age 6 years.
- More common in boys than girls
- More common in children with a family history of a first-degree family member: 50% chance a parent also had it
- Common in comorbidities of attention-deficit hyperactivity disorder

Signs and Symptoms:

- Bedwetting
- Constipation
- Encopresis
- Severe stress

Differential Diagnoses:

- Diabetes mellitus
- Obstructive sleep apnea
- Encopresis or constipation
- Urinary tract infection
- Child abuse
- Renal disease
- Diabetes insipidus

Diagnostic Studies:

- Thorough history: Previously dry for 6 months, daytime incontinence, constipation, severe recent stress
- Thorough physical examination: Genital examination, neurologic examination
- Urinalysis as screening tool for renal disease
- Stool and bladder diary

Treatment (Both Pharmacologic and Nonpharmacologic):

- Discuss expectations with parents. A supportive home environment is needed.
- Educate that this is not caused by a physical abnormality. Children should not be punished for it. Nocturnal enuresis often resolves by itself.
- Combination therapy is the most beneficial:
  - Initial therapy: Education and reassurance
    - Void regularly during the day and before bed.
    - Limit fluids during the evening.
    - Avoid high-sugar and caffeinated beverages.
    - Diaper and pull-up use routinely will interfere with motivation.
    - Motivational therapy (reward system, sticker chart)
  - If no improvement after 6 months
    - Enuresis alarms (long-term treatment)
    - Desmopressin (short-term treatment): Initial dose 0.2 mg, titrated up to 0.4 mg; taper when discontinuing
  - If no improvement after 3 months
    - Refer to urology

Kawasaki Disease

Description of the Disease: Kawasaki disease (KD), a vasculitis with a predilection for the coronary arteries, is one of the most common pediatric vasculitides and the most common cause of acquired heart disease in developed countries. KD is the widespread inflammation of medium-sized muscular arteries.

Epidemiology/Etiology:

- Obscure etiology
- Genetic predisposition
  - Children of parents with KD have a twofold risk.
  - Siblings have a 10-fold risk.
- Acute illness resolves, but coronary artery lesions occur in 3% to 5% of children treated with intravenous immunoglobulin and 25% untreated children.

Signs and Symptoms:
- Prodrome of respiratory or gastrointestinal symptoms
- Systematic inflammation combined with mucocutaneous inflammation
- Fever: >38.5°C, minimally responsive to antipyretics, may be intermittent
- Bilateral nonexudative conjunctivitis (>75% of cases)
- Erythematous lips and oral mucosa (90% of cases)
- Polymorphous rash (70% to 90% of cases): Usually begins the first few days
- Peripheral changes of extremities: Erythema, edema, and desquamation (50% to 85% of cases)
- Cervical lymphadenopathy (at least one note >1.5 cm in diameter) (25% to 70% of cases)
- Cardiac manifestations: Tachycardia, gallop sounds, muffled heart tones
- Coronary artery aneurysms > 10 days after illness
- Cold, pale, cyanotic digits (young infants)
- Arthritis of large joints
- Diarrhea, vomiting, abdominal pain
- Irritability
- Cough, rhinorrhea
- Decreased appetite

Differential Diagnoses:
- Infectious exanthema
- Viral gastroenteritis
- Viral upper respiratory tract infection
- Pneumonia
- Meningitis
- Adenovirus
- Streptococcal pharyngitis
- Measles
- Stevens–Johnson syndrome
- Epstein–Barr virus
- Echovirus
- Toxic shock syndrome
- Rocky Mountain spotted fever
- Systemic juvenile idiopathic arthritis

Diagnostic Studies:
- Clinical diagnostic criteria of fever lasting 5 days or more without another cause and at least four of the following five: bilateral bulbar conjunctival injection, oral mucous membrane changes (injected lips or pharynx, or strawberry tongue), peripheral extremity changes, polymorphous rash, cervical lymphadenopathy
- Refer to emergency department if suspected

Treatment (Both Pharmacologic and Nonpharmacologic):
- Refer to emergency department.
- Intravenous immune globulin (IVIG) 2 g/kg infused over 8 to 12 hours one time
- Aspirin 80 to 100 mg/kg daily divided into four doses
- Echocardiogram for baseline and to evaluate cardiac involvement
- Observe for 24 hours after initial therapy to evaluate resolving symptoms
- On follow-up, monitor for recurring symptoms, repeat echocardiogram at 2 to 6 weeks
- Activity restrictions
- Postpone live vaccines for at least 11 months after IVIG is administered.

School-Age Case Presentation

Seven-year-old Danny has type 1 diabetes for 1 year now and is being seen in your office accompanied by his father with the chief complaint of a sore throat, fever, and a rash. He has been sick for the past 24 hours, which started with a sore throat and 101° fever. On the first evening, he began developing a rash on his cheeks, neck, back, chest, and abdomen which now seems to be spreading to his arms. Danny states his belly hurts at times but no diarrhea or vomiting. He has been drinking but his eating has diminished. His father is concerned since before the symptoms began he had shrimp and was wondering if it could be connected. During the visit, his father also, noted that he worried that Danny has been "very hyper" and "boisterous" at home and is wondering if he could be developing ADHD.

Past Medical History: Type 1 diabetes, controlled, history of otitis externa

Medications:
5.5 units of Lantus insulin once daily
5 to 8 units daily of Novolog for meal coverage
Allergy: None

Immunizations: All immunizations are up to date.

Family History:
Mother: +ADHD;
Maternal grandmother: Has history of type 1 diabetes (well controlled)
Father: Healthy
Paternal grandfather: + hypertension; +high cholesterol (both controlled on medications)
Sibling sister (age 5): Healthy

Social History:
In grade 2, performs well in school
Denies any recent travel
Has one pet dog

Previous Diagnostic Data:
FBS: (done 1 month ago) 84 mg/dL (normal blood sugar range 5 to 11 years of age: 70 to 180 mg/dL)
HbA1c: 6% (normal for 6 to 12 is <8%)
Urinalysis: WNL: negative for ketones and sugar

Review of Systems/Health Promotion:
Constitutional: + tiredness + chills, states "feels sick"
HEENT: **Head:** Denies headache, dizziness; **Ears:** Denies ear pain; **Eyes:** Denies eye pain or discharge; **Nose:** Denies runny nose or nasal stuffiness; **Throat:** Sore throat: "hurts to eat and swallow," cold drinks and popsicles makes it feel better
Neck: Feels bumps in neck, denies stiff neck
Respiratory: Denies wheezing, cough, or shortness of breath
Cardiovascular: Denies chest pain
Gastrointestinal: States belly hurts off and on, drinking normally, not eating as well as prior to being ill
Integumentary: Rash is slightly itchy, makes him "feel hot"; scalp began itching 1 day prior to development of symptoms

Physical Examination:
Vital Signs: Temperature = 101.4°F   Pulse = 102   Respirations = 20   BP = 104/70   Weight = 54 lb
General/Psych: Appears flushed, quiet, yawning a lot, cooperative with examination
HEENT: **Head:** Normocephalic. **Eyes:** PERRLA, Sclera white, conjunctivae without redness. **Ears:** TMs intact, pearly gray, landmarks visible bilaterally. **Nose:** Turbinates slightly swollen and deep pink, no discharge noted, no nasal flaring. **Throat:** Buccal mucosa moist, Pharynx reddened, Tonsils +3 B/L with some exudate, tongue whitish coating with reddened raised papillae
Neck: + anterior cervical adenopathy, has full ROM without pain
Thoracic/Lungs: No retractions noted, CTA bilaterally; Respirations = 20
Cardiovascular: RRR without murmur, rubs, clicks; apical rate = 102
Abdomen: + BS all four quadrants, soft, nontender, no organomegaly
Skin: Warm to touch, slightly raised maculopapular rash noted on neck, trunk, arms, and upper thighs, rash appears almost linear and darker in antecubital folds of arms.

Case Study Review Questions

1. Considering the patient's rash, fever, and sore throat, what is your differential diagnoses?

   a. Scarlet fever
   b. Streptococcal pharyngitis
   c. Fifth disease
   d. Measles
   e. Rubella
   f. Kawasaki disease
   g. Toxic shock syndrome
   h. Drug reaction

2. What diagnostic studies should be ordered by the nurse practitioner at this time? What is the rationale for each?

   a. Rapid Antigen Detection Test (RADT) for Group A streptococci (Rapid Strep Test) (positive results: 99% specificity and 90% sensitivity)
   b. If negative, perform throat culture (back-up cultures in children if negative are recommended by the Infectious Diseases Society of America)
   c. Finger stick for blood glucose level (to determine management of diabetes)

3. If the patient's RADT is positive, what is your final diagnosis? What is the mainstay treatment for this diagnosis?

   This patient's diagnosis is scarlet fever.
   Treatment recommended by the Infectious Diseases Society of America:
   Penicillin V: 250 mg p.o. two to three times daily for 10 days.
   If allergic:
   First-generation cephalosporin (for those not anaphylactic) for 10 days, clindamycin or clarithromycin for 10 days, or azithromycin for 5 days (Shulman et al., 2012)
   Acetaminophen can be given as an antipyretic and analgesic.

4. What would be an appropriate way to address and diagnose this father's concern about his son's behaviors?

   Danny's father needs to be educated in the signs/symptoms required for a true diagnosis of ADHD.

   Danny must meet six of the following criteria symptoms set by the *Diagnostic and Statistical Manual of Mental Disorder*, fifth edition (*DSM-V*). Symptoms must exist for at least 6 months, and seen in two settings (both home and school):
   • Fidgety with hands and/or feet; squirms
   • Inability to sit still or remain in chair during appropriate times

   • Excessive energy
   • Talks nonstop
   • Unable to play quiet games or board games
   • Easily distracted
   • Loses interest rapidly in a task
   • Often forgetful or losing things
   • Difficulty organizing tasks and activities
   • There are also a variety of checklist assessments such as ADHD Rating Scale IV (5 to 17) and the Conners Comprehensive Behavior Rating Scales (6 to 17 years) to help confirm diagnosis.

5. Danny's office blood sugar is 180 mg/dL. What must you consider with his illness and his insulin management?

   Sick day management centers around five principles. Adapting these principles to Danny,

   1. Reinforce: Never stop insulin even if appetite is diminished, in fever entities without GI involvement (i.e., vomiting and diarrhea). Glucose level will usually increase. Add supplemental rapid-acting insulin according to glucose and ketone results (in fever entities). Danny's glucose is fine at this time and no additional insulin is needed.
   2. Increase blood glucose and ketone testing to at least every 3 to 4 hours.
   3. Encourage hydration through water, salty foods, and liquids (chicken soup, broths, water, simple carbs such as rice and crackers). If blood sugar levels fall below 180, add sugary drinks such as Gatorade, Kool-Aid, flat colas, or ginger ale.
   4. Treat underlying illness.
   5. Review a written sick management plan with Danny's dad and Danny with the goal of minimizing diabetic ketoacidosis or hypoglycemia.

6. Since every office visit should be an opportunity for patient education, what anticipatory guidance should you promote in the school-age child?

   According to the Bright Futures Anticipatory Guidelines by the American Academy of Pediatrics, children and parents should be assessed in areas of school adaptation, especially in the area of bullying; mental health and the encouragement of building self-esteem and independence; physical health and expected body changes; proper nutrition and physical activity; oral health; and safety especially playground, sports and careful monitoring/limitations in screen use (i.e., computers, iPads, TV, and video gaming).

Common School-Age Diagnoses

Diabetes Mellitus: Type 1

Description of the Disease: Diabetes mellitus is a chronic illness in children and young adults involving glucose intolerance due to a lack of insulin being produced by the pancreas. This in turns leads to symptoms of hyperglycemia.

Epidemiology:
- Most common childhood chronic illness
- 15% of children living in the United States
- Highest in Caucasian incidence while Chinese have the lowest
- Peak appearance of symptoms is usually at 5 to 9 years of age and again at puberty.
- Increasing in prevalence

Etiology:
- Related to the self-destruction of the β-cells of the pancreas, responsible for the production of insulin
- Possible genetic component
- Possibly an autoimmune process due to various environmental, bacterial, viral, and dietary (gluten and cow's milk) triggers

Risk Factors:
- Diabetes in first-degree relatives
- Presence of genetic markers: HLA, DR3, B8, B15

Signs and Symptoms:
- Classic three "Ps": Polyuria, polydipsia, polyphagia
- Enuresis in a previously toilet-trained child
- Weight loss
- Delay in growth
- Fatigue and decrease in activity level
- Blurry vision
- *Monilia* candidiasis infection
- If initial signs/symptoms are missed, may exhibit signs/symptoms of diabetic ketoacidosis:
  - Lethargy
  - Headache
  - Abdominal pain
  - Vomiting
  - Fruity odor of breath
  - Decreased heart rate and increased BP

Differential Diagnoses:
- Diabetes mellitus type 2 (increasing incidence due to obesity in children)
- Pancreatitis
- Endocrine tumors
- Salicylate poisoning
- Steroid therapy
- Renal glucosuria

Diagnostic Studies:
- Serum glucose level
  - Fasting: >126 mg/dL (on two occasions)
  - Nonfasting: >200 mg/dL
- Urine for glucose and ketones
- HbA1C
- C-peptide insulin level
- Chem Profile: Attention to electrolytes and BUN
- Lipid levels

Treatment:
- Mainstay of care involves insulin therapy (cornerstone), nutritional counseling, and prevention of complications. Referral to endocrinologist recommended for management.

Pharmacologic:

- Insulin therapy: Tailored to HbA1C and blood glucose levels
  - Targeted HbA1C: <7.5
  - Blood glucose levels:
    - Before meals: 90 to 130 mg/dL
    - Bedtime/overnight: 90 to 150mg/dL
- First-line insulin regimen in children: Basal–bolus combination
  - Basal/long acting: Glargine (Lantus), detemir (Levemir) one or two injections per day
    - Onset 3 to 4 hours; peaks 6 to 18 hours; lasts 18 to 26 hours
  - Rapid acting: Lispro (Humalog) /Aspart (NovoLog)/ Glulisine (Apidra) given prior to meals
    - Onset: 10 minutes; peaks 1 to 2 hours; lasts 4 hours
  - In children, an initial daily dose will be 0.5 to 1 units/kg/day divided evenly between basal and bolus.
- Insulin injection devices
  - Syringes
  - Pen devices
  - Automatic injection devices
  - Pumps

Nonpharmacologic:

- Self-monitoring blood glucose (SMBG): Before meals (breakfast, lunch, dinner) and bedtime (may need to increase times during periods of illness and exercise)
- Monitor and educate on signs/symptoms and management of hypoglycemia and hyperglycemia.
- Dietary education: Refer to nutritionist or diabetic educator; important to stress well-balanced diet and limited amounts of sweets; ADA diet recommended
- Educate on sick day plans and how to adjust insulin accordingly
  - Five principles of sick day management of children with diabetes (Brink et al., 2014)
    - Do not stop insulin (this can increase the risk of diabetic ketoacidosis).
      - Insulin is usually increased or decreased depending on blood glucose and ketone levels
      - Rapid insulin is used supplemental according to results.
      - Supplemental rapid insulin dosage is usually 0.05 to 0.1 unit/kg or 5% to 10% of total daily dosage of insulin
    - Blood sugars and ketones should be monitored more closely during illnesses. (3 to 4 hours; GI illnesses may need every 1 to 2 hours depending on severity.)
      - Illnesses with fever tend to elevate blood sugars.
      - Gastrointestinal illnesses tend to lower blood sugars.
    - Maintain hydration with water and salt:
      - Sick day management at home should include:
        - Chicken soups and broths
        - Sports drinks such as Gatorade and Pedialyte can be given as well as other sugary drinks (Kool-Aid, flat colas, flat ginger ale) if sugars are falling below 180 mg/dL
        - Easy digestible carbohydrates such as rice, crackers, etc.
      - Treat underlying illness.
    - Review sick management plan with parent and child at each office visit.
  - Encourage participation in some type of exercise program, since exercise has been linked to improved insulin sensitivity.
  - Monitor laboratories:
    - HbA1C: Every 3 months
  - Microalbuminuria: Yearly after diagnosed for 5 years or after age 12 (American Diabetes Association, 2014)
  - Important to encourage to maintain ideal body weight
  - Patient visits every 3 months (important to monitor growth, signs/symptoms of neuropathy, injection sites, feet [after age 12])

Attention-Deficit Hyperactive Disorder

Description of the Disease: Attention-deficit hyperactivity disorder (ADHD) is a behavior disorder manifesting as short attention span, hyperactivity, and impulsiveness.

Epidemiology:
- Affects up to 7% of school-age children
- Prevalent more in males than females (5:1); girls may display less hyperactivity.
- Up to 50% have a comorbid mental or behavior condition
- American Academy of Pediatrics Guidelines extends diagnosis between ages 4 and 18.
- Increase in new cases diagnosed is 3% of school-age children yearly.

Etiology:
- Unknown
- Possible a neurochemical imbalance causing abnormal uptake of dopamine

Risk Factors:
- Family history
- Possibly associated with fetal exposure to smoking and drug/alcohol abuse prenatally

Signs and Symptoms:
- Must meet six of following criteria symptoms set by the *DSM-V*; symptoms must be for at least 6 months, starting prior to the age of 12 and seen in two settings (home and school) (American Psychological Association, 2013).
  - Fidgety with hands and/or feet; squirms
  - Inability to sit still or remain in chair during appropriate times
  - Excessive energy
  - Talks non-stop
  - Unable to play quiet games or board games
  - Easily distracted
  - Loses interest rapidly in a task
  - Often forgetful or losing things
  - Difficulty organizing tasks and activities

Differential Diagnoses:
- Learning disability
- Hearing or vision disorder
- Mental health issues: Anxiety disorder, bipolar disorder
- Developmental disorder: Asperger syndrome, autism
- Tourette syndrome
- Inadequate parenting skills (poor discipline rules)

Diagnostic Studies:
- Must meet criteria set by *DSM-V*
- Must be observed in at least two settings
- ADHD Rating Scale IV (5 to 17)
- Conners Comprehensive Behavior Rating Scales (6 to 17 years)
- NICHQ Vanderbilt Assessment Scales (for parent and teacher)

Treatment:
Pharmacologic:
- Stimulants: First-line treatment for school-age children
  - Short acting: Duration 3 to 6 hours (may need more than one dosage for the day)
    - Methylphenidate (MPH) (Ritalin) $\geq$ 6 years.
    - Dextroamphetamine/amphetamine (Adderall) $\geq$ 6 years.
    - Dexmethylphenidate (Focalin) $\geq$ 3 years.
  - Intermediate acting: 6 to 10-hour duration
    - Methylphenidate CD (Metadate CD) $>$ 6 years.
    - Methylphenidate SR (Ritalin CD) $\geq$ 6 years.
  - Long acting: Lasts 10 hours
    - Dexmethylphenidate XR
    - MPH transdermal patch
    - Lisdexamfetamine 30 mg daily, can titrate 10 mg weekly till maximum dose of 70 mg
  - Stimulants are listed as controlled substances. Please follow state prescriptive privilege laws.
  - Monitor for side effects of stimulants: diminished appetite, growth suppression, elevated BP and heart rate, etc.

- Nonstimulants: Only to be used if stimulants are contraindicated or no response from stimulants
- American Academy of Pediatrics recommends a stepwise approach starting with atomoxetine (Strattera) → guanfacine (Intuniv) → clonidine ER (Kapvay). Only approved for children > 6 years

Nonpharmacologic:
- Parent and teacher behavior modification coexists with pharmacologic treatment. (In preschoolers, parent/teacher behavior modification is first line of treatment.)
- Educate on proper parenting skills, utilizing time outs, proper reprimands for disobeying rules.
- Monitor height and weight every 6 months while on stimulants due to diminished appetite and possible growth suppression.
- Monitor BR and heart for possible changes due to small risk of cardiovascular events.

Precocious Puberty

Description of the Disease: Early development of secondary sex characteristics before the age of 8 in girls and 9 years of age in boys.

Pathophysiology of Puberty:
- Reactivation of the hypothalamic–pituitary–gonadal (HPG) axis: Hypothalamus releases GnRH → pituitary releases FSH/LH → in females causes ovarian follicular development and the production of estrogens and in males causes the testes to release testosterone, in addition to the adrenal cortex role in androgen production → development of secondary sex characteristics.
- Also causes rapid linear growth with closure of the skeletal growth plate halting growth.

Epidemiology:
- 1 in 5,000 children affected
- Affects girls more than boys (3:1)
- Can be seen in infancy

Etiology:
- Majority of cases are of idiopathic entity
- Classified as:
  - Central precocious puberty (true) caused by:
    - CNS tumors (associated more with male precocious puberty)
    - Primary hypothyroidism
    - Chronic adrenal insufficiency
    - McCune–Albright syndrome
    - Head injury or radiation to the head
    - Congenital adrenal hyperplasia
  - Peripheral precocious puberty
    - Genetic factors: Deficiency of MKRN3; seen in genetically linked diseases such as neurofibromatosis
    - Ovarian/testicular tumor
    - Exogenous estrogen (girls)
    - Exogenous androgen

Risk Factors:
- Ethnicity: Affects African-Americans more frequently, seen in adoptive children
- Nutritional status: Moderate obesity (severe obesity may cause delayed puberty)
- Head trauma
- Exposure to exogenous estrogen (i.e., plant-derived phytoestrogens), mother's oral contraceptives, some cosmetic products containing estrogen derivatives
- Exposure to testosterone or hCG, that is, father's topical testosterone products
- Exposure to other endocrine disturbers (i.e., bisphenol A (BPA), phthalates)

Signs and Symptoms:
- In girls:
  - Earlier than normal thelarche (breast development)
- In boys:
  - Earlier than normal testicular enlargement (usually first sign in boys)
  - Earlier than normal penis enlargement

- In both:
  - Rapid initial increase in height (usually first sign in girls)
    - Due to advancing bone age (however this causes the growth plates to close stopping growth in height, and may leave child short in stature)
  - Appearance of axillary and pubic hairs
  - Oily skin, possible onset of acne
  - Body odor

Differential Diagnoses:
- Pseudoprecocious puberty or a benign variant of puberty; may have only premature thelarche, adrenarche, or pubarche, but no sperm or egg production
- Congenital adrenal hyperplasia
- Primary hypothyroidism
- McCune–Albright syndrome

Diagnostic Studies:
- Based on clinical signs, that is, observed breast development
- Laboratory confirmation of:
  - Rising levels of LH
  - ↑ estradiol levels in girls
  - ↑ testosterone levels in boys
- Bone age x-ray (shows advanced bone age)
- May need MRI if CNS tumor is suspected
- May need pelvic or testicular ultrasound if ovarian or testicular tumor suspected

Treatment:
  Pharmacologic:
- Referral to pediatric endocrinologist for GnRH analog therapy to suppress puberty
  - Leuprolide 22.5 mg to 30 mg IM every 3 months
  - Histrelin 50 mg subdermal implant for 1 year
  - Nafarelin acetate 1,600 mcg/day INTRANASALLY by two sprays into each nostril in the morning and two sprays into each nostril in the evening

  Nonpharmacologic:
- Surgical intervention if tumor is involved
- Monitor for side effects of medications.
- Emotional and psychological support is needed since appearance change is not occurring in friends, may display anxiety or depressive symptoms.

Common Communicable Diseases in School Age

Group A β-Hemolytic Streptococcus Pharyngitis (Strep Throat)/ Scarlatina (Scarlet Fever)

Description of the Disease:
- Strep throat is a bacterial infection caused by the GABHS organism producing inflammation of the pharynx and tonsils.
- Scarlet fever is a bacterial infection attributed to GABHS pyogenes and is characterized by a sore throat and classic rash.

Epidemiology:
- Predominately seen in 5- to 12-year-olds
- Occurs equally in males and females
- GABHS accounts for 20% to 30% of cases of acute pharyngitis (strep throat) in children, scarlet fever develops in 10% of these cases.
- Higher incidence in winter and spring

Etiology:

- Exposure to the GABHS organism is the underlying etiology of both strep throat and scarlet fever.
- In scarlet fever, GABHS generates enzymes and toxins that destroy red blood cells. The toxins released by GABHS produces the classic "scarlet" rash.
  - Although scarlet fever is mostly associated with GABHS pharyngitis, it can occur after GABHS-infected wound or burn.
- Onset of symptoms

Risk Factors:

- Age (rarely seen in under 2)
- Strep throat
- Wounds and/or burns
- Crowded environment (schools, day care)

Signs and Symptoms:

- Fever
- Sore throat—throat and tonsils are erythematous; may or may not have exudate
- May have symptoms of nausea, vomiting, and abdominal pain
- Cervical adenopathy
- Usually lack of upper respiratory symptoms such as cough or runny nose

Classic to Scarlet Fever:

- "Sandpaper-" textured rash: Begins on neck and axillary areas, then extends to the trunk, and then to the extremities. Skin creases in the flexor surface of the elbow, axillary, knees and groin area become redder than the remaining rash (Pastia lines)
- May display initially bright red cheeks before the classic rash develops
- Strawberry tongue (initial white coating of the tongue is replaced by visible, red, slightly enlarged papillae causing the tongue to look like a strawberry)
- As rash fades, a peeling of skin occurs that can last for weeks.

Differential Diagnoses:

Strep Throat:

- Pharyngitis
- Upper respiratory infection
- Infectious mononucleosis
- Epiglottitis

Scarlet Fever:

- Fifth disease
- Measles, rubella, rubeola
- Kawasaki disease
- Toxic shock syndrome
- Drug reaction

Diagnostic Studies:

- RADT for Group A streptococci, throat swab; if positive, treat; if negative, do throat culture
- Throat culture for Group A streptococci remains gold standard.

Treatment:

Pharmacologic:

- Penicillin or amoxicillin is the drug of choice for those nonallergic (Shulman et al., 2012)
  - Children under 12: Penicillin V 250 mg in two to three divided dosages for 10 days
  - Children over 12: Penicillin V 250 mg four times a day Or 500 mg twice a day
  - Amoxicillin 25 mg/kg (max 500 mg) twice daily for 10 days.
- If allergic to penicillin, the Infectious Disease Society of America suggests a first-generation cephalosporin (for those not anaphylactic sensitive to penicillin) for 10 days; clindamycin is an acceptable alternative for 10 days, as well as clarithromycin for 10 days or azithromycin for 5 days (Shulman et al., 2012)
- Can give antipyretics (acetaminophen) for fever

Nonpharmacologic:

- Contagious for 24 hours after start of antibiotics

- Organism can remain on toothbrushes. Recommend either vigorous rinsing after use during course of treatment or replacing in 3 days after starting antibiotics.
- Supportive measures: encourage fluids, education on preventing spread, progression of disease, that is, peeling of the skin

Varicella

Description of the Disease: Commonly known as "chicken pox," this highly contagious childhood illness is caused by the varicella-zoster virus. It is characterized by the presentation of multiple pruritic lesions ranging from papules, vesicles, and crusts.

Epidemiology:
- Marked decrease in incidence since vaccine has been made available
- Occurs mainly in winter and early spring
- Mainly seen in children under 10
- Once disease process ends, virus lays dormant within the sensory ganglia of the spinal cord where it can recur in older life in the form of shingles.

Etiology:
- Varicella-zoster virus
- Transmitted by droplet and/or direct contact of lesions
- Incubation about 1 to 3 weeks; contagious 48 hours prior to the development of the rash until all lesions have crusted

Risk Factors:
- Exposure to an infected individual
- Not being immunized or having had a history of varicella
- Immunosuppressed individuals

Signs and Symptoms:
- Prodromal:
  - Low-grade fever
  - Malaise
  - Headache
  - Diminished appetite
- Exanthem:
  - Papules usually start on head or face, progressing rapidly to the trunk and extremities.
  - Lesions go through stages: papule → vesicle → ruptured vesicle → crusts.
  - Various lesion stages can be seen in one area.
  - Lesions can occur anywhere on the body such as in the mouth, nose, and on the genitals.
  - Lesions are extremely pruritic.
  - Outbreaks usually occur for 2 to 4 days.

Differential Diagnoses:
- Insect bites
- Impetigo
- Small pox
- Drug reactions
- Coxsackievirus (i.e., hand–foot–mouth disease)

Diagnostic Studies:
- None indicated; diagnosed by clinical presentation

Treatment:
Pharmacologic:
- Varicella vaccine: CDC recommends two doses of the vaccine between 12 and 15 months and 4 to 6 years of age.
- Acetaminophen for fever
- Do not give ASPIRIN to children infected with varicella due to high incidence of Reye's syndrome
- Antipruritics:
  - Diphenhydramine, 1.25 mg/kg every 6 hours
  - Hydroxyzine, 0.5 mg/kg every 6 hours
  - Loratadine, children 2 to 5 years of age: 5 mg once daily. Children over 6 years: 10 mg

- Anitvirals such as Acyclovir are not recommended for healthy children. Recommended within 24 hours in children who are on chronic steroid or inhaled steroid therapy, premature infants, children with chronic lung disorders and chronic skin disorder. IV Acyclovir is recommended for any child who is immunosuppressed.
  - Acyclovir: 20 mg/kg per dose orally four times daily (maximum daily dose is 800 mg)

Nonpharmacologic:
- Promote comfort: Cornstarch or oatmeal baths (Aveeno), calamine lotion
- Promote general hygiene measures to prevent infection: good hand washing, daily tepid or cool baths, change clothes daily.
- Keep nails short to avoid scratching open lesions: may suggest child wear gloves.
- Isolate child from others till all lesions have crusted over.
- Encourage fluids.
- Monitor for complications: cough, high fever, lethargy, neck pain

Pediculosis

Description of the Disease: Commonly known as lice infestation. Pediculosis is the presence of ectoparasites on the body, head, and/or pubic area.

Epidemiology:
- Mainly seen in the 5- to 12-year-old age group
- Head and body lice are more common in this group while pubic pediculosis is seen more in adults (usually associated with sexual activity)
- Common in both males and females with girls having a higher incidence
- Less common in African-Americans possible due to hair texture
- Affects all socioeconomic classes

Etiology:
- Pediculus humanus capitus (head lice)
- Pediculus humanus corporis (body lice)
- Phthirus pubis (pubic lice)
- Survives on body by feeding on human blood
- Adult lice last about 9 to 10 days. Each louse lays approximately 10 eggs (nits) daily.
- Nits are female eggs and can survive up to 3 weeks after removal from host.
- Transmission is by direct contact.

Risk Factors:
- Crowded conditions (schools, camps, day care)
- In children, it should not be associated with poor hygiene.
- Sharing of combs, hats, hair ties, etc.
- Laying on infected sheets, pillows, stuff animals

Signs and Symptoms:
- Itching (can be severe and associated with all three types)
- Pediculosis of the head:
  - Presence of nits (pearly white minuscular orbs) which are attached to the hair shaft and difficult to remove
  - Often seen behind ears and base of scalp
- Pediculosis of the body:
  - Usually can see 'bite' marks and excoriation in areas of infestation, mainly in warmer areas such as the axillae, groin, waist
  - May see actual lice in seams of clothing
- Pediculosis of the pubis (usually not seen in children, if so may be a red flag for child abuse)
  - Excoriated areas: lower abdomen, genitals, and thighs. May see pinpoint bluish "bite" marks
  - Can spread to other hairy parts of body such as the eyebrows
  - In adolescence, may see nits in pubic hair

Differential Diagnoses:
- Dandruff
- Scabies
- Atopic dermatitis
- Scabies

Diagnostic Studies:
- Diagnosed by clinical presentation
- Visualization of live lice (head and body: 1 to 2 mm long with 6 legs, reddish-brown to black in color; pubic: 1 to 2 mm, brownish, crab-like appearance) or nits (use of magnifying glass or fine-tooth comb)
- Wood's lamp: Nits produce a fluorescence.

Treatment:

Pharmacologic: (CDC, 2013)
- **Head:**
  - OTC treatments should be tried initially:
    - Permethrin 1% (Nix) (only kills live lice)
      - Least toxic
      - Apply for 10 minutes; rinse; can repeat in 7 to 10 days on day 9 since not completely ovicidal
      - Approved for use in children older than 2 months
    - Pyrethrins with piperonyl butoxide (only kills live lice)
      - Do not use in children with allergies to chrysanthemums; also may exacerbate ragweed allergies
      - Apply for 10 minutes; rinse; can repeat on day 9 since not completely ovicidal
    - Approved for use in children 2 months and older
  - Prescription treatment (if OTC treatment fails)
    - Benzyl alcohol 5%
      - Apply 10 minutes; rinse; repeat; can repeat after 7 days
      - Approved for use in children older than 6 months
    - Malathion (0.5%)
      - Known to be highly flammable; avoid using hair dryer, curling iron on hair; do not smoke near child.
      - Apply for 10 to 12 hours; rinse; can repeat in 7 to 9 days if live lice are seen.
      - Approved for use in children older than 6 months
    - Lindane (1%)
    - Use is no longer recommended by the American Academy of Pediatrics.
- **Body:**
  - Guidelines for the choice of the pediculicide are the same as for head lice. (CDC, 2013)
- **Pubic:** (CDC, 2013)
  - Permethrin 1%, pyrethrins with piperonyl butoxide, or malathion (0.5%)
    - If eyelashes are infected, do not use pediculicides; use ophthalmic-prescribed petroleum jelly on lashes up to q.i.d. for 10 days (suffocates lice)

Nonpharmacologic:
- According to the Academy of Pediatrics, no restriction from school is necessary due to head lice and recommends abandoning no-nits rule.
- Control measures:
  - Wash in hot water or dry-clean all items that have had lice contact: Hats, scarfs, sheets, pillow cases, towels
  - Stuffed animals and nonwashable items placed in sealed bag for 2 weeks
  - Submerge all brushes and combs in hot water for 10 minutes.
  - Can remove nits with fine-tooth comb; empty nits can remain on hair shaft 2 weeks or more.

Scabies

Description of the Disease: Scabies is a parasitic infection of the skin caused by a mite. This common infestation causes intense itching.

Epidemiology:
- Estimated 300 cases worldwide and approximately 1 million in the United States
- Affects all ages, gender, socioeconomic groups
- Associated often with overcrowded or close living conditions

Etiology:
- Caused by *Sarcoptes scabiei*
- Highly contagious via skin-to-skin contact; infected clothing and bedsheets may transmit mites but is stated to be uncommon.

- Males and female mate on skin surface → males die post mating → female mites burrow into warm skin areas where they deposits eggs (up to 4 eggs per day), feces, and saliva → causing itching and local hypersensitivity response → when eggs mature into mites, they exit and repeat the cycle. Cycle takes approximately 2 to 3 weeks.

Risk Factors
- Close or crowded conditions, that is, schools, camps, hospitals, nursing homes
- Immunocompromised patients

Signs and Symptoms:
- Usually appears 4 to 10 weeks after exposure
- Intense itching, especially at night
- Small vesicles and papules
- Burrows may be visible on skin
- Common areas of infestation are between fingers (finger webs), wrists, waistband area of the trunk, groin, under breasts and areola, axillae, and bottom of the buttocks, but rarely above neck.

Differential Diagnoses:
- Insect bites (especially flea bites)
- Dermatitis (atopic, contact)
- Pediculosis

Diagnostic Studies:
- Diagnosis made by clinical presentation
- Microscopic scrapings of infested area may show eggs, feces, or mites
- Burrow ink test

Treatment:
Pharmacologic:
- Permethrin 5% cream
  - Can be used over the age of 2 months.
  - Apply and massage into skin from head to soles of feet.
  - Leave on for 8 to 14 hours and then rinse completely.
  - Usually only one treatment is needed.
  - Treat entire family.
- Benadryl, Claritin, Allegra OTC for itch

Nonpharmacologic:
- Clothing, bedding, towels, and toys should be washed with hot soapy water.
- Stuffed animals and nonwashable items should be placed in sealed bag for 1 week.

Otitis Externa

Description of the Disease: Otitis externa, commonly known as swimmer's ear is the inflammation of the ear's auditory canal and in some cases the pinna.

Epidemiology:
- Seen mostly in warm weather months, warmer climates
- Seen in all ages; incidence peaks in children ages 7 to 12
- Equal incidence in males and females
- Prevalence is 10% risk of being diagnosed in one's lifetime.

Etiology:
- 90% of cases are bacterial; common organisms:
  - *Pseudomonas aeruginosa* (most common)
  - *S. aureus*
- Fungal
  - Aspergillus (prominent fungi etiology)
  - Candidiasis
- Loss of protective cerumen from overcleaning ears
- Disruption of the protective surface of the ear canal (cerumen and acidity) → susceptibility for organism entry → infectious process occurs with inflammation, resultant pus, swelling, and pain of the canal and pinna.

Risk Factors:
- Swimming or continuous moisture in the ears
- Skin conditions such as eczema, seborrhea, psoriasis
- Overcleaning ear canals resulting in removal of protective wax
- Ear plugs and ear buds
- Narrow ear canals
- Ear canal trauma, that is scratch, laceration, foreign object
- Hearing aids

Signs and Symptoms
- Otalgia agitated by pulling on the pinna or pushing on the tragus
- Feeling of fullness of ear
- Itching often a precursor of pain (itching may be seen in fungal origins)
- Otorrhea (purulent in most bacterial infections; can be white, stringy, and thick in fungal infection)
- Canal erythema and edema
- Diminished hearing

Differential Diagnoses:
- Otitis media with tympanic membrane (TM) perforation
- Allergic reaction to topical otic antibiotics
- Eczema
- Contact dermatitis
- Foreign body
- Malignant otitis externa (rapid progression of symptoms and tissue involvement)
- Mastoiditis

Diagnostic Studies:
- None indicated, diagnosed by clinical presentation.
- Culture of discharge (not required)
- Microscopic evaluation for evidence of fungal infection (hyphae)

Treatment:
   Pharmacologic: (Rosenfeld et al., 2014)
- Topical antimicrobial otic drops: First-line treatment for uncomplicated acute otitis externa
  - Ciprofloxacin 0.2%, hydrocortisone 1.0%
    - Recommended over the age of 1 year
    - Three drops in affected ear twice daily for 7 days
  - Ciprofloxacin 0.3%, dexamethasone 0.1%
    - Recommended over the age of 6 months
    - Four drops in affected ear twice daily
  - Ofloxacin 0.3%
    - Recommended over the age of 6 months
    - Instill five drops once daily for 7 days
  - Neomycin, polymyxin B, hydrocortisone
    - Recommended for children over 2
    - Do not use if TM is perforated
    - Instill three drops three to four times a day for 10 days
    - Known to cause contact sensitivity
- Educate parents to proper instillation:
  - Be sure bottle is warmed by rolling or holding in hands. Instillation of cold liquids can cause dizziness.
  - Instill drops while child is laying on side and ensure that child remains in that position for 5 minutes.
  - If canal is severely swollen, may need to insert an ear wick.
- May need oral antibiotics if suspected TM perforation, cellulitis of the auricle, fever
- Analgesics for pain depending on severity; most respond to acetaminophen or ibuprofen.
- 1:1 parts of isopropyl alcohol and white vinegar can help restore acidity of the canal post swimming as prevention or as an early treatment for swimmer's ear.

   Nonpharmacologic:
- Keep ear canals dry.
- When showering, use inserted cotton ball coated with petroleum jelly during treatment phase to keep water out.

- Avoid use of earplugs, earbuds, or earphones during treatment.
- Limit hearing aid use.
- Do not use cotton swabs at any time.

Adolescent Case Presentation

Jane, a 15-year-old Caucasian female, presents with her mother to the office for a sports physical for track and field hockey. She offers no major complaints other than feeling a bit more tired than usual. Her mother is concerned about daughter's "skinniness." As you review the chart, you note that the patient has had a 10 lb. weight loss within the past 6 months. Her last physical examination was 3 years ago. Last office visit was 6 months ago for gastroenteritis and dehydrations symptoms. The patient voices no concern about her weight loss and feels she is still heavier than her friends.

Past Medical History: Unremarkable

Medications: None

Allergy: Erythromycin (rash)

Social:
Home: Lives with parents and 2 younger siblings; feels safe
Education: 10th grade; B average student.
Activities: Babysits, runs track, and plays field hockey
Drugs: + EOTH (weekends); + marijuana (1 to 2 times/month); denies any other drug use
Diet: Acknowledges weight loss from dieting
Suicidal Ideation: Denies thoughts of suicide
Sex: + Sexual activity past 6 months; uses condoms "most of the time," only one sexual partner

Last Menstrual Period: 3 months ago; onset of menses at age 13

Immunizations:
TDAP last given age 10
MCV4 last given at age 12
HPV first dose given at age 12
No record of influenza
All infancy immunizations were given. Hepatitis B, IPV, MMR, and varicella are all up to date.

Family History: Unremarkable; negative for heart disease, Marfan syndrome, or sudden unexplainable death

Previous Diagnostic Data:
Laboratory data from 6 months ago: Electrolytes and CBC were all WNL.
Spinal x-ray (3 year prior) shows 10° thoracolumbar curve.

Review of Systems/Health Promotion:
Constitutional: Denies fevers, fatigue
HEENT: **Head:** Denies head injury, concussion, or headaches. **Eyes:** Denies visual changes, eye problems, does not wear glasses. **Ears:** Denies ear pain or hearing difficulties. **Nose:** Denies nasal congestion. **Throat:** Denies sore throats, + history of cold sores
Neck: Denies neck pain, swollen lymph nodes
Respiratory: Denies shortness of breath, cough, wheeze, or history of asthma
Cardiovascular: Denies chest discomfort or pain
Gastrointestinal: Denies n/v/d; follows mostly vegetarian diet with occasional white meat (turkey, chicken), no dairy, no wheat products due to "makes her feel fat"; denies reflux or GI pain with exercise
Musculoskeletal: Denies previous fractures, sprains, tendon injuries, muscle cramps, joint pain, + occasional back discomfort, + history of mild scoliosis
Neurology: Denies seizures, numbness, tingling
Genitourinary: Denies any kidney or urinary problems
Female Reproductive: LMP- 3 months ago; states periods have "always been irregular"; + sexually active, uses condom most of the time for birth control
Integumentary: Denies rashes, open sores, nail problems; + acne on face and upper back

Physical Examination:

Vital Signs: Temperature = 98.2°F   BP = 112/66   HR = 56 bpm   RR = 12   Height: 5 ft 3 inches   Weight = 100 lbs   BMI = 17.7

Tanner Stage: V

General/Psych: AAO times three; appropriate and cleanly dressed; thin stature, quiet but cooperative; accompanied to visit by mom

Skin: Dry, cool to touch, open and closed comedones on cheeks, jawline, and forehead, a few open comedones noted on back, none on chest; few pustules noted <10; no cystic or papular lesions; + notable amount of soft hair on arms

HEENT: **Head:** Normocephalic. **Eyes:** Vision: 20/20 PERLA, EOM intact. **Ears:** No drainage, TMs pearly gray bilaterally. **Nose:** Patent, turbinates slight pallor, no discharge, septum intact and midline. **Mouth/Throat:** Buccal mucosa somewhat pale, teeth with no signs of wear or decay, Pharynx pink, tonsils +1, uvula midline

Thoracic/Lungs: CTA B/L, no wheezing noted

Breast: Tanner stage V

Cardiovascular: Rate 54, regular $S_1 S_2$, no murmurs, PMI @ 5ICS MCL

Abdomen: Scaphoid, soft, nontender, +BS, no masses, no hepatomegaly, no splenomegaly.

Musculoskeletal: Gait steady; full range of motion in all joints of the upper and lower extremities; muscle strength 5/5 all four extremities; spine shows mild lumbar-thoracic "C" curve measuring 12°

Neurologic: Upper and lower extremity reflexes +2; Romberg; cranial nerves II-XII intact

Genitalia: No lesions, discharge, or rashes noted

Case Study Review Questions

1. When obtaining a psychosocial history from an adolescent, what set of questions is crucial to ask in order to assess risky behavior?

   > Both the AMA and The AAP recommend using the HEEADSSS assessment questions as a proficient way to assessing a teen's life and the risk of unhealthy behaviors. HEEADSSS is the mnemonic for Home, Education, Eating habits, Activities, Drug, Suicidality, Sex, and Safety.

2. It was noted by the American College of Preventative Medicine that immunization compliance is only 24% among adolescence. In looking at the documented immunizations what immunizations will Jane need at this visit?

   > According to the immunization guidelines of the Center for Disease Control, Jane will need the following immunizations:
   >
   > 1. Tetanus and diphtheria toxoids and acellular pertussis (TDAP) vaccine (34% of recorded pertussis cases occurred among adolescents in middle and high school.)
   > 2. Human papillomavirus (HPV) vaccine Dose #2 (The Advisory Committee on Immunization Practices advises catch-up vaccinations for HPV until the age of 26.)
   > 3. Influenza immunization (if during flu season)

3. After performing Jane's History and Physical, you note a variety of problems you must address before approving her for sports. What is your immediate priority?

   > Addressing the issue of amenorrhea is immediate priority due to the primary cause of this entity.

4. What are the two top differential diagnoses for this problem in this particular patient?

   > 1. Pregnancy
   > 2. Hormonal imbalance related to possible weight loss, stress, or female athletic triad syndrome.

5. Through private conversation with the patient, you conclude that this teen has an eating disorder. What diagnostic tests would you order for this patient considering all her needs?

   > 1. Urine in office pregnancy test (r/o pregnancy)
   > 2. FSH, LH, prolactin level, TSH (r/o hormonal causes of amenorrhea)
   > 3. Fasting glucose (r/o diabetes as a cause for amenorrhea)
   > 4. CBC, (r/o other diagnoses for weight loss and fatigue)
   > 5. Chemistry profile (assess electrolytes, BUN, which can be abnormal in eating disorders), serum HCG (if in-office pregnancy test is negative)
   > 6. EKG: To r/o cardiac involvement due to possible electrolyte disturbance and in lieu of bradycardia
   > 7. Posteroanterior (PA) x-rays of the full spine (monitor scoliosis since there was an increase in size.)

6. What is the mainstay treatment for anorexia?

> A nonpharmacologic approach is the mainstay of treatment for anorexia, centering on psychotherapy (individual and family therapy); nutritional counseling, and in-office medical management.

7. Jane, at this time, is most concerned about her acne and how it is starting to affect her appearance. How would you initially treat her and what is your rationale?

> Using classification by the American Academy of Dermatology, Jane's acne can be classified as mild. Initial treatment involves prescribing either benzoyl peroxide or topical retinoids (tretinoin, adapalene, and tazarotene). If inadequate response or extensive areas of comedonal acne persist, a combination topical therapy of benzoyl peroxide + topical antibiotic (erythromycin or clindamycin gel) can be prescribed.

8. Jane's participation in sports is denied at this time due to her anorexia. In closing this office visit, what anticipatory guidance should you promote in the adolescent age group?

> According to Bright Futures, anticipatory guidance for the adolescent is set in three stages: Early adolescence (11 to 14 years), middle adolescence (15 to 17 years), and late adolescence (18 to 21 years). All three stages mainly center on addressing the following topics:
>
> Encouraging proper physical development and eating habits; fostering family connectedness and academic success; promoting emotional well-being through stress reduction and appropriate coping mechanisms; reducing risky behaviors by open discussion of alcohol, tobacco, water pipe (hookah) smoking, drugs; safe sex; preventing injury, especially car safety, and forms of violence (guns, bullying, dating violence).

Common Adolescent Diagnoses

Acne Vulgaris

Description of the Disease: Acne vulgaris is a common adolescent skin condition occurring on the back, face, and chest characterized by increased sebum secretion and plugging of sebaceous follicles. Comedones are the characteristic lesion of acne.

Pathophysiology:
- Multifactorial: Stimulation of sebaceous follicles + sebum production + abnormal desquamation of the keratinocytes → follicular plugging → bacterial colonization of *Propionibacterium acnes* (*P. acnes*) → inflammatory and noninflammatory lesions

Epidemiology:
- One of the most common dermatologic problems is primary care.
- Affects between 79% and 95% of adolescents with its highest incidence between 16 and 18 years of age
- Males are more commonly affected in the adolescent age group.
- Multifactorial etiology: Hormones, genetics

Etiology/Risk Factors:
- Age
- Hormones
- Medications (lithium, phenytoin, systemic corticosteroids, anabolic steroids)
- Genetic disposition
- Environment: Hot, humid weather
- Comedogenic cosmetics and greasy hair products can aggravate
- Diet: No relationship with chocolate, pizza, soda, etc.
- Stress: Newer studies show correlation between stress and acne.
- Can be associated with androgen excess and polycystic ovary disease

Signs and Symptoms:
- Mixture of noninflammatory (open and closed comedones) and inflammatory lesions (papules, pustules, cysts, and nodules)
- Lesions seen commonly on face, upper back, and chest
- Classified by the American Academy of Dermatology:
  - Mild: Open (blackhead) and closed (whitehead) comedones plus a few papules and pustules (less than 10)
  - Moderate: Mixture of open and closed comedones, papules, and pustules (between 10 and 40) and a few nodules
  - Severe: Mixture of open and closed comedones papules, pustules, multiple nodules, and cysts

Differential Diagnoses:
- Acne rosacea
- Folliculitis
- Drug-induced acne
- Periorbital dermatitis

Diagnostic Studies:
- Diagnosis made by clinical presentation
- May need culture to r/o bacterial folliculitis
- May need hormone testing if polycystic ovary disease is suspected

Treatment
- Geared to stages with focus to decrease sebum production, prevent comedone formation, suppress *P. acnes*, and reduce inflammation

Pharmacologic:
- Mild: (Initial) Benzoyl peroxide *or* topical retinoids (tretinoin, adapalene, and tazarotene)
  - Inadequate response or extensive comedonal acne: Try combination topical therapy: benzoyl peroxide + topical antibiotic (erythromycin or clindamycin gel) Or benzoyl peroxide + topical retinol Or a combination of all three (topical retinoid, topical antibiotic, and benzoyl peroxide)
  - Note acne may initially worsen at start of topical retinoids.
- Moderate: Topical therapy, as stated above plus oral antibiotics: Dapsone 5% gel may be considered as an alternative to topical antibiotics and benzoyl peroxide. Oral antibiotic treatment can last up to 12 weeks.
  - Tetracycline and its derivatives
    - Tetracycline 500 mg b.i.d. (3 to 6 weeks); once effective can be reduced to 250 mg b.i.d. (can be used as alternate-day dosing if improvement is noted)
    - Minocycline 100 mg b.i.d. (3 to 6 weeks); once effective can be reduced to 50 mg b.i.d.
    - Doxycycline 50 to 100 mg q.i.d. or b.i.d.
  - Erythromycin 250 mg q.i.d. (use if the above are contraindicated, high rate of resistance)
  - Sulfamethoxazole-trimethoprim (SMX-TMP) 160 to 800 mg b.i.d. (not usually used as first- or second-line treatment)
  - Oral contraceptives may be second alternative for female patients with moderate to severe acne: can take for 3 to 6 months used with topical acne regimen.
- Severe: Systemic antibiotics and/or oral isotretinoin (can be initiated in primary care if office is competent in its prescribing or refer to dermatology)
  - All must sign a "I Pledge" contract (www.ipledgeprogram.com) to protect fetal exposure from isotretinoin due to its strong teratogen effects and to assure proper follow-ups during treatments.
  - Complete blood count, liver function tests, and lipids, especially triglycerides, at baseline and then every 4 to 6 weeks until therapy is completed
  - Females must have a pregnancy test prior to beginning treatment, then monthly during treatment, then 1 month posttreatment.
  - Treatment usually lasts 4 to 5 months
  - Must monitor for mood alteration such as depression and suicidal ideation

Nonpharmacologic:
- Avoid facial scrubs which can aggravate acne conditions.
- Ordinary face washing once or twice daily with mild soap and water.
- Avoid squeezing and popping pustules and papules to prevent further skin irritation and scarring.
- Avoid oil-based makeup, skin creams, and hair products.
- Well-balanced diet and plenty of fluids to keep skin hydrated while undergoing treatment
- Studies have suggested correlation between stress and acne, teaching stress reduction strategies may have its advantage.

Adolescent Depression

Description of the Disease: Depression is a generalized feeling of being sad or "down" for an extended amount of time without direct cause, such as in grief. It is the most common mental health issue seen in adolescents.
- *Diagnostic and Statistical Manual of Mental Disorders,* fifth edition, text revision (*DSM-V-TR*) classifies three forms of depression.

- Major depressive disorder (MDD) has depressed mood but needs to meet five of the eight major symptomatology associated with MDD for at least 2 weeks.
- Dysthymia: Milder symptoms than MDD but longer duration, at least a year
- Adjustment disorder: Depressed mood usually related to exposure to outside stressor (occurs up to 3 months after stressor and lasts only about 6 months)

Epidemiology:
- Approximately 5% to 8% of adolescents have been affected with a MDD.
- Average age of first episode is 13 to 15 years.
- Early adolescence equal incidence; late adolescence 2:1 female to male
- Suicide is the third most common cause of death among adolescents.
- Average of 26% of high-school students thought seriously about killing themselves with 10% actually having a plan.

Etiology:
- No one cause singled out. Linked to many possible causes:
  - Genetics
    - More common in those with a positive family history especially first-degree relative
  - Neurochemical causes:
    - Serotonin depletion
    - Neurotransmitter-uptake defect
      - Norepinephrine
      - Dopamine
  - Psychosocial causes:
    - High levels of stress

Risk Factors:
- Family history (first-degree relative)
- Female
- History of childhood behavior issues (ADHD)
- History of chronic illness
- High levels of stress
  - Family crisis
  - Sexual abuse
  - Neglect
- Significant loss (death of a close relative or friend, parental divorce)
- History of previous depressive episode or mental health issue

Signs and Symptoms:
- Similar to that of adults (MDD is diagnosed based on five of the following symptoms: changes of patterns in sleeping and/or eating, lack of concentration, fatigue, loss of interest in favorite things, somatic complaints, suicidal ideation, sense of guilt, or low self-esteem.)
- Additional signs:
  - Drop in grades
  - Impulsivity
  - Personality changes: Agitation and Irritability[1]
  - Substance abuse
  - Withdrawal from friends

Differential Diagnoses:
- Other psychiatric disorders: Bipolar disorder, posttraumatic stress disorder
- Other depressive disorders such as premenstrual dysphoric disorder (PMDD) in female adolescents; dysthymia
- Substance abuse
- Endocrine disorders: Hypothyroidism, diabetes mellitus
- Grief reaction

---

[1] Irritability is the most common symptom of depression in adolescence.

Diagnostic Studies:
- Use of Depression Scales:
  - U.S. Preventive Services Task Force recommends screening all children over the age of 12.
    - ○ Patient Health Questionnaire for Adolescents (PHQ-A).
    - ○ Beck Depression Inventory-Primary Care Version (BDI-PC).
    - ○ Children's Depression Inventory (CDI)
- Verbal assessment of the use of drugs and EOTH
- Laboratory studies to rule out any physical cause for symptomatology
  - Urine or serum toxicology report
  - TSH

Treatment:

Pharmacologic:
- Selective serotonin reuptake inhibitors (SSRIs)
  - Fluoxetine has been cited by the U.S. Preventive Services Task Force Recommendation as being efficacious.
    - ○ Fluoxetine 10 mg p.o. daily (usual starting dose with titration in increments of 10 mg until maximum dose of 60 mg)
  - Citalopram is another alternative with good efficacy.
    - ○ Citalopram 10 mg p.o. daily (usual starting dose with titration in increments of 10 mg until maximum dose of 60 mg)
- Monitor for risk of suicidal ideations since increased risk has been noted with use of SSRIs.
- Most medication regimens are continued for 4 to 9 months.

Nonpharmacologic:
- Psychotherapy (cognitive behavioral therapy [CBT] and interpersonal therapy)
- Encourage exercise program as exercise has both direct and indirect positive effects on depression.
- Frequent follow-up is suggested for 2 to 3 months after treatment is completed due to the potential of relapse.
- Assessing and educating parents regarding the potential of suicide

Adolescent Idiopathic Scoliosis

Description of the Disease: Adolescent idiopathic scoliosis is a musculoskeletal disorder in children 10 years and older involving vertebral rotation and a lateral curvature of the spine that measures greater than 10°.

Epidemiology/Etiology:
- 85% of detected scoliosis is idiopathic scoliosis, meaning having no cause.
- Develops after the age of 10
- 2% to 4% of the population is affected.
- Incidence: Equal among boys and girls; girls more likely to have larger curves and greater progression
- Unknown etiology but recent research suggests genetics may be a factor as well as biomechanical and hormonal causes.
- Seen at the onset of growth spurts during preadolescence; so adolescence screening should begin at age 10.
- Other causes of structural scoliosis: Cerebral palsy, Marfan syndrome, Arnold–Chiari malformation, polio, syringomyelia, muscular dystrophy, spinal tumors
- Classifications based on onset: infantile (birth to 3 years of age), juvenile (3 to 10 years of age), adolescent (in children older than 10 years of age), or adult

Signs and Symptoms:
- Mainly asymptomatic
- Physical observation of unequal heights of the shoulders or hip
- One arm may hang lower
- Prominent shoulder blade
- Unequal rib prominences
- Normally does not cause back pain; if complaints of significant pain, r/o other diagnosis, that is, tumor.

Differential Diagnoses:
- Postural or functional scoliosis due to leg-length discrepancy
- Structural scoliosis due to neuromuscular problem or spinal deformity

Diagnostic Studies:
- Mixed opinions regarding routine school screening (USPTF against and AAP pro)
- Adams forward bend test
- Scoliometer measurement increases sensitivity.
  - Measurements greater than 10° need radiologic follow-up.
- Spinal radiography: Standing A-P and lateral views (Cobb angle measurement)
- Spine MRI for atypical presentation, especially with back pain

Treatment (Pharmacologic and Nonpharmacologic):
- For curves 10° to 20°: observation every 3 to 4 months with spinal x-ray every 6 months to 1 year
- Curves greater than 20 should be referred to an orthopedic specialist for monitoring.
- Curves between 25° and 40°: Milwaukee bracing
- Over 40°: Surgery

Amenorrhea

Description of the Disease: Absence of menstruation flow
- Primary amenorrhea is the absence of menstruation by the age of 16 with secondary sex characteristics or by 14 without any signs of sexual development.
- Secondary amenorrhea is the absence of menstrual flow once menstruation has started for three cycles or 6 months.

Epidemiology:
- Primary amenorrhea: 0.3% of females with 60% due to structural development issues; 40% is hormone related
- Secondary amenorrhea: 3% to 4% of females
- 44% of competitive athletes experience secondary amenorrhea (female athlete triad)

Etiology:
- Primary amenorrhea:
  - Structural anomalies of the ovaries, uterus, hymen: Imperforated hymen, Müllerian agenesis, absence of the vagina and/or uterus
  - Gonadal dysfunction (most common cause) related to genetic disorders
    - Turner syndrome
  - Hypothalamus and pituitary disorders
    - Tumors
    - Hyperprolactinemia
    - May see functional hypothalamic amenorrhea from stress, eating disorders, excessive exercise
  - Thyroid disorders
  - Constitutional delay of puberty (no direct cause found, menses is delayed for up to 2 years—usually a family history of delayed puberty)
- Secondary:
  - Pregnancy (most common cause)
  - Breast-feeding
  - Hormonal imbalance
    - Hypothalamic-pituitary disruption (stress, significant weight loss, eating disorders, competitive athletics, excessive exercise)
    - Thyroid disorders
    - Hypothalamic and pituitary disorders: Tumors
- Medications (oral contraceptives, Depo-Provera, danazol, systemic steroids, antipsychotics, antidepressants, cocaine, chemotherapy)
- Structural
  - Polycystic ovary disease
  - Asherman's syndrome (results from uterine surgery)
- Chronic illnesses
  - Uncontrolled diabetes mellitus

Risk Factors:
- Primary
  - Family history of delayed amenorrhea

- Secondary
  - Excessive exercise (athletes, dancers)
  - High levels of stress
  - Anorexia and bulimia

Signs and Symptoms:
- Absence of menses
- Physical characteristics associated with chromosomal disorders: Such as in Turner's syndrome (short stature, short toes and fingers, webbed neck, widely spaced nipples)
- Signs of pregnancy
- Signs and symptoms associated with various etiology (i.e., hirsutism and acne with PCOS; galactorrhea and headaches with pituitary tumors; signs/symptoms of hypothyroidism or hyperthyroidism)
- Weight disturbances
  - Underweight (may be associated with anorexia, bulimia, and female athlete triad)
  - Overweight (may be associated with PCOS)

Differential Diagnoses:
- See Etiology

Diagnostic Studies:
- Serum hCG (pregnancy test)
- FSH, LH
- Prolactin level
- TSH
- Fasting glucose (r/o diabetes)
- Pelvic ultrasound to determine if any structural cause
- Primary amenorrhea: Consider chromosome analysis if genetic abnormality is suspected.
- If all diagnostic tests are within normal limits and pregnancy is excluded, may do progesterone challenge test.
  - Medroxyprogesterone acetate 10 mg p.o. for 5 to 10 days or one dose of progesterone in oil 100 to 200 mg IM
    ○ Spotting or bleeding up to a week or two afterward is positive challenge test (correlation to + estrogen being present but anovulatory)
    ○ Negative results consider low estrogen levels causing anovulation or structural outlet flow alteration.
  - If no menses after 6 months, consider bone density to r/o osteoporosis

Treatment:
- Dependent upon etiology
- Refer all patients with primary amenorrhea to gynecologist.
- Refer all patients with negative progesterone testing to gynecologist.

Pharmacologic:
- Replacement of progesterone
  - Oral contraceptives
  - Medroxyprogesterone acetate 10 mg p.o. for 10 days each month until cycle is reestablished
- Calcium supplement 800 to 1,200 mg of calcium with 400 mg vitamin D or increasing dietary sources of calcium

Nonpharmacologic:
- Decrease exercise
- Nutritional counseling:
  - Increase weight if significant weight loss—a 5 to 10 lb increase may reestablish cycle.
  - Decrease weight if obesity is a concern.

Eating Disorders: Anorexia, Bulimia, and Binge Eating

Description of the Disease: Eating disorders are the interplay of multifactorial etiologies that result in either under or over nutritional conditions of the body.

Eating disorders fall into three groups: Anorexia nervosa (anorexia), bulimia, and binge eating
- Anorexia is psychosocial disorder in which there is an obsession to be thin through excessive exercise, dieting, or starvation.
- Bulimia is periods of binge eating followed by purging via self-induced vomiting, use of laxatives, diarrhea, and/or exercise to avoid weight gain.
- Binge eating is the overconsumption of food, which leads to obesity.

Epidemiology:
- Average onset of eating disorders is 12- to 13-year-olds.
- Females > males;
- 10% of those adolescents with eating disorders are males.
- These three disorders affect approximately 3% of the teen population:
  - Anorexia: 0.5% of the adolescent population
  - Bulimia: 1% to 2% of the adolescent population
  - Binge eating: 1.6% of the adolescent population
- 79% of teens with eating order have underlying mental health issues (i.e., depression, anxiety, suicidal ideation)
- Anorexia is associated with the highest mortality rate of all mental health diagnoses.
- Binge eating is the most common eating disorder.

Etiology:
Multifactorial
- Biologic factors:
  - Tendency to run in families—research shows possibility of a genetic link
  - Questionable biochemical imbalance (serotonin, leptin)
- Psychological:
  - Low self-esteem
  - Perfectionist personality
  - Obsessive–compulsive behavior
  - Stress
  - Poor body image
- Social:
  - Peer pressure
  - Anorexia and bulimia—associated with American culture idolizing "thinness"
  - Troubled relationships

Risk Factors:
- Gender: Girls more than boys
- Age: Seen as early as 8, peaks between 13 and 14 and then 17 and 18
- Family history: Tendency to run in families
- Athletes (sports, gymnastics)
- Artistic activities (dancers, models, actors)

Signs and Symptoms:
- Initially may not have apparent signs of symptomatology
- Diagnostic criteria set by the *DSM-V*

Anorexia Nervosa	Bulimia	Binge Eating Disorder
• Continuous weight loss • Thin body appearance • Cold intolerance • Amenorrhea • Fine hair growth on back or face (Lanugo) • Thinning hair • Brittle nails • Dry, dull, flaky skin • Speaks continuously of dieting or looking fat • Fear of gaining weight • Overly concerned about appearance and weight • Low pulse and BP • Fatigue • May wear baggy or excessive clothes to hide weight. • As anorexia progresses: 　◦ Cardiac abnormities 　◦ Osteoporosis 　◦ Electrolyte imbalances 　◦ Abnormal liver function test	• Binge-eating habits • Uses restroom frequently after eating • Fluctuations in weight up to 10 lb • Swelling around cheeks (due to enlarged parotid glands) • Teeth erosion and dental caries (due to vomitus acidity) • Calluses or small abrasions on knuckles from self-induced vomiting (Russell sign) • Facial capillaries or subconjunctival hemorrhages of the eye • Signs/symptoms of electrolyte disturbances: weakness • Fatigue, cardiac irregularities • Chief complaint of acid reflux or esophagitis • Decreased gag reflex • Laboratory abnormalities: 　◦ Hypokalemia, hyponatremia 　◦ Elevated serum bicarbonate	• Weight normal or overweight • Reported episodes of excessive eating even when not hungry • Reports of eating extremely fast • Complaints of abdominal discomfort due to fullness • Experiences guilt after binge episodes • Binging occurs at least once a week for 3 mo

Differential Diagnoses:
- Gastrointestinal illnesses (malabsorption syndromes, inflammatory bowel diseases)
- Malignancies
- Hormonal imbalances (hyperthyroidism, adrenal insufficiency, diabetes mellitus)
- Other psychiatric disorders: Depression, obsessive–compulsive disorder
- Substance abuse

Diagnostic Studies:
- All adolescents should be prescreened for an eating disorder. The SCOFF questionnaire and EAT-26 are two validated tools to use.
- Performed initially to r/o other causes. Laboratories usually will remain normal until electrolytes/fluid imbalance or malnutrition
  - CBC (may indicate anemia)
  - Urinalysis (evaluates kidney function)
  - Thyroid panel (r/o thyroid disorder as cause)
  - Serum amylase (elevations noted with severe vomiting)
  - Chemistry profile (r/o diabetes as cause; evaluates electrolytes, liver and kidney functions)
  - EKG (detects cardiac abnormalities due to malnutrition and electrolyte imbalances)

Treatment:
- If adolescent has signs and symptoms of severe malnutrition or is below 75% weight for height, hospitalization is required. Hospitalization is recommended for adolescents not improving during outpatient treatment.
- Otherwise can be managed as outpatient

Anorexia:
- **Nonpharmacologic**: Mainstay of treatment is threefold: refer for psychotherapy (individual and family therapy); nutritional counseling, and in-office medical management. Preferred treatment is seeking outpatient treatment center.
  - In office medical management:
    ○ Weekly weights: Weights should be done in underwear and/or patient gown.
    ○ Weekly urine specific gravity (detects dehydration or water loading for weight gain)
    ○ Laboratory work as needed (CBC and Chemistry profile)
    ○ Monitor for anxiety, depression, and suicidal tendencies
    ○ Provide psychological and emotional Support—takes 2 to 3 years to get in remission with only a 50% success rate
    ○ Restrict activities in beginning to conserve calorie burning
    ○ Expected weight gain is 1 to 2 lb a week
    ○ Encourage three supervised meals/day
- **Pharmacologic**:
  - Only if needed to treat coexisting anxiety or depression (may need lower dosage adjustment due to low body weight and impaired liver/kidney function)

Bulimia:
- **Nonpharmacologic**: Mainstay of treatment is CBT and family therapy, in addition to nutritional counseling; majority of cases treated without the need for hospitalization
  - In-office medical management: Determined by the severity and any noted complications; usually biweekly till stable
    ○ Monitor weight. Since weight can be within normal range, weekly weigh-ins are not necessary. Watch for major fluctuations.
    ○ Laboratories as needed
    ○ Monitor for associated psychological problems (depression and/or anxiety)
    ○ Supervised meals and bathroom visits up to 2 hours after meals
    ○ Provide psychological and emotional support
    ○ If weight is within normal range, can participate in a healthy form of exercise
- **Pharmacologic**:
  - Fluoxetine has been shown to be effective in the management of bulimia.
    ○ Dosage: 20 mg p.o. daily, can be increased if needed to recommended dosage of 60 mg p.o. daily
    ○ Monitor for complications and suicidal tendencies
  - Do not prescribe bupropion due to increased incidence of seizures in bulimia.

Binge Eating:
- **Nonpharmacologic:**
  - CBT has seen a 50% improvement rate.
  - Interpersonal therapy (IPT) has also had some success rate.
  - Nutritional counseling
- **Pharmacologic:**
  - Lisdexamfetamine, first ADA-approved drug, for moderate to severe binge eating
  - Antidepressants (SSRIs) for treatment of coexisting anxiety or depression
  - Anticonvulsive drugs (such as Topamax) have been used off label with some effectiveness.

Infectious Mononucleosis

Description of the Disease: Often referred as the kissing disease, mononucleosis is viral infection characterized by fever, fatigue, sore throat, and lymphadenopathy.

Epidemiology and Etiology:
- 90% of cases are caused by the Epstein–Barr virus (EBV); cytomegalovirus (CMV) has been a causative factor in a few cases.
- Peak incidence is between the ages of 15 and 24: by adulthood 90% of individuals have been infected with EBV.
- Transmission is via oropharyngeal secretions; saliva can be infectious for up to 18 months.
- Incubation is 4 to 6 weeks after exposure.
- Splenomegaly occurs in 15% to 65% of cases.

Risk Factors:
- Exposure to infected individual's saliva such as kissing, sharing eating utensils, glasses, and food
- Droplet exposure of an infected individual, that is, coughing, sneezing

Signs and Symptoms:
- Fatigue
- Pharyngitis[2]
- Tonsillitis
- Pharynx often displays enlarged white or grayish-green exudate on tonsils.
- Lymphadenopathy[2] (commonly posterior cervical lymph node involvement)
- Fever[2]
- Headache
- Splenomegaly (occurs in 15% to 65% of cases)
- Hepatomegaly (noted in 10% of cases)

Differential Diagnoses:
- Streptococcal pharyngitis
- CMV
- Human immunodeficiency virus (HIV)
- Viral syndrome
- Toxoplasmosis

Diagnostic Studies:
- CBC with differential shows leukocytosis and atypical lymphocytes > 10%.
- Monospot test (heterophile antibody test) (sometimes can be negative if done too soon)
- EBV IgM ad IgG
- Rapid group A β strep culture, if negative send culture.
- Liver function test

Treatment:

Pharmacologic:
- Supportive care: Analgesics, acetaminophen, or NSAIDS
- Antibiotics if concurrent infection (avoid amoxicillin and ampicillin due to association with the development of a skin rash)

---

[2]Classic triad symptoms.

Nonpharmacologic:
- Saline gargles for sore throat
- Rest
- Avoid strenuous exercise and contact sports for 6 to 8 weeks and until symptom free.
- Monitor for complications: ruptured spleen, upper airway obstruction, meningitis, and encephalitis.

Osgood-Schlatter Disease (Tibial Tubercle Apophysitis)

Description of the Disease: The swelling and inflammation of the tubercle tuberosity due to stress/pull on the patellar tendon insertion site at that point; often associated with rapid growth and repetitive or excessive movement (i.e., exercise, sports)

Epidemiology: (Zayas, 2010)
- Seen in preadolescence during growth spurt or early adolescence (11 to 15); girls may demonstrate it as early as age 9.
- Affects boys more than girls (3:1)
- Commonly seen among sports participants (28%): Only 4.5% of nonparticipants
- Can occur bilaterally in up to 30% of cases

Etiology:
- Overuse of the quadriceps muscle in activities that involve running, jumping, kicking, and/or kneeling causes a pull of the patellar tendon at the insertion site (apophysis) on the tibia resulting in inflammation of the apophysis or apophysitis.
- Bone ossification of the tibia has not been completed causing its susceptibility.
- Repeated tension can actually cause small avulsions of the site.
- May lead to hypertrophic ossification as micro avulsions heal resulting in a bump at the tuberosity site

Risk Factors:
- Sport activities with running, jumping, and kicking motions, such as soccer, basketball, track
- Kneeling activities such as gardening

Signs and Symptoms:
- Pain while participating in repetitive activity
- Pain is found to subside with rest.
- Pain on palpation of the tibial tuberosity area
- Swelling of affected area may be noted.
- + Pain with extension of the knee against resistance

Differential Diagnoses:
- Avulsion fracture
- Patellar–femoral syndrome
- Patellar tendonitis
- Tumor
- Infection

Diagnostic Studies:
- Usually not required; diagnosis is based on clinical findings.
- Can order AP and lateral (with slight internal knee rotation) x-ray of the knee
  - R/o other pathology
  - Radiographs may show swelling of area and/or micro fragmentation of area to verify diagnosis.

Treatment:
Pharmacologic:
- Ibuprofen or acetaminophen for pain management

Nonpharmacologic:
- Mainstay of treatment is conservative.
- Rest and limitation of activity depending on severity
  - If moderate or severe symptomatology, limit sports participation
- Ice is used in all stages, especially after activity.
- Use of knee pad (Osgood-Schlatter band/pad)
- Physical therapy for quadriceps and hamstring strengthening

Sports-related Concussions (Mild Traumatic Brain Injury)

Description of the Disease: A concussion is direct impact to the head or part of the body that the force is transferred to the head. Concussions can cause patients physical, cognitive, sleep, or emotional symptoms. To denote the seriousness of this injury, concussions are not being diagnosed as mild-traumatic brain injury (MTBI).

Epidemiology:
- In United States over 300,000 sports-related concussions; 130,000 are between the ages of 5 and 18.
- 8.9% of all high school athletic injuries
- Overall, males have the greater occurrences than females.
  - However, incidence is greater in girls than boys playing similar sports (may be skewed since boys are less likely to report symptoms).
- MVA accidents are the number one cause of MTBI, followed by sports.

Etiology:
- Outside force either directly to the head or indirectly to the body causes brain movement against the skull resulting in a neuronal—metabolic dysfunction within the brain causing cascade of symptoms.
- Contact sports: Higher incidence
- Top five concerning sports: football, boys' ice hockey, boys' lacrosse, girls' soccer, and girls' lacrosse (Marar, McIlvain, Fields, & Comstock, 2012)

Risk Factors:
- Organized sports participation
- Contact sports: Highest risk
- Recreational activities

Signs and Symptoms:
- May or may not have loss of consciousness (approximately up to 10% lose consciousness)
- Physical: Headache, dizziness, photophobia, or other visual changes, nausea, and vomiting
- Cognitive changes: Difficulty concentration, confusion, memory impairment either before or after occurrence, slowness in processing questions or thoughts
- Emotional: Sadness, irritability, anxiety, or nervousness
- Sleep disturbances: Increased daytime fatigue and sleepiness, difficulty falling or staying asleep

Differential Diagnoses:
- Intracranial hemorrhage
- Head contusion
- Headache disorder

Diagnostic Studies:
- Immediate sideline evaluation involves assessment of ABCs and the use of Standardized Assessment of Concussion (SAC), which measures cognitive function or The Sports Concussion Assessment Tool 3 (SCAT3) if a health provider/medical trainer is available.
- A head CT is the gold standard during the first 24 to 48 hours if any loss of consciousness, vomiting, severe headache, change in mental status, or signs of skull fracture.
- If a CT scan is not available, a skull radiograph or MRI is an acceptable option.
- Neuropsychological testing has been beneficial in detecting deficits and is recommended by the CDC Heads Up Program.
- Spinal films, especially neck films, may be considered to r/o associated vertebral fracture if suspected.

Treatment:

Nonpharmacologic:
- In-office treatment consists of frequent observation and monitoring
- Moderate to severe cases will most likely be seen and treated by emergency medicine or a specialist.
- Any athlete with a suspected concussion should be unable to return to play for the remainder of the day and until evaluated by a health care provider.
- Office evaluation should consist of frequent monitoring; symptom reduction should occur in 3 to 5 days. Most symptoms take about 7 to 10 takes for resolution.
  - Cognitive symptom monitoring by the SCAT3 or another valid tool is helpful in monitoring improvement.
- If signs and symptoms are not diminishing or worsening, refer to MTBI specialist
- Signs of worsening conditions include a constant headache, slurred speech, repeated episodes of dizziness, extreme irritability, vomiting more than two times, change in gait, change in sleeping habits, change in

pupil reactivity, convulsions, change in vision, weakness in extremities, tinnitus, or bloody or watery fluid from nose or ears (DeRosea et.al, 2010).
- Rest and instruction in activity modification is a key to recovery.
  - Physical or cognitive exertion is to be limited during recovery, especially for the first 24 to 48 hours. This means no sports, gym, exercising, heavy lifting. Cognitive exertion means avoidance of homework, classroom work, video gaming, and computer work.
  - Activity can begin slowly as symptoms improve. Each step should be tolerated for at least 3 to 5 days without symptoms
    - ○ Physical activity: Beginning with light aerobic activity → mild training drills for sports, that is, running, skating → noncontact drills → full training → game play. Continuous monitoring must be made during phases; if symptoms return, physical rest is once again initiated.
    - ○ Cognitive activity recovery begins with half day of schooling for 3 days progressing to full days. Classroom and homework may need modification to still allow for rest.
  - Initiate primary prevention education to prevent reoccurrence, that is, protective equipment, helmets, seat belts, etc.

Tanner Stages

Definition: A way to monitor sexual development

Epidemiology:
- Can begin as early as 8 years of age with African-American girls maturing earlier, followed by Hispanics and Latinos, then Caucasians

Girls

Tanner Stage	Pubic Hair	Breasts
I	Prepubescence: No growth	Prepubescence: No glandular tissue growth; elevation of papillae
II[a]	Sparse, lightly pigmented, and straight; along labia majora	Breast bud stage[b]: Small mound of breast tissue; areola increases in size
III	Darker and curly, moderate in amount, extends upward, limited to the mons	Breast and areola grow bigger—no separation in contour
IV	Darker, curly, course, and abundant (but not full adult size) triangular—not spread to thighs	Areola and papillae form a second mound above breast tissue
V	Adult appearance, hair extends to thighs	Adult appearance, areola recedes to meet remaining breast tissue—smooth contour; nipple protrudes

[a]Breast budding can begin as early as age 8.
- Development before age 8 is considered precocious puberty.
- No secondary sex characteristics by age 12 to 13 are considered delayed puberty.

[b]First visible sign of puberty is breast enlargement (thelarche) → growth spurt → menarche (follows in approximately 3 years after development of breast buds)

Boys

Tanner Stage	Pubic Hair	Penis/Scrotum
I		No change
II[a]	Sparse, lightly pigmented and straight; along the base of penis	Scrotum and testes[b] enlarge. Scrotal skin changes: thins, pinkish-reddish color
III	Darker and coarser, begins to curl	Enlargement of the length of penis; scrotum and testes continue to grow
IV	Almost adult like, course, curly, and abundant—hair does not extend to thighs	Scrotum and testes still continue to grow and darken; penis continues to grow in length and circumference
V	Adult appearance—hair extends to thighs	Adult appearance

[a] Can begin as early as age 9
- Development before age 9 is considered precocious puberty.
- No secondary sex characteristics by age 12 to 13 is considered delayed puberty.

[b] First visible sign of puberty is testicular enlargement.
- Secondary sex characteristics later than age 14: delayed puberty

Review Section

Review Questions

1. John is 16 years of age and presents to the office with symptoms of sore throat, fever, fatigue, and posterior cervical adenopathy. His CBC shows leukocytosis and atypical lymphocytes ≥10%. Your treatment includes:

   a. penicillin V 500 mg p.o. t.i.d. for 10 days.
   b. oseltamivir 75 mg p.o. b.i.d. daily for 5 days.
   c. famciclovir 500 mg p.o. every 8 hours for 7 days.
   d. acetaminophen, saline gargles, no contact sports.

2. In the initial management of an adolescent with anorexia, all of the following are recommended as first-line treatment except:

   a. nutritional counseling.
   b. fluoxetine 20 mg p.o. daily.
   c. psychotherapy.
   d. in-office management of weight, urine specific gravity, observation for concurrent depression, and/or anxiety.

3. The diagnosis of ADHD in a school-age child can be confirmed only if which of the following criteria are met?

   a. Symptoms have occurred for the past 3 months.
   b. Symptoms have been seen either school or at home.
   c. Must display at least six inattentive or hyperactive–impulsive symptoms.
   d. Symptoms need to be present before the age of 6.

4. Kelly is 6 years old and has type 1 diabetes that is controlled by insulin. Which parental educational pearl is true regarding the management of her diabetes during illness?

   a. If Kelly experiences a fever or an infection, her insulin needs most likely will increase.
   b. When Kelly experiences symptoms of gastroenteritis (vomiting and diarrhea), withhold all insulin for 24 hours to prevent hypoglycemia and resume once symptoms have stopped and Kelly gets back to her regular dietary intake.
   c. Since Kelly is young and appetite is often diminished with illness, her blood glucose level only needs to be checked in the morning and night during times of illness.
   d. During mild illnesses, Kelly should be encouraged to continue the same insulin amount but consume a higher-caloric diet to promote healing.

5. Four-year-old Trina has a history of asthma. Her grandmother brings her in for her 6-month follow-up. During history taking, you note that Trina is on a short-acting β$_2$-agonist as needed. According to her grandmother she has been having coughing "attacks" almost 3 to 4 days a week and is using her inhaler with a spacer at least 6 times a week. Grandmom notes she mostly sleeps through the night but may wake up occasionally coughing but this does not occur every night or every week. Knowing this your next step in Trina's asthma management is:

   a. prescribe a long-acting β-agonist daily, in addition to p.r.n. use of her short-acting β$_2$-agonist.
   b. note that Trina has level 1, mild intermittent asthma and continue the use of the short-acting β$_2$-agonist along with a second-generation antihistamine.
   c. prescribe a low-dose inhaled corticosteroid daily, in addition to p.r.n. use of her short-acting β$_2$-agonist.
   d. note that Trina has moderate persistent asthma and according to guidelines needs to be referred to a asthma specialist for management.

6. A 3-year-old male with no significant medical history is in your clinic with complaints of nasal congestion, and pressure in his left ear for the past 3 days. He has a decreased appetite, coughing during the night, and his temperature this morning was 38.2°C. No medications have been tried. What would your treatment be for this patient?

   a. A 10-day course of amoxicillin 90 mcg/kg/day
   b. A 10-day course of amoxicillin–clavulanate 90 mg/kg/day
   c. A 10-day course of amoxicillin 45 mcg/kg/day
   d. Watchful waiting with a follow-up in 48 hours

7. A 4-month-old patient is in your office with parental concerns of a diaper rash for the past week. The mother states "It is getting worse and it is causing her pain." On evaluation, you notice beefy red satellite lesions extending to the inner thighs and stomach. Which treatment would be the most appropriate for this patient? Select all that apply.

   a. Mupirocin (Bactroban) topical twice a day for 5 days
   b. Nystatin cream three times a day for 5 days
   c. Hydrocortisone cream 2.5% topically twice a day for 5 days
   d. A barrier paste with every diaper change
   e. Allow the skin to dry after diaper changes
   f. Start using rubber or plastic pants over the diaper

8. An 8-month-old female presents to an urgent care clinic where you are working with a chief complaint of a cough. Her father states she has had a runny nose for 3 days, but tonight she has a barky cough.

   On physical examination you note, vital signs: HR 110, RR 40, temperature 98.7°F, BP not obtained

   She is pink, anterior fontanel open and flat, no nasal flaring, no retractions, +nasal congestion, OP clear, tonsils +1, lungs clear to auscultation, S1, S2, no murmur, pulses +2, well perfused.

   What treatment would you provide to this patient?

   a. Since she has a stridor, she is at risk for respiratory distress and should be evaluated in the emergency department.
   b. Prescribe amoxicillin 90 mcg/kg/day to treat the infection.
   c. Administer one dose of dexamethasone 0.6 mg/kg in the office to prevent worsening symptoms.
   d. Administer albuterol 1.25 mL via nebulizer to open up the airway.

9. You are evaluating a 2-year-old male with presenting symptoms of nasal congestion, a sore throat, a cough, and a low-grade fever. On physical examination you note both eyes to be tearing with injected conjunctiva with minimal yellow exudate. His father is concerned with his "pink eye." As the nurse practitioner, which treatment would you consider the most appropriate? Select all that apply.

   a. Cool compresses three times a day
   b. Preservative-free artificial tears four times a day for comfort
   c. Fluoroquinolone drops three times a day for 7 days
   d. Corticosteroid drops twice daily for 7 days
   e. Refer to ophthalmology immediately for management
   f. Educate on good hand washing and transmission prevention

10. A 3-year-old male has been having intermittent abdominal pain with episodes of relief, bloody mucous stools, and vomiting. He is being evaluated in the urgent care division of the emergency department where you are the nurse practitioner. What would be the best treatment for him?

   a. Order an abdominal flat-plate radiograph to assess for gastritis.
   b. Refer to radiology and surgery for an air contrast enema.
   c. Immediately order a CT of the abdomen to an acute abdomen.
   d. Discharge home with BRAT diet and hydration therapy

Answers with Rationales

1. (d) acetaminophen, saline gargles, no contact sports.

   Rationale: John is displaying classic symptoms of infectious mononucleosis, which is caused by the Epstein–Barr virus and treated symptomatically. Contact sports should be avoided due to possible splenomegaly that occurs in up to 50% of cases.

2. (b) fluoxetine 20 mg p.o. daily.

   Rationale: Mainstay treatment for anorexia is nonpharmacologic treatment. Fluoxetine is prescribed for the management of bulimia.

3. (c) Must display at least six inattentive or hyperactive–impulsive symptoms.

   Rationale: According to the *DSM-V*, the diagnosis of ADHD can only be made in a school-age child if six or more symptoms of inattention and/or hyperactivity–impulsivity occur at BOTH school and home; have been present for at least 6 months; and were present before the age of 12.

4. (a) If Kelly experiences a fever or an infection, her insulin needs most likely will increase.

   Rationale: Illnesses cause stress on the body, resulting in increased cortisol levels, which ultimately raise blood glucose level; therefore, during illness most likely more insulin will be needed. It is recommended that more-than-normal blood glucose testing be done at this time often as many as every 2 to 4 hours. Withholding insulin is to be avoided.

5. (c) Prescribe a low-dose inhaled corticosteroid daily, in addition to her p.r.n. use of her short-acting β_2-agonist.

   Rationale: Trina is exhibiting signs of mild persistent asthma, which means symptoms are occurring more than twice a week but less than daily and nighttime symptoms are less than once a week. Guideline recommendations state for level 2 asthma (mild persistent) to prescribe a low-dose inhaled corticosteroid daily or as an alternate a leukotriene modifier such as montelukast.

6. (d) Watchful waiting with a follow-up in 48 hours

    Rationale: For patients above 2 years of age with mild otalgia and temperatures <39°C, the treatment of choice is watchful wait for 48 to 72 hours. Within 24 hours of diagnosis, the majority of children's symptoms resolve. Antibiotics should be administered diligently to prevent antibiotic resistance.

7. (b) Nystatin cream three times a day for 5 days
    (d) A barrier paste with every diaper change
    (e) Allow the skin to dry after diaper changes

    Rationale: This is *Candida* diaper dermatitis and should be treated with nystatin, a barrier paste, and allowing the skin to dry after diaper changes. Mupirocin would not treat the yeast. Hydrocortisone cream 1% would be appropriate, but 2.5% is too strong for the genital area. Using rubber or plastic pants is a risk factor to cause diaper dermatitis, so not a treatment option.

8. (c) Administer one dose of dexamethasone 0.6 mg/kg in the office to prevent worsening systems.

    Rationale: Her physical examination is consistent with mild croup. She does not need to report to the emergency department. Croup is usually caused

by parainfluenza type 1, so an antibiotic would not help. Dexamethasone would be appropriate to administer. Albuterol treats the lower airway, not the upper airway, which is affected in croup.

9. (a) Cool compresses three times a day
    (b) Preservative-free artificial tears four times a day for comfort
    (f) Educate on good hand washing and transmission prevention

    Rationale: All of his symptoms are consistent with adenovirus. He has viral conjunctivitis. Symptomatic care with cool compresses and preservative-free artificial tears are the appropriate management. Antibiotic drops are not recommended and corticosteroid drops are contraindicated. If he does not heal in 7 days he could be referred to ophthalmology. Transmission prevention is also important since viral conjunctivitis is contagious.

10. (b) Refer to radiology and surgery for an air contrast enema.

    Rationale: His diagnosis is intussusception. Air contrast enema is diagnostic and the treatment of choice. The other answers are incorrect.

Suggested Readings

Advisory Committee on Immunization Practices. (2010). FDA licensure of bivalent human papillomavirus vaccine (HPV2, Cervarix) for use in females and updated HPV vaccination recommendations from the Advisory Committee on Immunization Practices (ACIP). *Morbidity and Mortality Weekly Report (MMWR), 59*(20), 626–629.

Altman, C. A. (2015). Congenital heart disease (CHD) in the newborn: Presentation and screening for critical CHD. In *UpToDate*, Waltham, MA: UpToDate.

American Academy of Pediatrics. (2012). Policy statement: Breastfeeding and the use of human milk. *Pediatrics, 129*(3), e827–e841.

American Academy of Pediatrics. (2016). *Bright futures*. Retrieved from www.brightfutures.aap.org

American Academy of Pediatrics and American Academy of Family Physicians, Subcommittee on Management of Acute Otitis Media. (2004). Diagnosis and management of acute otitis media. *Pediatrics, 113*(5), 1451–165.

American Academy of Pediatrics: Subcommittee on Attention-Deficit/Hyperactivity Disorder, Steering Committee on Quality Improvement and Management. (2011). ADHD: Clinical practice guideline for the diagnosis, evaluation, and treatment of attention-deficit/hyperactivity disorder in children and adolescents. *Pediatrics, 128*(5), 1007–1022. doi:10.1542/peds.2011-2654.

American College of Preventative Medicine. (2010). *Adolescent depression—enhancing outcomes in primary care: A clinical reference.* 1–32. Retrieved from http://www.acpm.org/?AdDepresTTClinicians

American College of Preventative Medicine. (2010). *Adolescent wellness exam: Overcoming reluctance on both sides by building rapport using every opportunity to promote healthy choices.* Retrieved from http://www.acpm.org/?adWellnessTimetool

American Diabetes Association. (2014). Standards of medical care in diabetes. *Diabetes Care, 38*(S1), S1–S94.

American Psychiatric Association. (2013). *Diagnostic and statistical manual of mental disorders* (5th ed.). Washington, DC: American Psychiatric Association.

AspectsIn, C., & Saccomano, S. J. (2013). Infectious mononucleosis. *Clinician Reviews, 23*(6), 42. Retrieved from http://go.galegroup.com/ps/i.do?id=GALE%7CA336176313&v=2.1&u=drexel_main&it=r&p=AONE&sw=w&asid=362e9d55cbc55bd65ab20e80db42e72f

Brink, S., Joel, D., Laffel, L., Lee, W. W. R., Olsen, B., Phelan, H., & Hanas, R. (2014). Sick day management in children and adolescents with diabetes. *Pediatric Diabetes, 15*(S20), 193–202. doi:10.1111/pedi.12193.

Burns, C. E., Dunn, A. M., Brady, M. A., Starr, N. B., & Blosser, C. G. (2013). *Pediatric primary care* (5th ed.). Philadelphia, PA: Elsevier Saunders. http://brightfutures.aap.org/tool_and_resource_kit.html

Cash, J. C., & Glass, C. A. (Eds.). (2011). *Family practice guidelines* (2nd ed.). New York, NY: Springer Publishing Company.

Center for Disease Control and Prevention. (2006). Preventing tetanus, diphtheria, and pertussis among adolescents: Use of tetanus toxoid, reduced diphtheria toxoid and acellular pertussis vaccines. *MMWR, 4,* 55(RR03), 1–34. Retrieved from http://www.cdc.gov/mmwr/preview/mmwrhtml/rr5503a1.htm

Centers for Disease Control and Prevention. (2010). WHO growth standards are recommended for use in the U.S. for infants and children 0 to 2 years of age. Retrieved from http://www.cdc.gov/growthcharts/data/who/grchrt_girls_24lw_9210.pdf

Centers for Disease Control and Prevention. (2013). *Parasites: Head lice.* Retrieved from www.cdc.gov.ezproxy2.library.drexel.edu/parasites/lice/head/index.html

Center for Disease Control and Prevention. (2015). *Recommended immunization schedule for persons aged 0 through 18 years.* Retrieved from http://www.cdc.gov/vaccines/schedules/hcp/child-adolescent.html

Chen, S. (2015). Measles. *Medscape Drug and Diseases.* Retrieved from http://emedicine.medscape.com/article/966220-overview

Cohen, J. I. (2012). Epstein–Barr virus infections, including infectious mononucleosis. In D. L. Longo, A. S. Fauci, D. L. Kasper, S. L. Hauser, J. Jameson, & J. Loscalzo (Eds.), *Harrison's principles of internal medicine* (18th ed.). New York, NY: McGraw-Hill. Retrieved from http://accessmedicine.mhmedical.com.ezproxy2.library.drexel.edu/content.aspx?bookid=331&Sectionid=40726937

Committee on Quality Improvement, Subcommittee on Developmental Dysplasia of the Hip. (2000). Clinical practice guideline: Early detection of developmental dysplasia of the hip. *Pediatrics, 105*(4), 896–905.

Corona, M., McCarty, C., & Richardson, L. (2013). Screening adolescents for depression, *Contemporary Pediatrics, 30*(7), 24–30. Retrieve from http://contemporarypediatrics.modernmedicine.com/contemporary-pediatrics/content/tags/depression/screening-adolescents-depression?page=full

DeRosea, M., Grimes, M., Mahoney, J., Ruthman, M., King, S.K., Levin-Dorobo, L., . . . Smessaert, L., (Eds.). (2010). *Pediatric clinical practice guidelines & policies: A compendium of evidence-based research for pediatric practice* (10th ed.). Elk Grove Village, IL: American Academy of Pediatrics.

Duderstadt. (2014). *Pediatric Physical exam: An illustrated handbook.* St. Lewis, MO: Mosby/Elsevier.

DynaMed. (2014). *Precocious puberty.* Ipswich, MA: EBSCO Information Services. Retrieved from http://search.ebscohost.com.ezproxy2.library.drexel.edu/login.aspx?direct=true&site=DynaMed&id=113862

Eichenfield, L., Krakowski, A., Piggott, C., Del Rosso, J., Baldwin, H., Friedlander, S., Levy, M., . . . Thiboutot, D. (2013). Evidence-based recommendations for the diagnosis and treatment of pediatric acne. *Pediatrics, 131*(3), S163–S186. doi:10.1542/peds.2013-0490B

Ferri, F. (2014). *2015 Ferri's clinical advisor: 5 books in 1.* Philadelphia, PA: Elsevier/Mosby.

Frankowski, B. L., & Bocchini, J. A. (2010). Clinical report - head lice (from the American Academy of Pediatrics). *Pediatrics, 126*(2), 392–403.

Friedman, A. D. (2013). Wilms tumor. *Pediatric in Review, 34*(7), 328–330.

Funari, M. (2013). Detecting symptoms, early intervention, and preventative education: Eating disorders & the school-age child. *NASN School Nurse, 28*(3), 162–166. doi:10.1177/1942602X12473656.

Gan, M. J., Albanese-O'Neill, A., & Haller, M. J. (2012). Type 1 diabetes: Current concepts in epidemiology, pathophysiology, clinical care, and research. *Current Problems in Pediatric and Adolescent Health Care, 42*(10), 269–291.

Garzon, D. L., & Figgemeier, M. E. (2011). Dying to be thin: Identifying and managing eating disorders. *The Nurse Practitioner, 36*(10), 45–51. doi:10.1097/01.NPR.0000405157.98547.90.

Hagan, J. F., Shaw, J. S., & Duncan, P. M. (2008). Adolescence. In J. F. Hagan, J. S. Shaw, & P. M. Duncan (Eds.), *Bright futures: Guidelines/health supervision of infants, children, and adolescents* (3rd ed.). Elk Grove Village, IL: American Academy of Pediatrics. Retrieved from: https://brightfutures.aap.org/pdfs/Guidelines_PDF/18-Adolescence.pdf

Halstead, M. E., Walter, K. D., & The Council on Sports Medicine and Fitness. (2010). Sport-related concussion in children and adolescents. *Pediatrics, 126*(3), 597–615. doi:10.1542/peds.2010-2005

Hollier, A., & Hemsely, R. (2011). *Clinical guidelines in primary care: A reference and review book.* Lafayette, LA: Advanced Practice Education Associates.

Horne, J. P., Flannery, R., & Usman, S. (2014). Adolescent idiopathic scoliosis: Diagnosis and management. *American Family Physician, 89*(3), 193.

Hresko, M. T. (2013). Idiopathic scoliosis in adolescents. *The New England Journal of Medicine, 368*(9), 834–841.

Huffaker, M. F., & Phipatanakul, W. (2015). Pediatric asthma. *Immunology and Allergy Clinics of North America, 35*(1), 129–144. doi:10.1016/j.iac.2014.09.005

International Hip Dysplasia Institute. (2012). *Developmental dysplasia of the hip (DDH).* Retrieved from http://hipdysplasia.org/developmental-dysplasia-of-the-hip/

Kaneshiro, N. K. (2013). *Bronchiolitis.* Retrieved from http://www.nlm.nih.gov/medlineplus/ency/article/000975.htm

King, J. (2009). Infectious mononucleosis: Update and considerations. *The Nurse Practitioner, 34*(11), 42–45. doi:10.1097/01.NPR.0000363593.26568.66

Kletter, G. B., Klein, K. O., & Wong, Y. Y. (2015). A pediatrician's guide to central precocious puberty. *Clinical Pediatrics, 54*(5), 414–424. doi:10.1177/0009922814541807.

Kolon, T. F., Herndon, C. D. A., Baker, L. A., Baskin, L. S., Baxter, C. G., Cheng, E. Y., . . . Barthold, J. S. (2014). *Evaluation and treatment of cryptorchidism: American Urological Association Guideline.* Retrieved from https://www.auanet.org/education/guidelines/cryptorchidism.cfm

Koning, S., van der Sande, R., Verhagen, A. P., van Suijlekom-Smit, L. W. A., Morris, A. D., Butler, C. C., . . . van der Wouden, J. C. (2012). Interventions for impetigo. *The Cochrane Database of Systematic Reviews, 1,* CD003261.

Kroger, A. T., Sumaya, C. V., Pickering, L. K., Atkinson, W. L., National Center for Immunization and Respiratory Diseases, & Texas A&M Health Science Center. (2011). General recommendations on immunization: Recommendations of the Advisory Committee on Immunization Practices. *Recommendations and Reports, 60*(RR02), 1–60.

Larson, N. (2011). Early onset scoliosis: What the primary care provider needs to know and implications for practice. *Journal of the American Academy of Nurse Practitioners, 23*(8), 392–403. doi:10.1111/j.1745-7599.2011.00634.x.

Levin, M. J., & Weinberg, A. (2013). Infections: Viral & rickettsial. In W.W. Hay, M. J. Levin, R. R. Deterding, & M. J. Abzug. (Eds.), *Current diagnosis & treatment: Pediatrics* (22nd ed.). New York, NY: McGraw-Hill. Retrieved April 3, 2015 from http://accessmedicine.mhmedical.com.ezproxy2.library.drexel.edu/content.aspx?bookid=1016&Sectionid=61606752

Maisels, M. J. Clune, S., Coleman, K., Gendelman, B., Kendall, A., McManus, S., & Smyth, M. (2014). The natural history of jaundice in predominantly breastfed infants. *Pediatrics, 134*(2), e340–e345.

Marar, M., McIlvain, N. M., Fields, S. K., & Comstock, R. D. (2012). Epidemiology of concussions among United States high school athletes in 20 sports. *The American Journal of Sports Medicine, 40*(4), 747–755. doi:10.1177/0363546511435626.

McInerny, T. K., Adam, H. M., Campbell, D. E., Kamat, D. M., & Kelleher, K. J. (Eds.). 2009. *American Academy of Pediatrics: Textbook of pediatric care.* Elk Grove Village, IL: American Academy of Pediatrics.

McLean, H. Q., Fiebelkorn, A. P., Temte, J. L., Wallace, G. S., & Centers for Disease Control and Prevention. (2013). Prevention of measles, rubella, congenital rubella syndrome, and mumps, 2013: Summary recommendations of the advisory committee on immunization practices (ACIP). *Morbidity and Mortality Weekly Report: Recommendations and Reports, 62*(RR-04), 1–34.

Miller, S. (2013). *Undescended testicle.* Retrieved from http://www.nlm.nih.gov/medlineplus/ency/article/000973.htm

Muchowski, K. E. (2014). Evaluation and treatment of neonatal hyperbilirubinemia. *American Family Physician, 89*(11), 873–878.

National Center for Immunization and Respiratory Diseases, Division of Bacterial Diseases. (2009). *Otitis media: Physician information sheet (pediatrics).* Retrieved from http://www.cdc.gov/getsmart/campaign-materials/info-sheets/child-otitismedia.html

National Center for Injury Prevention and Control, Centers for Disease Control and Prevention. (2014). *Concussion and mild TBI.* Retrieved from http://www.cdc.gov/headsup/providers/tools.html

National Institute of Health. (2007). *National asthma education and prevention program. Expert panel report III: Guidelines for the diagnosis and management of asthma.* Bethesda, MD: National Institutes of Health; National Heart, Lung, and Blood Institute. NIH Publication No. 07-4051. Retrieved from http://www.nhlbi.nih.gov/files/docs/guidelines/asthsumm.pdf

Neely, E. K., & Crossen, S. S. (2014). Precocious puberty. *Current Opinion in Obstetrics & Gynecology, 26*(5), 332.

Newell, C. (2010). Early recognition of eating disorders. *Practice Nurse, 39*(12), 20.

Olive, A. P., & Endom, E. E. (2015). Infantile hypertrophic pyloric stenosis. In W. J. Klish, J. L. Singer, & A. G. Hoppin(Eds.), *UpToDate.* Waltham, MA: UpToDate.

Perrine, C. G., Sharma, A. J., Jefferds, M. E. D., Serdula, M. K., & Scanlon, K. S. (2010). Adherence to vitamin D recommendations among US infants. *Pediatrics, 125*(4), 627–632.

Potter, P. C. (2010). Current guidelines for the management of asthma in young children. *Allergy, Asthma & Immunology Research, 2*(1), 1–13. doi:10.4168/aair.2010.2.1.1.

Richards, A., & Guzman-Cottrill, J. A. (2010). Conjunctivitis. *Pediatrics in Review, 31*(5), 196–208.

Richardson, B. (2006). *Practice guidelines for pediatric nurse practitioners.* St. Louis, MO: Elsevier.

Rosenfeld, R. M., Schwartz, S. R., Cannon, C. R., Roland, P. S., Simon, G. R., Kumar, K. A., . . . Robertson, P. J. (2014). Clinical practice guideline: Acute otitis externa. *Otolaryngology–Head and Neck Surgery, 150*(1), S1–S24.

Shulman, S. T., Bisno, A. L., Clegg, H. W., Gerber, M. A., Kaplan, E. L., Lee, G., . . . Van Beneden, C. (2012). Clinical practice guideline for the diagnosis and management of group A streptococcal pharyngitis: 2012 update by the infectious diseases society of America. *Clinical Infectious Diseases, 55*(10), 1279–1282.

Shimose, L., & Munoz-Price, L. S. (2013). Diagnosis, prevention, and treatment of scabies. *Current Infectious Disease Reports, 15*(5), 426–431. doi:10.1007/s11908-013-0354-0

Steering Committee on Quality Improvement and Management, Subcommittee on Febrile Seizures. (1996). Practice parameters: The neurodiagnostic evaluation of the child with a first simple febrile seizure. *Pediatrics, 97*(5), 769–772.

Steering Committee on Quality Improvement and Management, Subcommittee on Febrile Seizures. (2008). Febrile seizures: Clinical practice guidelines for the long-term management of the child with simple febrile seizures. *Pediatrics, 121*(6), 1281–1286.

Stevens, D. L., Bisno, A. L., Chambers, H. F., Dellinger, E. P., Goldstein, E. J. C., Gorbach, S. L., . . . Wade, J. C. (2014). Practice guidelines for the diagnosis and management of skin and soft tissue infections: 2014 update by the infectious diseases society of America. *Clinical Infectious Diseases, 59*(2), 147.

Subcommittee on Diagnosis and Management of Bronchiolitis. (2006). Clinical practice guideline: Diagnosis and management of bronchiolitis. *Pediatrics, 118*(4), 1774–1793.

Thapar, A., Collishaw, S., Pine, D. S., &Thapar, A. K. (2012). Depression in adolescence. *Lancet. 379*(9820), 1056–1067.

Turiy, Y. (2012). Evaluation of a newborn with a murmur. *Journal of Pediatric Health Care, 27*(3), 226–229.

Turner, T. L. & Palamountain, S. (2014a). Infantile colic: Clinical features and diagnosis. In M. Augustyn, & M. M. Torchia (Eds.), *UpToDate.* Waltham, MA: UpToDate.

Turner, T. L. & Palamountain, S. (2014b). Infantile colic: Management and outcome. In M. Augustyn, & M. M. Torchia (Eds.), *UpToDate.* Waltham, MA: UpToDate.

U.S. Preventive Services Task Force. (2009). *Screening and treatment for major depressive disorder in children and adolescents.* Retrieved from: http://www.uspreventiveservicestaskforce.org/uspstf09/depression/chdeprrs.htm

Well, D. (2013). Acne vulgaris: A review of causes and treatment options. *The Nurse Practitioner, 38*(10), 22–31. doi:10.1097/01.NPR.0000434089.88606.70

Witherington, T. L., & Trotter, S. (2012). New primary care guidelines for pediatric attention-Deficit/Hyperactivity disorder. *The Journal for Nurse Practitioners, 8*(7), 573. doi:10.1016/j.nurpra.2012.05.012.

Woods, C. R. (2013). Croup: Approach to management. In S. L. Kaplan, & C. Armsby (Eds.), *UpToDate.* Waltham, MA: UpToDate.

Woods, C. R. (2015). Croup: Clinical features, evaluation, and diagnosis. In S. L. Kaplan, G. Redding, & C. Armsby (Eds.), *UpToDate.* Waltham, MA: UpToDate.

World Health Organization. (2009). Weekly epidemiological record: Measles vaccines: WHO position paper. 35(84). 349–360. Retrieved from www.polioeradication. org/Portals/0/Document/Aboutus/Governance/ IMB/14IMBMeeting/8.5_14IMB.pdf

World Health Organization. (2015). Measles: Fact sheet N°286. Retrieved from http://www.who.int/mediacentre/factsheets/ fs286/en/

Yetman, R. J. (2015). The child with pediculosis capitis. *Journal of Pediatric Health Care, 29*(1), 118–120. doi:10.1016/j. pedhc.2014.09.002

Zayas, F. (2010). Osgood Schlatter's syndrome (tibial tubercle apophysitis). In W. Micheo (ed.), *Musculoskeletal, sports, and occupational medicine.* New York, NY: Demos Medical Publishing.

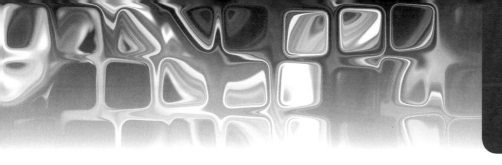

Chapter 16

Professional Issues for the Adult-Gero and Family Nurse Practitioner (Advanced Practice Registered Nurse)

Al Rundio

Scope and Standards of Practice

Standards of practice published by the American Nurses Association and American Academy of Nurse Practitioners

Describes standards, practice settings, professional conduct, and role
- Clinician
- Educator
- Consultant
- Collaborator
- Researcher

Does not confer authority to perform acts or prescribe
- Scope of practice: dictated by State Boards of Nursing and Nurse Practice Acts
- Scope of practice varies from state to state.
- Do not anticipate "across the board" scope mandates.
- Rights and privileges dictated by the scope of practice and state law.

Pursuant to Practice
- Dynamic environment
- Increasing awareness
- Duty
- Breach of duty
- Vigilance in preventing liability
- Safe practice

Legal Issues in Health Care

THE DEFINITION OF LAW

- Types of law
  - Public versus private
  - Criminal versus noncriminal
  - Case versus code based

Public versus Private

- Public law—constitutional law, criminal law, and administrative law
  - Defines citizen to government relationship
- Private law = civil law
  - Defines citizen to citizen relationships
    Includes
    - ○ Personal responsibilities about things we own
    - ○ Injuries we inflict or avoid
    - ○ Contracts we make or break

Public Law

- Constitutional law, criminal law, and administrative law
- Defines citizen to government relationship

Private Law = Civil Law

- Defines citizen to citizen relationships
- Personal responsibilities about things we own
- Injuries we inflict or avoid
- Contracts we make or break

Criminal versus Noncriminal

Criminal Law

- Federal or state government
- Prosecuting an offense against society
- Attempts to deprive personal liberty or life
- Requires proof beyond a reasonable doubt

Noncriminal or Civil Law

- Disputes between two parties
- Often settled with exchange of money
- Requires convincing a jury that complaint is true with relevant example
- Medical or nursing malpractice is an example.

Case versus Code based

Case Law or Common Law

- Created by judges
- Nonstatutory

Code Law—Collection of Laws

- Created by legislation

LEGAL TERMINOLOGY

- Res judicata
- Stare decisis
- Respondeat superior
- Charitable immunity
- Res ipsa loquitor
- Tort

Res Judicata

- The thing has been decided

Stare Decisis

- To stand by that which is decided

Quinlan Case Study—Karen Ann Quinlan is a New Jersey case that dates back to mid-1970s. She was on a ventilator in a persistent vegetative state. Her parents decided that they wanted the ventilator discontinued. As this was relatively new technology, ventilators were not discontinued. This case went to the New Jersey State Supreme Court, who ruled that the ventilator could be discontinued. The course decision was based on a couple of factors. One factor was the US Constitution and the right to privacy, that individuals in their own home have the right to make decisions. Another factor was that of surrogate decision making, that individuals can make decisions on behalf of another person when that person does not have decision-making capacity. In this case, Karen Ann Quinlan's parents were the decision makers.

This case relates to stare decisis in that it set the stage for discontinuing ventilators in New Jersey for those patients where the chance of survival is nil.

Respondeat Superior
- Let the master speak
- Vicarious liability
- Borrowed servant doctrine
- Captain of the ship rule

Darling Case Study—The Darling case is a 1960s case. It centers on a young patient being treated by a contracted physician at a hospital. The physician was not an employee of the hospital. The patients suffered a preventable situation and there was a resultant lawsuit. The hospital tried to claim that they were not responsible as the physician was not one of their employees. The court ruled differently as under the principle of respondeat superior an agency is responsible for those individuals who provide care in said agency even if they are not employees. The Darling case was the basis for The Joint Commission's first chapter on Medical Staff Credentialing in the Joint Commission Manual.

This case illustrates that one in a supervisory capacity or one who has a higher credential than another staff member, for example, an APRN compared to an RN, can be held accountable for another's care or lack of care. This really relates to peer review and how action must be taken when one is not competent.

Carlino Case Study—Carlino was a young girl, who was hospitalized in a southern New Jersey hospital with appendicitis. An appendectomy was performed by a general surgeon on the hospital's staff. There was a complication and the patient required more surgeries. After 2 months of hospitalization, the patient was transferred to a tertiary hospital in Pennsylvania, where she died a couple of days after transfer. A lawsuit resulted, and it was the first time in the nation that an entire medical staff was sued. The basis of the suit was respondeat superior and lack of peer review. The medical staff knew that this physician was incompetent, yet they did nothing to curtail his privileges, supervise his care, etc.

Cases such as this one can set precedent for future cases, that is attorneys looking to sue an entire medical staff rather than the incompetent provider themselves.

Charitable Immunity
- Protection of charitable (nonprofit) hospitals
- Immunity is never absolute.
- Negligent conduct can nullify the CI doctrine.
- Examples: Willful, wanton, gross, or reckless behaviors
- Only seven states apply charitable immunity doctrine to health care.

Flagiello Case Study—Mrs. Flagiello was a patient at a tertiary hospital in Pennsylvania. She inadvertently sustained an injury in the hospital, which should not have occurred. There was a lawsuit. Based on the concept of charitable immunity, the first-level court and the intermediate appellate court ruled in favor of the hospital. This case then went to the Pennsylvania Supreme Court, which ruled in favor of Mrs. Flagiello, thus nullifying the concept of charitable immunity in this state.

Res Ipsa Loquitor
- The thing speaks for itself
- Health-care examples

Tort
- Law includes negligence and professional negligence.
- Law protects others from unreasonable and foreseeable risks of harm.

- A civil wrong other than breach of conduct
- Law provides a remedy for injured person to seek damages.
- Civil, noncriminal decision relating to injuries that occur as a result of a breach of a duty owed to the injured party

Requirements for a tort claim
- Defendant has a duty to the plaintiff—defendant breached this duty.
- Harm or injury resulted from the breach of this duty
- Example: Negligence

Negligence and Professional Negligence
- Conduct that falls below standard established by law—protection from unreasonable risk harm
- Includes concept of foreseeability
- Includes things that we do, that is procedures
- Includes things that we omit to do but should have done
- Professional negligence or professional malpractice
- Conduct of professionals that falls below professional standard of due care
- Conduct of care falls below standard minimum of special knowledge and ability
- Failure to exercise the standard of care that a reasonably prudent person would exercise in a similar situation

What Is in Your Job Description?
- One's job description is often used to determine the "standard of care" owed to a plaintiff in a lawsuit.
- The court may use an APRNs job description to measure a nurse's action or inaction in a civil suit.

Malpractice Liability Insurance
- APRNs may be covered to a certain extent by their employer's insurance.
- Employer-based coverage is a good starting point.
- *But*, be aware of the policy and specific provisions and acquire your own individual policy as well.

Factors to Consider
- The type of nursing that you normally perform
- The dollar amount of the average awards in your particular geographic area
- The type of nursing care you normally provide
- The propensity for lawsuits against nurses in that geographic area

Types of Malpractice Liability Insurance Products
- After examining your risk and your coverage, if you find that it is inadequate, you need to obtain coverage for your areas of exposure.
- May need to purchase a personal policy or increase coverage of an existing personal policy

Different Types of Policies
- "Claims made"—provides coverage only for claims *filed* during the policy term; "occurrence policy"—provides coverage for an incident that occurs during the time the policy is in effect, regardless of when the claim is filed
- "Tail" coverage—protects against claims that occur after nurses drop their "claims-made" insurance and discontinue coverage
- "Prior acts" or "nose" coverage—protects those purchasing insurance for the first time for acts occurring prior to the insurance

Intentional Torts
- Are you covered for "intentional torts"?—Some policies may cover certain acts of negligence, but may exclude intentional torts (i.e., battery, false imprisonment, defamation, and intentional infliction of emotional distress).

What about Intentional Torts?
- Why do you need to be covered for intentional torts?—Important because, unlike a claim for negligence, plaintiff's suing for an intentional tort may be seeking punitive damages

Standards of Care
- What is the standard of care for the APRN?
- What an ordinary, prudent, and reasonable APRN would do in the same or a similar situation?

Anatomy of a Malpractice Case
- Duty to provide care
- Breach the duty.
- A tort is committed.
- An untoward outcome results.
- Events were foreseeable.

Events are foreseeable is critical when looking to see if a potential lawsuit exists.

Philadelphia Case Study—Mrs. J was a psychic. She was having headaches. Her physician ordered a CT scan of her head. A few months postprocedure she claimed that she lost her psychic ability and sued for a large amount of money. The trial court awarded her $1 million for loss of her psychic ability. This court decision was overturned at the intermediate appellate court as loss of psychic ability secondary to having a CT scan done could not be foreseen.

Tarasoff Case Study—Tarasoff was a young woman who was dating someone. She broke the engagement off. Her former boyfriend was being cared for by a psychologist. He told the psychiatrist that he was going to kill Tarasoff. The psychologist reported that to his supervisor, who advised him that he would take care of this. Nothing was done, and Ms. Tarasoff was murdered by her former boyfriend.

The events in this case were foreseeable and both the psychologist and his supervisor had the duty to forewarn Ms. Tarasoff. Many states changed legislation following this case, where the duty to forewarn a person when someone makes a terroristic threat supersedes the confidentiality of the patient.

Standards of Care
- Regional
- National

Professional Negligence Claims against APRNS
- Based almost exclusively on personal injury
- Resulted from various types of negligent conduct
- Involved product liability and most recently complimentary/alternative health care options

Failure to:
- Order appropriate medications and other treatments.
- Order a treatment or procedure according to standards of care.
- Document a patient's condition, treatment, and response to treatment.

Case Examples

Expert Witness: Cases Settled
- Wiggins versus Correctional Medical Services 1994 Albuquerque, New Mexico: case settled out of court for nominal sum for improper assessment, documentation, and transport.
- Villagran versus Correctional Medical Services 1999 Las Vegas, Nevada: case settled out of court for failure to communicate pertinent CT scan results.
- Family versus County Justice Facility 1988 Atlantic County, New Jersey: case settled out of court for minimal sum for improperly performed CPR.
- Nofer versus Substance Abuse Treatment Center 2005 Morristown, New Jersey: case settled in court for $1.5 million for plaintiff's improper assessment, lack of communication, and failure to protect patient.

Contract Law
- Promises made
- Enforcement once a legal right is created
- Application in health care—Nurse employer, nurse manager, nurse practitioner, nurse entrepreneur

- A contract is voluntary agreement for the benefit of two or more individuals—legally qualified **consents**.
  - Verbal
  - Written
  - Implied

Informed consent
- Informed consent is the process that a provider explains to a competent patient of what procedure is going to be done, why it is being done, the potential risks and complications, and alternatives to the procedure.

Other Legal Issues
- Sexual harassment
- Comparable worth

Other Legal Issues
Discrimination
- Affirmative action (Civil Rights Act of 1964)
- Title VII of Civil Rights Act of 1964
- The Age Discrimination in Employment Act of 1967

Defenses
- Untimely filing of the case: Files after the statute of limitations runs out
- Assumption of risk: The plaintiff knew "it" was dangerous, had facts about the danger, and chose to take on the danger.
- Immunity from suit: Common one is "Good Samaritan act."

Harm to a Patient Can Arise from Intentional or Nonintentional Acts:
- Intentional acts of harm can include defamation, invasion of privacy, assault and battery, false imprisonment, or infliction of emotional distress.
- Nonintentional acts of harm can include omission or negligence

Consensus Model for APRNS

LACE
- L = Licensure—granting of authority to practice
- A = Accreditation—formal review and approval by a recognized agency of education's degree programs or certification programs
- C = Certification—formal recognition of knowledge, skills, and experience demonstrated by the achievement of standards identified by the profession
- E = Education—formal preparation of APRNs in graduate degree–granting or postgraduate certificate programs

Requirements for APRNs
- Completed accredited graduate level education program in one of four roles of CRNA, CNM, CNS, CNP
- Passed national certification that measures APRN role and population-based competencies
- Acquired advanced clinical knowledge and skills to provide direct care to patients (defining factor for all APRNs is that significant component of education and practice focuses on the direct care of individuals)
- Practice builds on RN competencies.
- Greater depth/breadth of knowledge
- Greater synthesis of data
- Increased complexity of skills and interventions
- Greater role autonomy
- Educationally prepared to assume responsibility/accountability for the following:
  - Health promotion/maintenance
  - Assessment, diagnosis, management of patient problems
  - Use and prescription of pharmacologic and nonpharmacologic interventions
  - Clinical experience with sufficient depth and breadth
- Licensed as independent practitioner to practice as APRN in role of CRNA, CNM, CNS, or NP
- APRN title required to be used (*Note:* Each state must pass legislation to change titling)
- Role and population included.
- Specialty title may be used.
- Example: John Doe, MSN, APRN, AGPCNP

For entry into practice and regulatory purposes, APRN education must conform to the following:
- Be through a formal graduate or postgraduate accredited institution.
- Comprehensive, at graduate level
- Prepare graduates to practice as CRNA, CNM, CNS, or NP across at least one population foci (neonatal, pediatric, adult-gero, gender-specific, or psych–mental health).

For entry into practice and regulatory purposes, APRN education must comprise the following:
- Include at least three separate comprehensive graduate-level courses:
  - Advanced physiology/pathophysiology
  - Advanced health assessment
  - Advanced pharmacology
- May also include preparation in a specialty area of practice, but it must build upon the APRN role and population focused competencies.
  - Build upon role and population-focused competencies.
  - Represent a focused area of practice.
    - Specific population subset
    - Specific patient needs
      - Disease states
      - Body system
  - Developed, recognized, monitored by the profession (not regulatory agencies)
  - Preparation cannot replace role-/population-focused education.
  - Crossover roles and populations.
  - Title may not be used in lieu of licensing title, which includes role and population.
  - Competencies must be assessed separately from role and population competencies.

New roles or populations that include a unique or significantly differentiated set of competencies from the current roles and populations may evolve over time.

To be recognized, criteria must be met the following:
- Education standards, core competencies
- Accredited graduate, postgraduate educational programs
- Certification program that meets accreditation standards

Specific Criteria for Each Prong of Regulation
- Licensure
- Accreditation
- Certification
- Education

Target Date: December 31, 2015
- Current certification examinations: ANP; ACNP; Gero was retired in 2015.
- New examinations begin implementation in 2013.
- The certification does not "retire"—only the examinations retire.
- One must maintain current certification through the continuing education option.
- Should current certification expire, the APRN would have to meet the eligibility requirements of the new examination.

Grandfathering
- When states adopt new eligibility requirements for APRNs, currently practicing APRNs will be permitted to continue practicing within the states(s) of their current licensure.
- If APRN applies for endorsement by another state, they will need to meet new criteria OR criteria in place when they became licensed.
- American Association Colleges of Nursing (AACN) created the Doctor of Nursing Practice (DNP)
- Essentials document written by AACN in 2006
- Recommended that DNP be entry level into Advanced Practice by 2015
- The first group to formally adopt this recommendation is the American Association of Nurse Anesthetists (AANA). Nurses that enter a nurse anesthesia program in 2022 must graduate in 2025 with a DNP or DNAP (Doctor of Nurse Anesthesia Practice).
- For other APRNs, each state must adopt legislation to enact the DNP as entry level into practice.

APRN Regulatory Model

Speciality Certification

by Professional Association, i.e.,
International Nurses Society on
Addictions ANCB Board
Certification in Addictions Nursing

Population Foci

Family, Adult-Gero,
Women's Health—Gender
Specific, Neonatal, Pediatric,
Psych–Mental Health

APRN Role

CRNA, CNM, CNS
NP (Acute or Primary Care)
New Role Not Yet Defined

Ethics

Definition

- Ethics is a discipline in which one attempts to identify, organize, analyze, and justify human acts by applying certain principles to determine the right thing to do in a given situation.

Ethical Premise for Nursing Practice

- Help regain health.
- Help maintain health.
- Help attain a maximum potential.
- Help the dying.

Ethical Theories

Act Utilitarianism (Teleologic)
- Focus is on the consequence of the actions. The approach here is to do good.
- Or to provide the greatest amount of happiness for the greatest number of people or the least amount of harm to the greatest number of people.

Libertarianism (Egoism)

This position maintains a focus on the individual person. This position seeks a solution that is best for that person. The rights of each member of society are paramount.

Formalism (Deontologic or Egalitarianism)

Focus of this theory is centered on the rules that govern a situation.

- Democratic principles are emphasized.
- Concepts of quality and comparable worth are paramount.

Universality is the major theme guiding or directing the decision-making process.

Humanitarianism (Fairness)

- Democratic principles are emphasized.
- Concepts of quality and comparable worth are paramount.
- Universality is the major theme guiding or directing the decision-making process.

Humanitarianism (Fairness)

- Focus of this theory is concerned with the distribution of benefits and burden in society.
- Concepts of fair opportunity, basic needs, and individual needs are emphasized.
- Fairness may not be the same as equality.

Rawlsian

- Focus of this theory is that the least advantaged should not be hurt.
- The overriding principle is justice. Each person is entitled to quality and access to medical care.

Naturalistic

- Focus of this theory is "it is what it ought to be." That is, if you have a terminal illness, you are meant to die.
- The major principle here is utmost rationality.

Consequential

- Focus of this theory is scientism, that is, scientific and objective data guide the ethical decision making process.
- No feelings enter into the equation.
- Basis is rationality.

Ethical Decision-Making Model

- Identify the problem.
- Tease out the ethical problem/dilemma.
- Gather objective and subjective data.
- Look at alternatives.
- Study the consequences of alternatives.
- Select the most appropriate alternative.
- Compare the selected alternative with your own value/values system.

The Role of APRNs in Ethics

- Acquire knowledge of ethical theory.
- Assess the ethical situation at hand.
- Implement the decision-making model/process.
- Identify the specific theory in use.

Landmark Cases

Karen Ann Quinlan—New Jersey case—Courts not needed for ethical decisions; permitted surrogate decision-making; based on right to privacy in US Constitution

Nancy Ellen Jobes—New Jersey case—Reaffirmed Quinlan decision with other types of artificial interventions (tube feedings).

Nancy Beth Cruzan—Missouri case—Patient Self-Determination Act

Terri Ann Schiavo—Florida case—Demonstrated importance of communication and consensus; legal rights and surrogate decision-making

Nancy Beth Cruzan Tombstone

Note the three dates on Nancy Beth's tombstone.

Ethical Issues Today
- Conflicts and dilemmas

Ethical Encounters
- Advance directives and right to live/die
- Euthanasia
- Do not resuscitate orders
- Rights of a dying patient
- Use of life-sustaining equipment
- Lack of respect for patient's dignity
- Stem cell research
- HIV and AIDS
- A nurse with HIV
- A patient with HIV

Ethical Encounters
- Human cloning
- Research on the mentally ill
- Research on embryos
- Patient autonomy and the Patient Self-Determination Act (1990)
- Organ donation issues
- Incompetent health-care providers—a peer, a nurse, a physician
- Operative issues
- Inadequate consents

CPT Coding: Evaluation/Management Guidelines and Reimbursement for APRNs

Regulatory Payers
- Government Agency: Medicare and Medicaid
  - Established in 1965 under the Lyndon Baines Johnson Administration
  - Federally mandated health insurance program for the aged and disabled persons
  - Medicare has four parts.
  - Part A covers inpatient hospital care and up to 20 days (at 100% reimbursement) and the next 80 days (at 80% reimbursement) in a nursing home if the patient has had a minimum of a three night stay in an acute care hospital setting with a valid diagnosis within 30 days of being admitted to the nursing home. Also covers home health visits (when skilled nursing is required) and hospice care.
  - Part B—Available to all persons covered under Part A
  - Covers outpatient care such as health provider office visits, physical therapy, laboratory and radiology services, some durable medical equipment (DME), and some preventative services.
  - Part C is the Medicare Advantage Plans.
  - Part D is the prescription drug plan.
  - Prescription Drug Plan covers up to $270,000 per year. After coverage limit is reached, the patient falls into the "doughnut hole." Patient then pays up to $435,000 out of pocket. When this amount is reached, patient is out of the "doughnut hole," and Medicare covers prescription costs again.
  - The Patient Protection and Affordable Health Care Act (2010) will eventually close the "doughnut hole" in Medicare Part D.
  - Legislation in August 1997 expanded direct reimbursement for nurse practitioners in all geographic regions.
  - Primary care provider reimbursement is calculated on a resource-based relative value scale system [RBRVS].

Medicaid
- Authorized in 1965 as Title XIX of Social Security Act
- Federal and state funded program administered by each state
- Eligibility based on financial need

- Covered services include: Hospital and physician services, laboratory and radiographic services, nursing home care, home health care, prenatal and preventive services, and medically necessary transportation
- States can choose to cover additional services.
- Omnibus Budget Reconciliation Act (OBRA) 89 mandated Medicaid reimbursement for certified pediatric and family nurse practitioners beginning July 1, 1990.
- Many states have additional provisions for nurse practitioner reimbursement not identified in federal statutes.

Fee for Service—becoming obsolete. Unit of payment is per visit/procedure.
- Commercial insurers
- Self-Insured institutions
- Managed care organizations
  - Managed care deals with aggregates. Connects patients, providers, sponsors, and third-party payers. Controls type, level, and frequency of treatment. Designed to control cost while assuring quality. Providers do not dictate price; assume financial risk.
  - HMOs (Health Maintenance Organizations)
  - POS (Point of Service Plans)
  - PPO (Preferred Provider Organization)
  - IPA (Independent Professional Association and/or Independent Physician or Provider Association)
  - Case management deals with individuals. Balances quality and cost over the course of an illness. Standardized use of resources. Encourages collaboration among disciplines. Manages the patient prehospital, intrahospital, and posthospital discharge. Manages the continuum of care.
- These programs cover the majority of health-care costs in the United States.

Capitation
- More and more plans are moving to a capitated form of reimbursement.
- Under capitation, a primary care provider is reimbursed a set dollar amount each month for the covered person. The dollar amount provided by the insurance company is usually based on risk stratification, for example, the more comorbidities that the patient has the greater the dollar amount. Generally the dollar amounts are not great, for example, $10.00 per member per month regardless of how many times the patient accesses services. It is estimated that more and more will reimburse primary care with a capitated form of reimbursement.
- The result is that more financial risk is shifted to the provider. The goal of the provider is to keep the patient well and out of the practice as the practice is reimbursed whether the patient accesses services or not.

The Bottom-Line Money
- How dollars that you as an NP generate for the practice will improve your chances of maintaining a position?

Coding and Reimbursement Common Procedural Terminology
- Common procedural terminology (CPT) coding identifies the services rendered rather than the diagnosis on the claim. It is similar to *ICD-9* and *ICD-10* coding. ICD code sets also contain procedure codes, but these are only specific to the inpatient setting.
- CPT is identified by the Centers for Medicare and Medicaid Services (CMS) as Level 1 of the Health Care Procedure Coding System (HCPCS).
- The American Medical Association (AMA) developed the CPT. This coding system is maintained by an AMA CPT Editorial Board.
- What is the CPT Code Set?
  - Developed by the AMA
  - Listing of descriptive terms and five-digit numeric codes for reporting medical services and procedures performed by HC providers
- What is its purpose?
  - Provides universal language to accurately designate office and diagnostic services > Serves as a means of consistent nationwide communication

How to Locate a CPT Code?
- Alphabetic Index organized in main terms
- Four primary classes
  - Listing of descriptive terms and five-digit numeric codes for reporting medical services and procedures performed by HC providers

- What is its purpose?
  - Provides universal language to accurately designate office and diagnostic services
  - Serves as a means of consistent nationwide communication

How to Locate a CPT Code?

- Alphabetic Index
  - Organized in main terms
- Four Primary Classes
  - Procedure
  - Service
  - Anatomic sites or organs
  - Condition: Synonyms, eponyms, and abbreviations

Principles and Requirements of Quality Chart Documentation

- Record must be thorough and legible.
- States the reason for the encounter (chief complaint).
- Relevant history
- Assessment/impression/diagnosis
- Details of the management of the patient's condition
- Date and legible identity of the author
- Rational for ordering diagnostic and other ancillary services
- Identify risk factors of the condition(s) and treatment(s).
- Document patient progress, response to, and changes in treatment and revision of diagnosis.
- Opinions of other providers who have been consulted
- CPT and *ICD-10* codes supported by documentation

ICD 10 Coding Overview

- Coding is now alphanumeric not just numeric
- Became effective in 2015
- There is much greater specificity and clinical information, for example under ICD-9, a fractured wrist could be billed. Now the wrist that is fractured must be specified, for example, left fractured wrist.
- Improves ability to measure health care services
- More sensitivity when refining grouping and reimbursement methodologies
- Enhances the ability to conduct public health surveillance
- Decreases the need to include supporting documentation with claims
- Enhances payment for services rendered
- Facilitates evaluation and monitoring of medical processes and outcomes
- Accommodates emerging diagnoses and procedures
- Diagnoses and procedures precisely identified

Evaluation/Management Guidelines

- These are used for reimbursement and are available at www.cms.hhs.gov or through Medicare.
- Seven components
  - Nature of the presenting problem
  - History
  - Physical examination
  - Medical decision-making
  - Counseling
  - Coordination of care
  - Time

History of Present Illness (HPI)

- Chronologic description of the development of the patient's present illness from symptom/sign or from previous encounter.
- Elements:
  - Location
  - Duration
  - Modifying factors
  - Quality
  - Associated signs and symptoms

  - Context
  - Timing
  - Severity

Review of Systems (ROS)
  - Responses:
    - None
    - Pertinent
    - Extended
    - Complete
  - Inventory of body systems obtained through a series of questions seeking to identify signs and symptoms that the patient may be experiencing or has experienced.

Past, Family, and/or Social History (PFSH)
  - Consists of three areas:
    - Past history
    - Family history
    - Social history

Documentation of the Examination
  - Physical examination is an assessment of the patient's organ and body systems.
  - Four categories:
    - Problem focused
    - Expanded problem focused
    - Detailed
    - Comprehensive

Medical Decision-making Complexity
  - Four types:
    - Straight-forward
    - Low complexity
    - Moderate complexity
    - High complexity

New versus Established Patients
Evaluation and Management: New patient 99203 (Outpatient)
  - Chief complaint (CC): Nasal congestion and swollen eyelids
  - HPI: 58-year-old female new to my practice comes in today with increased nasal congestion for about 2 weeks. She states the problem is sometimes quite severe and is worse when she goes outside. She is concerned she may be developing seasonal allergies. She says the congestion is often associated with swollen eyelids and watery eyes and can last for several hours at a time.
  - Medications: HCTZ 12.5 mg p.o. daily
  - Past Medical History (PMH): HTN, nonsmoker
  - ROS:
    - Ears, nose, mouth, and throat: Negative for epistaxis, sore throat, or decreased hearing.
    - Pulmonary: negative for cough, hemoptysis, SOB
  - Physical Examination:
    - General: No acute distress, conversant, looks younger-than-stated age
    - Vital signs: BP: 130/72   Pulse: 88   RR: 16   Temperature: 98.6
    - Head: Normocephalic, no sinus tenderness, or submandibular lymphadenopathy
    - Neck: Supple without lymphadenopathy; trachea midline; eyes: anicteric with moist, pale conjunctiva
    - Nose: Normal noninjected nasal mucosa, with normal septum: pale, swollen turbinates
    - Oropharynx: No ulcerations or pharyngeal edema
    - Ears: Patent external canals with pearly TMs and normal hearing acuity
    - Lungs: Clear to air bilaterally
    - Cardiovascular: Regular rhythm
    - Extremities: No edema
  - Assessment: Allergic rhinitis 477.9 (unspecified) >Essential HTN 401.9 (unspecified)
  - Plan: OTC acetaminophen and diphenhydramine, saline nasal flushes, patient was instructed to avoid decongestants with phenylpropanolamine due to the risk of exacerbating her HTN.

Time-Based Example of Established Office Visit 99213

- CC: Muscle weakness
- Interval History: The patient is here today to discuss the risks and benefits of statin medication for dyslipidemia with LDL of 160. She states she has muscle weakness and wants to know if she really needs to continue this medication.
- Physical Examination:
  - General: No acute distress, conversant, looks younger-than-stated age.
  - Vital signs: BP 124/72, HR 84, RR 18
  - Lungs: Clear to air bilaterally
  - Cardiovascular: regular rate and rhythm, no peripheral edema
- Laboratory information: LDL 92
- Impression: Disorders of lipid metabolism 272.4 (other and unspecified hyperlipidemia)
- Plan: Continue pravastatin 20 mg p.o. daily; RTO in 6 months with LFTs and lipid panel
- Time: I spent 20 minutes face to face with this patient; over 50% of the time was devoted to counseling and/or coordination of care. We discussed the side effect and risks of statin medications in primary prevention of cardiovascular events. All questions were answered and the patient understands the risks involved.

Consultation versus Referral

- A consultation is a request by one HC provider for the advice or opinion of another HC provider regarding the evaluation and/or management of a specific problem. It is usually one specialty to another specialty
- A referral is the transfer of care from one HC provider to a second HC provider when the second HC provider assumes responsibility for treatment of the patient.

Present Reimbursement Policy

- NPs presently receive 85% of a physician's rate. There are many organizations that would like to see this changed.

Research Categories

- Applied
- Basic
- Case study
- Descriptive
- Developmental
- Experimental
- Field
- Historical
- Laboratory
- Longitudinal
- Qualitative

Nursing Research

- Epistemology—The study of knowledge acquisition. When we refer to nursing epistemology, we are concerned with knowledge acquisition that will improve/enhance nursing practice.
- All research begins with a question.
- Review of the literature.
- Refine the question.
- Define the methodology.
- Conduct the study.
- Analyze the findings.
- Discuss the results.

Types of Research

- Quantitative
- Qualitative
- In quantitative research, the researcher creates a framework or design to provide a plan for answering the research question.

- Design includes a plan, structure, and strategy.
- Purpose of a research design: Aid in the solution of research problems—Maintain control

Quantitative Research

- Experimental
- Quasi-experimental
- The three essential elements of experimental design are as follows:
  - Manipulation—The researcher does something to at least some of the participants in the research.
  - Control—The experimenter introduces one or more controls over the experimental situation.
  - Randomization—The experimenter assigns participants to different groups on a random basis.

Quasi-Experimental

- Designs were developed to provide alternate means for examining causality in situations which were not conducive to experimental control.
- Designs have been developed to control as many threats to validity as possible in situations where at least one of the three elements of true experimental research is lacking (i.e., manipulation, randomization, control group).
- Most are adaptations of experimental designs where one of the three elements is missing. An example could be where the researcher uses groups (control and treatment) which have evolved naturally in some way rather than being randomly selected. This is a quasi-experimental approach using nonequivalent control groups.

Qualitative Research

- Investigation of human experiences in naturalistic settings
- Studies are guided by research questions.
- Five basic elements
  - Identifying the phenomena
  - Structuring the study
  - Gathering the data
  - Analyzing the data
  - Describing the findings
- Purpose is to describe—understand or explain phenomena or culture.
  - Can be utilized to create solutions to practical problems
- Types of Qualitative Research:
  - Phenomenology
  - Ethnography
  - Grounded theory
  - Case study
  - Focus group
  - Descriptive exploratory
  - Historical

Research Terms

- Population—The group or sample that is selected to be studied
- For statistical purposes, usually written as an "n"

Validity

- Addresses the degree to which an instrument actually measures what it is intended to measure appropriately and assesses the characteristic or construct it is intended to measure
- Addresses whether an instrument really measures what it sets out to measure or, instead, measures some other related variable
- Internal validity asks whether the independent variable really made the difference or the change in the dependent variable.
- External validity deals with possible problems of generalization of the investigation's findings to other populations and other environmental conditions.
- What conditions and types of subjects will lend themselves to the same results?

Reliability

Refers to the degree of consistency with which an instrument measures whatever it measures.

- Maximizes the true component of a score and minimizes the error component
- Reliability is equated with stability, consistency, dependability.

- Sample specific
- Not an enduring property of an instrument

Sensitivity

- The sensitivity of a test refers to how many cases of a disease a particular test can find. A very sensitive test is likely to give a fair number of false-positive results, but almost no true positives will be missed. A numerical value can be calculated for a test's sensitivity that represents the probability of it returning a "true" value for samples (i.e., patients) from the population of interest (i.e., samples from patients who do in fact have the disease in question); this is often described as a test's "positivity in disease."
- Numerically, sensitivity is the number of true positive results (TP) divided by the sum of true positive and false negative (FN) results, that is sensitivity $= TP/(TP + FN)$. These tests are utilized to *screen* for disease.

HIV is very likely to be present in the person being tested (true positive), and the result is not likely to be due to some error in the test. A numerical value can be calculated for a test's specificity that represents the probability of it returning a "false" value for samples (i.e., patients) from the population of interest (i.e., samples from patients who are in fact healthy); this is often described as a test's "negativity in health."

Specificity—Numerically, specificity is the number of true negative results (TN) divided by the sum of true negative and false positive (FP) results, that is specificity $= TN/(TN + FP)$. These tests are utilized to *confirm* a disease.

Types of Samples

- Random sampling—All members of the population have an equal chance of being selected in the sample population. Avoids research bias
- Convenience sampling—Acquiring the sample by selecting those participants who are readily available, for example, staff nurses who attend an in-service program.
- Purposive sampling—The researcher establishes certain criteria and the subjects are then selected according to the predetermined criteria.
- Quota sampling—Allows a maximum number of participants
- Snowball sampling—Participants in the sample recruit other individuals. Used in difficult-to-obtain sample populations, that is drug addicts. May contribute to research bias

Ethical Issues in Research

- Nuremberg trials of Nazi Germany set the tone for the conduct of future research on human subjects.
- Department of Health and Human Services has guidelines.

Consent—Must be informed, detailed in layman's terms at a reading level that is appropriate for the subjects. Must state that subjects can withdraw from the research program at any time without being penalized

- Minors sign an "assent."

Institutional Review Board

- Purpose of Institutional Review Board (IRB)
- Composition of IRB
- IRB review cycles
- Expedited review

Evidence-Based Practice

"Evidence-based practice is the conscientious us of current best evidence in making decisions about patient care." (Sackett, Straus, Richardson, Rosenberg, & Haynes, 2000; as cited in Melnyk & Fineout-Overholt, 2005, 2011, 2014).

- Systematic search
- Critical appraisal of the most relevant evidence that attempts to answer a burning clinical question
- One's own clinical expertise
- Patient preferences and values

Another Way to View EBP

- The six steps of EBP are described as follows:
- Create a spirit of inquiry.
- The need for information to be placed into a clinically relevant, answerable question
- Systematic retrieval of best evidence available
- Critical appraisal of evidence for validity and clinical relevance

- Application of critically appraised evidence in clinical practice
- Evaluation of outcomes

Evidence-Based Practice

- Today, 75% of health-care encounters are not based on evidence. Thus, we have a long way to go to make EBP a reality!!!

Documentation

- If not documented, it is not done.
- Must be clear and concise, state pertinent facts not the provider's subjectivity
- Must meet regulatory and payer requirements

Documentation Methods

- The handwritten record dictation systems
- Electronic record systems
- PDAs
- Electronic records
- The World Wide Web

Other Issues

- DNP education
- AACN initiative
- Proposed that the DNP be the entry level into advanced practice by 2015

Suggested Readings

American Association Colleges of Nursing. (2006). *The Essentials of Doctoral Education for Advanced Nursing Practice.* Washington, DC.

American Medical Association. (2015). *CPT codes.* Retrieved January 2, 2015 from http://www.ama-assn.org/ama/pub/physician-resources/solutions-managing-your-practice/coding-billing-insurance/cpt.page.

Buppert, C. (2011). Three Frequently Asked Questions about Malpractice Insurance. *The Journal for Nurse Practitioners.* 7(1),16–17.

Melynk, B. M., & Fineout-Overholt, E. (2005). *Evidence based practice in nursing and health care: A guide to best practice* (1st ed., p. 6). Philadelphia, PA: Wolters Kluwer Lippincott.

Melynk, B. M., & Fineout-Overholt, E. (2011). *Evidence based practice in nursing and health care: A guide to best practice* (2nd ed., p. 6). Philadelphia, PA: Wolters Kluwer Lippincott.

Melynk, B. M., & Fineout-Overholt, E. (2014). *Evidence based practice in nursing and health care: A guide to best practice* (3rd ed., p. 6). Philadelphia, PA: Wolters Kluwer Lippincott.

Polit, D., & Beck, C. T. (2011). *Nursing research: Generating and assessing evidence for nursing practice* (9th ed.). Philadelphia, PA: Wolters Kluwer Lippincott.

Rundio, A. (2012). *The nurse manager's guide to budgeting & finance.* Indianapolis, IN: Sigma Theta Tau International.

Page numbers followed by *f*, *t* and *b* indicate figures, tables and boxes, respectively.